# Tumors of the Pancreas



## Atlas of Tumor Pathology

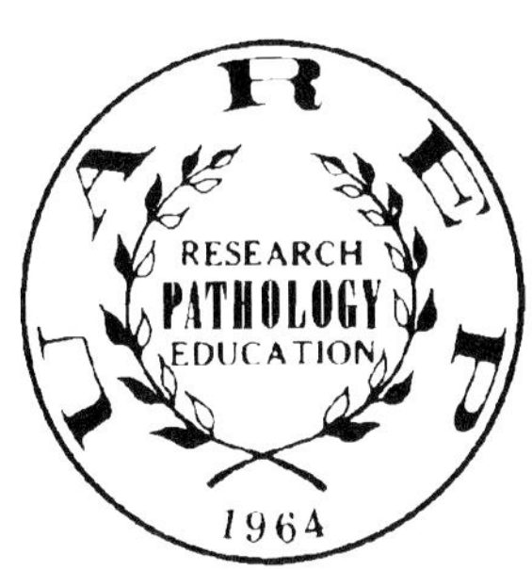


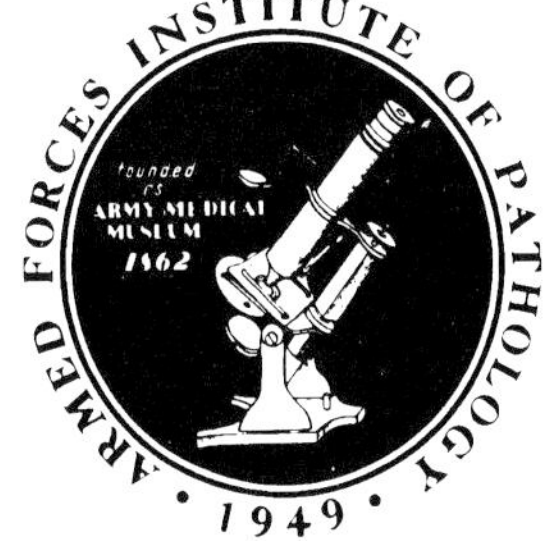


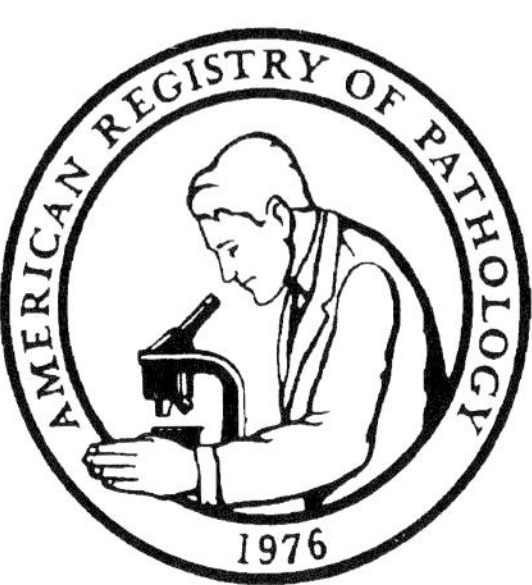

ATLAS OF TUMOR PATHOLOGY

Third Series
Fascicle 20

# TUMORS OF THE PANCREAS

by

**ENRICO SOLCIA, M.D., Ph.D.**
Professor of Pathology and Research Director
Department of Human Pathology and Genetics
University of Pavia and IRCCS Policlinico San Matteo
I-27100 Pavia, Italy

**CARLO CAPELLA, M.D., Ph.D.**
Professor of Pathology and Chairman
Department of Clinical and Biological Sciences
University of Pavia at Varese
I-21100 Varese, Italy

**GÜNTER KLÖPPEL, M.D., Ph.D.**
Professor of Pathology and Chairman
Institute of Pathology
University of Kiel
D-24105 Kiel, Germany

Published by the
ARMED FORCES INSTITUTE OF PATHOLOGY
Washington, D.C.

Under the Auspices of
UNIVERSITIES ASSOCIATED FOR RESEARCH AND EDUCATION IN PATHOLOGY, INC.
Bethesda, Maryland
1997

Accepted for Publication
1995

---

Available from the American Registry of Pathology
Armed Forces Institute of Pathology
Washington, D.C. 20306-6000
ISSN 0160-6344
ISBN 1-881041-29-8

# ATLAS OF TUMOR PATHOLOGY




THE LIBRARY
IC SCHOOL OF MEDICINE
AT ST. MARY'S

## EDITORS' NOTE

The Atlas of Tumor Pathology has a long and distinguished history. It was first conceived at a Cancer Research Meeting held in St. Louis in September 1947 as an attempt to standardize the nomenclature of neoplastic diseases. The first series was sponsored by the National Academy of Sciences-National Research Council. The organization of this Sisyphean effort was entrusted to the Subcommittee on Oncology of the Committee on Pathology, and Dr. Arthur Purdy Stout was the first editor-in-chief. Many of the illustrations were provided by the Medical Illustration Service of the Armed Forces Institute of Pathology, the type was set by the Government Printing Office, and the final printing was done at the Armed Forces Institute of Pathology (hence the colloquial appellation "AFIP Fascicles"). The American Registry of Pathology purchased the Fascicles from the Government Printing Office and sold them virtually at cost. Over a period of 20 years, approximately 15,000 copies each of nearly 40 Fascicles were produced. The worldwide impact that these publications have had over the years has largely surpassed the original goal. They quickly became among the most influential publications on tumor pathology ever written, primarily because of their overall high quality but also because their low cost made them easily accessible to pathologists and other students of oncology the world over.

Upon completion of the first series, the National Academy of Sciences-National Research Council handed further pursuit of the project over to the newly created Universities Associated for Research and Education in Pathology (UAREP). A second series was started, generously supported by grants from the AFIP, the National Cancer Institute, and the American Cancer Society. Dr. Harlan I. Firminger became the editor-in-chief and was succeeded by Dr. William H. Hartmann. The second series Fascicles were produced as bound volumes instead of loose leaflets. They featured a more comprehensive coverage of the subjects, to the extent that the Fascicles could no longer be regarded as "atlases" but rather as monographs describing and illustrating in detail the tumors and tumor-like conditions of the various organs and systems.

Once the second series was completed, with a success that matched that of the first, UAREP and AFIP decided to embark on a third series. A new editor-in-chief and an associate editor were selected, and a distinguished editorial board was appointed. The mandate for the third series remains the same as for the previous ones, i.e., to oversee the production of an eminently practical publication with surgical pathologists as its primary audience, but also aimed at other workers in oncology. The main purposes of this series are to promote a consistent, unified, and biologically sound nomenclature; to guide the surgical pathologist in the diagnosis of the various tumors and tumor-like lesions; and to provide relevant histogenetic, pathogenetic, and clinicopathologic information on these entities. Just as the second series included data obtained from ultrastructural (and, in the more recent Fascicles, immunohistochemical) examination, the third series will, in addition, incorporate pertinent information obtained with the newer molecular biology techniques. As in the past, a continuous attempt will be made to correlate, whenever possible, the nomenclature used in the Fascicles with that proposed by the World Health Organization's International Histological Classification of Tumors. The format of the third series has been changed in order to incorporate additional items and to ensure a consistency of style throughout. Close cooperation between the various authors and their respective liaisons from the editorial board will be emphasized to minimize unnecessary repetition and discrepancies in the text and illustrations.

To its everlasting credit, the participation and commitment of the AFIP to this venture is even more substantial and encompassing than in previous series. It now extends to virtually all scientific, technical, and financial aspects of the production.

The task confronting the organizations and individuals involved in the third series is even more daunting than in the preceding efforts because of the ever-increasing complexity of the matter at hand. It is hoped that this combined effort—of which, needless to say, that represented by the authors is first and foremost—will result in a series worthy of its two illustrious predecessors and will be a suitable introduction to the tumor pathology of the twenty-first century.

**Juan Rosai, M.D.**
**Leslie H. Sobin, M.D.**

## ACKNOWLEDGMENTS

The authors are extremely grateful to the many colleagues in the fields of pathology and clinical medicine who over the years have provided interesting material for consultation, permitted us to use their material for illustrative purposes, and provided follow-up information. Unfortunately, they are too many to list but where their material has been used they have been properly acknowledged.

We would like to thank the anonymous referees of the Armed Forces Institute of Pathology (AFIP) who reviewed the chapters of the Fascicle, for their most helpful constructive criticisms. The cooperation and guidance of Drs. Juan Rosai, Ronald DeLellis, and Leslie Sobin are especially appreciated.

We are deeply indebted to the staff, present and past, of the Departments of Pathology at the Academic Hospital Jette, Free University of Brussels, Belgium, and the University Hospitals of Pavia and Varese, Italy, where the authors have worked over the years. We are especially grateful to Drs. Philipp U. Heitz, Daniel Longenecker, Fausto Sessa, Guido Rindi, Federica Bosi, Stefano LaRosa, Bernard Maillet, Fabienne Rickaert, and Giuseppe Zamboni, for helpful collaboration and discussion. Ms. Nicole Buelens and Ms. Ursula Domscheit are thanked for the excellent slides and photographs they contributed, and Ms. Hilde Lox and Ms. Giovanna Vassallo for their secretarial help. We also wish to express our appreciation to the editorial staff, Ms. Dian Thomas, Mr. Andrew Male, Ms. Audrey Kahn, and Mr. Ken Stringfellow, for their assistance in the preparation of the Fascicle.

**Enrico Solcia, M.D.**
**Carlo Capella, M.D.**
**Günter Klöppel, M.D.**


**Dedication:**

**To our families.**

Permission to use copyrighted illustrations has been granted by:

American Society for Investigative Pathology:
Am J Pathol 1993;143:685–98. For figure 4-101.

Churchill Livingstone:
Pancreatic Pathology, 1984. For figures 4-32, 4-42, 4-106, 7-9, 7-11.

CRC Press:
Endocrine Pathology of the Gut and Pancreas, 1991. For figures 8-3 through 8-9, and 8-11.

Field & Wood:
Progr Surg Pathol 1980;1:119–33. For figure 5-1A.

Karger:
Digestion 1988;41:185–200. For figure 5-52.

Lippincott-Raven:
Am J Surg Pathol 1989;13:766–75. For figure 8-2.
Am J Surg Pathol 1990;14:503–13. For figure 5-47E.
The Pancreas: Biology, Pathobiology, and Disease, 1993. For figure 4-45.

Springer-Verlag:
Atlas of Exocrine Pancreatic Tumors, 1994. For figure 7-24.
Virchows Arch [A] 1988;412:255–66. For figure 5-19.
Virchows Arch 1994;424:13–7. For figures 4-8 through 4-10.
Virchows Arch 1994;424:485–90. For figure 4-105.

WB Saunders:
Developmental Anatomy. For figures 1-1.
Gastroenterology 1991;101:512–9. For figure 4-41.
Radiol Clin N Am 1989;27:105–19. For figure 4-44.

Contents

# TUMORS OF THE PANCREAS

## INTRODUCTION

The second series Fascicle on pancreatic tumors from the Armed Forces Institute of Pathology (AFIP) included only neoplasms of the exocrine pancreas (7). In this third series Fascicle, both exocrine and endocrine tumors are discussed, as they were in the first series Fascicle (10). Thus, all neoplastic diseases of the pancreas are covered in a single book. This is important because: 1) there is often a need to differentiate between endocrine tumors and nonendocrine tumors such as solid pseudopapillary tumor (17) or acinar cell carcinoma (15); 2) there exist mixed exocrine-endocrine tumors (9) and undifferentiated (small) cell carcinomas (19); 3) diagnostic procedures at the clinical, radiologic, and pathologic levels often overlap; 4) surgical therapy may overlap; and 5) there is common embryology and vascular and nerve supply of the two components of pancreatic tissue which are better dealt with together.

The general classification of tumors of the exocrine pancreas adopted by A.L. Cubilla and P.J. Fitzgerald in the second series Fascicle has been retained. Most of the literature published in the last decade confirms the value of their work. However, recent studies of relatively large series of less common tumors, using histochemical markers, electron microscopy, and newly developed technologies, allows us to provide important information on the natural history and clinicopathologic profile of pancreatic tumors (14–17, 23,24), as well as discussing new diagnostic tools. New tumor entities, like intraductal tumors, are introduced, based on the mounting evidence of their consistent occurrence and special behavior (5,11,16). On the other hand, the individuality of some tumor types tentatively considered by Cubilla and Fitzgerald, as for instance the so-called microadenocarcinoma (variety of acinar cell carcinoma?), remains questionable.

The long period of time between the first series Fascicle (1959) and the current one and the resulting increase in knowledge in the field of pancreatic endocrinology forced the authors to provide an entirely new layout for endocrine tumors. Most of the pertinent morphologic literature of the last three decades was devoted more to the improvement of diagnostic criteria through hormones and endocrine marker immunohistochemistry, electron microscopy, and new technologies (1,3,13,18), than to the definition of tumor behavior through follow-up studies. Still, several studies of endocrine tumors before and after surgery, with careful postoperative follow-up, have been published. Although sometimes the description of the macroscopic and microscopic morphology of such tumors has been superficial, nevertheless these studies allow correlation of hormone-characterized tumor diseases with tumor prognosis and, to some extent, tumor morphology. This is important for reconstructing tumor behavior. Indeed, a combination of careful investigation of endocrine syndromes and tumor morphology and hormone histochemistry results in prediction of tumor behavior (20). With the present lack of reliable, extensively investigated and unquestionably proven morphologic signs of malignancy, this remains the simplest and most rewarding approach to the problem of assessing pancreatic endocrine tumor behavior. Consequently, in addition to tumor morphology, special attention has been given to the clinicopathologic profile of each functionally characterized tumor type.

We include a chapter dealing with the contribution of cytology and needle biopsy, in conjunction with improved radiologic and endoscopic tools, to the preoperative (and intraoperative) diagnosis of pancreatic tumors. The practical relevance of this approach to pancreatic tumor diagnosis is important in the appropriate choice of surgical therapy for tumors other than ductal cancer.

## REFERENCES


1. Bordi C, Pilato FP, D'Adda T. Comparative study of seven neuroendocrine markers in pancreatic endocrine tumors. Virchows Arch [A] 1988;413:387–98.
2. Broughan TA, Leslie JD, Soto JM, Herman RE. Pancreatic islet cell tumors. Surgery 1986;99:671–8.
3. Buffa R, Rindi G, Sessa F, et al. Synaptophysin immunoreactivity and small clear vesicles in neuroendocrine cells and related tumors. Mol Cell Probes 1987;1:367–81.
4. Capella C, Polak JM, Buffa R, et al. Morphologic patterns and diagnostic criteria of VIP-producing endocrine tumors. A histologic, histochemical, ultrastructural and biochemical study of 32 cases. Cancer 1983;52:1860–74.
5. Conley CR, Scheithauer BW, van Heerden JA, Weiland LH. Diffuse intraductal papillary adenocarcinoma of the pancreas. Ann Surg 1987;205:246–9.
6. Creutzfeldt W. Endocrine tumors of the pancreas. In: Volk BW, Arquilla ER, eds. The diabetic pancreas. New York: Plenum Publishing, 1985:543–86.
7. Cubilla AL, Fitzgerald PJ. Tumors of the exocrine pancreas. Atlas of Tumor Pathology, 2nd Series, Fascicle 19. Washington, D.C.: Armed Forces Institute of Pathology, 1984.
8. Danforth DN Jr, Gorden P, Bruman MF. Metastatic insulin-secreting carcinoma of the pancreas: clinical course and the role of surgery. Surgery 1984;96:1027–37.
9. Eusebi V, Capella C, Bondi A, Sessa F, Vezzadini P, Mancini AM. Endocrine-paracrine cells in pancreatic exocrine carcinomas. Histopathology 1981;5:599–613.
10. Frantz VK. Tumors of the pancreas. Atlas of Tumor Pathology, 1st Series, Fascicles 27 and 28. Washington D.C.: Armed Forces Institute of Pathology, 1959.
11. Furukawa T, Takahashi T, Kobari M. Matsuno S. The mucus-hypersecreting tumor of the pancreas. Development and extension visualized by three-dimensional computerized mapping. Cancer 1992;70:1505–13.
12. Guillausseau PJ, Guillausseau C, Villet R, et al. Les glucagonomes. Aspects cliniques, biologiques, anatomopathologiques et therapeutiques (revue general de 130 cases). Gastroenterol Clin Biol 1982;6:1029–41.
13. Heitz PU, Kasper M, Polak JM, Kloppel G. Pancreatic endocrine tumors. Hum Pathol 1982;13:263–71.
14. Hoorens A, Lemoine NR, McLellan E, et al. Pancreatic acinar cell carcinoma. An analysis of cell lineage markers, p53 expression and Ki-ras mutations. Am J Pathol 1993;143:685–98.
15. Klimstra DS, Heffess CS, Oertel JE, Rosai J. Acinar cell carcinoma of the pancreas. A clinicopathological study of 28 cases. Am J Surg Pathol 1992;16:815–37.
16. Morohoshi T, Kanda M, Asanuma K, Klöppel G. Intraductal papillary neoplasms of the pancreas. A clinicopathologic study of six patients. Cancer 1989;64:1329–35.
17. Morohoshi T, Kanda M, Horie A, et al. Immunocytochemical markers of uncommon pancreatic tumors: acinar cell carcinoma, pancreatoblastoma, and solid cystic (papillary-cystic) tumor. Cancer 1987;59:739–47.
18. Mukai K, Grotting JC, Greider MH, Rosai J. Retrospective study of 77 pancreatic endocrine tumors using the immunoperoxidase method. Am J Surg Pathol 1982;6:387–99.
19. Reyes CV, Wang T. Undifferentiated small cell carcinoma of the pancreas: a report of five cases. Cancer 1981;47:2500–2.
20. Solcia E, Sessa F, Rindi G, et al. Classification and histogenesis of gastroenteropancreatic endocrine tumors. Eur J Clin Invest 1990;20(Suppl 1):572–81.
21. Stabile BE, Passaro E Jr. Benign and malignant gastrinoma. Am J Surg 1985;149:144–50.
22. Thompson NW, Vinik AI, Eckhauser FE. Microgastrinomas of the duodenum. A cause of failed operations for the Zollinger-Ellison syndrome. Ann Surg 1989;209:396–404.
23. Warshaw AL, Compton CC, Lewandrowsky K, Cardenosa G, Mueller PR. Cystic tumors of the pancreas. New clinical, radiologic, and pathologic observations in 67 patients. Ann Surg 1990;212:432–45.
24. Yamaguchi K, Enjoji M. Cystic neoplasms of the pancreas. Gastroenterology 1987;92:1934–43.
25. Zollinger RM, Ellison EC, O'Dorisio TM, Sparks J. Thirty years' experience with gastrinomas. World J Surg 1984;8:427–35.


✧✧✧

# 1
# THE NORMAL PANCREAS

## EMBRYOLOGY AND DIFFERENTIATION

The pancreatic primordia first appear during the fifth week of gestation as two evaginations, one dorsal and one ventral, to the primitive intestine at the level of the distal part of the foregut (5–7). The dorsal rudiment arises caudal to the stomach, at the same level and just opposite the hepatic diverticulum. The ventral rudiment arises in the inferior angle formed by the hepatic diverticulum and the duodenum, slightly caudal to the dorsal bud (fig. 1-1). During the sixth week the primitive intestine and its derivatives turn 90° clockwise, so that the dorsal primordium extends into the left side of the abdomen while the ventral primordium lies on the right side. In addition to this axial rotation, which involves all derivatives of the distal part of the foregut, the ventral pancreas migrates dorsally first, then to the left side, together with the primordium of the common bile duct to which it remains attached. At the end of this process, the ventral pouch adheres to the dorsal aspect of the originally dorsal (now left-sided) pancreas, at a site which in the adult pancreas corresponds to the posterior part of the pancreatic head. The common bile duct and ventral pancreatic duct, which first appear during the eighth week, pass independently through duodenal mesenchyme

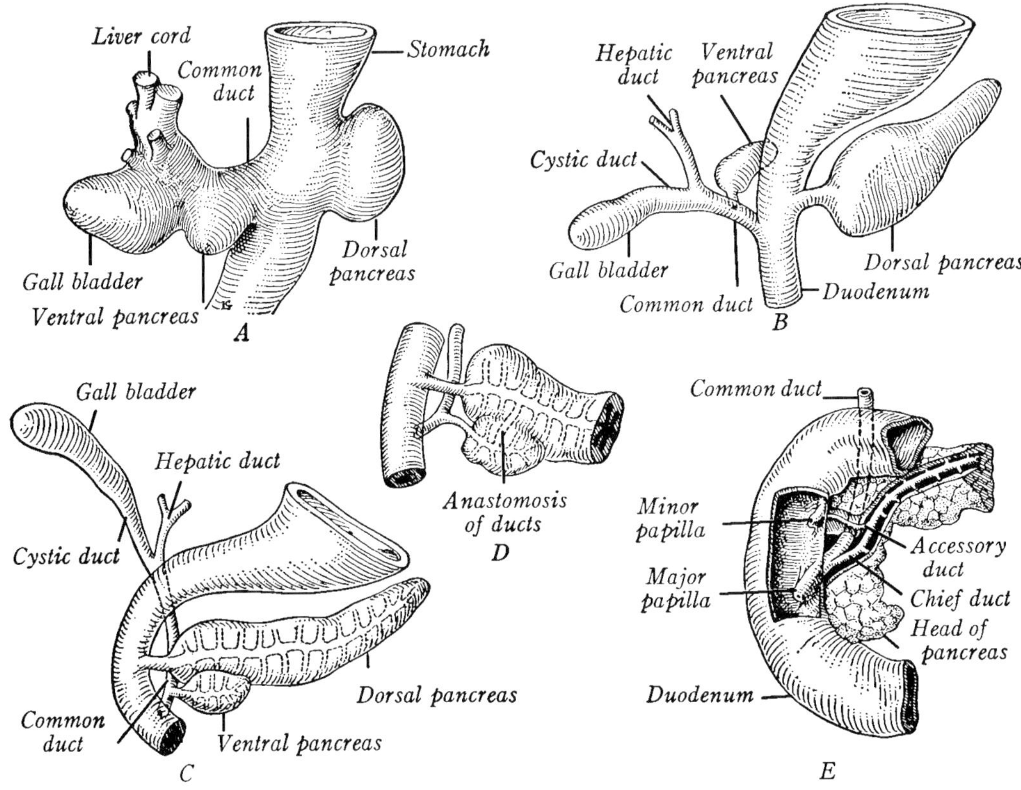


Figure 1-1
DEVELOPMENT OF THE HUMAN PANCREAS
Models shown are viewed from the left side: (A) At 6 mm (X83); (B, C, D) at 8 mm, 12 mm, and 16 mm, respectively (X42); and (E) at birth (X1). (Fig. 221 from Arey LB. Developmental anatomy, revised 7th ed. Philadelphia: W.B. Saunders, 1974.)

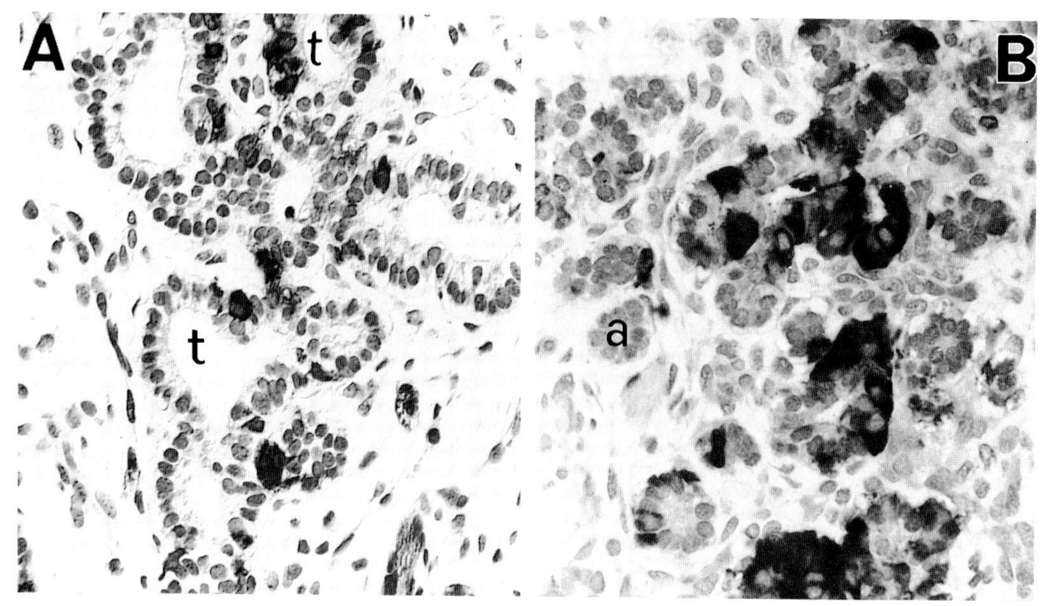


Figure 1-2
DEVELOPING PANCREAS IN A 10-WEEK-OLD FETUS
Primary tubules with scattered endocrine cells (A, synaptophysin immunoperoxidase-hematoxylin stain) or forming buds (B, chromogranin A immunoperoxidase-hematoxylin stain) represent primitive islets with chromogranin reactive cytoplasm or acini with unstained cytoplasm.

and enter the ampulla of Vater. The dorsal pancreatic duct penetrates the duodenal wall cephalad to the ampulla and major papilla, at a site in which a minor papilla may or may not form. Fusion of the ventral and dorsal primordia, which occurs during the sixth or seventh week of development, entails in most cases anastomosis of the respective ducts: the distal and midpart of the main (Wirsung) pancreatic duct results from the dorsal duct, while its proximal part up to the ampulla of Vater derives from the ventral main duct.

The proximal part of the dorsal main duct may form the accessory Santorini duct which opens into the duodenum through the minor papilla, or it may become a tributary to the Wirsung duct. A patent accessory duct is found in 85 percent of infants but only in 40 percent of adults, suggesting that secondary obliteration of the duodenal outlet of the accessory duct occurs in a large proportion of adults (3). Failure of duct fusion may leave the original ventral and dorsal ducts as two independent excretory systems, so-called pancreas divisum, a condition that occurs in 5 to 10 percent of people and predisposes to chronic pancreatitis. Interestingly, the duct system of the head immediately surrounding the intrapancreatic tract of the main bile duct and the Wirsung duct, which undergoes complex remodeling during embryogenesis, is the site of the highest incidence of ductal adenocarcinoma.

Histologically, the earliest primordia consist of a system of small primary tubules formed by undifferentiated epithelial cells immersed in a loose connective tissue matrix (4,5). Endocrine cells first appear during the eight week as single elements scattered at the base of these tubules. Immunohistochemical tests show the appearance of A, B, and D cells at about the same time, with pancreatic polypeptide (PP) cells following a few days later. From 10 to 13 weeks clusters of epithelial cells bud off from the tubules either at their distal end (terminal buds) or along their course (paratubular buds) (2). In some paratubular buds, cells poor in glycogen develop secretory granules of an endocrine nature; these primitive islets are penetrated later by a capillary bed. The remaining paratubular buds and all the terminal buds become primitive acini, formed by larger cells with abundant glycogen, increased cytoplasmic basophilia due to scattered ribosomes and progressively developing ergastoplasma, and a few zymogen granules (figs. 1-2–1-4).

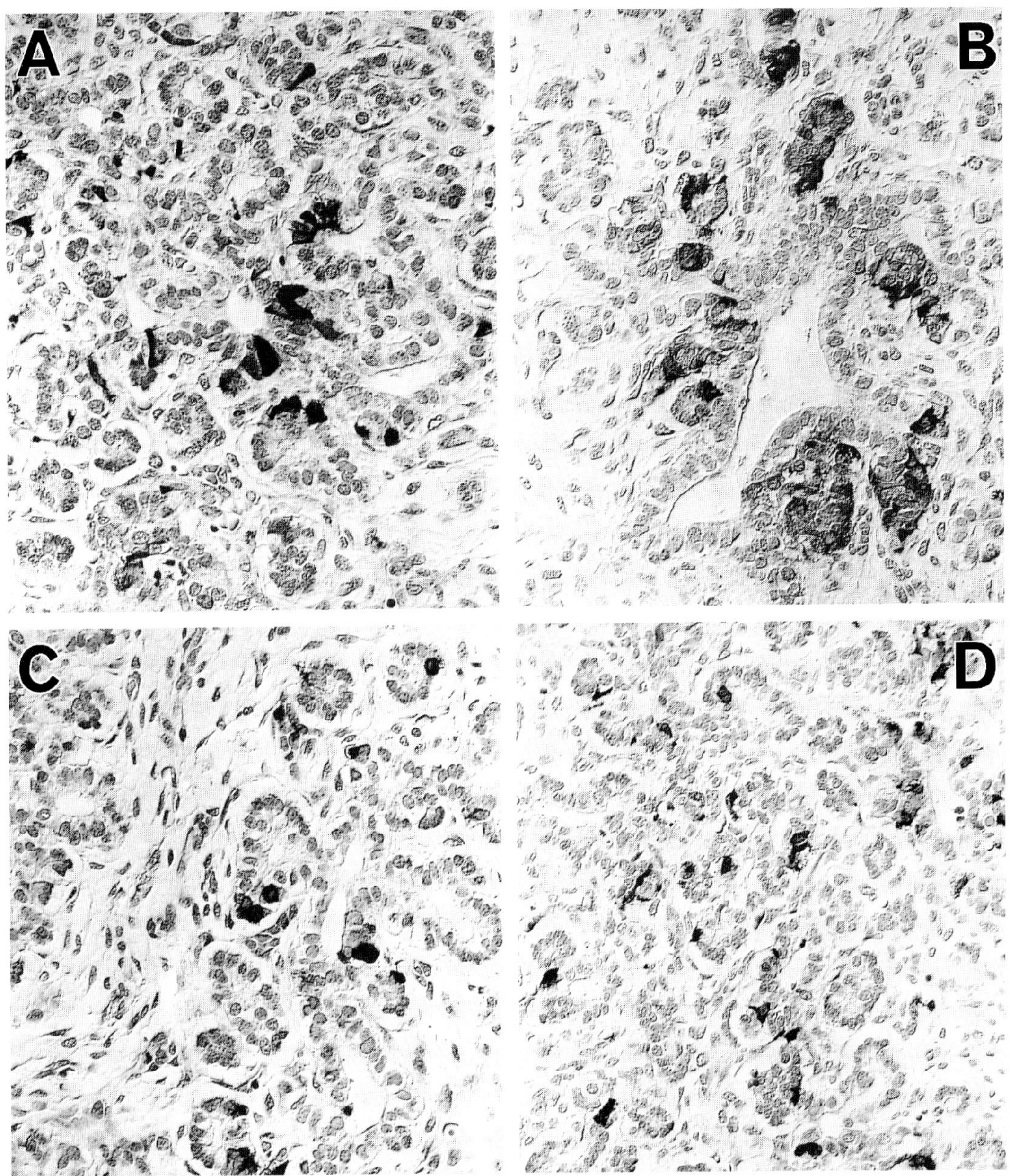


Figure 1-3

DORSAL POUCH OF DEVELOPING PANCREAS IN A 10-WEEK-OLD FETUS

Individual or clustered insulin (A), glucagon (B), pancreatic polypeptide (C), and somatostatin (D) cells are stained with specific hormone antibodies in primary tubules or their buds (X28,000).

Cells located at the center of some acini (centroacinar) or bordering the preterminal or intercalated ductules remain small and glycogen rich, with clear cytoplasm devoid of secretory granules, thus retaining the immature pattern of primary duct cells. The common origin of early islets, acini, and centroacinar cells from the same primary ductules is important, given the occurrence of ductular cells inside islet cell tumors and of islet cells inside centroacinar-ductular or acinar cell tumors.

Between 12 and 15 weeks (early fetal period) the parenchyma organizes into lobules. The developing main duct branches into interlobular

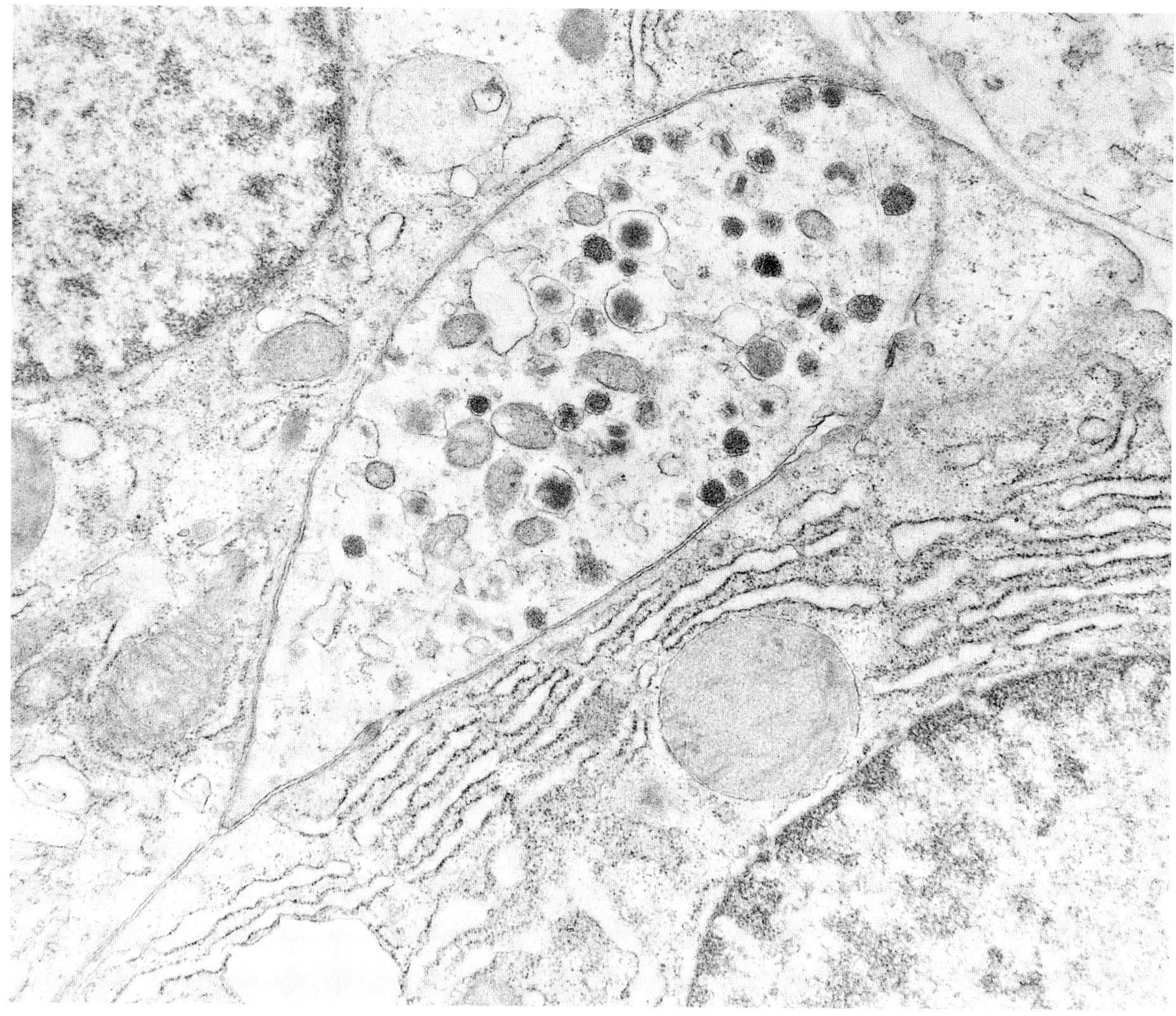

Figure 1-4
ULTRASTRUCTURE OF DEVELOPING PANCREAS IN A 38/39-WEEK-OLD FETUS
An acinar cell with well-developed rough endoplasmic reticulum (bottom right), an islet B cell with partly vesicular and crystalline beta granules (center), and a primitive ductule cell with a few scattered reticulum cisternae are seen in this 170-mm long fetus (X28,000).

(lobar) ducts and branches of these become the intralobular ducts or ductules. They terminate as centroacinar cells adjacent to acinar cell clusters, organized either as blind-ending acini or as tubular acini (1). Due to the growth of the terminal buds, newly formed acini accumulate at the periphery of the lobules while most islets, which originate from paratubular buds, accumulate in the center of the lobules, surrounded by tubuloacinar structures. The low columnar or cuboidal cells of the intralobular ducts differ from the small attenuated cells forming the intercalated-centroacinar ductules, as well as from the tall columnar cells of lobar (extralobular, interlobular) and main ducts. Juxtaluminal mucus granules and irregular, long luminal microvilli are present in the epithelial cells of the interlobular or main ducts, but are absent in the intralobular ducts and centroacinar cells.

Secreted mucin stratifies on the luminal surface of interlobular and main ducts to form a thin continuous layer that is reactive with Alcian blue and the high iron diamine (HID) technique for sulfomucins. The reactivity of most nonendocrine adenocarcinomas using these methods supports their histogenetic and phenotypic relationship to large extralobular ducts (11). Developmental studies delineate two distinct ductal compartments: the mucinous cells lining the main and interlobular ducts, which, together with the metaplastic changes, form the main component of papillary-mucinous tumors, mucinous cystic tumors, and duct cell carcinomas, and the ductulo-centroacinar (intralobular) compartment, to which serous cystic and solid-pseudopapillary tumors are closely related (9,12). Acinar and islet cells are embryologically related to the ductulo-centroacinar cells, with which they form the lobule. This may explain the frequent admixture of such intralobular cell types inside pertinent tumors.

During gestation islet cells of A, B, D, and PP types are formed along intralobular and intercalated ductules; islet cell neogenesis remains active in these ductules throughout gestation and up to the early postnatal period (10), while it ceases in the lobar or main ducts. A few "primary" islet cells originating from that part of the primary duct epithelium that later develops into larger ducts, may remain within interlobular connective tissue. After the fifth month such islets undergo degeneration and disappear (6). Islet A and D cells, which are more abundant in the fetal than adult pancreas, tend to segregate from B cells in some fetal islets: the so-called mantle islets have multiple strata of A and D cells enveloping a compact central nucleus of B cells; the bipolar islets have non-B and B cells clustering at opposite poles of the islet. The abundant islets at the posteroinferior part of the head, known to be of ventral pouch origin, produce PP cells, some B cells, and very few D or A cells (8). Such PP-rich islets are irregular in shape and size, and have a distinctive trabecular arrangement of columnar cells.

During fetal development the mesenchymal component, which is of splanchnic mesodermal origin and represents up to 50 percent of total pancreatic volume at first, progressively decreases so that in the newborn it corresponds to about one fourth of the total pancreatic volume. The mesenchymal tissue has an essential role in the modulation of growth and differentiation of the epithelial component, independent of the blood vessels and nerves running in it (4).

## PANCREAS OF NEWBORNS AND INFANTS

The pancreas of the newborn differs in many respects from the adult pancreas. Differences in the amount and distribution of the endocrine component are especially important in the diagnosis of neonatal nesidioblastosis.

The newborn pancreas is prominently lobulated due to the thickness of the connective tissue septa. This stroma represents 28 percent of pancreatic volume in newborns (14), compared to about 10 percent in adults. In newborns, the islet volume is about 10 percent of the total pancreatic tissue (compared to 1 to 2 percent in the adult gland) or about 15 percent of the epithelial component of the pancreas. The total islet weight is estimated to be 0.3 g while the maximum diameter of the islets range between 85 and 210 μm. In addition to the well-formed islets situated in the central part of the lobules, numerous endocrine cell clusters and even single endocrine cells are scattered in the exocrine tissue, especially at the periphery of the lobules. These extrainsular clusters and cells form a considerable proportion of the total endocrine component in the newborn pancreas, whereas they account for less than 10 percent of endocrine tissue in the adult pancreas.

The larger islets in the newborn pancreas have the same ribbon-lobular appearance as most regular islets in the adult pancreas. The prevalent, centrally grouped B cells are surrounded by A and D cells distributed at the islet periphery or along the capillaries, at the border of intrainsular ribbons and lobules (fig. 1-5). The smaller islets and cell clusters are compact; they are frequently associated with intralobular ductules. Only a few mantle or bipolar islets typical of fetal pancreas are found in the newborn. Budding-off of endocrine cells from the epithelium of interlobular or main ducts is rare. Islets dispersed in the interlobular spaces (the so-called septal islets) are infrequent, although, when present, they may be quite large (13). As in the adult pancreas, islets of the posteroinferior head are irregular in size and shape, and are mostly (70 to 80 percent) composed of columnar PP cells arranged in parallel, monolayered trabeculae separated by thin strands of vascular stroma (15).

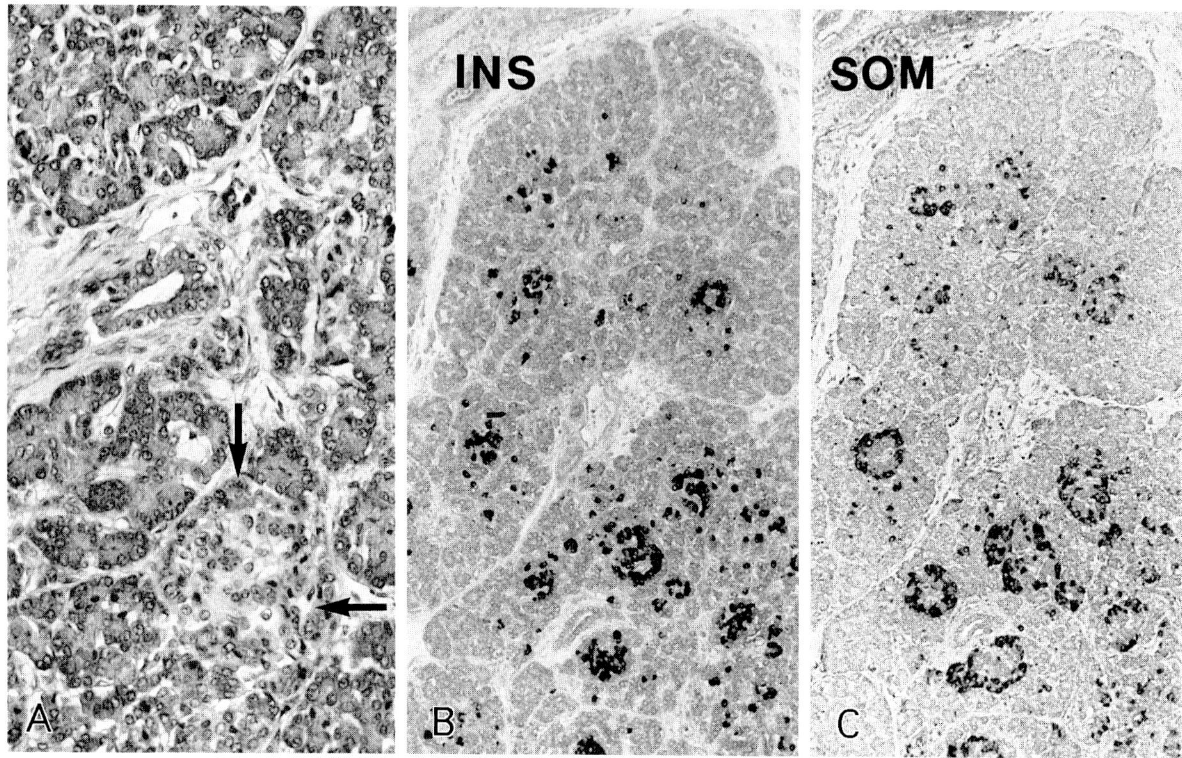


Figure 1-5
PANCREAS OF A NEWBORN

The illustration shows well-lobulated pancreatic tissue with an islet (arrows) at the periphery of a lobule (A). Immunostaining for insulin (INS) and somatostatin (SOM) reveals the presence of small islet cell clusters in addition to well-formed islets which show insulin cells in the center and somatostatin cells in the periphery.

The exocrine pancreas undergoes an accelerated expansion during early postnatal life. As a consequence, the volume density of the endocrine and stromal components decreases rapidly. The endocrine tissue is only 5 to 7 percent of the epithelial component in infants up to 6 months of age, and the connective tissue is about 20 percent of the total gland volume. The number of small cellular clusters and scattered single cells decreases considerably while the budding of endocrine cells from ductular epithelium is nearly completely discontinued (14).

## ADULT PANCREAS

### Gross Anatomy

**General Topography.** The pancreas is a retroperitoneal, yellow-white, firm, distinctly lobulated organ weighing approximately 100 g in adult males and 85 g in adult females (19). It is enveloped by retroperitoneal connective tissue which forms a poorly defined capsule. The dimensions of the pancreas are generally reported as between 15 to 25 cm in length, 1.4 to 4 cm in thickness, and 3 to 9 cm in height (34). Surgical access to the pancreas is difficult since it lies transversely in the retroperitoneum behind the stomach and transverse colon, with the head inserted into the duodenal C loop and the tail extending to the hilus of the spleen (fig. 1-6). The neck of the gland lies between the celiac trunk above and the superior mesenteric artery below.

The pancreas is divided into four parts: head, neck, body, and tail. The head is the thicker part of the organ and borders the duodenum, the common bile duct, the pancreatico-duodenal vessels, the vena cava, and the right renal artery and vein. The uncinate process of the head extends upwards from the lower border to pass behind the neck and the superior mesenteric vessels; it inserts between the portal vein and the inferior vena cava (59).

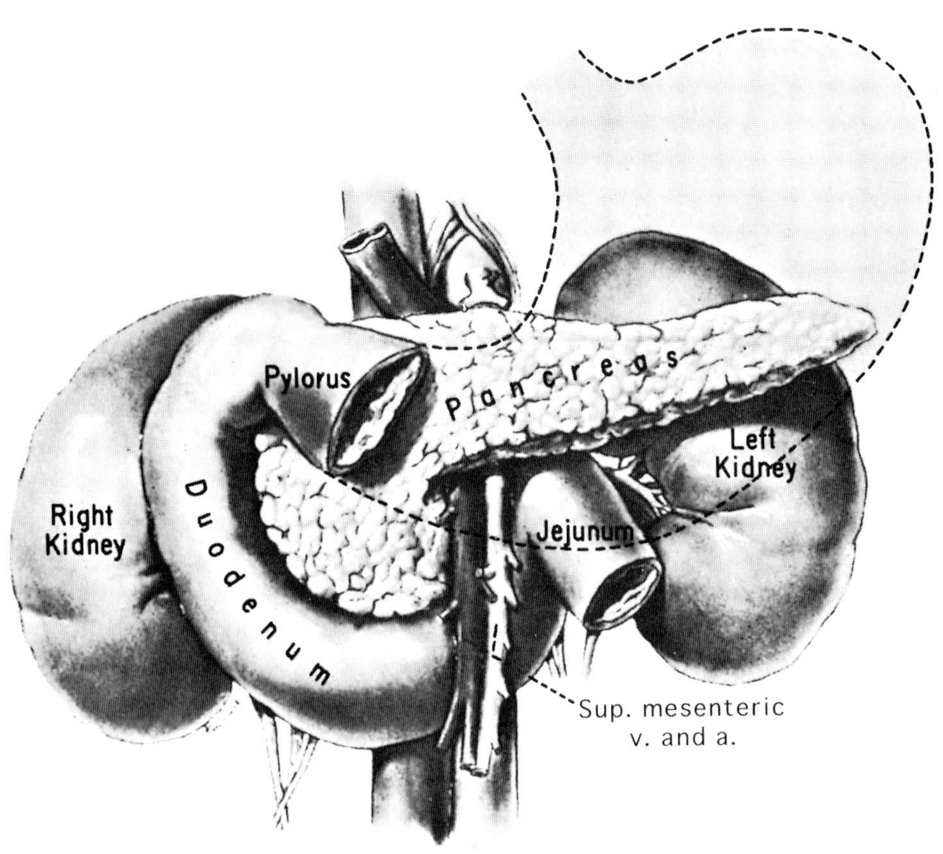


Figure 1-6
GROSS ANATOMY OF THE HUMAN PANCREAS
Topography of the pancreas and its neighboring structures. (Fig. 25 from Fascicle 19, Second Series.)

The superior mesenteric vessels sometimes indent the uncinate process to form a groove called the pancreatic notch. The body and tail of the organ are elongated and extend to the left anterior to the aorta, left kidney, and left adrenal gland, and posterior to the stomach from which they are separated by the lesser peritoneal sac.

The duct of Wirsung is the main pancreatic duct; it opens into the duodenum at the papilla of Vater. It drains the major part of the gland and begins in the tail by the convergence of several small ducts (secondary ducts) (fig. 1-7). Its course is horizontal in the tail and body; in the head, it moves posteriorly and inferiorly to form an arch (convex to right). It often receives a large secondary duct which drains the posteroinferior part, including the uncinate process. The diameter of the duct of Wirsung averages 3 mm, varying from 1.8 to more than 9 mm (18). The accessory pancreatic duct of Santorini, which embryologically corresponds to the head part of the dorsal duct, is present in 99 percent of people. This duct drains the anterosuperior part of the head and may open into the duodenum at a minor papilla, about 2 cm cephalad to the papilla of Vater. It may also anastomose with the duct of Wirsung, near the neck of the pancreas. Obliteration of duodenal outlet of the accessory duct is found in 15 percent of infants and 60 percent of adults. In such cases the accessory duct becomes a tributary of the Wirsung duct.

**Blood Supply.** The arterial supply of the pancreas consists of numerous anastomoses between different vessels and many anatomic variations. The main blood supply derives from the celiac trunk and the superior mesenteric artery (fig. 1-8) (36,58). The anterior and the posterior pancreatico-duodenal arcade, formed by the

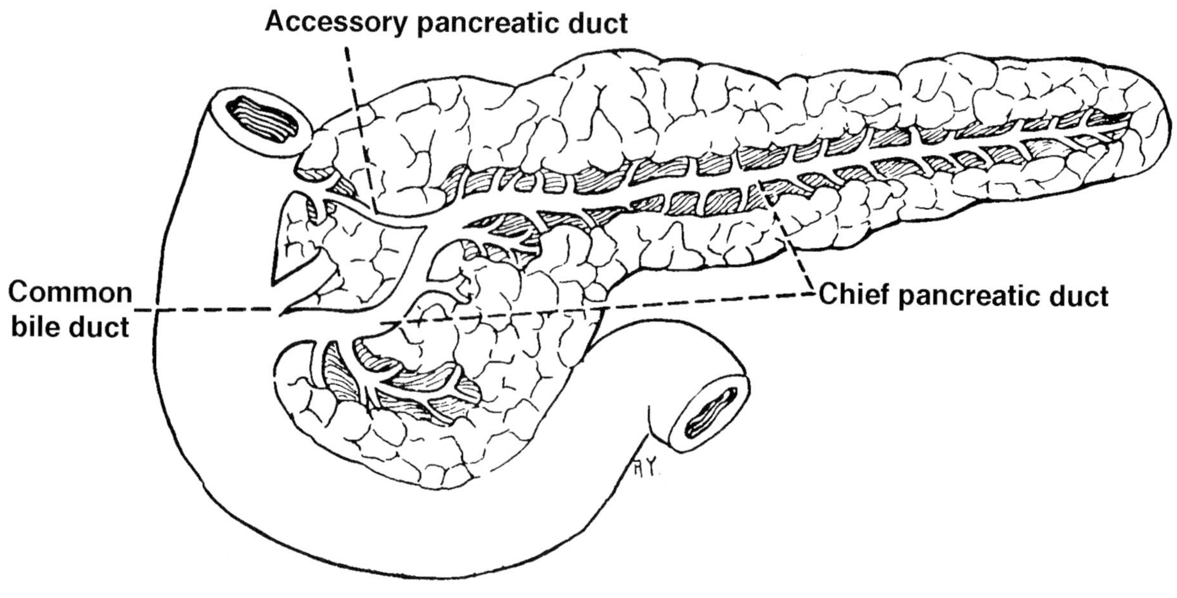


Figure 1-7
GROSS ANATOMY OF THE HUMAN PANCREAS: DUCTAL SYSTEM
Schematic view of the ductal system of the pancreas. (Fig. 28 from Fascicle 19, Second Series.)

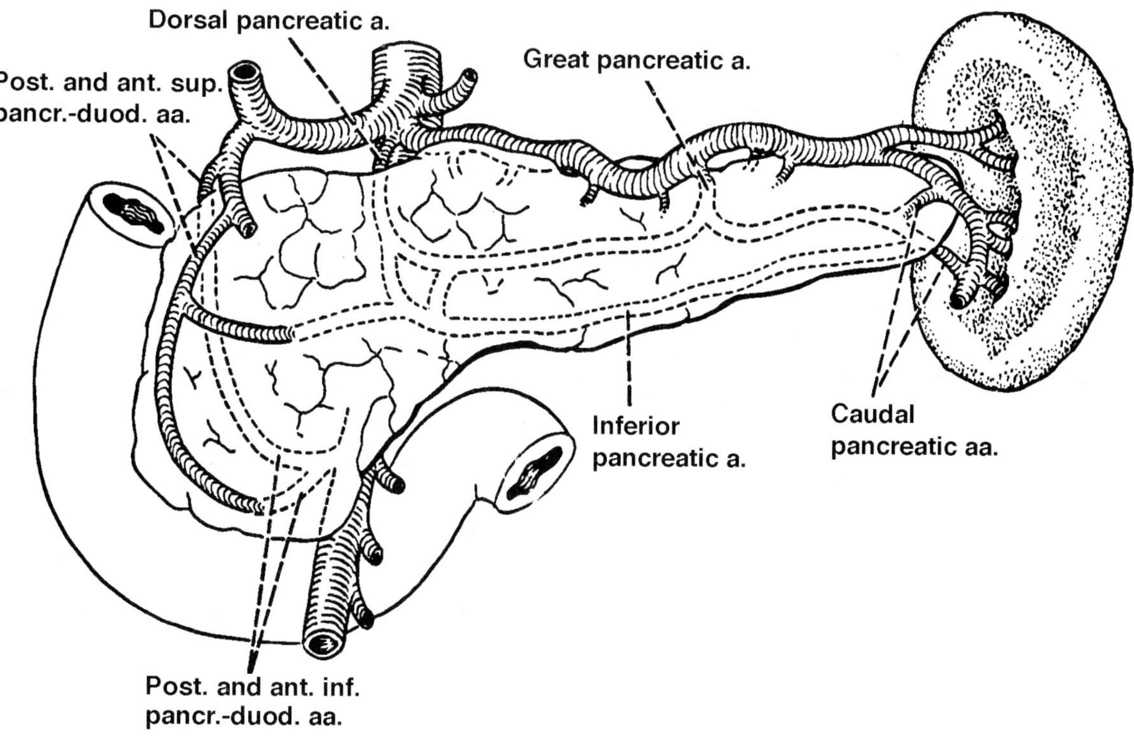


Figure 1-8
GROSS ANATOMY OF THE HUMAN PANCREAS: ARTERIAL SYSTEM
Principal arteries of the pancreas and their anastomoses. (Fig. 26 from Fascicle 19, Second Series.)

anastomosis of the anterior and posterior branches of the superior and inferior pancreatico-duodenal arteries, supply the head and the duodenum. The neck, uncinate process, and body are supplied by the dorsal pancreatic artery, which may be a branch of the celiac, hepatic, splenic, or superior mesenteric arteries, and by the inferior pancreatic artery which is a continuation of the left branch of the dorsal pancreatic artery. In addition, the splenic artery supplies the pancreas with as many as nine branches. A large branch of the splenic artery, the great pancreatic (pancreatica magna) artery, contributes, within the pancreas, a left and right branch often oriented along the course of the duct of Wirsung. The tail is supplied by branches of the splenic artery or the left gastroepiploic artery; these constitute the caudal pancreatic arteries.

Venous drainage is through the hepatic portal vein, which forms from the superior mesenteric and splenic veins. The veins of the pancreas correspond to the relative arteries and follow the same course (27). They are particularly abundant along the large pancreatic ducts. The splenic vein courses to the right in a groove on the posterior surface of the pancreas and in its course receives small collaterals draining the gland. The pancreatico-duodenal veins drain into the superior mesenteric vein, which passes ventral to the uncinate process and joins the splenic vein behind the neck of the pancreas to form the hepatic portal vein.

Since the major veins and arteries of the pancreas course posteriorly to the Wirsung duct, the ducts can be opened surgically through an anterior approach, avoiding serious hemorrhage (59). The intrinsic blood supply of the pancreas is well developed and assures a functional relationship between the endocrine and exocrine tissues. The branches of the pancreatic arteries supply interlobular arteries that course into the connective tissue septa; there is a single intralobular artery for each lobule.

The islets receive their blood supply via short arterioles. Since the capillaries of the islets are often wider than those in the exocrine part of the pancreas, it is inferred that the capillary pressure is higher in the islet vessels than in the neighboring exocrine vessels. Where islet-exocrine connections exist, the direction of flow should be from the islets to the exocrine tissue. Centrifugal flow from the islets and endocrine-exocrine connecting vessels has been demonstrated by cinematography and injection techniques (30,35). This flow ensures passage of hormone-rich blood from the endocrine to the exocrine tissue. In the absence of islets, the intralobular arteries end directly in a capillary network among the acini.

**Lymphatic Drainage.** The peripheral lymphatic plexi of the pancreas are formed by periacinar and perilobular lymphatic capillaries coursing next to blood capillaries in the interstitial connective tissue. At the surface of the pancreas they drain into valved channels that run through the interlobular septa (26). Superficial lymphatics can be subdivided into five main collecting trunks and lymph node groups (fig. 1-9) (22,23): superior, inferior, anterior, posterior, and splenic.

*Superior.* These afferent vessels drain lymph from the upper part of the pancreas into the suprapancreatic lymph nodes situated at the upper margin of the head and body. These are called superior head (SH) and superior body (SB) lymph nodes, respectively (fig. 1-9). Infrequently, some lymph passes to the nodes of the gastropancreatic fold or to the hepatic chain.

*Inferior.* These lymphatic channels drain the lower half of the head and body of the pancreas and end in the inferior pancreatic group of lymph nodes that are mainly located at the inferior border of the head (IH) and body (IB) of the gland. They may also be connected with the superior mesenteric and left lateroaortic lymph nodes. Rarely, a collecting trunk drains into a lumbar trunk directly, a situation that may explain the presence of systemic metastases from a pancreatic cancer in the absence of hepatic metastases.

*Anterior.* The collecting trunks course along the anterior surface of the head of the pancreas and terminate in the pyloric (Py) nodes, anterior pancreaticoduodenal (APD) nodes, and some mesenteric lymph nodes near the jejunum (Je).

*Posterior.* These collecting lymphatic channels run along the posterior surface of the head of the pancreas. They lead into the posterior pancreaticoduodenal (PPD) lymph nodes, the common bile duct (CBD) nodes, the right lateroaortic nodes, and to some lymph nodes at the origin of the superior mesenteric artery. The PPD group drains most of the lymph flowing from the ampulla of Vater and the common bile duct.

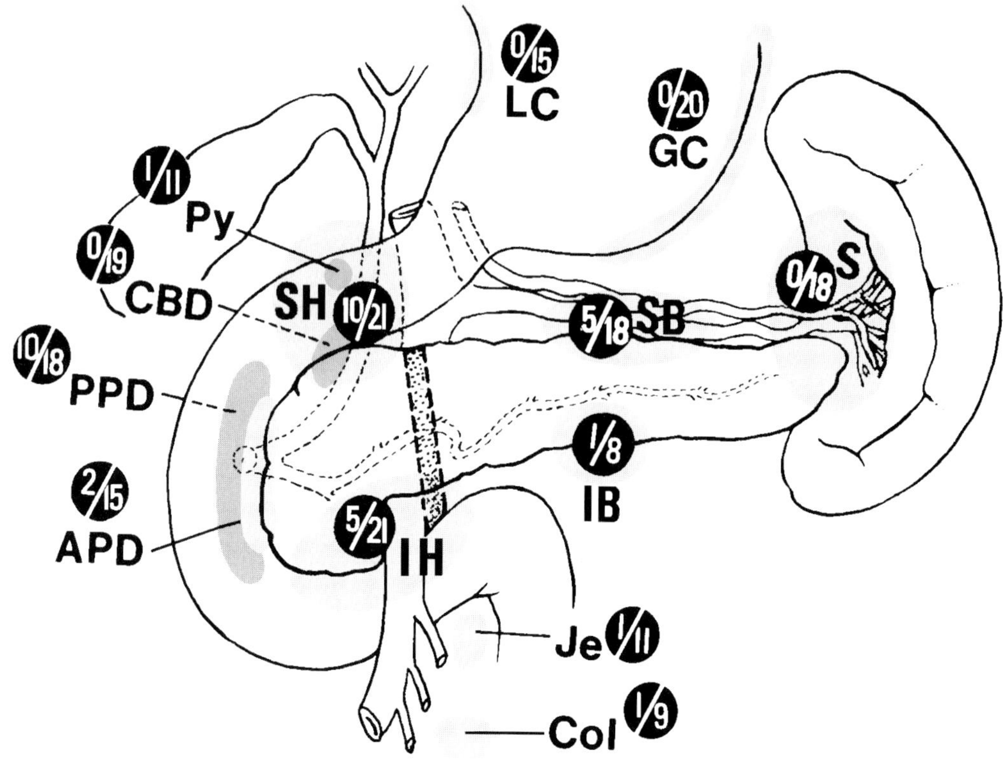


Figure 1-9

GROSS ANATOMY OF THE HUMAN PANCREAS: LYMPHATIC SYSTEM

Lymph node grouping (with results from dissection specimens of 21 cancers of the head of the pancreas). Denominator indicates the number of patients in whom lymph nodes of that group were found and the numerator indicates the number of patients in whom lymph nodes contained cancer, microscopically verified. The symbols represent the following groups of lymph nodes: SH = superior head; IH = inferior head; PPD = posterior pancreaticoduodenal; APD = anterior pancreaticoduodenal; SB = superior body; IB = inferior body; S = splenic; GC = greater curvature; LC = lesser curvature; PY = pylorus; CBD = common bile duct; Je = jejunum; and Col = colon. (Fig. 27 from Fascicle 19, Second Series.)

*Splenic.* These lymphatics drain the lymph from the tail of the pancreas to the S group of lymph nodes (formed by the superior lymph nodes of the tail of the pancreas), the phrenicolienal ligament nodes, and those at the hilus of the spleen. A few lymphatics, however, drain into the superior and inferior lymph nodes of the body of the pancreas. In addition, a recent study based on the frequency of lymph node involvement in cases of carcinoma of the head of the pancreas demonstrated that the main lymphatic pathway from the head of pancreas to the para-aortic lymph nodes is via lymph nodes around the superior mesenteric artery (40).

**Nerve Supply.** The pancreas is innervated by both vagal and sympathetic nerves. In addition, the organ is supplied by afferent fibers that course either with sympathetic or vagal branches. Innervation of the head of the pancreas is greater than in the tail.

The vagus fibers are part of the regulatory system that controls exocrine and endocrine secretory activity as well as capillary blood flow of the pancreas. Vagal efferent fibers originate from cell bodies located in the vagal dorsal nucleus. Fibers are carried by both right and left vagi to the celiac plexus, then to the interlobular septa of the pancreas where they synapse with small ganglia. The postganglionic neurons forming these ganglia have numerous nerve endings that are distributed to acinar cells, islet cells, and smooth muscle cells in the ducts (54).

Sympathetic innervation originates from neurons located in the lateral grey column of segments 5 to 10 of the thoracic spinal cord. Sympathetic fibers reach the celiac ganglia through the greater splanchnic nerve and synapse with these ganglia. Postganglionic fibers course along the hepatic, splenic, and superior mesenteric arteries and innervate the pancreatic vessels. In addition to pancreatic arteries and arterioles, pancreatic veins are also innervated by sympathetic fibers. Direct vasomotor control of these vessels and arteriolar vessels regulates blood flow through the pancreas.

A major portion of the pancreatic fibers of the vagus nerve are visceral afferent. These fibers are implicated in duodenal-pancreatic reflex mechanisms, but are not involved in the transmission of pain from the pancreas, which occurs by afferent sympathetic fibers. Afferent sympathetic fibers enter the spinal cord at the same levels as the efferent ones.

### Histology and Cytology

The pancreas is a composite exocrine-endocrine gland: the prevalent exocrine portion forms up to 84 percent of the pancreatic volume, blood vessels and duct cells represent about 4 percent, and the endocrine component is only 2 percent. The rest (about 10 percent) is formed by extracellular matrix (32). The lobule is the morphologic unit of pancreatic parenchyma. It is mostly composed of acini (fig. 1-10) separated by thin, incomplete connective tissue septa harboring blood vessels, lymphatics, nerves, and interlobular ducts (19,34). Recent studies based on retrograde injections of silicone rubber into the duct system and reconstruction using light microscopic analysis have shown that the relationship between ducts and acini within the lobule is complex (16). Not all acini are spheroidal and not all acini are at the end of intercalated ducts. Acini may be cylindrical or irregular. They may be formed on the side of a duct, crossed by a duct, or interpolated between ducts. Lumina may form anastomotic loops surrounded by combinations of acinar and ductular cells. This three-dimensional organization and the abundance of anastomosing tubular structures formed by ductular cells within the lobules may explain why these structures become well evident in conditions like chronic pancreatitis, conditions associated with acinar cell atrophy (16).

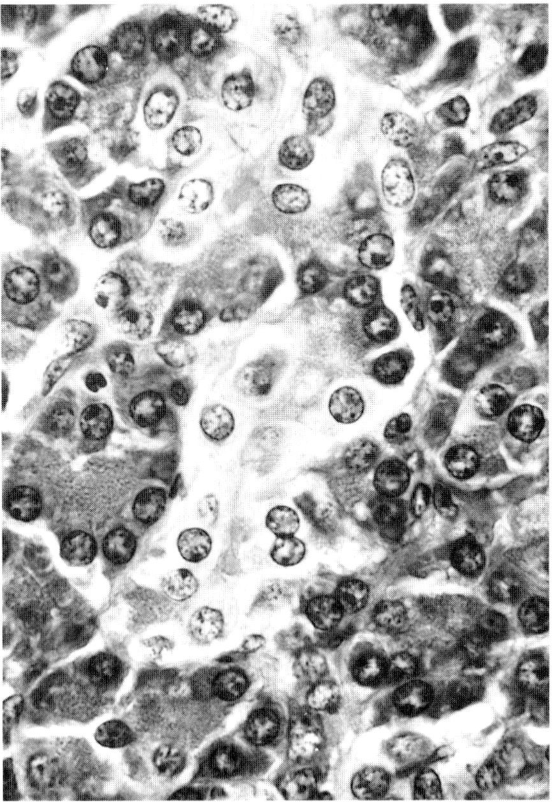

Figure 1-10
HISTOLOGY OF THE
HUMAN ENDOCRINE PANCREAS
Part of a lobule showing several acini. Cells with clear cytoplasm (centroacinar and ductal cells) stand out of a background of basophilic acinar cells.

The adult human exocrine pancreas has four major types of cells: 1) the exocrine acinar cells, organized in acini, which provide the enzymes involved in digestion; 2) the centroacinar-ductular cells which secrete fluid rich in bicarbonate; 3) the mucin-secreting cells which form interlobular and main ducts; and 4) connective tissue cells which form the interstitial tissue. The main distinctive markers of these cells are listed in Table 1-1.

**Acinar Cells.** More than 80 percent of the pancreas is composed of acinar cells. By light microscopy, these cells are large and pyramidal; their base sits on basal lamina that is composed of type IV collagen, laminin, and fibronectin (32). The apical cytoplasm of acinar cells contains characteristic eosinophilic, periodic acid–Schiff

Table 1-1

**HISTOCHEMICAL AND IMMUNOHISTOCHEMICAL MARKERS OF NORMAL PANCREATIC CELLS**

| | Mucin Stains | | | Immunohistochemical Markers | | | | | | |
|---|---|---|---|---|---|---|---|---|---|---|
| **Cell Types** | **PAS*** | **AB** | **HID** | **DuPan 2** | **CFTR** | **TRYP** | **CK8,18** | **CK7,19** | **CK4** | **SYN** |
| Ductal | +/– | + | + | + | + | – | + | + | + | – |
| Ductular | – | – | – | +/– | + | – | + | + | – | – |
| Centroacinar | – | – | – | – | +/– | – | + | + | – | – |
| Acinar | – | – | – | – | + | + | + | – | – | – |
| Endocrine | – | – | – | – | – | – | + | – | – | + |

*PAS - periodic acid-Schiff; AB - Alcian blue; HID - high iron diamine; DuPan 2 - antigen normally found in pancreatic duct cells; CFTR - cystic fibrosis transmembrane conductance regulator protein; TRYP - trypsinogen; CK - cytokeratin; SYN - synaptophysin.

(PAS)-positive zymogen granules. The basal region of the cell is characterized by intense basophilia due to the presence of a rough endoplasmic reticulum. The nucleus is round and generally located at the base of the cell (fig. 1-10).

Electron microscopy shows a rough endoplasmic reticulum that is extensively developed and mainly located in the infranuclear and paranuclear regions of the cytoplasm. Between the cisternae are mitochondria and free polyribosomes (40). The nuclei are prominent with clearly defined nucleoli. Above the nucleus and in the central portion of the cells are elements of the Golgi complex. The Golgi complex consists of three to five stacks of flattened saccules bound by smooth surface unit membranes and numerous vesicles. Located at the inner concave side of the complex (the trans or maturing face) are immature zymogen granules or condensing vacuoles (41).

In the apex of acinar cells are numerous spherical, mature storage granules, each bound by a smooth surface unit membrane and containing electron-dense material (fig. 1-11). At the luminal surface, the apical plasmalemma of the cell projects microvilli into the duct lumen. The microvilli have a core formed by bundles of microfilaments anchored to the filamentous network beneath the apical plasma membrane (terminal webs). Immunohistochemical investigations have demonstrated that villin, an actin-binding protein that plays a major role in the morphogenesis of microvilli, is located at the apical surface of the acinar cells (25). The cells are joined together by occluding junctions (zonula occludens) close to the luminal space, desmosomes (zonula adherens) at the level of terminal web, and spot desmosomes (macula adherens) at the lower parts of the lateral plasma membrane (41).

The main function of acinar cells is the production of enzymatically inert digestive proenzymes (trypsinogen 1, 2, and 3; chymotrypsinogen A and B; procarboxypeptidase A1 and A2; procarboxypeptidase B1 and B2; proelastase 1 and 2; kallikreinogen; prophospholipase A; lipase; and amylase). All these precursors are transformed into active forms by an activating cascade process which begins in the duodenal lumen (49). Immunohistochemical analysis of the pancreas at the electron microscopic level shows no qualitative specialization between acinar cells as regards secretory products (43). In an investigation of the cellular distribution of nine enzymes, Bendayan et al. (17) found ultrastructural labeling of all the enzymes in every cell, with progressively increasing concentrations from the reticuloendoplasmic region (RER) to the Golgi zone, and from this zone to the granules. This distribution reflects the pathway of the process of synthesis: protein precursors are first synthesized in the polyribosomes in the

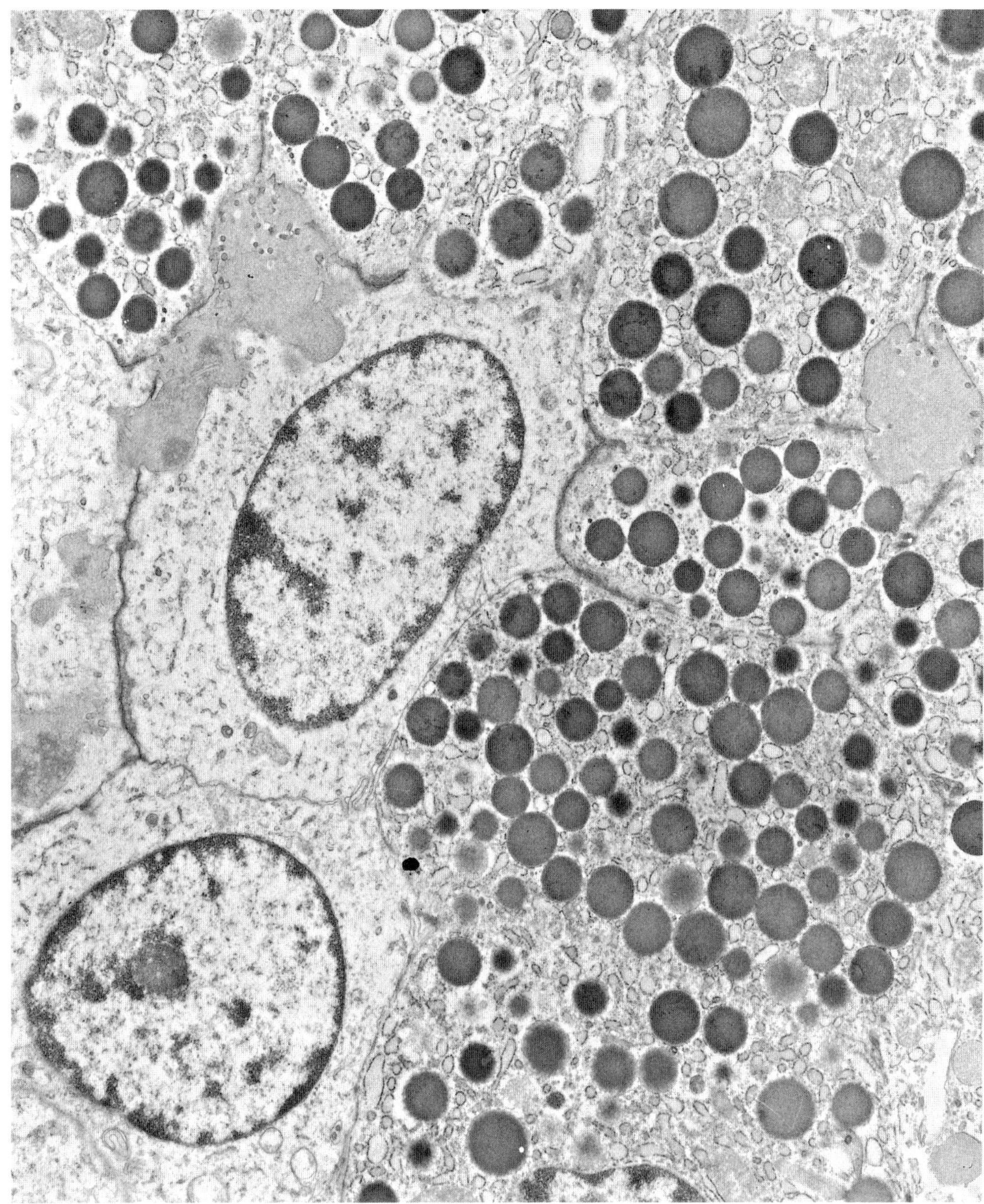

Figure 1-11
NORMAL PANCREAS: CENTROACINAR AND ACINAR CELLS
Two centroacinar cells with electron-lucent cytoplasm, poor in organelles, surrounded by acinar cells rich in zymogen granules (X11,200).

RER, they are then segregated into cisternae of RER, and transported to the Golgi apparatus where concentration of proteins results in the formation of zymogen granules, in which all proenzymes are packaged together (51). The final step in this pathway consists of the discharge of zymogen granules into the acinar lumen by a complex mechanism called exocytosis. This step implies the movement of zymogen granules to the cell apex where fusion of the limiting membranes occurs. As a consequence, the stored products are delivered to the acinar lumen.

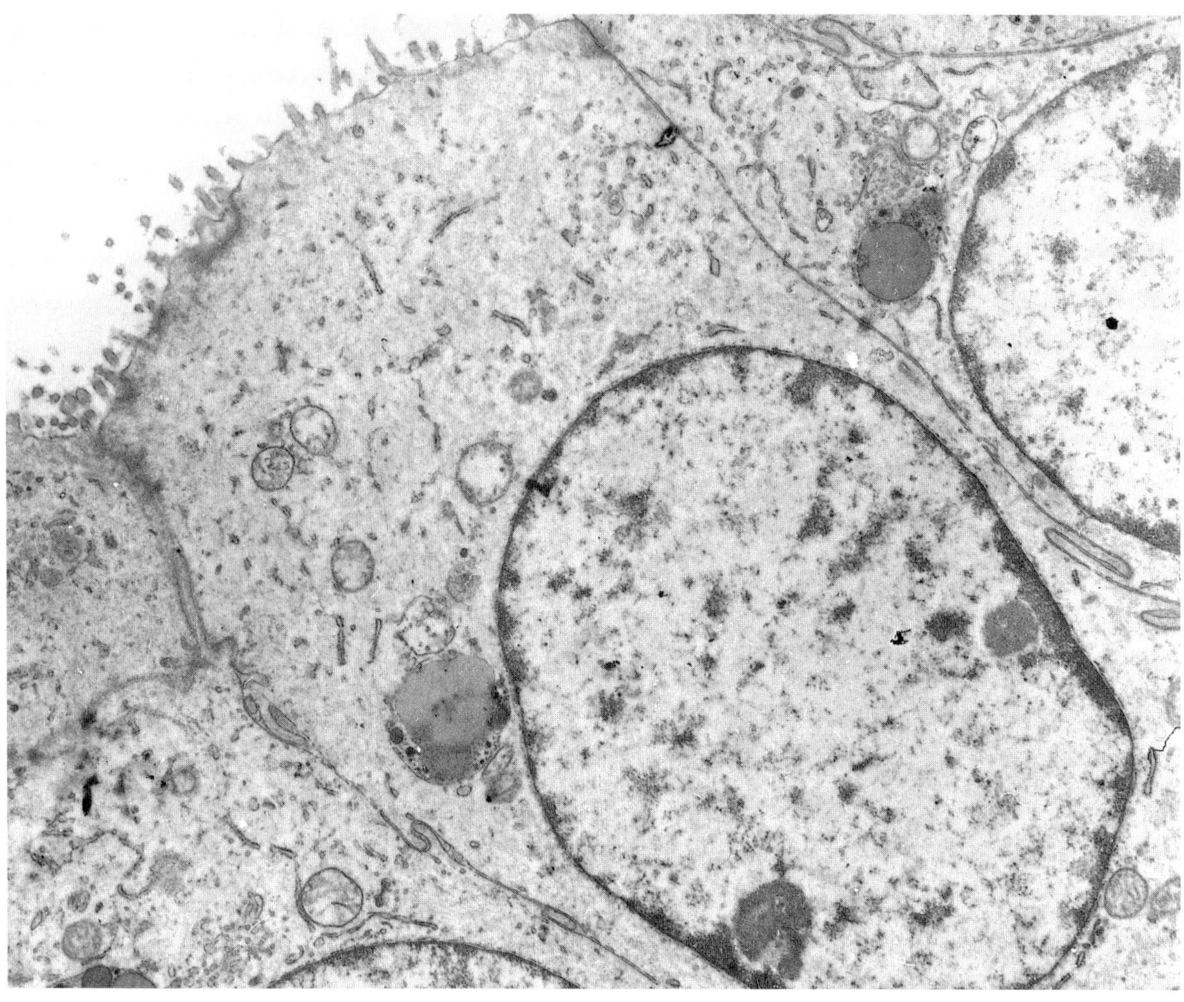

Figure 1-12
NORMAL PANCREAS: DUCTULAR CELLS
Ductular cells with a clear cytoplasm, some mitochondria, and several elongated endosomes (X28,000).

In the normal pancreas, acinar cells express cytokeratins 8 and 18, whereas ductal and centroacinar cells express cytokeratins 7, 8, 18, and 19 (52).

**Centroacinar Cells, Intercalated Ducts, and Intralobular Ducts.** Centroacinar cells are small, round to elongated cells lying in the center of the acinus. They are easily distinguished by their pale staining in histologic sections (fig. 1-10). The clear appearance of their relatively scant cytoplasm reflects the paucity of organelles (fig. 1-11). Occasional centroacinar cells, however, are mitochondria-rich and have a finely granular acidophilic cytoplasm (42). Intercalated duct cells are similar to centroacinar cells and possess a small number of microvilli (fig. 1-12). Their nuclei are round, and smaller and lighter staining than those of acinar cells. The cytoplasm is less electron dense and has a large number of mitochondria. Numerous smooth vesicles are present within the Golgi area and in the vicinity of both the apical and the lateral plasma membrane, sometimes fusing with these membranes. Many intercalated duct cells possess a single cilium, which forms a junction with a basal body in the supranuclear region of the cytoplasm. With increasing duct size, the cells become more columnar. The initial part of an intralobular duct is formed by cuboidal cells that are continuous with the acinar unit. The intralobular ducts are also lined by cells with a clear cytoplasm, relatively few organelles, and elaborated interdigitations at the lateral and basal plasma membranes.

The centroacinar and ductular cells are mainly engaged in electrolyte, fluid, and bicarbonate metabolism. Immunohistochemical studies localize carbonic anhydrase mainly in intralobular duct cells of the human pancreas (56). Protein synthesis is minimal and no stored mucus is demonstrated within the cytoplasm of ductular cells by PAS, Alcian blue, and other mucin stains, or by electron microscopy.

**Interlobular Ducts and Major Ducts.** Interlobular ducts have a mucinous, low columnar epithelium which becomes taller in the ducts of Wirsung and Santorini. The mucins in the epithelium of interlobular ducts are mainly sulfated and stain strongly with Alcian blue at pH 1.0 as well as with high iron diamine (HID) (Table 1-1). As duct size increases, the sulfate groups decrease and increasing amounts of neutral mucins and sialomucins are detected (50). DuPan-2 antigen, primarily a marker of pancreatic ductal epithelium, is only occasionally found in ductular cells, while N-terminal gastrin-releasing peptide (N-GRP)–related antigen (53) and carbonic anhydrase are regularly found in both ductal and ductular epithelial cells. Marino et al. (45) identified the cystic fibrosis transmembrane conductance regulator (CFTR) as a pancreatic duct cell marker. Antibodies against synthetic peptide sequences of CFTR stain the apical regions of duct cells but not acinar cells. Ultrastructurally, pancreatic large duct cells contain juxtaluminal dense granules with a homogeneous inner structure (fig. 1-13) and, along their luminal borders, irregularly distributed microvilli containing microfilaments with long cytoplasmic roots (53).

Gel-forming mucus covers the epithelial surface of the ducts and probably acts as a defensive barrier. In addition, it provides a medium in which electrolytes, enzymes, and other secretions are trapped and mixed (29).

**Islets of Langerhans.** Although most pancreatic endocrine cells are found in the islets of Langerhans, a small proportion (less than 10 percent) are present in extrainsular sites, distributed either singly or in small groups among ductal cells or the paraductular acinar cells (21,31). These cells are most easily found in the small ducts and are mainly represented by PP and glucagon cells. A few serotonin or enterochromaffin (EC) cells are located in the epithelium of large ducts (20).

The pancreatic islets scattered in the tail, body, and anterior part of the head are well-demarcated, round to ovoid aggregates of lightly staining cells arranged into partly delineated ribbons or lobules (ordinary or regular islets) (fig. 1-14). The islets concentrated in the posterior part of the head are irregular in shape and size, and are mainly formed of parallel, thin trabeculae of perpendicularly oriented cells, mostly PP (irregular or PP-rich islets) (fig. 1-15). The islets are embedded in reticulum and collagen fibers but they lack a true capsule. The majority of ordinary islets measure between 75 and 225 μm in their greater diameter (33). They are evenly distributed throughout most of the pancreas and morphometric studies have failed to demonstrate substantial differences in endocrine cell mass between the body and the tail of the pancreas. The islets form compact masses penetrated throughout, but not divided, by a complex system of anastomosing sinusoids (33) to form a ribbon-microlobular type of endocrine structure. The capillaries of the islets are lined by layers of endocrine cells, most of which are in direct contact with the vessels, either directly or through cytoplasmic processes (33).

On the basis of their vascularity two subtypes of regular islets can be distinguished: the compact type and the ribbon type (33). Compact islets are usually smaller, and have a centrally located capillary (vas afferens) from which vasa efferentia radiate to the islet periphery. Ribbon islets are generally larger; the vas afferens is located in the islet cortex and ramifies into anastomosing sinusoids and then into short vasa efferentia.

The irregular, PP-rich islets reach 400 to 500 μm in size, and this, coupled with a frankly trabecular structure, facilitates their misinterpretation as hyperplastic or dysplastic islets. They are confined to the posterior part of the head, which corresponds to about 10 percent of the whole pancreas, and derive from the ventral primordium during the embryogenesis. Thus they are separated from the anterior part of the head by a thin strip of adipose and connective tissue (44).

The islets are innervated by both sympathetic and parasympathetic nerve fibers which course alongside the blood vessels. In addition, the islets

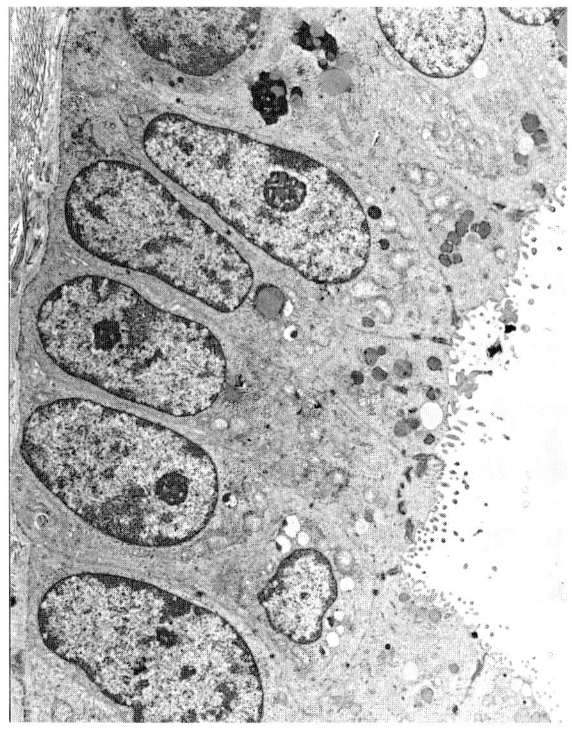

Figure 1-13
SECONDARY INTERLOBULAR DUCT

Columnar cells containing juxtaluminal mucin granules with a homogeneous dense inner structure and irregularly distributed microvilli along the luminal borders (X5,000).

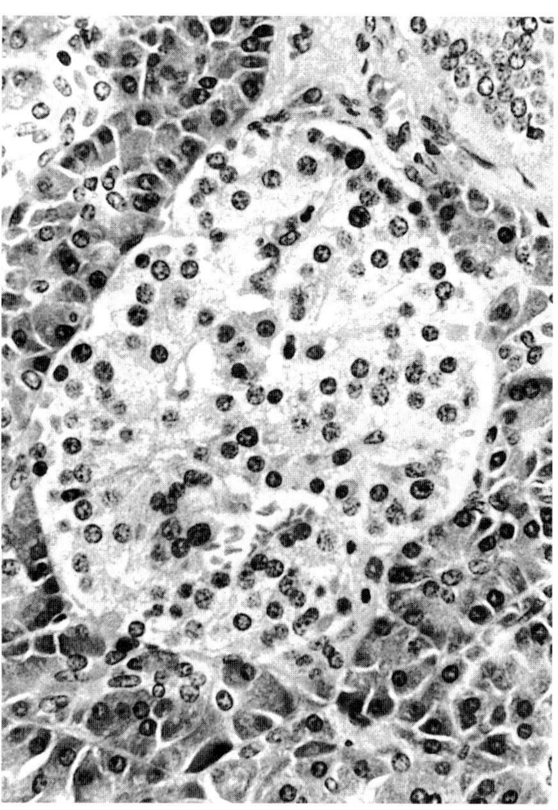

Figure 1-14
ADULT PANCREAS: ORDINARY TYPE ISLET

This islet with regular contour and compact shape is characteristic of islets rich in B cells.

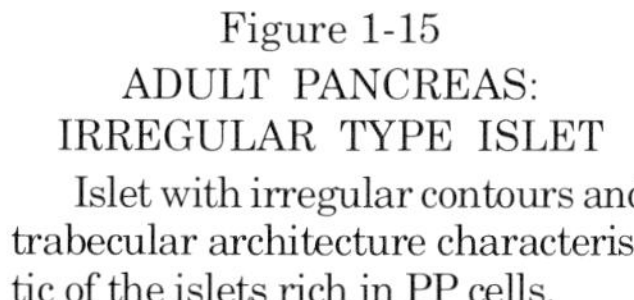

Figure 1-15
ADULT PANCREAS:
IRREGULAR TYPE ISLET

Islet with irregular contours and trabecular architecture characteristic of the islets rich in PP cells.

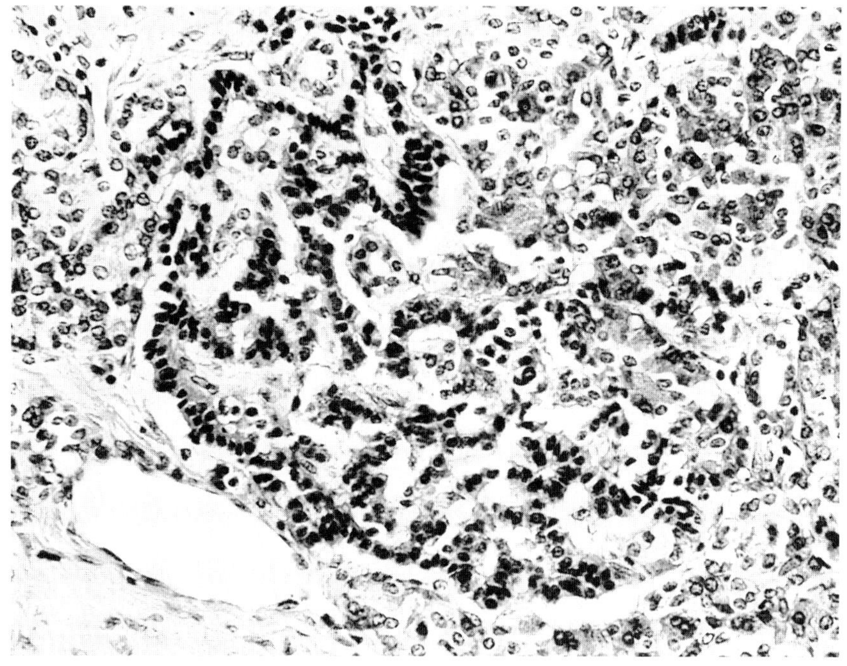

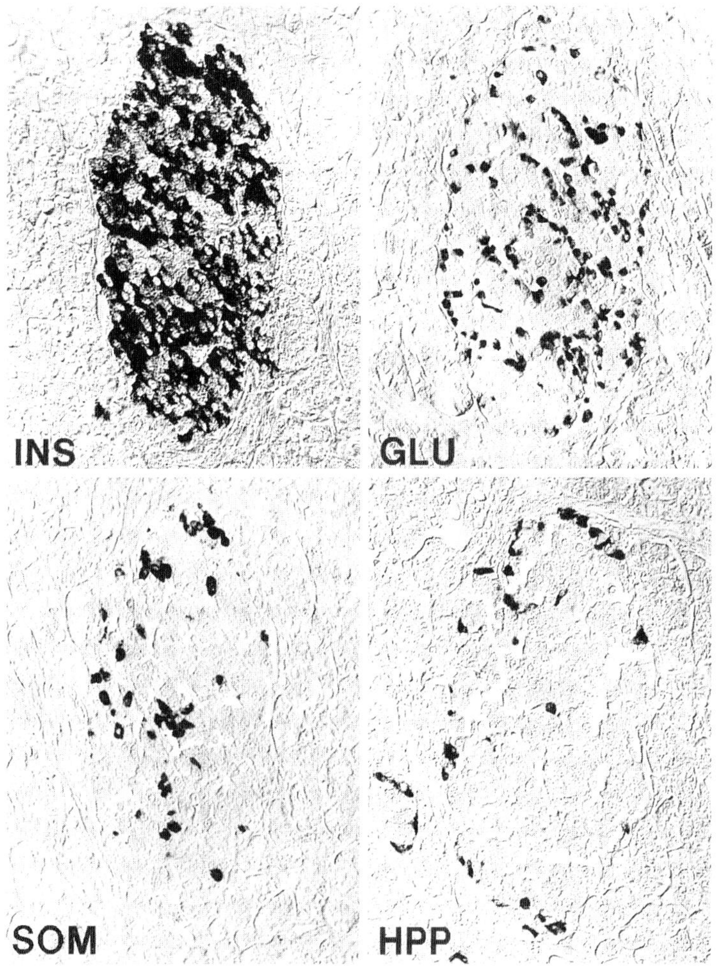


Figure 1-16
DISTRIBUTION OF ISLET CELL TYPES IN ORDINARY TYPE ISLET OF ADULT PANCREAS

Immunostaining for insulin (INS), glucagon (GLU), somatostatin (SOM), and PP (HPP) in ordinary type islet of the pancreatic tail (Nomarski optic).

possess a rich network of peptidergic fibers which originate from the ganglia of the intrinsic autonomic nervous system; these fibers are neuroregulators involved in the local control of the endocrine function of the pancreas (57).

There are four major cell types that have been definitively identified in the islets: glucagon-producing A (alpha) cells, insulin-producing B (beta) cells, somatostatin-producing D (delta) cells, and pancreatic polypeptide–producing PP cells (figs. 1-16, 1-17). The B cells are the most numerous of the islet cell types, corresponding to 60 to 70 percent of cells in the regular islets and 20 to 30 percent of those in the irregular islets of the posterior head (31). They synthesize, store, and secrete insulin. Direct evidence of the presence of insulin in the pancreatic B cell is demonstrated by immunoperoxidase antibody techniques for both insulin (fig. 1-16) and proinsulin. Ultrastructurally, the secretory granules of B cells have either a crystalline or compact finely granular core (fig. 1-18). Crystalline granules contain mainly insulin while compact core granules are considered immature and contain proinsulin that has not been cleaved enzymatically to form insulin (47). The granules measure between 225 and 375 nm. In addition to insulin, they contain chromogranin A and islet amyloid polypeptide (IAPP) (24,39). The function of these peptides is not well known. Chromogranin A is a precursor of other biologically active peptides such as betagranin (37); IAPP may have a role in glucose metabolism and in the development of type 2 diabetes (38).

A cells constitute less than 5 percent of the islet cells derived from the ventral primordium and 15 to 20 percent of the rest of the islets (31). Previous histochemical techniques such as phosphotungstic

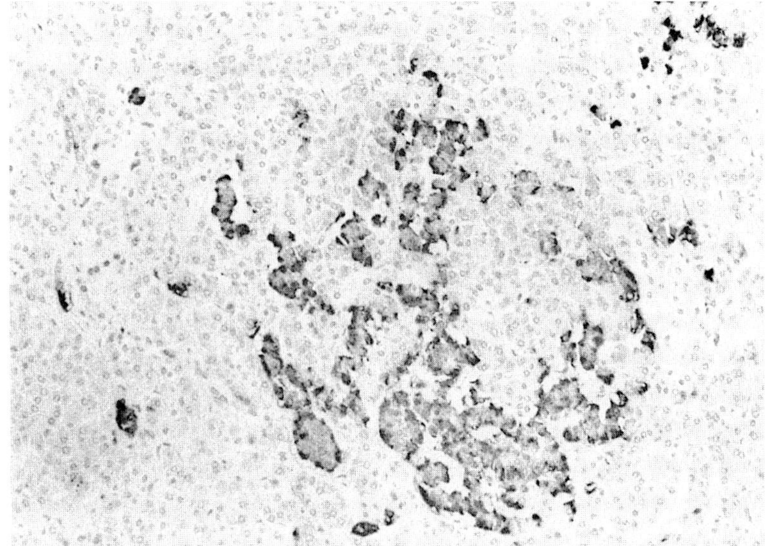

Figure 1-17
ISLET RICH IN PP CELLS
Immunostaining for human PP in an islet of the posterior part of the pancreatic head.

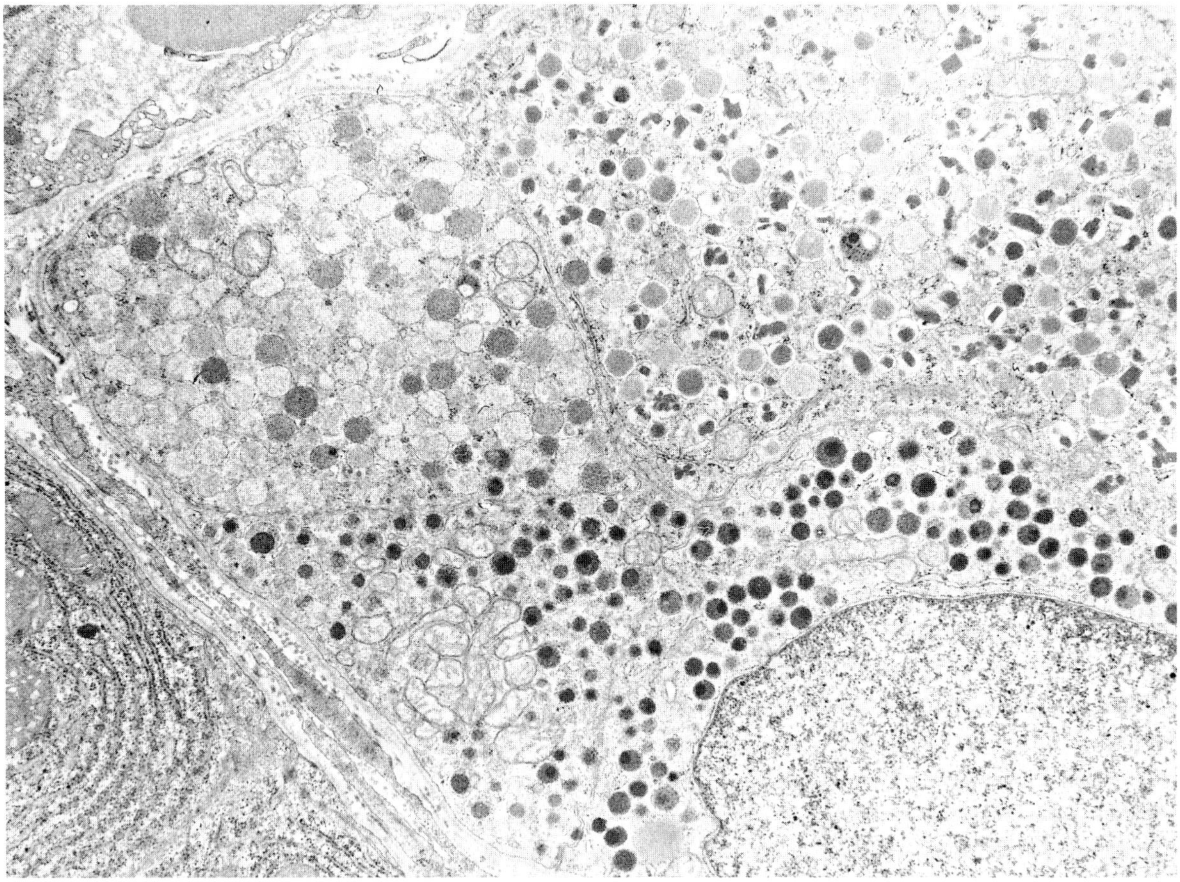

Figure 1-18
ULTRASTRUCTURE OF ADULT PANCREATIC ISLET CELLS
A glucagon cell (bottom), insulin cell (upper right), and somatostatin cell (left) are seen. Note the fenestrated capillary vessel at the upper left corner.

acid hematoxylin, Bodian, and Grimelius silver stains were not specific for the identification of A cells. Currently, immunohistochemical techniques using specific C-terminal glucagon sera are used to demonstrate A cells (fig. 1-16). Ultrastructurally, A cells exhibit characteristic 180- to 300-nm secretory granules with a central or eccentrically located, round, compact, highly electron-dense core, and a pale granular halo (fig. 1-18). The dense argyrophobic core stores mainly glucagon, glucagon-37, and the major proglucagon fragment (MPGF) while the pale argyrophilic halo stores mainly chromogranins and glicentin-related pancreatic peptide (GRPP) (48,55).

D cells represent 5 percent of the islet cell population in the posterior head of the pancreas (46) and 5 to 10 percent in the rest of the islets (31). In human pancreatic islets the D cells are mainly distributed at the islet periphery, with some also scattered among the central B-cell clusters. D cells have both short processes that contact adjacent endocrine cells and long processes that extend to intrainsular capillaries (33). The anatomic position of D cells within the islets and their different cell processes permit the somatostatin secreted by these cells to modulate insulin and glucagon release from the A and B cells by paracrine as well as endocrine influences (33). D cells do not react with Grimelius silver techniques but stain with alcoholic silver solutions. Somatostatin is stored in secretory granules measuring 170 to 220 nm in diameter. Their cores are of moderate and uniform density.

PP cells constitute the major population (around 70 percent) of the irregular islets of the posterior part of the head (fig. 1-17) but account for only 2 to 5 percent of the endocrine cells in the rest of the islets. Ultrastructurally, PP cells of the posterior part of the head differ from those of the rest of the pancreas: PP cells of the ventrally derived pancreas have fairly large (mean diameter, 208 nm) granules of variable shape, density, and inner structure, resembling those of the "F cells" of the dog uncinate pancreas (28); PP cells of the dorsally derived part of the pancreas have small (mean diameter, 138 nm), mostly round, homogeneous, granules with a fairly dense core and a closely applied membrane. Both cell types appear to contain the same peptide hormone.

## REFERENCES

### Embryology and Differentiation


1. Akao S, Bockman DE, Lechene de la Porte P, Sarles H. Three dimensional pattern of ductuloacinar association in normal and pathological human pancreas. Gastroenterology 1986;90:661–8.
2. Conklin JL. Cytogenesis of the human fetal pancreas. Am J Anat 1962;111:181–93.
3. Dawson W, Langman J. An anatomical-radiological study on the pancreatic duct pattern in man. Anat Rec 1961;139:59–68.
4. Githens S. Development of duct cells. In: Lebenthal E, ed. Human gastrointestinal development. New York: Raven Press, 1989:669–83.
5. Lebenthal E, Lev R, Lee PC. Prenatal and postnatal development of the human exocrine pancreas. In: Go VL, Gardner JD, Brooks FP, Lebenthal E, DiMagno EP, Scheele GA, eds. The exocrine pancreas: biology, pathobiology, and diseases. New York: Raven Press, 1986:33–43.
6. Liu HM, Potter EL. Development of the human pancreas. Arch Pathol 1962;74:439–52.
7. Moore KL. The developing human. 3rd ed. Philadelphia: WB Saunders, 1982:234–5.
8. Paulin C, Dubois PM. Immunohistochemical identification and localization of pancreatic polypeptide cells in the pancreas and gastrointestinal tract of the human fetus and adult man. Cell Tissue Res 1978;188:251–7.
9. Pellegata NS, Sessa F, Renault B, et al. K-ras and p53 gene mutation in pancreatic cancer: ductal and nonductal tumors progress through different genetic lesions. Cancer Res 1994;54:1556–60.
10. Rahier J, Falt K, Müntefering H, Becker K, Gepts W, Falkmer S. The basic structural lesion of persistent neonatal hypoglycaemia with hyperinsulinism: deficiency of pancreatic D cells or hyperactivity of B cells? Diabetologia 1984;26:282–9.
11. Sessa F, Bonato M, Frigerio B, et al. Ductal cancers of the pancreas frequently express markers of gastrointestinal epithelial cells. Gastroenterology 1990; 98:1655–65.
12. Sessa F, Solcia E, Capella C, et al. Intraductal papillary-mucinous tumors represent a distinct group of pancreatic neoplasms: an investigation of tumor cell differentiation and K-ras, p53 and c-erB-2 abnormalities in 26 patients. Virchows Arch 1994;425:357–67.

**Pancreas of Newborns and Infants**

13. Gossens A, Heitz PU, Klöppel G. Pancreatic endocrine cells and their non-neoplastic proliferations. In Dayal Y, ed. Endocrine pathology of the gut and pancreas. Boca Raton: CRC Press, 1991:69–104.
14. Rahier J, Wallon J, Gepts W, Haot J. Localization of pancreatic polypeptide cells in a limited lobe of the human neonate pancreas: remnant of the ventral primordium? Cell Tissue Res 1979;200:359–66.
15. Rahier J, Wallon J, Henquin JC. Cell populations in the endocrine pancreas of human neonates and infants. Diabetologia 1981;20:540–6.

**Adult Pancreas**

16. Akao S, Bockman DE, Lechene de la Porte P, Sarles H. Three dimensional pattern of ductuloacinar associations in normal and pathological human pancreas. Gastroenterology 1986;90:661–8.
17. Bendayan M, Roth J, Perrelet, A, Orci L. Quantitative immunocytochemical localization of pancreatic secretory proteins in subcellular compartment of the rat acinar cell. J Histochem Cytochem 1980;28:149–60.
18. Birnstingl MA. Study of pancreatography. Br J Surg 1959;47:128–39.
19. Bockman D. Anatomy of the pancreas. In: Go VL, Gardner J, Brooks FP, Lebenthal E, Di Magno EP, Scheele GA, eds. The exocrine pancreas: biology, pathobiology and diseases. New York: Raven Press, 1993:1–8.
20. Capella C, Solcia E, Frigerio B, Buffa R, Usellini L, Fontana P. The endocrine cells of the pancreas and related tumors. Ultrastructural study and classification. Virchows Arch [A] 1977;373:327–52.
21. Chen J, Baithun SI, Pollock DJ, Berry CL. Argyrophilic and hormone immunoreactive cells in normal and hyperplastic pancreatic ducts and exocrine pancreatic carcinoma. Virchows Arch [A] 1988;413:399–405.
22. Cubilla AL, Fitzgerald PJ. Tumors of the exocrine pancreas. In: Atlas of Tumor Pathology, 2nd Series, Fascicle 19. Washington, D.C.: Armed Forces Institute of Pathology, 1984:34–6.
23. Cubilla AL, Fortner JG, Fitzgerald PJ. Lymph node involvement in carcinoma of the pancreas area. Cancer 1978;41:880–7.
24. Eiden LE. Is chromogranin a prohormone? Nature 1987;325:301.
25. Elsässer HP, Klöppel G, Mannherz G, Flocke K, Kern HF. Immunohistochemical demonstration of villin in the normal human pancreas and chronic pancreatitis. Histochemistry 1991;95:383–90.
26. Evans BP, Ochsner A. The gross anatomy of the lymphatics of the human pancreas. Surgery 1954;36:177–91.
27. Falconer CW, Griffiths F. The anatomy of the blood-vessels in the region of the pancreas. Brit J Surg 1950;37:334–44.
28. Fiocca R, Sessa F, Tenti P, et al. Pancreatic polypeptide (PP) cells in the PP-rich lobe of the human pancreas are identified ultrastructurally and immunocytochemically as F cells. Histochemistry 1983;77:511–23.
29. Forstner G, Forstner J. Mucus: biosynthesis and secretion. In: Go VL, Lebenthal E, Scheele GA, Brooks FP, Di Magno EP, Gardner JD, eds. The exocrine pancreas: biology, pathobiology, and disease. New York: Raven Press, 1987:283–6.
30. Fraser PA, Henderson JR. The arrangement of endocrine and exocrine pancreatic microcirculation observed in the living rabbit. Q J Exp Physiol 1980;65:151–8.
31. Goossens A, Heitz P, Klöppel G. Pancreatic endocrine cells and their non-neoplastic proliferations. In: Dayal Y, ed. Endocrine pathology of the gut and pancreas. Boca Raton: CRC Press, 1991:69–104.
32. Gorelick FS, Jamieson JM. Structure-function relationships of the pancreas. In: Johnson IR, ed. Physiology of the gastrointestinal tract. New York: Raven Press, 1981:773–83.
33. Grube D, Bohn R. The microanatomy of human islets of Langerhans with special reference to somatostatin (D) cells. Arch Histol Jap 1983;46:327–53.
34. Heitz PU, Beglinger C, Gyr K. Anatomy and physiology of the exocrine pancreas. In: Klöppel G, Heitz PH, eds. Pancreatic pathology. Edinburgh: Churchill-Livingstone, 1984:3–21.
35. Henderson JR, Daniel PM. A comparative study of the portal vessels connecting the endocrine and exocrine pancreas, with a discussion of some functional implications. Q J Exp Physiol Cogn Med Sci 1979;64:267–75.
36. Hollinshead WH. The thorax, abdomen, and pelvis. In: Anatomy for Surgeons, Vol. 2, 2nd ed. New York: Harper and Row, 1971.
37. Hutton JC, Peshavaria M, Johnston CF, Ravazzola M, Orci L. Immunolocalization of betagranin: a chromogranin A-related protein of the pancreatic B-cell. Endocrinology 1988;122:1014–20.
38. Johnson KH, O'Brien TD, Betsholz C, Westermark P. Islet amyloid, islet amyloid polypeptide, and diabetes mellitus. N Engl J Med 1989;327:313–8.
39. Johnson KH, O'Brien TD, Hayden DW, et al. Immunolocalization of islet amyloid polypeptide (IAPP) in pancreatic beta cells by means of peroxidase-antiperoxidase (PAP) and protein A-gold techniques. Am J Pathol 1988;130:1–8.
40. Kayahara M, Nagakawa T, Kobayashi H, et al. Lymphatic flow in carcinoma of the head of the pancreas. Cancer 1992;70:2061–6.
41. Kern HF. Fine structure of the human exocrine pancreas. In: Go VL, Gardner JD, Brooks FP, Lebenthal E, Di Magno EP, Scheele GA, eds. The exocrine pancreas: biology, pathobiology, and disease. New York: Raven Press, 1993:9–19.
42. Kodama TA. A light and electron microscopic study of the pancreatic ductal system. Acta Pathol Jap 1983;33:297–321.
43. Kraehenbuhl JP, Racine L, Jamieson JD. Immunohistochemical localization of secretory proteins in bovine pancreatic exocrine cells. J Cell Biol 1977;72:406–23.
44. Malaisse-Lagae F, Stefan Y, Cox J, Perrelet A, Orci L. Identification of a lobe in the adult human pancreas rich in pancreatic polypeptide. Diabetologia 1979;17:361–5.

45. Marino CR, Matovcik LM, Gorelick FS, Cohn JA. Localization of the cystic fibrosis transmembrane conductance regulator in pancreas. J Clin Invest 1988;88:712–6.
46. Orci L, Malaisse-Lagae F, Baetens D, Perrelet A. Pancreatic polypeptide-rich regions in the human pancreas [Letter]. Lancet 1978;2:1200–1.
47. Orci L, Ravazzola M, Storch MJ, Anderson RG, Vassalli JD, Perrelet A. Proteolytic maturation of insulin is a post-Golgi event which occurs in acidifying clathrin-coated secretory vesicles. Cell 1987;49:865–8.
48. Ravazzola M, Orci L. Glucagon and glicentin immunoreactivity are topologically segregated in the alpha granule of the human pancreatic A cell. Nature 1980;286:66–7.
49. Rinderknecht H. Pancreatic secretory enzymes. In: Go VL, Gardner JD, Brooks FP, Lebenthal E, Di Magno EP, Scheele GA, eds. The exocrine pancreas: biology, pathobiology, and disease. New York: Raven Press, 1986:163–83.
50. Roberts PF, Burns J. A histochemical study of mucins in normal and neoplastic human pancreatic tissue. J Pathol 1972;107:87–94.
51. Scheele GA, Kern HF. Cellular comportamentation, protein processing and secretion in the exocrine pancreas. In: Go VL, Lebenthal E, Di Magno EP, et al., eds. The exocrine pancreas: biology, pathobiology, and disease. New York: Raven Press, 1993:121–50.
52. Schussler MH, Skoudy A, Ramaekers F, Real FX. Intermediate filaments as differentiation markers of normal pancreas and pancreas cancer. Am J Pathol 1992;140:559–68.
53. Sessa F, Bonato M, Frigerio B, et al. Ductal cancers of the pancreas frequently express markers of gastrointestinal epithelial cells Gastroenterology 1990;98:1655–65.
54. Singh M, Webster PD. Neurohormonal control of pancreatic secretion. A review. Gastroenterology 1978; 74:294–309.
55. Solcia E, Fiocca R, Capella C, et al. Glucagon- and PP-related peptides of intestinal L cells and pancreatic/gastric A or PP cells. Possible interrelationships of peptides and cells during evolution, fetal development and tumor growth. Peptides 1985;6(suppl 3):223–9.
56. Spicer SS, Sens MA, Tashian RE. Immunocytochemical demonstration of carbonic anhydrase in human epithelial cells. J Histochem Cytochem 1982;30:864–73.
57. Sundler F, Alumets J, Hakanson R, Fahrenkrug J, Schaffalitzky de Muckadell O. Peptidergic (VIP) nerves in the pancreas. Histochemistry 1978;55:173–6.
58. Testut L, Latarjet A. Traite' d'anatomie humaine. 9th ed. Paris: Doin et Cie, 1948.
59. White TT. Surgical anatomy of the pancreas. In: Carey LC, ed. The pancreas. St.Louis: CV Mosby, 1973:3–16.


✧✧✧

# 2
# CLASSIFICATION OF PANCREATIC TUMORS

In the past, classification schemes for exocrine pancreatic tumors were either overly complicated or overly simplified. Some focused mainly on usual ductal adenocarcinoma while others were exaggerated by histologic details and principles. The World Health Organization (WHO) classification published in 1978 considered only well-known tumor entities and strictly differentiated between benign and malignant neoplasms (4). With increasing knowledge of pancreatic tumors, this practical classification became limited by tumors that were either not mentioned or inadequately considered. The classifications published by Morohoshi et al. in 1983 (7) and Cubilla and Fitzgerald in 1984 (3) attempted to correlate histologic type with prognosis; both classification systems followed the same histologic and histogenetic guidelines. Later classification systems followed more or less the same principles (2,5). Since our understanding of benign, malignant, and tumor-like lesions of the pancreas has further increased during recent years, revision of the current classifications is justified.

The scheme that we have adopted for this Fascicle follows that one recently proposed by the WHO (6). It was developed by a committee of pathologists from seven countries (see Acknowledgments). We fully anticipate that it will continue to be modified and improved after its publication, but it is presented at this time as the most current and, we hope, most widely accepted classification available.

A primary goal of a histologic tumor classification scheme is, in addition to staging and grading, assessing the prognosis of neoplasms. The major guideline is, therefore, the distinction of pancreatic exocrine tumors according to their biologic behavior. Neoplasms are broadly divided into benign (adenoma) and malignant (carcinoma) tumors. However, in recent years we have learned that this division is not a sharp but a rather gradual transition. We have added, therefore, a third category which we call "tumors of uncertain malignant potential," a borderline category analogous to that recognized for ovarian tumors. Included in this group are some mucinous cystic tumors, some intraductal papillary-mucinous tumors, and most solid-pseudopapillary tumors. These neoplasms are defined by their grade of dysplasia or potential to become malignant. Mucinous cystic tumors of uncertain malignant potential, for instance, exhibit moderate epithelial dysplasia but do not have severe changes of dysplasia-carcinoma in situ or destructive invasion of the stroma or adjacent pancreatic tissue. Solid-pseudopapillary tumor has a benign histologic appearance, but metastases may occur. Biologically, all these neoplasms are usually slow-growing lesions and have a benign outcome when adequately treated by complete resection. However, when inadequately treated or untreated, they may become frankly malignant and evolve into metastasizing neoplasms. As this behavior is difficult or even impossible to predict in an individual tumor on the basis of currently available morphologic and biologic features, we classify them as tumors with uncertain behavior or borderline malignant potential.

This classification does not group tumors on the basis of their phenotypic (histogenetic) derivation. However, whenever possible, the names given to tumors reflect their phenotypic characteristics consistent with differentiation towards the known epithelial cell types in the pancreas, i.e., duct cells (of mucinous ducts or serous ductules), acinar cells, and endocrine cells.

Problems in the classification of pancreatic endocrine tumors result from their peculiar clinicopathologic behavior. Morphologic atypia and infiltrative growth, two important morphologic criteria for establishing the malignant nature of most neoplasms, are too minimal to be of help in assessing endocrine tumors. The only exception is the rare small cell carcinoma (so called poorly differentiated neuroendocrine carcinoma), the marked anaplasia and aggressive behavior of which can easily be recognized in conventional histologic sections. Recently, some criteria for the evaluation and classification of well-differentiated endocrine tumors have been proposed (1). Metastases, macroscopic evidence of local invasion, invasion of perineural spaces or blood vessels, and tumor size greater than 3 cm, in decreasing order of reliability, have been accepted as indicative of malignancy. Size below 2 cm in the absence of invasive patterns and mitoses is considered suggestive of benign behavior. However, even with these criteria, the behavior of a relevant proportion of pancreatic endocrine tumors remains unpredictable. Thus, a borderline group of "tumors with uncertain malignant potential" should be included among endocrine tumors as well.

A majority of these tumors, when carefully investigated, are composed of more than one, and sometimes several, cell types (8). For this reason classifying pancreatic endocrine tumors by endocrine cell typing alone is of limited value in practice, unless correlated with clinical symptoms and hormone measurements in blood. It is known that pancreatic endocrine tumors are associated with well-defined hyperfunctional syndromes which determine the clinicopathologic profile and are usually more predictive of the tumor's natural history than are the purely morphologic findings (9). The use of a classification system based on endocrine syndromes is supported by the fact that most available follow-up studies of pancreatic endocrine tumors are syndrome based.

A system combining clinicopathologic features is therefore adopted for classifying endocrine tumors: all the morphologic and functional information necessary for precise diagnosis and appropriate treatment of these pleomorphic tumor diseases are covered. In particular, "functioning" tumors associated with various types of hyperfunctioning syndromes are separated from "nonfunctioning" tumors in which behavior can only be predicted by general criteria like association with local symptoms (signs of an expanding mass), size, angio-neuroinvasion, and gross invasion of peripancreatic tissues.

The classification scheme for pancreatic neoplasms used in this Fascicle follows.

## CLASSIFICATION OF PANCREATIC TUMORS

1. Primary Tumors
    - 1.1 Tumors of the exocrine pancreas
        - 1.1.1 Benign
            - 1.1.1.1 Serous cystadenoma
            - 1.1.1.2 Mucinous cystadenoma
            - 1.1.1.3 Intraductal papillary-mucinous adenoma
            - 1.1.1.4 Mature cystic teratoma
        - 1.1.2 Borderline (uncertain malignant potential)
            - 1.1.2.1 Mucinous cystic tumor with moderate dysplasia
            - 1.1.2.2 Intraductal papillary-mucinous tumor with moderate dysplasia
            - 1.1.2.3 Solid-pseudopapillary tumor
        - 1.1.3 Malignant
            - 1.1.3.1 Ductal adenocarcinoma
                - Mucinous noncystic carcinoma
                - Signet ring cell carcinoma
                - Adenosquamous carcinoma
                - Undifferentiated (anaplastic) carcinoma
                - Mixed ductal-endocrine carcinoma
            - 1.1.3.2 Osteoclast-like giant cell tumor
            - 1.1.3.3 Serous cystadenocarcinoma
            - 1.1.3.4 Mucinous cystadenocarcinoma—noninvasive; invasive
            - 1.1.3.5 Intraductal papillary-mucinous carcinoma—noninvasive; invasive (papillary-mucinous carcinoma)
            - 1.1.3.6 Acinar cell carcinoma
                - Acinar cell cystadenocarcinoma
                - Mixed acinar-endocrine carcinoma
            - 1.1.3.7 Pancreatoblastoma
            - 1.1.3.8 Solid-pseudopapillary carcinoma
            - 1.1.3.9 Miscellaneous carcinomas

- 1.2 Tumors of the endocrine pancreas
  - 1.2.1 Benign
    - 1.2.1.1 Well-differentiated adenoma
      - Insulinoma
      - Nonfunctioning adenoma
  - 1.2.2 Borderline (uncertain malignant potential)
    - 1.2.2.1 Well-differentiated nonangioinvasive tumor
    - 1.2.2.2 Insulinoma
    - 1.2.2.3 Gastrinoma, vipoma, glucagonoma, somatostatinoma, others
    - 1.2.2.4 Nonfunctioning tumor
  - 1.2.3 Low-grade malignant
    - 1.2.3.1 Well to moderately differentiated carcinoma
      - Insulinoma
      - Gastrinoma, vipoma, glucagonoma, somatostatinoma, others
      - Nonfunctioning carcinoma
  - 1.2.4 High-grade malignant
    - 1.2.4.1 Poorly differentiated carcinoma (i.e., small cell carcinoma)
      - Functioning or nonfunctioning
- 1.3 Nonepithelial tumors
  - 1.3.1 Benign soft tissue tumors
  - 1.3.2 Malignant soft tissue tumors
  - 1.3.3 Malignant lymphomas

2. Secondary Tumors
3. Tumor-like Lesions of the Exocrine Pancreas
   - 3.1 Chronic pancreatitis
   - 3.2 Miscellaneous inflammatory changes
   - 3.3 Cysts
     - 3.3.1 Pseudocyst
     - 3.3.2 Retention cyst
     - 3.3.3 Parasitic cyst
     - 3.3.4 Congenital cyst
     - 3.3.5 Para-ampullary duodenal wall cyst
     - 3.3.6 Enterogenous cyst
     - 3.3.7 Lymphoepithelial cyst
     - 3.3.8 Endometrial cyst
   - 3.4 Duct changes
     - 3.4.1 Squamous metaplasia
     - 3.4.2 Mucinous cell hypertrophy
     - 3.4.3 Ductal papillary hyperplasia
     - 3.4.4 Adenomatoid ductal hyperplasia
     - 3.4.5 Ductal dysplasia
   - 3.5 Acinar changes
   - 3.6 Heterotopic pancreas
   - 3.7 Heterotopic (ectopic) spleen
   - 3.8 Hamartoma and pseudotumor
   - 3.9 Pseudolipomatous hypertrophy
   - 3.10 Pseudolymphoma
4. Tumor-like Lesions of the Endocrine Pancreas
   - 4.1 Islet hyperplasia
   - 4.2 Nesidioblastosis
     - 4.2.1 Persistent neonatal hyperinsulinemic hypoglycemia
     - 4.2.2 Persistent hyperinsulinemic hypoglycemia in adults
   - 4.3 Dysplasia

## REFERENCES

1. Capella C, Heitz PU, Höfler H, Solcia E, Klöppel G. Revised classification of neuroendocrine tumors of the lung, pancreas and gut. Virchows Arch 1995;425:547–60.
2. Chen J, Baithun SI. Morphological study of 391 cases of exocrine pancreatic tumours with special reference to the classification of exocrine pancreatic carcinoma. J Pathol 1985;146:17–29.
3. Cubilla AL, Fitzgerald PJ. Tumors of the exocrine pancreas. Atlas of Tumor Pathology, 2nd Series, Fascicle 19. Washington, D.C.: Armed Forces Institute of Pathology, 1984.
4. Gibson JB. Histological typing of tumours of the liver, biliary tract and pancreas. International histological classification of tumors, No. 20. Geneva: World Health Organization, 1978.
5. Lack EE. Primary tumors of the exocrine pancreas. Classification, overview, and recent contributions by immunohistochemistry and electron microscopy. Am J Surg Pathol 1989;13(Suppl 1):66–88.
6. Klöppel H, Solcia E, Longnecker DS, Capella C, Sobin LH. Histological typing of tumors of the exocrine pancreas. International histological classification of tumors, 2nd ed. Berlin: Springer, 1996.
7. Morohoshi T, Held G, Klöppel G. Exocrine pancreatic tumours and their histological classification. A study based on 167 autopsy and 97 surgical cases. Histopathology 1983;7:645–661.
8. Mukai K, Grotting JC, Greider MH, Rosai J. Retrospective study of 77 pancreatic endocrine tumors using the immunoperoxidase method. Am J Surg Pathol 1982;6:387–99.
9. Solcia E, Sessa F, Rindi G, et al. Classification and histogenesis of gastroenteropancreatic endocrine tumors. Eur J Clin Invest 1990;20(Suppl 1):72–81.

✧✧✧

# 3
# GENERAL CONSIDERATIONS

**Tumor Phenotype and Diagnosis.** Three main cell lineages are found in the human pancreas: the duct cell, the acinar cell, and the endocrine cell; among ductal cells, the mucin-producing cell of large ducts is phenotypically distinct from the ductular-centroacinar serous cell. Their features and currently available markers are discussed in chapter 1. The cellular phenotype of the various tumors of the pancreas reflects, to a certain degree, their origin from (or differentiation along) one of these four cell lineages. This implies that cell lineage markers (see Table 1-1) can "cum grano salis" be also used to separate and categorize these tumors. Table 3-1 attempts to summarize the pattern of immunohistochemical markers used for diagnosing common tumors of the pancreas.

Recent studies concerning oncogene activation in pancreatic tumors have shown that the oncogene pattern is related to tumor phenotype (7). The K-*ras* oncogene is activated by point mutation at codon 12 in 70 to 90 percent of ductal adenocarcinomas, a figure which exceeds by far that observed in either acinar (8 percent) or endocrine tumors (0 percent). The p53 suppressor gene is mutated in 40 to 60 percent of ductal cancers and 8 percent of endocrine tumors but seems to play no significant role in acinar cell carcinoma or solid-pseudopapillary tumors (1,5, 7). Data on molecular events will most likely increase in the years to come and will probably lead to molecular marker constellations which may help to subdivide and further characterize pancreatic neoplasms.

**Incidence.** Pancreatic cancer is among the most frequent human neoplasms. In the abdomen it is second only to colorectal carcinoma in frequency. If pancreatic cancer is stratified according to the relative frequency of the various tumor types, it becomes clear that the high incidence can solely be attributed to the common occurrence of ductal adenocarcinoma: it accounts for at least 80 percent of all pancreatic tumors. If important variants of ductal adenocarcinoma, i.e., mucinous noncystic carcinoma (1 to 3 percent), adenosquamous carcinoma (3 to 4 percent), and undifferentiated (anaplastic) carcinoma (2 to 7 percent), are included, about 90 percent of pancreatic tumors are of duct type (2,3,6). The other tumor entities comprise only 8

Table 3-1

**DIFFERENTIAL IMMUNOHISTOLOGY OF EPITHELIAL PANCREATIC TUMORS**

| Tumor Type | CK8,18* | CK7,19 | CEA | M1 | TRYP | NSE | SYN | CG | AAT |
|---|---|---|---|---|---|---|---|---|---|
| Serous cystadenoma | + | + | – | – | – | – | – | – | – |
| Ductal adenocarcinoma | + | + | + | + | – | – | – | – | – |
| Mucinous cystic tumor | + | + | + | + | – | –§ | –§ | –§ | – |
| Intraductal papillary mucinous tumor | + | + | + | + | – | –§ | –§ | –§ | – |
| Acinar cell carcinoma | + | +** | – | – | + | –§ | –§ | –§ | + |
| Pancreatoblastoma | + | + | – | –/+ | + | –§ | –§ | –§ | – |
| Solid-pseudopapillary tumor | –† | –† | – | – | – | + | – | – | + |
| Endocrine tumor | + | +‡ | – | – | – | + | + | + | – |

*CK- cytokeratin; CEA - carcinoembryonic antigen; M1 - peptide core antigen of mucin in gastric superficial foveolar cells; TRYP - trypsinogen; NSE - neuron-specific enolase; SYN - synaptophysin; CG - chromogranin A; AAT-alpha-1-antitrypsin.

**Negative in about 20 to 30 percent of the cases.

†Usually negative.

‡Negative in most cases for CK7.

§Focal positivity possible.

to 10 percent: serous cystadenoma (1 percent), mucinous cystic tumor (2 percent), intraductal papillary-mucinous tumor (1 percent), acinar cell carcinoma (1 percent), pancreatoblastoma (less than 0.5 percent), solid-pseudopapillary tumor (1 percent), and endocrine tumor (2 percent). It must be emphasized, however, that these figures are rough estimates extrapolated from older studies (2,3,6) which are not entirely comparable with each other and do not include all the tumor entities known today.

**Age Distribution.** Cancer of the pancreas usually affects older patients. In our study of 325 patients with all kinds of pancreatic tumors, 80 percent were older than 40 years (4). This is due to the high relative frequency of ductal adenocarcinoma, which has its peak incidence between the ages of 60 and 80 years. Only 10 of 243 patients with ductal adenocarcinoma were younger than 40 years (range, 16 to 39 years). Of the 10, most occurred in the head of the pancreas and showed the same range of differentiation and a similar prognosis as in older patients. Tumors other than ductal adenocarcinoma are seen in 90 percent of patients younger than 40 years. Among these neoplasms, endocrine tumors are most common (approximately 50 percent), followed by solid-pseudopapillary tumors (approximately 30 percent), and other tumors such as mucinous cystic tumor, acinar cell carcinoma, pancreatoblastoma, serous cystadenoma, and nonepithelial tumors (together approximately 10 percent). If only tumors in children up to 15 years of age are considered, the spectrum is narrowed to pancreatoblastoma, acinar cell carcinoma, and solid-pseudopapillary tumor.

**Clinical Presentation.** Most cancers of the pancreas, including ductal adenocarcinomas of the pancreatic head, develop insidiously and only relatively late in the course present with abdominal pain, weight loss, or jaundice (8). A second group of tumors which include ductal adenocarcinomas of the body-tail region as well as acinar cell carcinomas and nonfunctioning endocrine tumors usually become clinically apparent through the development of metastases or the involvement of organs surrounding the pancreas. A third group, such as intraductal papillary-mucinous tumor, produce chronic pancreatitis-like symptoms. A fourth group, the functioning endocrine tumors, produce characteristic hormonal syndromes such as the hypoglycemia syndrome (insulinoma) or Zollinger-Ellison syndrome (gastrinoma). And a fifth group presents as an abdominal mass, with or without abdominal pain. This group includes mucinous cystic tumor and solid-pseudopapillary tumor. The specific approaches to the diagnosis of these various types of pancreatic neoplasm are discussed in a separate chapter on Diagnosis as well as in the various tumor chapters.

## REFERENCES.


1. Almoguera C, Shibata D, Forrester K, Martin J, Arnheim N, Perucho M. Most human carcinomas of the exocrine pancreas contain mutant c-K-ras genes. Cell 1988;53:549–54.
2. Chen J, Baithun SI. Morphological study of 391 cases of exocrine pancreatic tumours with special reference to the classification of exocrine pancreatic carcinoma. J Pathol 1985;146:17–29.
3. Cubilla AL, Fitzgerald PJ. Tumors of the exocrine pancreas. In: Atlas of Tumor Pathology, 2nd Series, Fascicle 19. Washington, D.C.: Armed Forces Institute of Pathology, 1984;220:162.
4. De Vuyst M, Rickaert F, De Roy G, Klöppel G. The spectrum of ductal adenocarcinomas and other tumors of the pancreas in patients younger than 40 years of age [Abstract]. Path Res Pract 1993;189:681.
5. Hoorens A, Lemoine NR, McLellan E, et al. Pancreatic acinar cell carcinoma. An analysis of cell lineage markers, p53 expression and Ki-ras mutations. Am J Pathol 1993;143:685–98.
6. Morohoshi T, Held G, Klöppel G. Exocrine pancreatic tumours and their histological classification. A study based on 167 autopsy and 97 surgical cases. Histopathology 1983;7:645–61.
7. Pellegata NS, Sessa F, Renault B, et al. K-ras and p53 gene mutations in pancreatic cancer: ductal and nonductal tumors progress through different genetic lesions. Cancer Res 1994;54:1556–60.
8. Warshaw AL, Fernandez-Del Castillo C. Pancreatic carcinoma. N Engl J Med 1992;326:455–65.

# 4
# TUMORS OF THE EXOCRINE PANCREAS

## SEROUS CYSTIC TUMORS

Cystic pancreatic tumors are formed of epithelial cells that produce serous fluid and show evidence of ductular differentiation. Most are benign and only exceptionally exhibit malignant features.

Serous cystic tumors have been well defined since they were separated from mucinous cystic neoplasms by Compagno and Oertel (9) and Hodgkinson et al. (16) in 1978. They are also known as *microcystic adenomas* or *glycogen-rich cystadenomas* (9). Recently, however, serous cystic tumors dissimilar to microcystic adenoma (12,22) as well as malignant serous neoplasms (39,40,41) have been reported. There are also reports of serous cystic tumors in children (34), which seem to differ in their gross features from microcystic adenoma. It appears, therefore, that this is a heterogeneous group of tumors which has to be further subdivided.

According to the above studies, the serous cystadenoma group consists at least of two types: microcystic adenomas and other tumors that have been described as macrocystic serous cystadenoma (22) or serous oligocystic and ill-demarcated adenoma (12). We include the latter under the term *serous oligocystic adenoma*; the term oligocystic is preferred to macrocystic because single cysts in microcystic adenomas may be the same size as those usually seen in the "macrocystic" type. A better discriminator is the number of cysts, which is much lower in oligocystic adenoma than in microcystic adenoma.

Apart from adenomas, there are rare malignant serous cystic tumors that metastasize or show evidence of local angioinvasion or perineural invasion. These tumors are called *serous cystadenocarcinomas*. It is not known whether serous cystadenomas have a malignant potential and develop into carcinomas or whether serous cystadenocarcinomas are an entirely separate tumor group.

Serous cystic tumors are composed of cells that exhibit the features of intralobular duct cells (ductular and centroacinar cells). This implies that they express, like all duct cells (29,31), cytokeratins 7, 8, 18, and 19 (1,12), but do not produce mucin as do interlobular duct cells (ductal cells). Instead of mucin granules the cytoplasm of the tumor cells contains abundant glycogen (1,6,12,21) which has also been found in fetal centroacinar cells (23). In an ultrastructural study of a serous microcystic adenoma, Nyongo and Huntrakoon (28) described not only cells with glycogen-rich cytoplasm but also cells that they considered to be myoepithelial. This finding was, however, not confirmed by other investigators (1,33). We have not identified myoepithelial cells in normal pancreatic ducts or serous cystadenomas, using actin as the immunohistochemical myoepithelial cell marker.

## SEROUS CYSTADENOMA

There are two types of serous cystadenoma of the pancreas: the common microcystic adenoma (9) and the infrequent oligocystic adenoma (12). In the subsequent sections the two variants are referred to as serous microcystic adenoma and serous oligocystic adenoma.

### Serous Microcystic Adenoma

**Definition.** This is a benign tumor composed of numerous small cysts arranged around a central stellate scar and lined by epithelial cells; there is evidence of ductular differentiation. Serous microcystic adenoma occurs predominantly in women. Synonyms include *microcystic adenoma* and *glycogen-rich cystadenoma* (9).

**General Features.** This is an uncommon tumor: it accounts for 1 to 2 percent of all exocrine pancreatic tumors (26). Approximately 350 cases have been reported to date (1,3,6,8–10,12, 15,16,20,30,33,35,36). The tumor occurs more often in women (70 percent) than men; the age at presentation is 66 years (range, 34 to 91 years) (1,6,9,10,12,15,30,33,35,36). The tumor has been reported in all races (9,36).

The etiology and pathogenesis of the tumor are unknown. The striking predilection for women suggests a role for sex hormones or genetic factors. The reported association with von Hippel-Lindau syndrome (retinal angiomatosis, cerebellar hemangioblastoma, renal carcinoma,

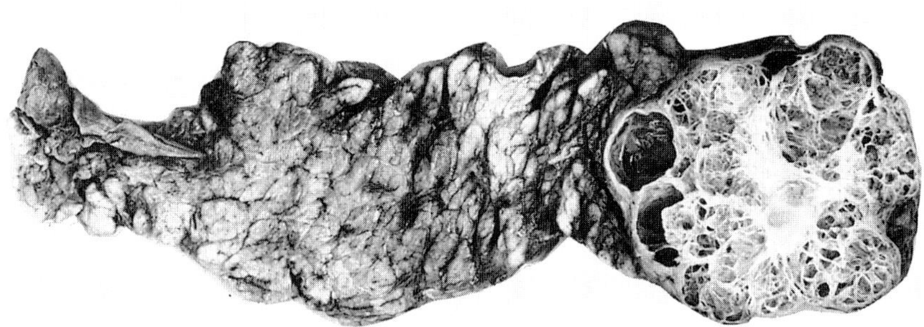

Figure 4-1
SEROUS MICROCYSTIC ADENOMA
Well-demarcated cystic lesion located in the tail of the pancreas, displaying a central stellate scar. The cysts are filled with a watery fluid and are separated by thin septa.

pheochromocytoma, renal and pancreatic cysts), which is transmitted as an autosomal trait with variable penetrance (9,27), remains to be clarified. Based on the descriptions and illustrations (4,5,9,17,27), it is uncertain whether the pancreatic lesions represent serous microcystic adenomas. According to our own experience, the typical polycystic transformation of the entire pancreas in von Hippel-Lindau syndrome (27,32) is a lesion that is distinct from microcystic adenoma and more closely related to the oligocystic variant of serous cystadenoma.

**Clinical Features.** One third of the tumors are either found incidentally on routine physical examination or at autopsy (12). Approximately two thirds of patients have symptoms related to local pressure effects of tumor mass, including abdominal pain or mass, nausea and vomiting, and weight loss (30). Jaundice due to obstruction of the common bile duct is unusual, even in tumors originating from the head of the pancreas. There is one case report describing an association with autoimmune hemolytic anemia and idiopathic thrombocytopenic purpura (Evan's syndrome) (11). Two patients with an associated pancreatic ductal adenocarcinoma have been reported (25). The occurrence of cystic lesions of the pancreas similar to serous microcystic adenomas has been reported in patients with von Hippel-Lindau syndrome (see above). Serous microcystic adenomas are frequently associated with cholelithiasis, diabetes mellitus, and extrapancreatic malignancies (10,16,30), but these associations seem to be coincidental and related to patient age.

All known serum tumor markers are normal. Plain abdominal roentgenograms may show calcifications in a few patients. Ultrasonography and computed tomography (CT) reveal a sharply demarcated, multilocular cyst, occasionally with a clearly recognizable central stellate scar and a sunburst type calcification (13,18,24,30,35). On angiography the tumors are usually hypervascular.

**Gross Findings.** Half to two thirds of the tumors occur in the body or tail; the remaining tumors are located in the head of the pancreas (1,9,10,12,33). The tumors are usually solitary, with diameters ranging from 1 to 25 cm in greatest dimension (average, 6 to 10 cm). In rare cases, the pancreas is diffusely involved by multiple tumors (9,19,20). The tumors present as well-circumscribed, slightly bosselated, round lesions. Their cut surface is polycystic and honeycomb-like, showing numerous tiny cysts ranging from 0.01 to 0.5 cm, with a few larger cysts of up to 2.0 cm in diameter (fig. 4-1). The cysts, which are filled with serous (clear watery) fluid, are separated by thin fibrous septa and arranged around a more or less centrally located, dense fibrous core from which fibrous trabeculae radiate to the periphery (central stellate scar). In tumors larger than 5 cm this scar may be calcified. The tumors are well demarcated from the adjacent pancreatic tissue. They are greyish yellow, with an occasional focus of hemorrhage in resected specimens.

**Microscopic Findings.** The tumors consist predominantly of small cysts with some admixed larger ones (fig. 4-2). At low magnification, the pattern of the cysts resembles a sponge. The cysts contain proteinaceous fluid and are lined by a single layer of cuboidal or flattened epithelial cells. Their cytoplasm is pale to clear (fig. 4-3) and only rarely eosinophilic. The cells have a

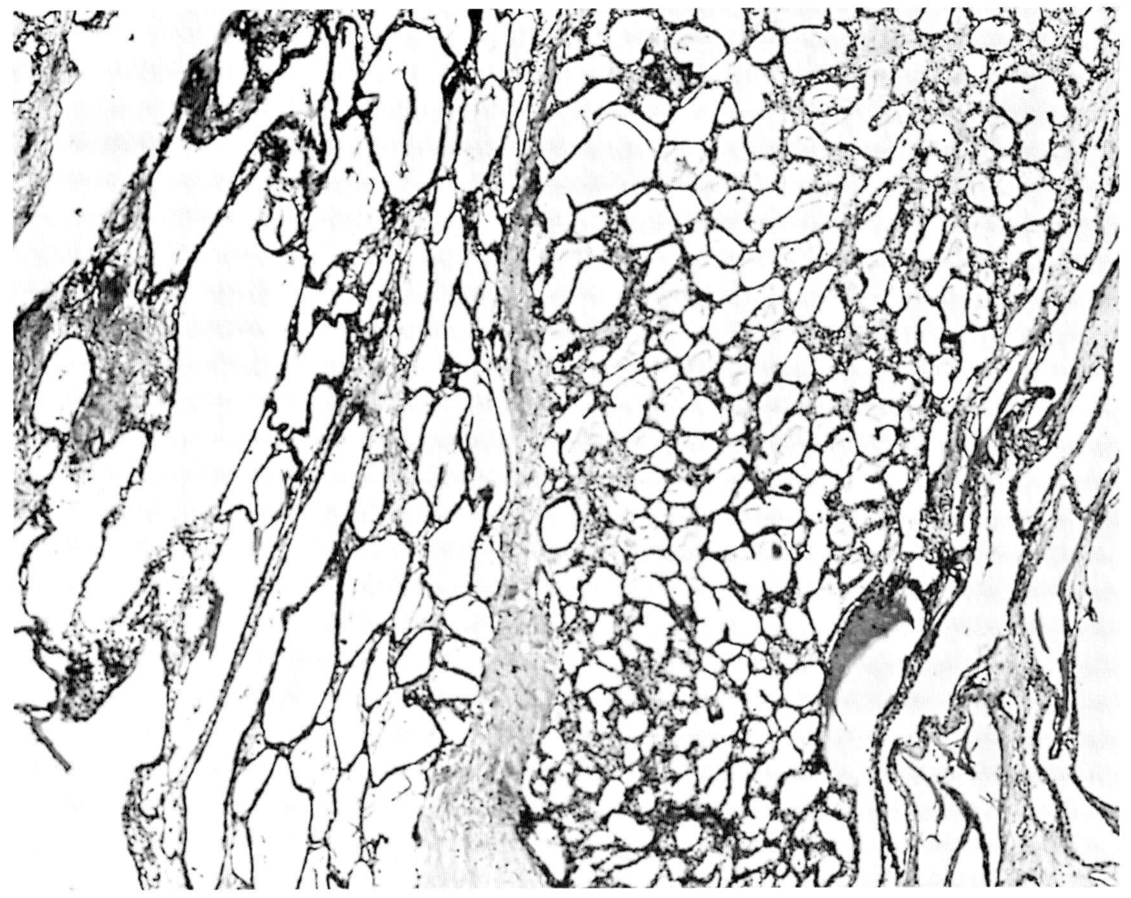

Figure 4-2
SEROUS MICROCYSTIC ADENOMA
There is considerable variation in the size of cysts. Cysts at right are more typical (small, uniform size). Large cysts are present at the left and right extremities. (Fig. 85 from Fascicle 19, Second Series.)

centrally located, round to oval nucleus with an inconspicuous nucleolus. The periodic acid–Schiff (PAS) stain without diastase digestion is positive due to the presence of intracytoplasmic glycogen (fig. 4-4), whereas stains for PAS following diastase digestion and Alcian blue are negative (6). Mitoses are absent and there is no cytologic atypia. Occasionally the tumor cells form intracystic papillary projections (fig. 4-5), usually without a fibrovascular stalk. The acellular stroma separating the cysts is thin, with only occasional larger hyalinized areas. The stroma may contain single islets of Langerhans, acini, ducts, nerves, or lymphocytic aggregates. Focally there may be also hemosiderin deposits, probably due to earlier hemorrhage, and calcifications. The central stellate core is composed of hyalinized tissue with a few clusters of minute cysts. The tumor tissue is well demarcated and usually separated by a fibrous band from the adjoining pancreatic parenchyma, but complete fibrous encapsulation is not a consistent feature (fig. 4-6). The peripheral fibrous tissue contains many large blood vessels.

**Immunohistochemical Findings.** The epithelial nature of these tumors is demonstrated by their positivity for epithelial membrane antigen and cytokeratins 7, 8, 18, and 19. In addition, the tumor cells may be focally positive for CA19-9 and B72.3. They are uniformly negative for carcinoembryonic antigen (CEA), trypsin, chromogranin A, synaptophysin, S-100 protein, desmin, vimentin, and factor VIII–related antigen (see Table 3-1) (1,12,15,33,36). They are also negative for actin (Capella C., unpublished observation, 1995).

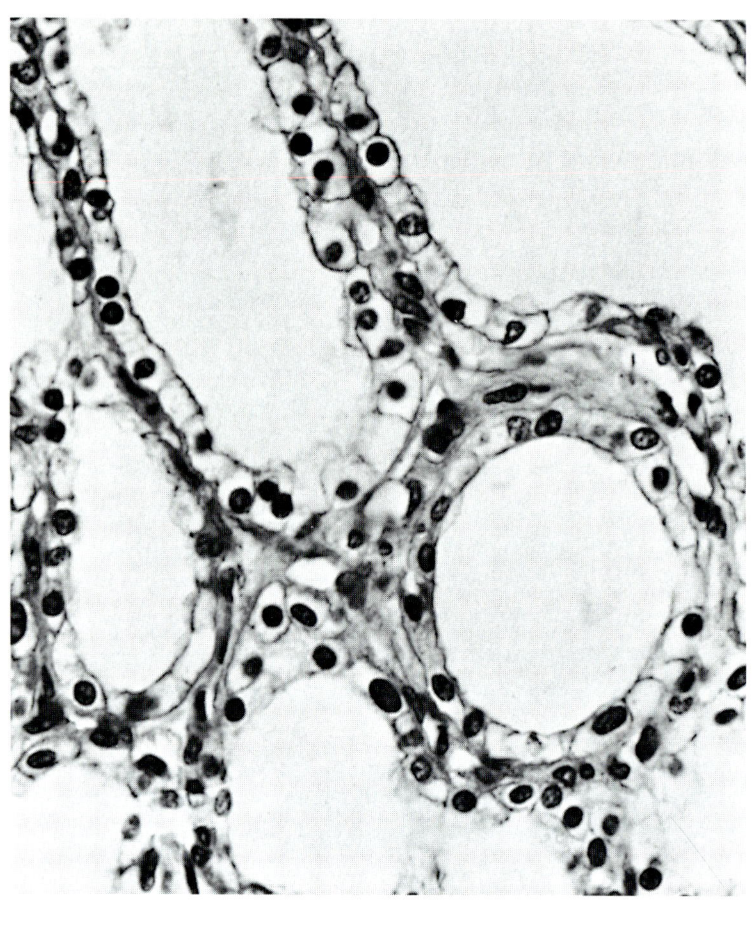

Figure 4-3
SEROUS MICROCYSTIC ADENOMA

Cuboidal cell with watery clear cytoplasm surrounding a spherical, densely staining nucleus. Special stains and electron microscopy reveal glycogen in the cytoplasm. There is relatively little stroma between the cysts and no significant staining of cyst content. (Fig. 86 from Fascicle 19, Second Series.)

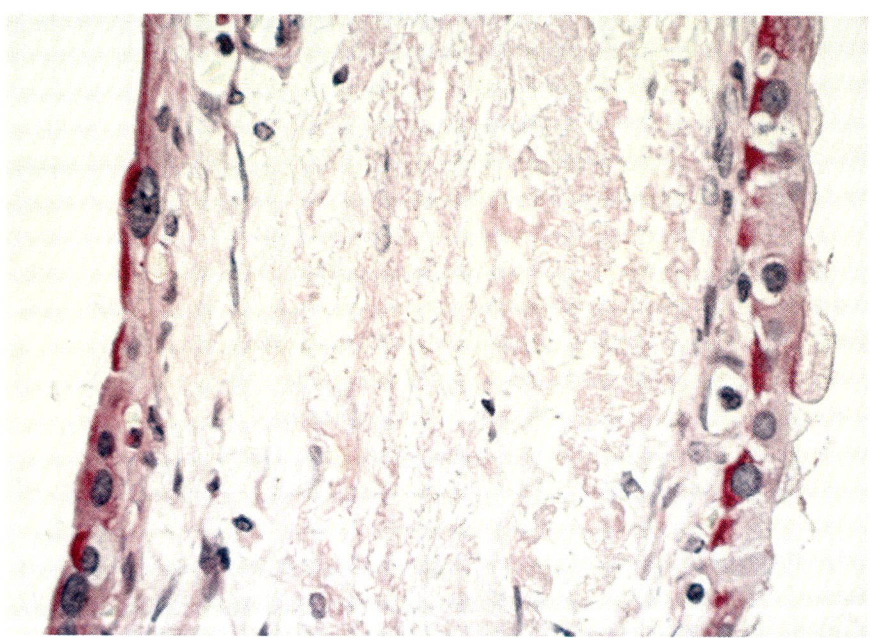

Figure 4-4
SEROUS
MICROCYSTIC ADENOMA

The tumor cells show cytoplasmic PAS positivity due to their glycogen content.

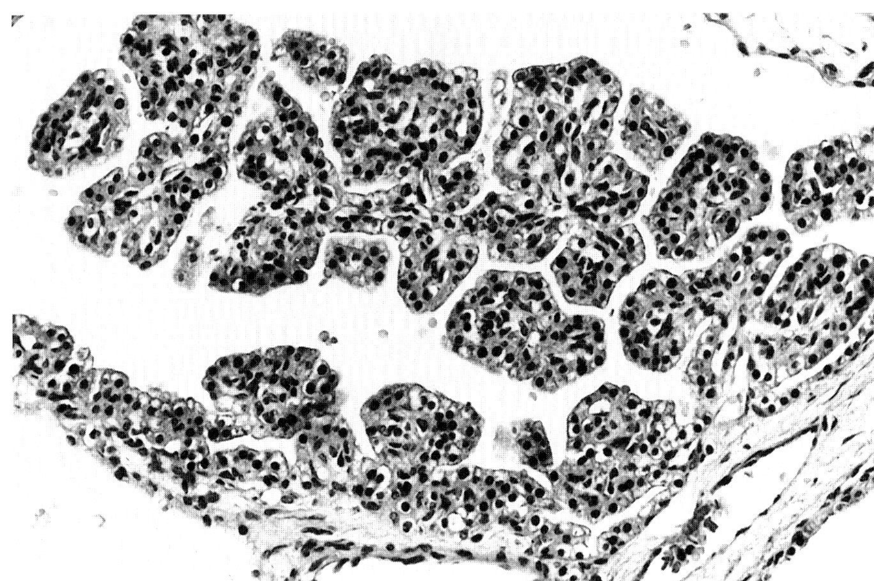

Figure 4-5
SEROUS
MICROCYSTIC ADENOMA
Intracystic papillary projection formed by regular cuboidal cells.

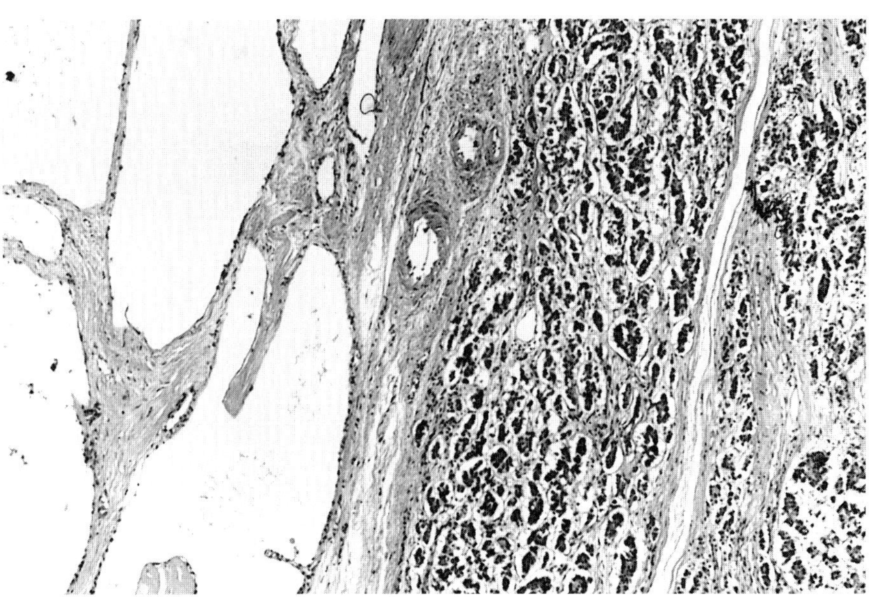

Figure 4-6
SEROUS
MICROCYSTIC ADENOMA
The cystic lesion is well demarcated from the adjoining pancreatic tissue by a small fibrous band containing some vessels.

**Ultrastructural Findings.** Electron microscopy demonstrates a single row of uniform epithelial cells lining the cysts and resting on a basement membrane (1,6,9,20,23,33). The apical surface shows poorly developed or no microvilli. The cytoplasm contains numerous glycogen granules but only a few mitochondria, short profiles of endoplasmic reticulum, lipid droplets, and multivesicular bodies (fig. 4-7). Golgi complexes are rarely identified. Zymogen granules and neurosecretory granules are absent. The tumor cells are connected by occluding junctions and belt desmosomes. The belt desmosomes are often in contact with intracytoplasmic filament bundles. Within the collagenous matrix of the stroma are fibroblasts, degenerated acinar cells, lymphocytes, and small vessels. Nyongo and Huntrakoon (28) described myoepithelial cells beneath some of the epithelial cells; this finding, however, has not been confirmed by others (1,33).

**Differential Diagnosis.** The differential diagnosis of serous microcystic adenoma includes all other cystic lesions of the pancreas as well as lymphangioma and renal cell carcinoma. Most

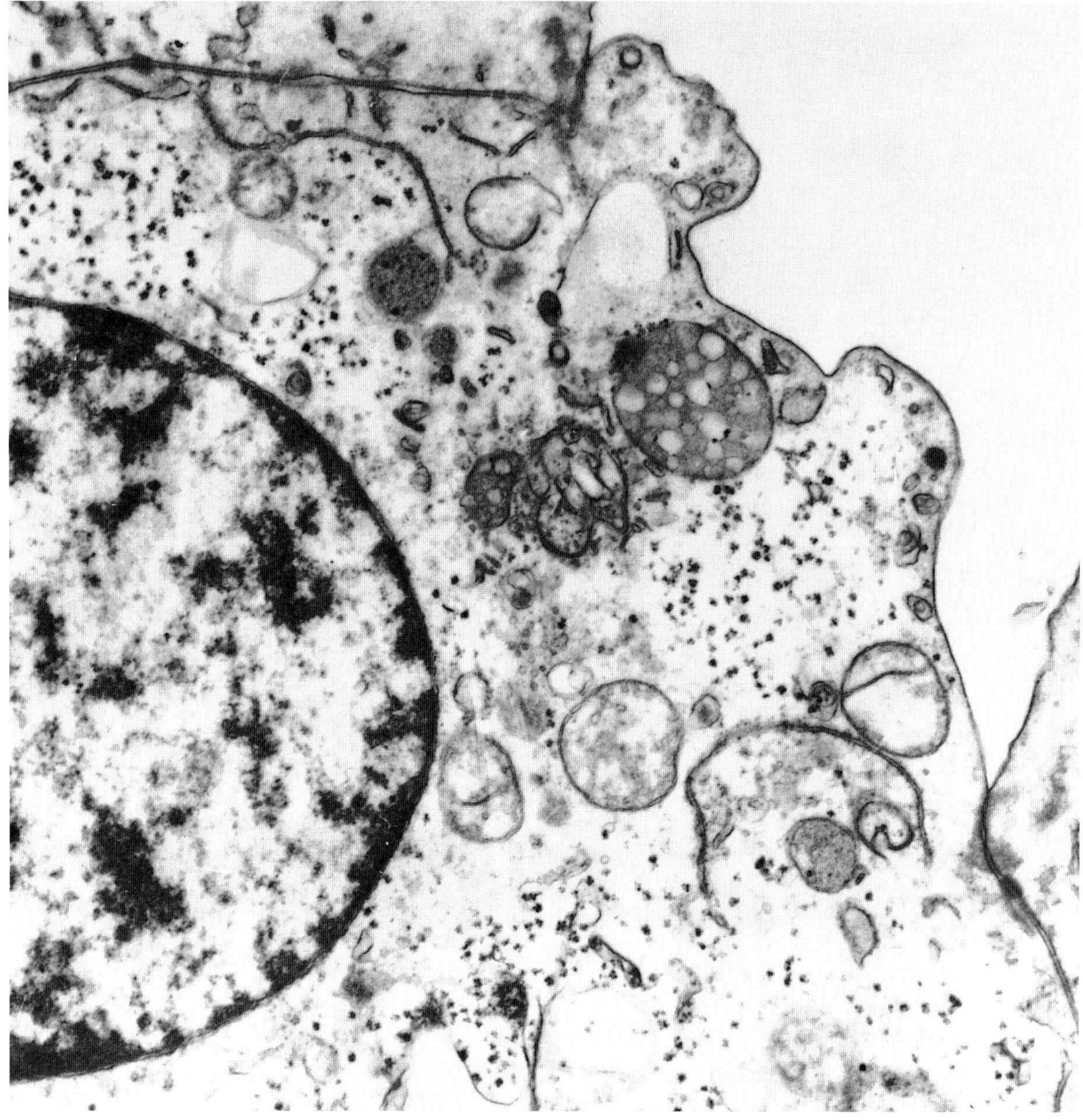

Figure 4-7
SEROUS MICROCYSTIC ADENOMA
The cytoplasm of the tumor cell contains multiple glycogen particles, some mitochondria, and multivesicular bodies. There are no microvilli at the apical surface (X12,800).

important is distinguishing serous microcystic adenoma from mucinous cystic neoplasms of the pancreas because of the malignant potential of the latter. Grossly, mucinous cystic neoplasms are unilocular or oligolocular lesions and contain viscous mucin, while serous microcystic adenomas are polycystic, have a central stellate scar, and contain watery fluid. Histologically, the columnar epithelium of the mucinous cystic neoplasms, which may show severe cellular atypia, stains for mucins and CEA, while the epithelium of serous microcystic adenoma does not. In the solid-pseudopapillary tumors of the pancreas the cystic changes result from degeneration of originally solid parts. Therefore these cystic spaces lack a single epithelial lining. Moreover, solid-pseudopapillary tumors occur predominantly in young women, while serous microcystic adenoma is a tumor of the elderly. Acinar cell cystadenocarcinoma is easily separated from serous microcystic adenoma by the absence of a central stellate scar and evidence of acinar cell differentiation. Lymphoepithelial cyst of the pancreas usually presents as an unilocular cystic lesion filled with keratinaceous material. Histologically, it is lined by keratinizing squamous epithelium which is supported by lymphoid tissue stroma. Lymphangioma shows relatively large cystic spaces lined by cells that are not glycogen rich; they are keratin negative and stain for factor VIII–related antigen. Renal cell carcinoma is characterized by small tubular structures composed of cells with nuclei that are often irregular in size and have distinct nucleoli. In addition, the tumor cells are often vimentin positive.

**Frozen Section Diagnosis and Cytology.** Clues for a correct frozen section diagnosis are the sponge-like pattern of the cystic lesion, the clear cytoplasm, and the uniform appearance of the lining epithelium. Fine-needle aspiration cytology is characterized by cellular sheets and strips of small cuboidal cells. The cells have central round nuclei and clear cytoplasm. Nuclear pleomorphism and conspicuous nucleoli are absent, but occasional intranuclear cytoplasmic inclusions and nuclear grooves may be seen (37).

**Treatment.** With rare exceptions (see Serous Cystadenocarcinoma) serous microcystic adenoma is benign. Surgical intervention either by resection or biliary bypass is only necessary when the tumors are symptomatic and the benefits of the operation outweighs its risk.

**Prognosis.** The prognosis of this tumor is excellent because there is only a minimal risk of malignant transformation and there are no related major complications.

## Serous Oligocystic Adenoma

**Definition.** This benign tumor is composed of only a few relatively large cysts lined by epithelial cells showing evidence of ductular differentiation. This definition includes macrocystic serous cystadenoma (22), serous oligocystic and ill-demarcated adenoma (12), and the cystadenomas observed in children (34). Whether these tumors indeed form one group remains to be established.

**General Features.** Serous oligocystic adenomas are much less common than serous microcystic adenomas. To date, such tumors have been described in nine adult patients (12,22) and four children (2,7,14,34). The tumor shows no sex predilection. Adults are usually 60 years and over (age range, 46 to 69 years; mean, 65 years); the tumor has been described in two male and two female infants, aged between 2 and 16 months.

The etiology of the tumor is not known. In children, it has been suggested that the tumors may be malformative processes and not true neoplasms because of the finding of cytomegalovirus infection in the adjacent pancreas in two cases (2,7). The histochemical and immunocytochemical features are the same as for serous microcystic adenomas, indicating that these epithelial neoplasms probably also derive from ductular cells (12).

**Clinical Features.** In most adult patients so far observed there were symptoms that led to the discovery and removal of the tumor. Most common was upper abdominal discomfort or pain. Two patients presented with jaundice, one of whom also had steatorrhea. In two other patients, the tumor was discovered incidentally during surgery for a duodenal ulcer. In infants, the tumors presented as a palpable abdominal mass.

**Gross Findings.** The tumors typically present as oligocystic neoplasms with a diameter of 4 to 10 cm (mean, 6 cm). Their cut surface reveals few (fig. 4-8), and occasionally only one, macroscopically visible cysts filled with watery clear or brown fluid. The cysts usually measure between 1 and 2 cm in diameter, but cysts as large as 8 cm have been reported (22). The irregularly arranged cysts, separated sometimes by broad septa, lie within a fibrous stroma that lacks a central stellate scar. The cysts and the supporting fibrous tissue may extend into the adjoining pancreatic tissue so that the tumors are ill-demarcated. Most tumors are located in the head and body of the pancreas. In the head they may obstruct the periampullary portion of the common bile duct.

**Microscopic Findings.** Serous oligocystic adenoma shows, in general, the same histologic features as serous microcystic adenoma. Occasionally, however, the lining epithelium may be

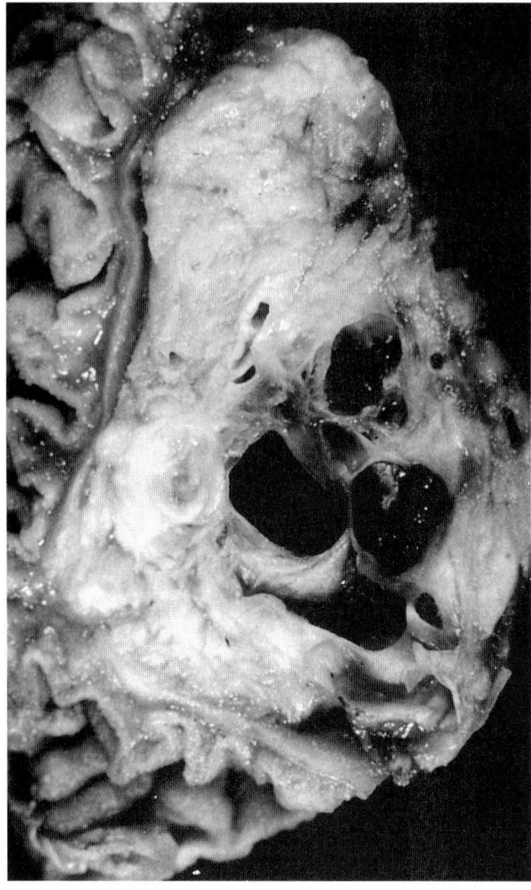

Figure 4-8
SEROUS OLIGOCYSTIC ADENOMA
This oligocystic lesion in the head of the pancreas shows a few cysts which are separated by thin as well as broad fibrous bands. The lesion lacks the central stellate scar and the sharp demarcation that are typical for the microcystic type of serous cystadenoma (compare with figure 4-1). (Fig. 2 from Egawa E, Maillet B, Schröder S, Mukai K, Klöppel G. Serous oligocystic and ill-demarcated adenoma of the pancreas: a variant of serous cystic adenoma. Virchows Arch 1994;424:13–7.)

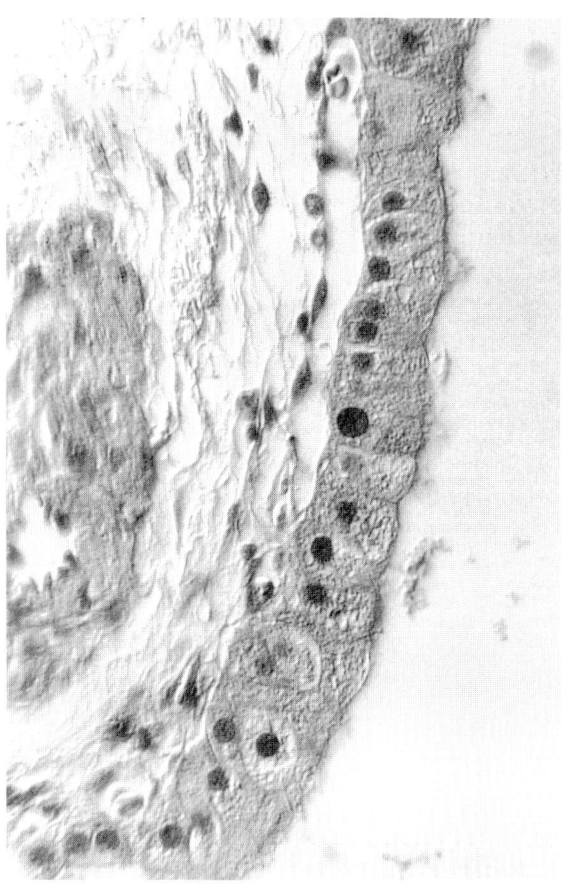

Figure 4-9
SEROUS OLIGOCYSTIC ADENOMA
Focally, the lining epithelial cells have a more columnar appearance and a granular (eosinophilic) cytoplasm. (Nomarski optic) (Fig. 3 from Egawa E, Maillet B, Schröder S, Mukai K, Klöppel G. Serous oligocystic and ill-demarcated adenoma of the pancreas: a variant of serous cystic adenoma. Virchows Arch 1994;424:13–7.)

more cuboidal and less flattened and the nuclei are generally larger. The cytoplasm is either eosinophilic (fig. 4-9) or clear due to the presence of glycogen. Mucin stains are all negative. Mitoses or cytologic atypia are lacking. The stromal framework is well developed and often hyalinized. Occasionally the tumor contains entrapped islets, single ducts, or nerves. The tumor border is not well defined and small cysts often extend into the adjoining pancreatic tissue (fig. 4-10). The immunohistochemical features are the same as for serous microcystic adenoma (12).

**Ultrastructural Findings.** Electron microscopic examination of one tumor revealed cytoplasmic features similar to those of serous microcystic adenoma (34). However, instead of glycogen granules this tumor had dense vacuoles 250 to 500 nm in diameter.

**Differential Diagnosis.** The main structural difference between serous oligocystic adenoma and serous microcystic adenoma is the oligocystic pattern and the absence of a central stellate scar in the former tumor. The criteria distinguishing serous oligocystic adenomas from other cystic tumors of the pancreas are in general the same as for serous microcystic adenoma. Since serous oligocystic adenoma may present as

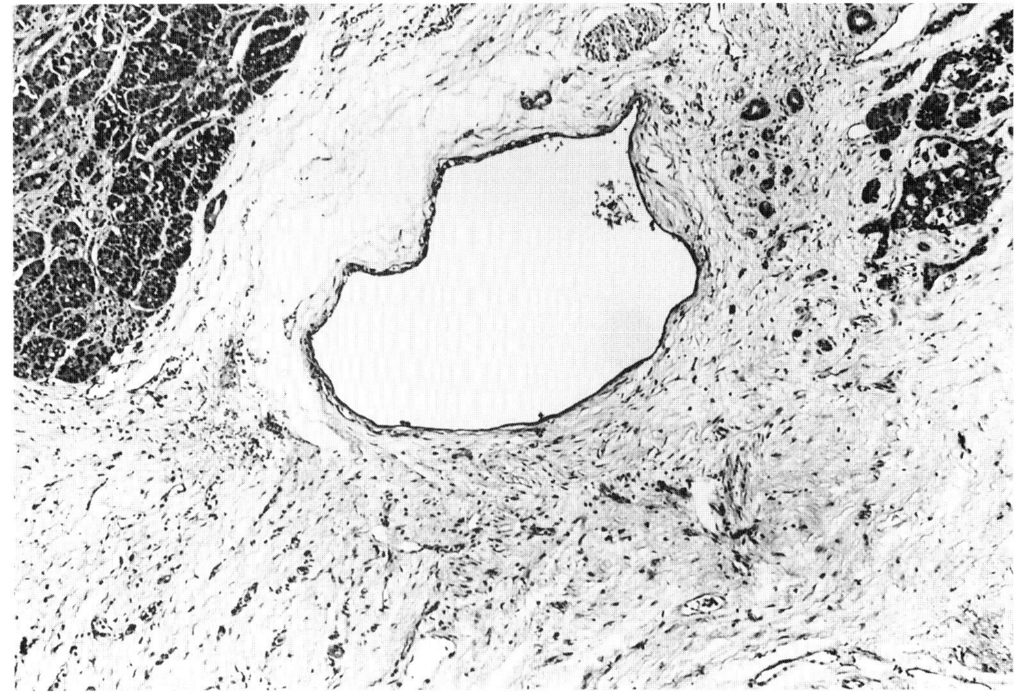

Figure 4-10
SEROUS OLIGOCYSTIC ADENOMA
The illustration shows a small cyst at the margin of the lesion extending into the adjacent pancreatic tissue. (Fig. 4B from Egawa E, Maillet B, Schröder S, Mukai K, Klöppel G. Serous oligocystic and ill-demarcated adenoma of the pancreas: a variant of serous cystic adenoma. Virchow Arch 1994,424:13–7.)

a unilocular cystic lesion filled with blood, difficulties may arise in distinguishing it macroscopically from a pseudocyst. However, microscopically, pseudocysts are lined by granulation tissue instead of epithelial cells.

**Treatment.** Lesions that are symptomatic may be removed by resection.

**Prognosis.** Mean follow-up of four patients for 2.9 years showed no tumor recurrence or malignant transformation (12).

## SEROUS CYSTADENOCARCINOMA

**Definition.** This is a malignant epithelial tumor showing evidence of ductular differentiation. Whether the nonmucinous, glycogen-poor cystadenocarcinoma described by Friedman (38) is a variant of serous cystadenocarcinoma is unclear; this tumor is described in more detail in the chapter on Miscellaneous Carcinomas.

**General Features.** So far only three cases have been reported (39,40,41). These patients were between 63 and 72 years of age; there were two women and one man. One patient was caucasian and two were from Japan. We recently saw a 71-year-old man with a metastasizing serous cystadenocarcinoma.

**Clinical Features.** One patient presented with bleeding from gastric varices due to tumor involvement of the wall of the stomach and the splenic vein. Two patients had an upper abdominal mass and one patient developed jaundice. Ultrasonography and CT revealed a hyperechoic mass. CEA and CA19-9 were normal or slightly increased.

**Gross Findings.** The pancreatic tumors had a spongy appearance (39,40,41). Their size varied between 10 and 12 cm. In one case, in addition to a large tumor which histologically showed perineural invasion, there were five smaller cystic tumors as well as an endocrine neoplasm (40). In another case the tumor invaded the spleen and metastasized to the gastric wall and liver (39). Liver metastases were also found in the third patient (41). In the patient seen by us, the

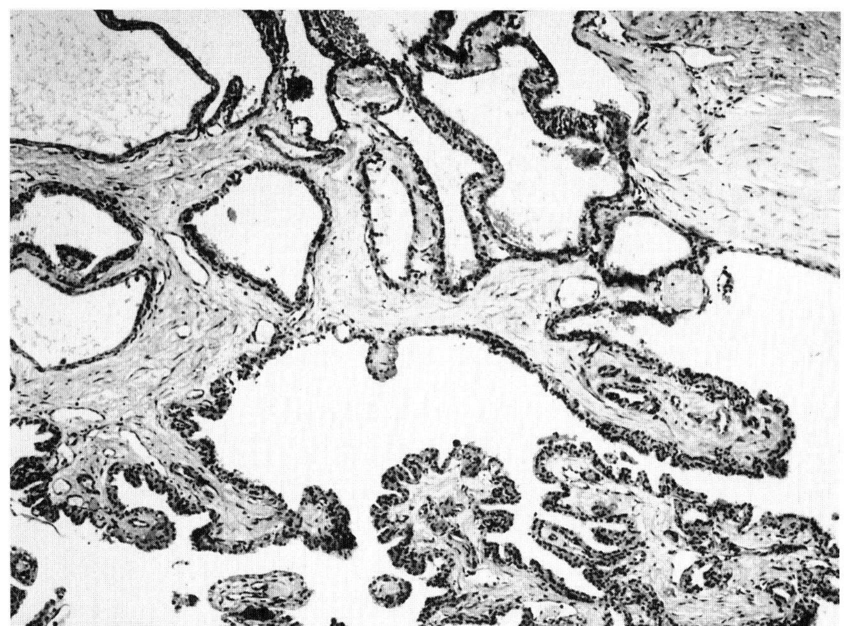

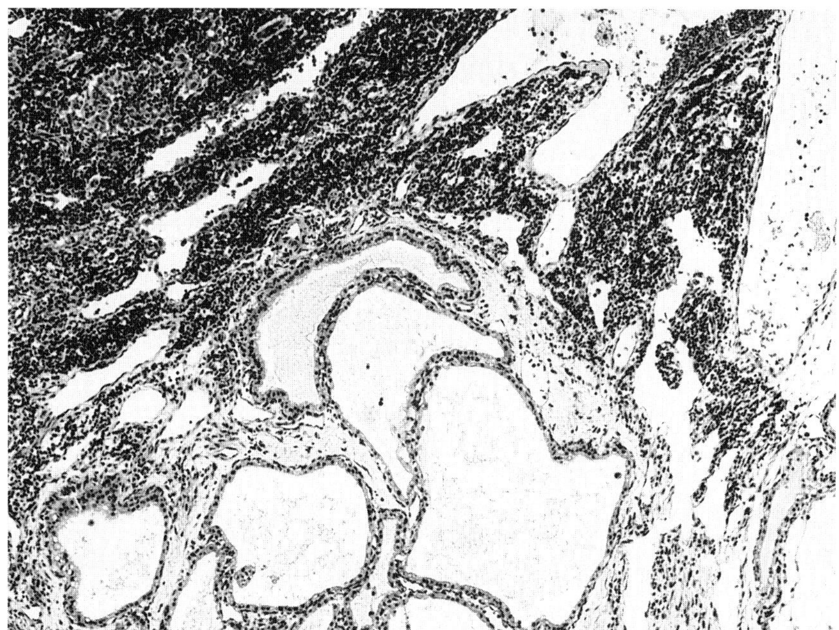

Figure 4-11
SEROUS
CYSTADENOCARCINOMA

Top: The histologic appearance of this metastasizing tumor in a 71-year-old patient is that of a serous microcystic adenoma. The tumor shows multiple cysts of varying size. Focally the cuboidal epithelium forms papillary projections. (Courtesy of Dr. Torsten Mattfeldt, Ulm, Germany.)

Bottom: Lymph node metastasis of the tumor shown in A.

tumor was in the head of the pancreas and metastasized to a regional lymph node.

**Microscopic and Ultrastructural Findings.** The histologic features in the primary tumor as well as in the metastases are consistent with those of serous microcystic adenoma (fig. 4-11), although focally, mild nuclear pleomorphism was found (39–41). One tumor showed neural invasion and aneuploid nuclear DNA content (40).

**Differential Diagnosis.** The tumors have to be separated from serous microcystic adenoma. This may be difficult or impossible on histologic grounds alone and may only be established by the absence or presence of metastatic deposits. Other tumors that have to be distinguished from serous cystadenocarcinoma are essentially those that have also been discussed for serous microcystic adenoma.

**Treatment and Prognosis.** From the reports available it seems that serous cystadenocarcinomas are slowly growing neoplasms and palliative resection may be helpful even in advanced stages (41).

## MUCINOUS CYSTIC TUMOR

**Definition.** Mucinous cystic tumor is a cystic pancreatic tumor formed of epithelial cells producing mucin; there is evidence of gastroenteropancreatic differentiation and an "ovarian-type stroma." It occurs almost exclusively in women. According to the degree of epithelial dysplasia, the tumor is classified as adenoma, borderline tumor, or carcinoma.

**General Considerations.** In 1978, Compagno and Oertel (50) separated mucinous cystic tumors from their serous counterparts. In their study of 41 cases, all the mucinous cystic tumors were considered potentially malignant based on the following observations: mucinous cystic tumors recur as cystadenocarcinomas after incomplete resection or internal drainage (46,50,62, 67,75,77,88) and they may contain benign columnar epithelium in combination with severe dysplasia or obvious invasive carcinoma (50,53, 93). Consequently, they introduced the term "mucinous cystic neoplasm with overt or latent malignancy" for all mucinous cystic tumors. This implies that all mucinous cystic tumors, regardless of their individual morphologic features, fall into one group without further differentiation. However, some small mucinous cystic tumors found incidentally at radiologic examination, surgery, or autopsy show no evidence of severe dysplasia even after complete histologic work-up (93). Without denying the basic concept that even the benign-looking tumors of this category have the potential to transform into carcinoma, we propose classifying mucinous cystic tumors of the pancreas according to their grade of dysplasia. These tumors represent a spectrum of lesions that include mucinous cystadenoma, mucinous cystic tumor of borderline malignant potential, and mucinous cystadenocarcinoma. This separation follows the classification of mucinous tumors of the ovary which closely resemble their pancreatic counterparts in biology and cell lineage differentiation (81,85). Tumors in the borderline category are characterized by epithelial dysplasia exceeding that of benign tumors, but lack the severe dysplasia-carcinoma in situ changes or frank stromal invasion seen in cystadenocarcinoma. It is also of interest to emphasize the striking resemblance of pancreatic mucinous cystic tumors to hepatobiliary cystadenomas and cystadenocarcinomas with "mesenchymal stroma" (91), both in regard to morphology and biology (42,63).

These tumors are almost exclusive to women, a feature that they share with their counterparts in the liver (91) and the retroperitoneum. And both pancreatic and hepatobiliary mucinous cystic tumors usually have an ovarian-type stroma which makes them comparable to ovarian mucinous tumors. Moreover, the same pattern of cell lineage differentiation is found in pancreatic and ovarian mucinous cystic tumors (81,85). It seems, therefore, that tumors of this type, regardless of whether they occur in the ovary, pancreas, liver, or retroperitoneum, have a common cellular origin which is determined by gender and characterized by differentiation towards gastroenteropancreatic cells (43,81).

**General Features.** This is an uncommon tumor of the pancreas. It accounts for approximately 2 to 2.5 percent of all exocrine pancreatic tumors (49,71). Von Segesser and Rohner (87) cited 300 published cases up to 1984; since 1978, 10 series of mucinous cystic tumors (including mucinous cystadenocarcinomas) have appeared in the literature (43,47,49–51,59,61,62,89,93). Mucinous cystadenocarcinomas are half as frequent (46), or even less (87), than mucinous cystadenomas. More than two thirds of the patients are women and the peak age occurs in the fifth decade (range, 20 to 82 years; mean, 49 years including cystadenocarcinomas). Men are usually older than women (mean, 70 years) (50). If only cases with benign histology or borderline malignancy are considered, the age range for women is 26 to 79 years (mean, 50 years) and for men 47 to 85 years (mean, 64 years) (47,51,59, 92,93). In the author's (G.K.) series of patients with mucinous cystic tumors, from which tumors lacking an ovarian-type stroma were excluded, all were women. Mucinous cystic tumors occur in all races (50,92,93).

The etiology of the tumor is not known, but the predilection for women suggests that genetic factors may be involved in its pathogenesis (see

General Considerations). Smoking does not seem to play a significant role (92). In hamsters treated with nitrosamine derivatives, neoplasms similar to human mucinous cystic tumors were seen (see Ductal Adenocarcinoma).

**Clinical Features.** The clinical presentation depends on the size of the tumor. Tumors smaller than 3 cm are either found incidentally on radiologic examination, at surgery, or at autopsy. Larger tumors produce symptoms that are usually due to compression of adjacent structures and are often accompanied by a palpable abdominal mass. The most frequent symptom is upper abdominal discomfort or pain which is intermittent or continuous. Rare symptoms are weight loss and weakness (50). The duration of the symptoms varies from a few days to many years. Jaundice due to obstruction of the common bile duct is unusual even in tumors originating from the head of the pancreas. An association with diabetes mellitus is frequent and could be related to replacement of pancreatic tissue by tumor.

Serum tumor markers such as CEA or CA19-9 are only occasionally elevated and may suggest the presence of a cystadenocarcinoma (93). Plain abdominal roentgenograms may demonstrate nodular calcifications in the capsule of the tumor and compression or displacement of the stomach, duodenum, or colon. Ultrasonography and CT reveal a sharply demarcated, hypoechoic or low density mass with one or more large loculations (58,69,89). An irregular thickening of the cyst wall and a solid component projecting into the cystic cavity suggests malignant transformation (58,69,89). Angiography generally demonstrates a hypovascular or avascular lesion with vessels stretched over the surface. Endoscopic retrograde cholangiography shows nonspecific bowing of the pancreatic duct around a mass but, with few exceptions (60), no communication with the neoplastic cystic cavity. Aspirated fluid from the cyst frequently contains high levels of CEA and CA19-9 and only low levels of amylase and elastase (71,84,95).

In rare cases, a Zollinger-Ellison syndrome due to the secretion of gastrin from gastrin-producing cells in the tumor has been reported (68).

**Gross Findings.** More than 80 percent of the tumors occur in the pancreatic body or tail (50, 51,92). The tumors are solitary, with diameters ranging from 2 to 35 cm in greatest dimension; average size is between 6 and 10 cm, with benign tumors usually smaller (less than 3 cm) than borderline or malignant ones (93). They present as well-circumscribed, rounded masses with a coarsely lobulated and glistening external surface. On cut section, there is a unilocular cyst containing a thick gelatinous mucinous material surrounded by a dense fibrous capsule of variable thickness (fig. 4-12). Occasionally, the tumors are multilocular and consist of several large cysts and some peripheral small cysts (fig. 4-13). The inner surface is smooth, but sometimes (especially in large and malignant tumors) shows papillary excrescences and solid nodules and protuberances (fig. 4-14). In some tumors the contents of the cysts are hemorrhagic. The tumor capsule may contain small focal calcifications, or it may adhere to adjacent organs. A fistula into the distal part of the duodenum has been described (56). Most tumors are embedded

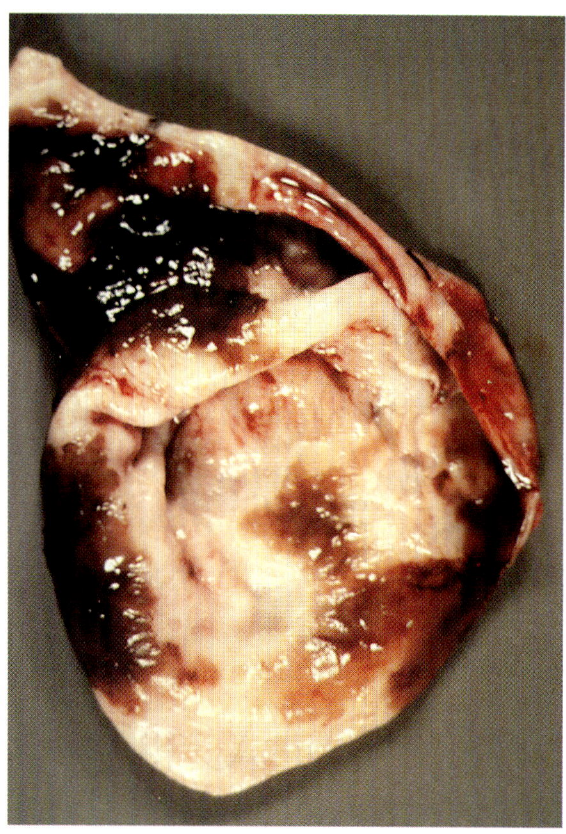

Figure 4-12
MUCINOUS CYSTIC TUMOR
The cut surface shows a unilocular cyst filled with gelatinous and partly hemorrhagic material.

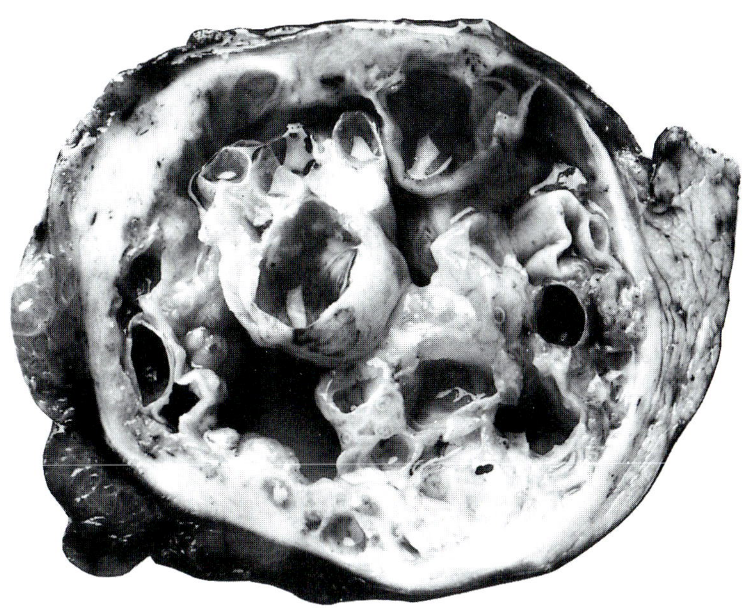

Figure 4-13
MUCINOUS CYSTIC TUMOR

This multiloculated cystic lesion (largest diameter 7 cm) from the tail of the pancreas is well demarcated. It contains mucinous material. The capsule shows nodular thickening. Uninvolved pancreatic tissue is seen at the right margin. (Courtesy of Dr. Klaus Riesner, Lüneburg, Germany.)

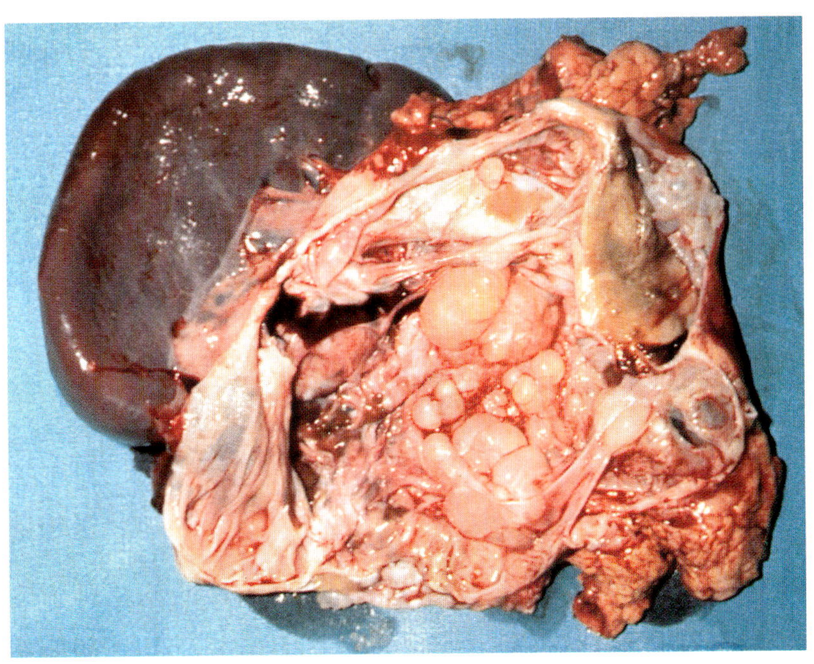

Figure 4-14
MUCINOUS CYSTADENOCARCINOMA

Tumor from the tail of the pancreas with adjacent spleen. The cut surface shows conspicuous, irregular, solid protuberances projecting into cystic cavities.

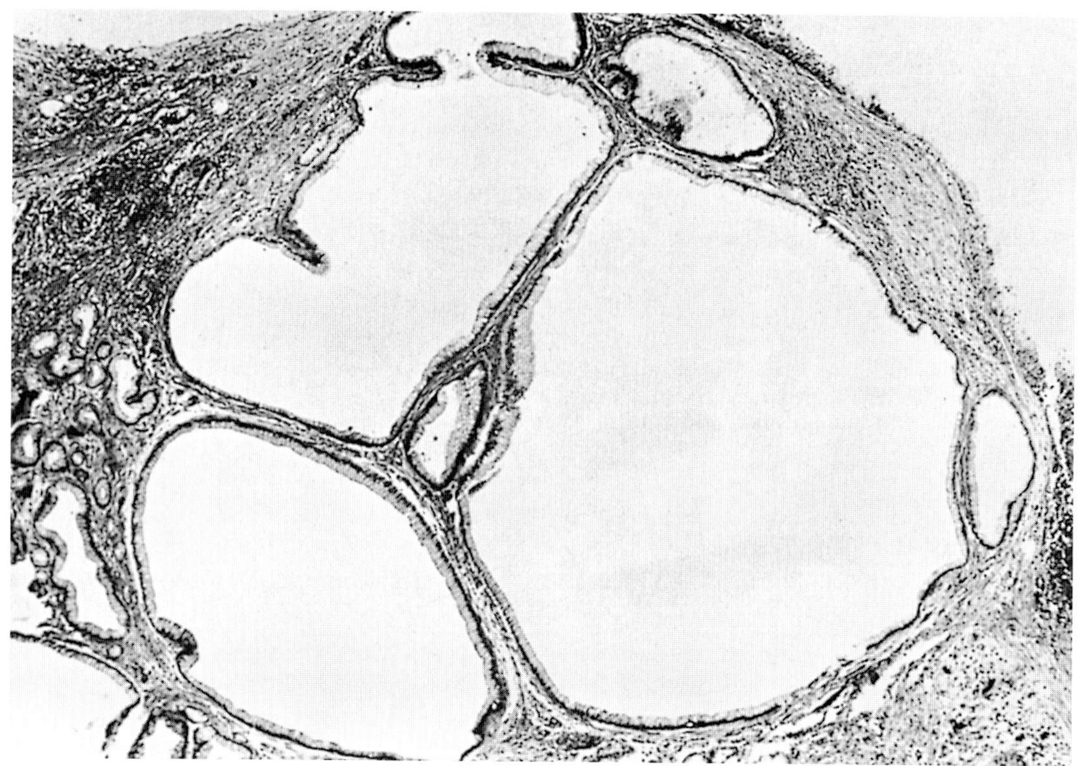

Figure 4-15
MUCINOUS CYSTIC TUMOR, ADENOMA
This mucinous cystadenoma from the tail of the pancreas shows varying sized cysts lined by tall columnar epithelium which looks benign. A few small papillae are present. (Fig. 88 from Fascicle 19, Second Series.)

in and have replaced pancreatic tissue which, in case of an obstruction of the pancreatic duct by the tumor, may be atrophic upstream of the obstructed duct. In some malignant tumors there is obvious invasion by carcinomatous tissue into the surrounding pancreatic parenchyma or adjacent organs such as the spleen, stomach, colon, duodenum, and common bile duct. A communication between the cyst and the pancreatic duct system is uncommon (60,89) and was only frequently observed in Yamada's series (92). Rarely, a tumor may be found attached to the pancreas by only a narrow tissue stalk. Some of the uncommon retroperitoneal or intrasplenic mucinous cystic tumors are thought to arise from heterotopic pancreatic tissue (57,70,83).

**Microscopic Findings.** Most of the cyst is lined by tall columnar cells (fig. 4-15), but large locules may be partially denuded of lining cells or have only flattened atrophic epithelium (fig. 4-16) (89). Where columnar epithelium is present, it is arranged in a single flat row or forms papillary or polypoid projections (fig. 4-17), pseudostratifications, and crypt-like invaginations. The columnar cells are characterized by basally located nuclei and abundant intracellular mucin which stains strongly with non-diastase digestible PAS and Alcian blue (pH 2.7 and pH 1.0). This staining pattern suggests the production and secretion of acidic mucin, with variable proportions of sulfomucins and sialomucins, and some neutral mucin (47,78). In most cases, cells with goblet-like morphology are found admixed with columnar cells (fig. 4-17). About half of the tumors also contain scattered argyrophil and argentaffin endocrine cells at the bases of the columnar cells (fig. 4-18) (43,44,50, 93). These cells are most numerous in areas with goblet-like cells (43,44).

The epithelium may vary from tumor to tumor but also within the same tumor or even the same cyst. The spectrum of differentiation ranges from histologically benign-appearing epithelium with only minimal variation from normal columnar

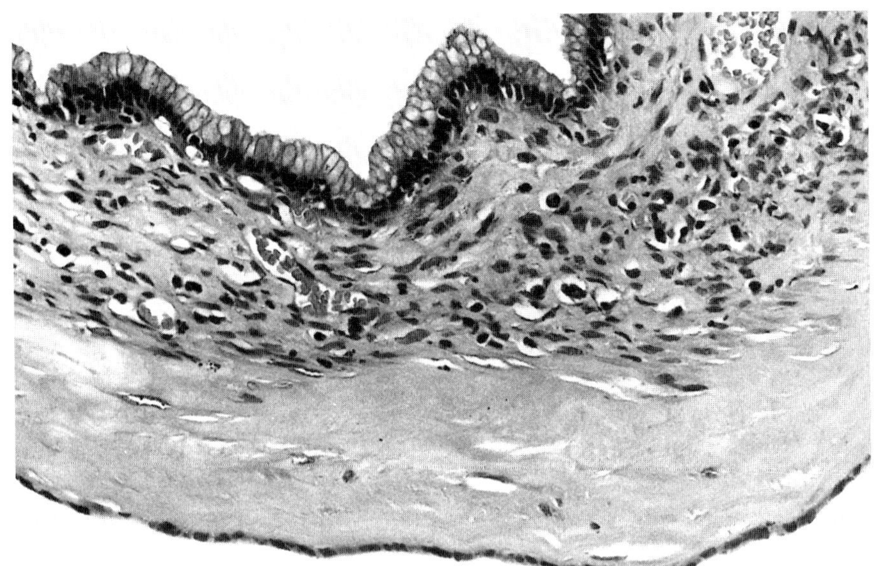

Figure 4-16
MUCINOUS CYSTIC TUMOR, ADENOMA

An intratumoral septum is lined by mildly dysplastic columnar epithelium on one side and atrophic epithelium on the other. Note the partly cellular, partly hyalinized ovarian-like stroma.

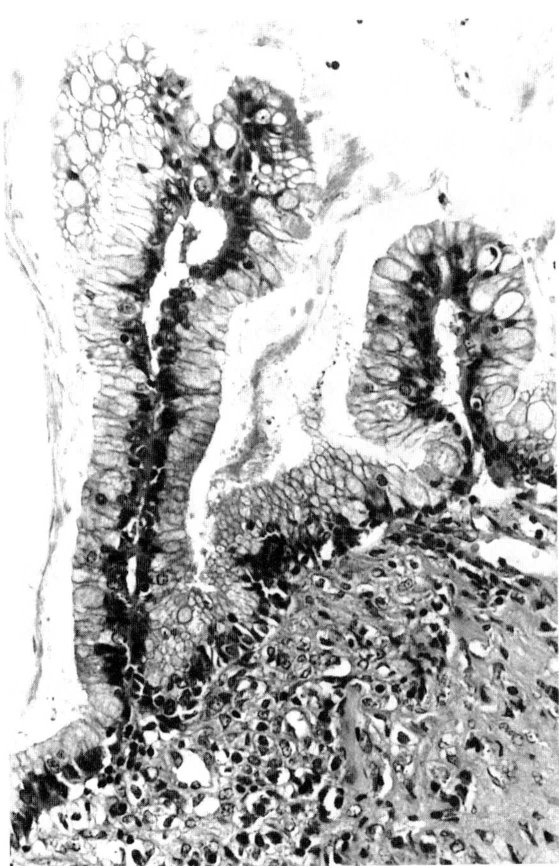

Figure 4-17
MUCINOUS CYSTIC TUMOR, BORDERLINE

The cyst-lining epithelium forms papillary projections with small tissue stalks. Note the tall columnar epithelium with considerable mucin in the apical cytoplasm and moderate nuclear atypia. Some columnar cells have a goblet-like appearance.

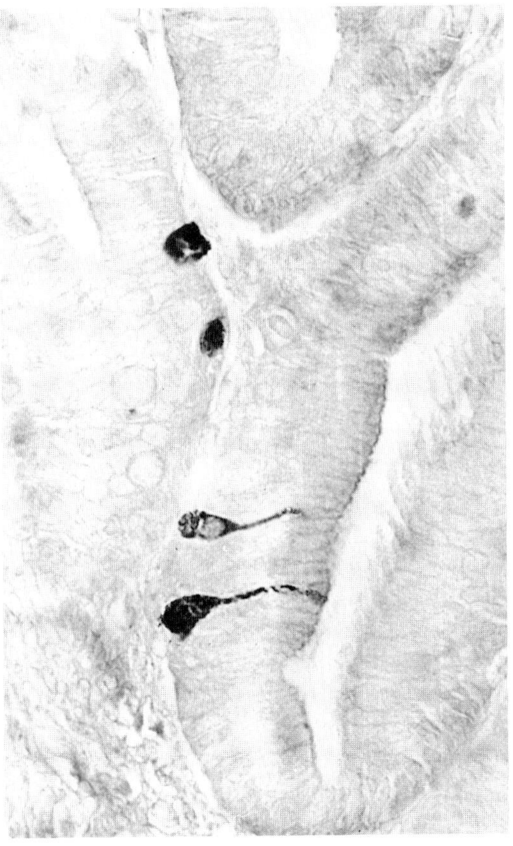

Figure 4-18
MUCINOUS CYSTIC TUMOR

The columnar epithelium contains scattered endocrine cells which immunostain for serotonin.

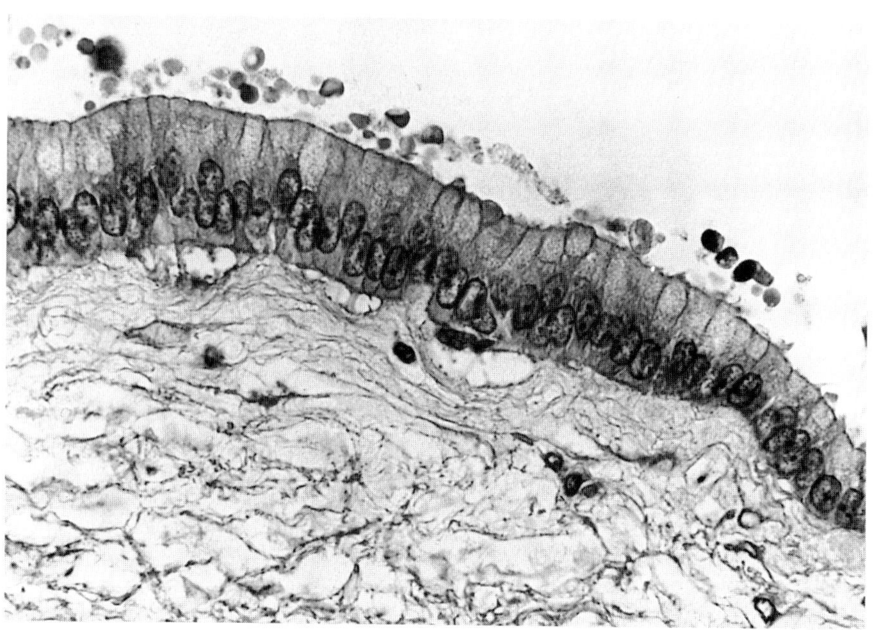

Figure 4-19
MUCINOUS CYSTIC TUMOR, ADENOMA

The lining epithelium consists of a single row of tall mucin-producing columnar cells with polarized nuclei of uniform size. This is considered mild dysplasia.

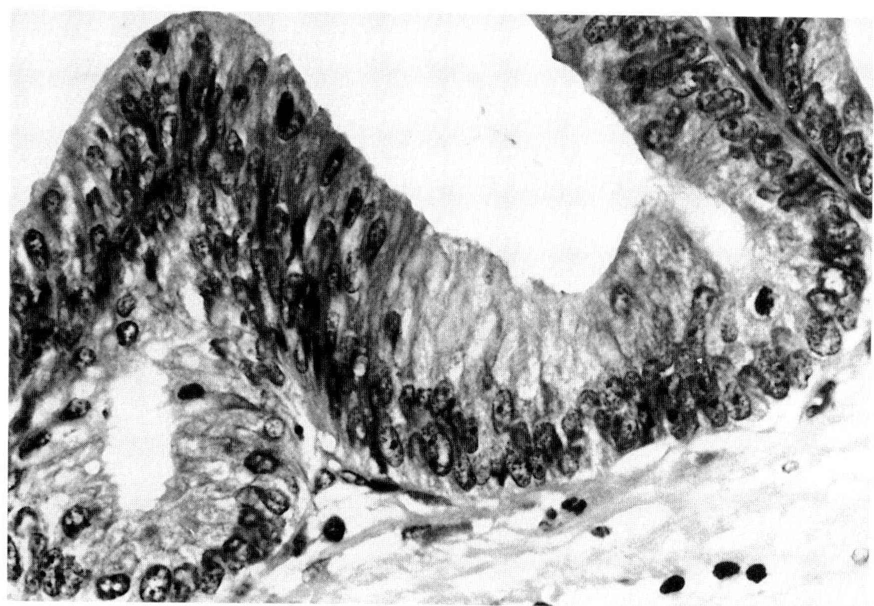

Figure 4-20
MUCINOUS CYSTIC TUMOR, BORDERLINE

Moderate dysplasia is indicated by a lining epithelium showing focal pseudostratification with crowding of enlarged nuclei. Note the mitotic activity.

epithelium (mild dysplasia) to moderately or severely atypical epithelium (moderate and severe dysplasia) and carcinoma in situ. Benign tumors (mucinous cystadenomas) show only mild epithelial dysplasia characterized by a slight increase in the size of the basally located nuclei and the absence of mitoses (fig. 4-19). Borderline tumors (mucinous cystic tumors of borderline malignant potential) exhibit moderate dysplasia, which can involve the entire epithelium or be focal. This dysplasia is characterized by cellular pseudostratification with crowding of atypical nuclei and mitoses (fig. 4-20). Most nuclei are still basally located but tend to be larger and more irregular in size than in mild dysplasia. They often have one or two conspicuous nucleoli. The epithelium often shows papillary projections or crypt-like invaginations, but unquestionable capsular and stromal invasion are, by definition, absent. Malignant tumors (mucinous cystadenocarcinomas)

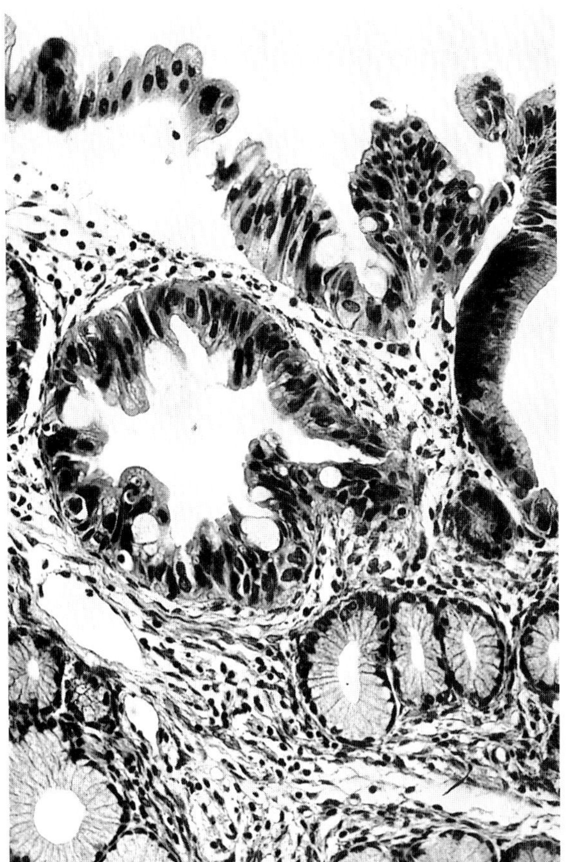
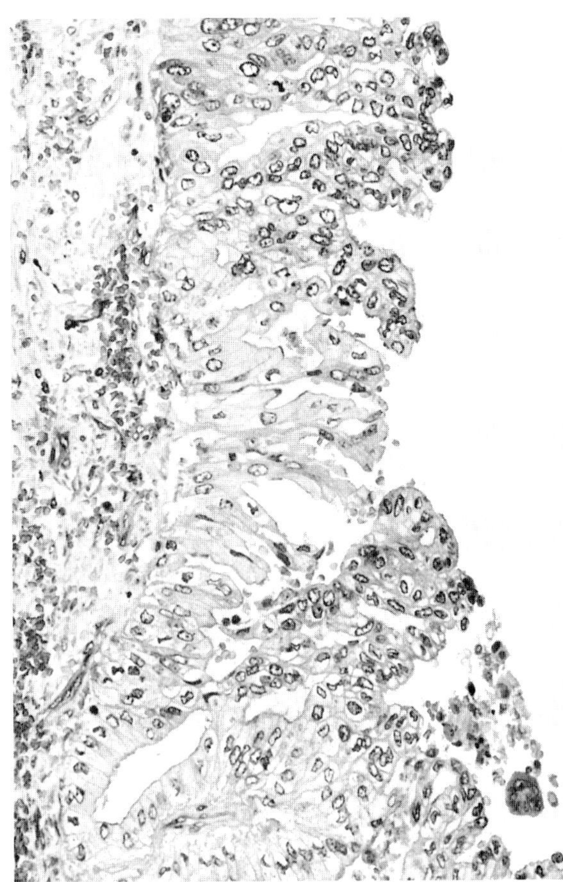

Figure 4-21
MUCINOUS CYSTADENOCARCINOMA

Left: Wall of a cyst lined by severely dysplastic epithelium. The large gland in the adjacent stroma is also lined by severely atypical columnar cells. The surrounding smaller glands still show a benign histology.

Right: Severely dysplastic epithelium forms small and irregularly shaped papillae.

have severe dysplasia-carcinoma in situ changes which are usually focal and may be detected only after careful search of multiple sections from different regions of the tumor (fig. 4-21, left). The epithelial cells show nuclear stratification, severe nuclear atypia, and frequent mitoses. Cellular mucin production is markedly reduced. The epithelium often forms papillae with irregular branching and budding (fig. 4-21, right). In areas with moderate or severe dysplasia, carcinomatous invasion of the stroma may occur.

The subepithelial stroma is characterized by a small inner layer of moderately to densely cellular mesenchyme, followed by a dense layer of collagenous connective tissue. The mesenchymal layer, which resembles ovarian stroma, consists of spindle-shaped cells with round to oval nuclei and capillaries (figs. 4-16, 4-22). The dense layer may contain microcystic daughter glands and, where it merges with the outer wall (fig. 4-23), scattered, normal-looking ducts and islets; lymphocytic aggregates; and large vessels. Apart from areas with typical stroma there may be regions displaying hemorrhage, calcification (fig. 4-24), and chronic inflammatory changes, sometimes with a foreign body–type reaction. This is often associated with mucin spillage from ruptured cysts (fig. 4-25). The adjoining pancreatic parenchyma is normal or may show fibrous atrophy due to obstruction of the main pancreatic duct by the tumor. Duct changes such as mucinous hypertrophy or ductal hyperplasia may occur in the nontumorous pancreas, but are not significantly associated with the tumor.

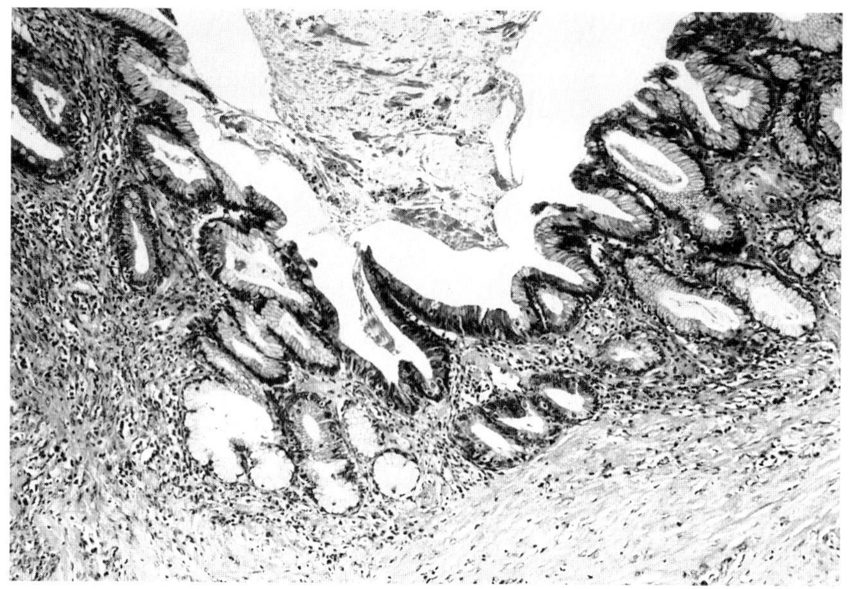

Figure 4-22
MUCINOUS CYSTIC TUMOR, BORDERLINE

Wall of a cyst with ovarian-like stroma. A subepithelial densely cellular layer is followed by a dense layer of collagenous connective tissue. Part of the epithelium is moderately dysplastic. In the cellular stroma are several small daughter glands.

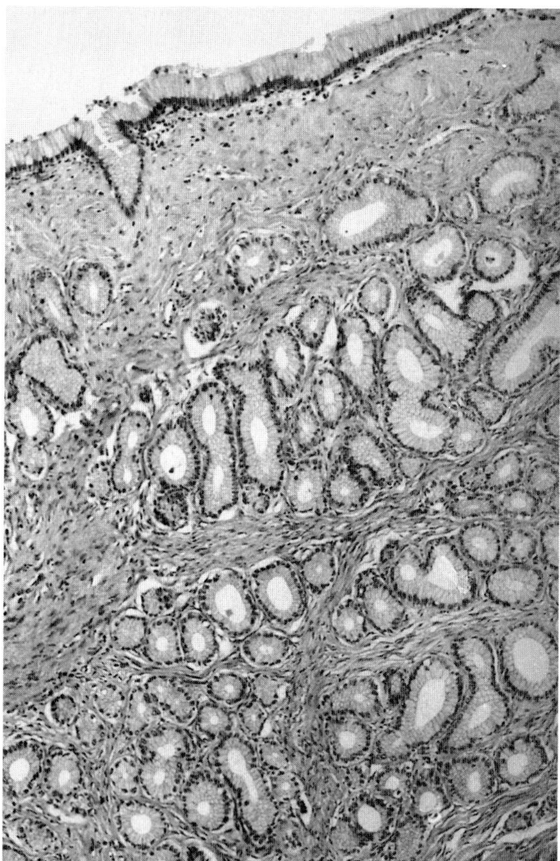

Figure 4-23
MUCINOUS CYSTIC TUMOR, ADENOMA

Wall of a cyst containing groups of associated glands. The lobular distribution of the glands as well as the benign histology of their epithelium excludes an invasive carcinoma component.

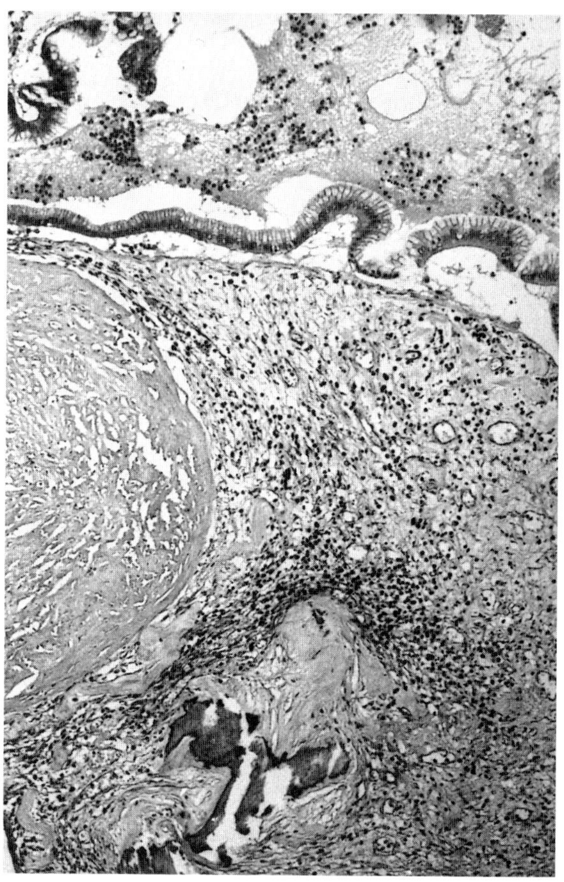

Figure 4-24
MUCINOUS CYSTIC TUMOR

Wall of a cyst with focal hyalinization and calcification in the cellular stroma.

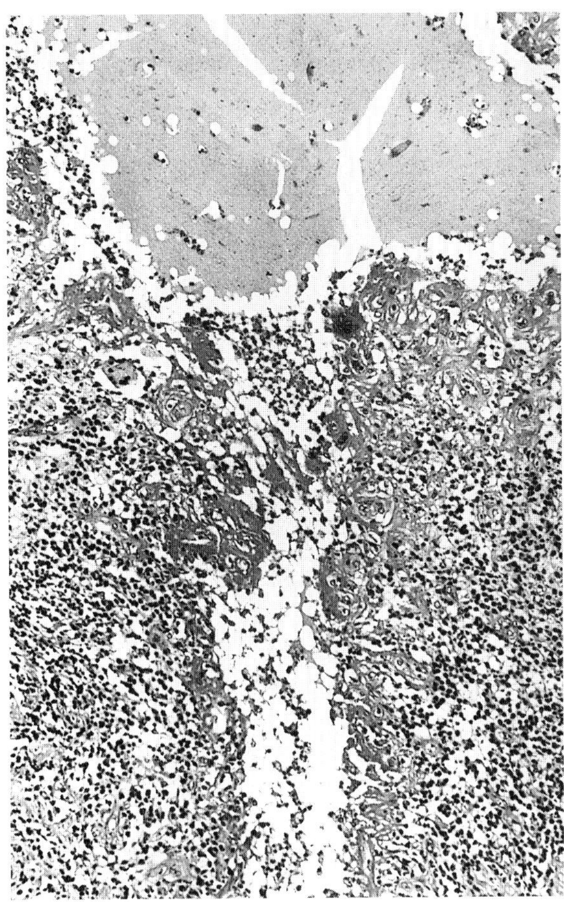

Figure 4-25
MUCINOUS CYSTIC TUMOR
This part of a cyst wall shows mucin spillage from a ruptured cyst causing chronic inflammation with a foreign body reaction.

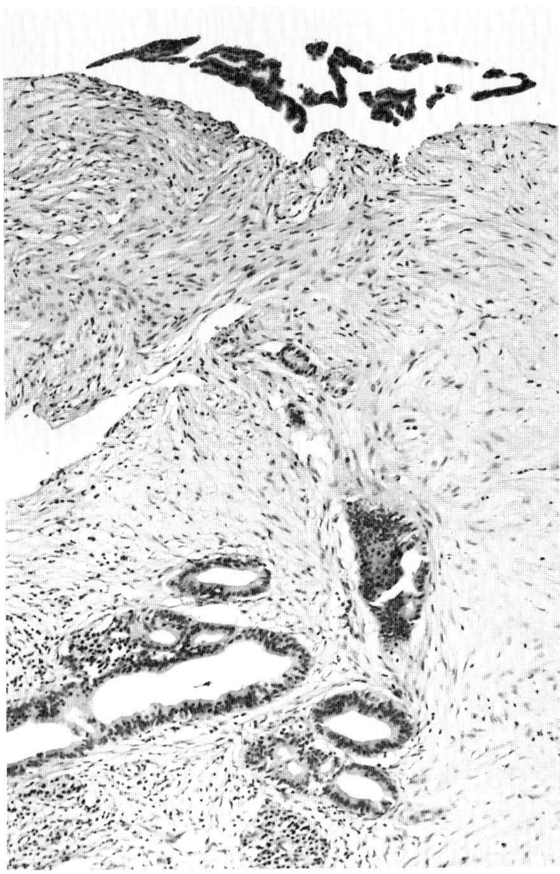

Figure 4-26
MUCINOUS CYSTADENOCARCINOMA
In this part of a cyst wall the lining epithelium is desquamated (top). In the depth of the wall are atypically structured glands invading the adjacent pancreatic tissue.

The presence of atypical glands in the stroma characterizes invasive mucinous cystadenocarcinoma. In some cases, stromal invasion by atypical glands is obvious; occasionally, however, the invading atypical glands may be difficult to distinguish from crypt-like invaginations or small daughter glands and cysts located in the subepithelial stromal layer (fig. 4-23). Gland architecture, cellular atypia, and depth of invasion are features that help in diagnosis (fig. 4-26). Invading atypical glands are recognized by their cribriform or irregular appearance (fig. 4-27), severe nuclear atypia, and infiltration into the outer layer of the capsule or the adjacent tissue. The invasive portions usually resemble ductal adenocarcinoma. Occasionally, however, the invading carcinoma component displays the features of adenosquamous carcinoma, undifferentiated (anaplastic) carcinoma, giant cell tumor of the osteoclastic type, or choriocarcinoma (50,73,76,96). Recent reports include a case of malignant fibrous histiocytoma and another with pseudosarcomatous nodules coexistent with mucinous cystic tumor and mucinous cystadenocarcinoma (76,86). We have seen a fibrosarcoma developing in the wall of a mucinous cystadenocarcinoma (fig. 4-28). These cases emphasize the resemblance of mucinous cystic tumors of the pancreas to ovarian mucinous tumors where mural nodules of similar histologic appearance have been reported (54,74).

**Immunohistochemical Findings.** The tumors are positive for epithelial membrane antigen and express cytokeratins 7, 8, 18, and 19 (59,93).

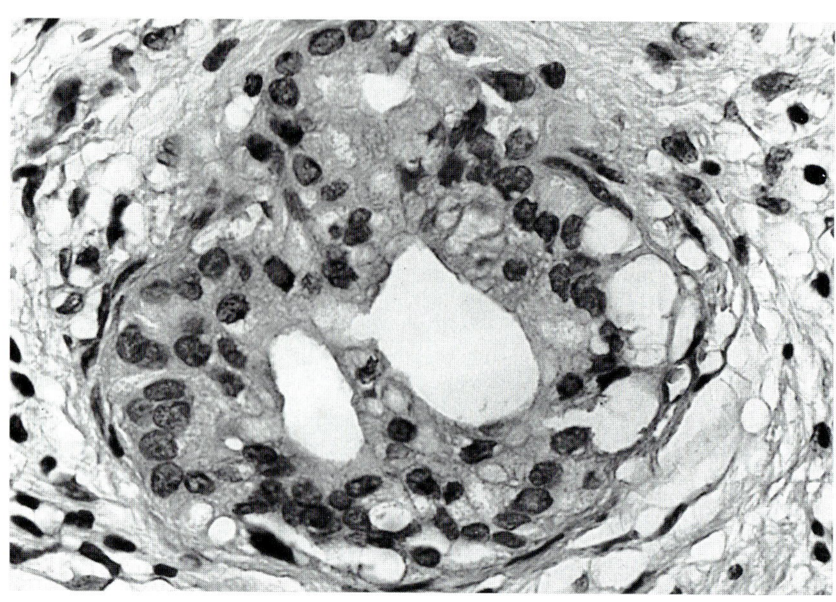

Figure 4-27
MUCINOUS CYSTADENOCARCINOMA

Atypical gland from the invasive component of a cystadenocarcinoma. Although nuclear atypia is only moderate, the cribriform architecture reveals the neoplastic nature of this gland.

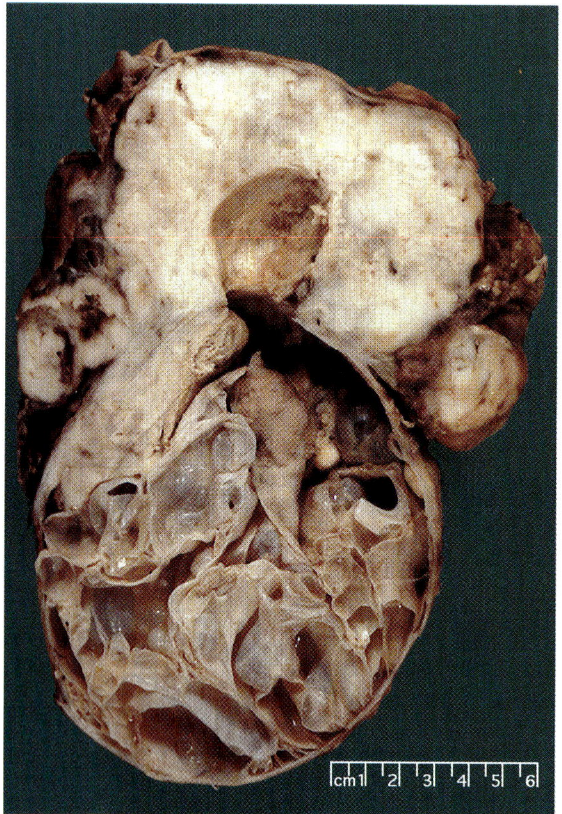


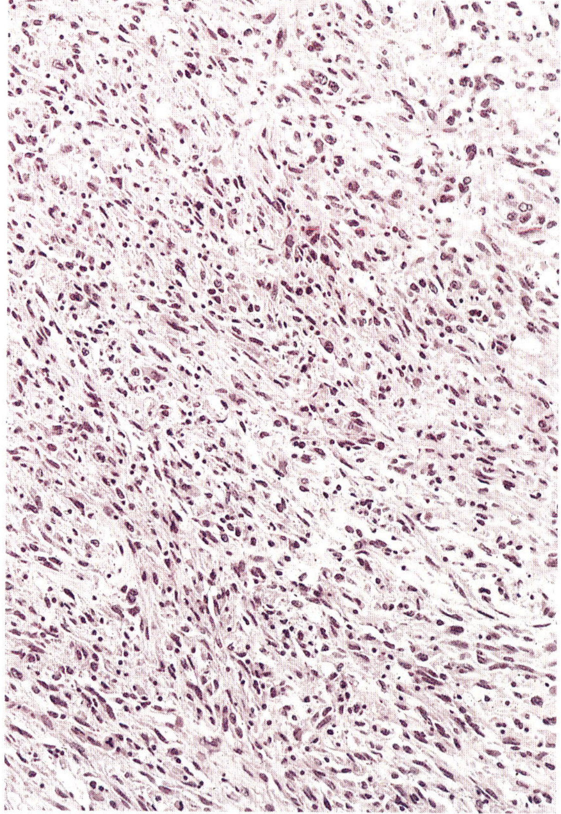

Figure 4-28
MUCINOUS CYSTADENOCARCINOMA

Left: Tumor from the tail of the pancreas in a 36-year-old woman showing a large cyst in combination with a solid tumor.

Right: Histologically the solid tumor proved to be a fibrosarcoma arising in the wall of a mucinous cystadenocarcinoma. (Courtesy of Dr. Reinhard Krüger, Koblenz, Germany.)

In addition, they are positive for M1 (gastric type mucin marker), CEA, and CA19-9, but negative for vimentin (45,59,81,93,95). CEA staining is linear at the apical surface of well-differentiated columnar cells and cytoplasmatic in cells with severe atypia (45,93). Endocrine cells are present in about 70 to 90 percent of the tumors, as demonstrated by staining for chromogranin A and neuron-specific enolase and expression most commonly of serotonin (followed by somatotatin, pancreatic polypeptide, and gastrin) (43,44,59,89).

**Ultrastructural Findings.** Electron microscopy of tumors with only mild to moderate dysplasia demonstrates columnar epithelial cells resting on a thin basement membrane. The cells may have well-developed microvilli at their apical surface as well as mucin granules in the apical portion of the cytoplasm (43).

**Differential Diagnosis.** The major problem is the differentiation of mucinous cystic tumor from pseudocyst. Much easier is the separation from intraductal papillary-mucinous tumor, serous cystadenoma, solid-pseudopapillary tumor, acinar cell cystadenocarcinoma, mucinous noncystic (colloid) adenocarcinoma, cystic endocrine tumor, and non-neoplastic cysts such as congenital and lymphoepithelial cysts.

*Pseudocysts.* These comprise 70 to 90 percent of all pancreatic cystic lesions (80,90) and are usually preceded by a history of alcoholic pancreatitis or trauma. Needle aspiration may yield fluid with a high amylase content, whereas in mucinous cystic tumors high CEA levels are found (84,95). Histologically, pseudocysts lack an epithelial lining, an ovarian-type stroma, and mucoid contents. Instead they are lined by granulation tissue with hemosiderin deposits and occasional foreign body reactions, and contain hemorrhagic-necrotic debris. However, the epithelial lining of mucinous cystic tumors may be partially absent due to exfoliation related to degenerative processes (89). Results obtained from a small biopsy should therefore be interpreted with some caution.

*Intraductal Papillary-Mucinous Tumor.* This tumor occurs in middle-aged and elderly patients of both sexes and is most frequently located in the head of the pancreas. In contrast, mucinous cystic tumors occur almost exclusively in women and are usually found in the body-tail region. Moreover, in intraductal papillary-mucinous tumors there is a cystic dilatation of the main pancreatic duct or one of its branches. Histologically, the tumor is characterized by intraductal papillary growth of mucin-producing columnar cells and does not form cysts separate from the duct system. The tumor cells, which also may show a wide range of differentiation from mild to severe dysplasia-carcinoma in situ, can not be differentiated from the epithelium of mucinous cystic tumors. However, the epithelium is not supported by an ovarian-like stroma but by pancreatic parenchyma with fibroatrophic changes. Those mucin-producing tumors that have been described in the head of the pancreas where they produce fistulas into the common bile duct and the duodenum and cause jaundice by mucinous biliary obstruction (52,65, 82) are most likely intraductal papillary-mucinous neoplasms involving the ampulla of Vater and the distal common bile duct (fig. 4-29).

*Serous Microcystic Adenoma.* This tumor is always polycystic and has a central stellate scar. Histologically, it has a cuboidal clear epithelium negative for CEA. The serous oligocystic adenoma shares the oligolocular appearance with mucinous cystic tumor, but shows the same histologic features as serous microcystic adenoma.

*Solid-Pseudopapillary Tumors.* The cystic changes of these tumors result from degeneration of solid tissue. Therefore the cystic spaces lack a one-layer epithelium and do not contain viscous mucin. Moreover, solid-pseudopapillary tumors affect predominantly adolescent girls and young women, whereas mucinous cystic tumors occur preferentially in middle-aged or older women.

*Acinar Cell Cystadenocarcinoma.* This tumor grossly shares the size and the oligolocular cystic appearance of mucinous cystic tumors. Histologically, however, it displays acinar cell differentiation and lacks mucin-producing columnar epithelium.

*Mucinous Noncystic Adenocarcinoma.* Also known as colloid carcinoma, this is a variant of ductal adenocarcinoma and is characterized by the production of much mucin without formation of cystic cavities. This type of carcinoma frequently forms the invasive component of intraductal papillary-mucinous carcinoma.

*Cystic endocrine tumors* have no mucoid contents and their cystic spaces are lined by cells with endocrine features. *Lymphoepithelial cysts* have columnar or squamoid epithelium supported by lymphatic tissue with a follicular pattern.

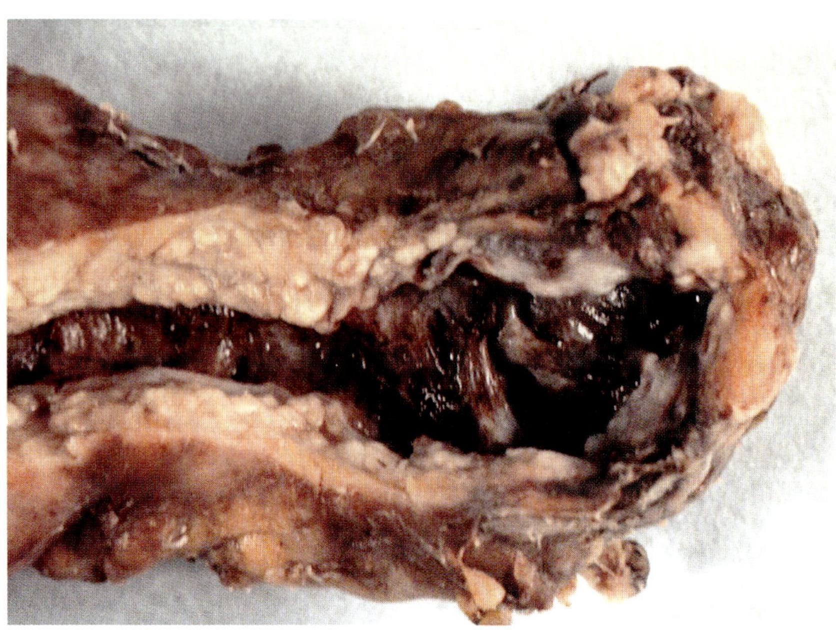

Figure 4-29
INTRADUCTAL PAPILLARY-MUCINOUS TUMOR

Left-sided pancreatectomy specimen with marked cystic dilatation of the main pancreatic duct in the tail of the pancreas due to mucin hypersecretion. Macroscopically, the duct wall shows no papillary projections.

If *adenomatoid hyperplasia of ducts* with mucinous hypertrophy is associated with some cystic duct dilatation, the distinction from a small mucinous cystadenoma may become a problem. In this case the best criterion to distinguish the two lesions is the ovarian-type stroma that characterizes the neoplasm.

**Frozen Section Diagnosis and Cytology.** Frozen section diagnostic features include the unilocular or oligolocular appearance of the cystic lesion, the lining of the cyst by tall columnar epithelium, the abrupt transition of well-differentiated columnar epithelium to atypical epithelium, and the uniformly dense and cellular (ovarian-type) structure of the subepithelial stroma. Fine-needle aspiration cytology is characterized by monomorphic populations of columnar cells and goblet-like cells, with a normal nuclear/cytoplasmic ratio, arranged in sheets and three-dimensional clusters. In addition, there may be groups of cells with loss of nuclear polarity and distinct nucleoli in enlarged nuclei (79,94). The latter feature is compatible with the diagnosis of cystadenocarcinoma (66).

**Spread, Metastasis, and Recurrence.** Invasive mucinous cystadenocarcinoma follows the same pathways of local spread, i.e., interstitial tissue, perineural sheaths, lymphatic channels, and peripancreatic fatty tissue, as the usual ductal adenocarcinoma. In addition, because of the frequent localization of these tumors to the body and tail of the pancreas, there may be direct invasion of the stomach wall, spleen, and colon. The first distant metastases are found in the regional parapancreatic lymph nodes and the liver. In patients with mucinous cystic tumors treated by drainage procedures, malignant transformation of the neoplasm occurs commonly in or near the drainage channel. There is to date no report describing pseudomyxoma peritonei in association with mucinous cystic tumor of the pancreas.

**Treatment.** Because of the difficulty in assessing the grade of dysplasia in a small biopsy of a mucinous cystic tumor and because these tumors may spontaneously transform into malignant invasive neoplasms, all mucinous cystic tumors have to be completely resected whenever possible. This includes tumors that appear histologically benign on biopsy or are asymptomatic and discovered incidentally. Resection should also be performed in biopsy-proven malignant tumors, because the chance to cure a patient by tumor removal is high if the tumor is found to be noninvasive. Internal (cyst-enteric anastomosis) or external drainage of cystic tumors should be avoided since there are many well-documented cases of apparently histologically benign mucinous cystic tumors which have recurred after drainage procedures as invasive cystadenocarcinomas (48,50,62).

**Prognosis.** The prognosis of a mucinous cystadenoma, borderline mucinous cystic tumor, and mucinous cystadenocarcinoma without invasion, regardless of the degree of cellular atypia, is excellent, if the tumor is completely removed (50,51,55,61,62,89). Incomplete resection or formation of tumor fistulas into adjacent organs almost inevitably leads to malignant transformation of the remaining tumor tissue and death of the patient from metastatic adenocarcinoma within months or a few years (46,50,62,67,75,77, 88). In Compagno and Oertel's (50) study, the mean interval between diagnosis and death in such cases was 30 months. The prognosis of mucinous cystadenocarcinoma with unquestionable invasion depends on the depth of invasion at the time of resection. Completely resected mucinous cystadenocarcinomas in which the invasive component is found to be limited to the tumor stroma and capsule probably have a much better prognosis than those tumors that already show carcinoma tissue beyond the tumor capsule within the surrounding tissues; although no current studies have tested this assumption, this is probably the reason that many resectable mucinous cystadenocarcinomas have a good prognosis with long-term survival (50,61,77,90). For mucinous cystadenocarcinomas that are not resectable because of advanced local invasion or distant metastasis, survival is similar to that of the usual ductal adenocarcinoma (50,90).

## INTRADUCTAL PAPILLARY-MUCINOUS TUMOR

**Definition.** This is an intraductal pancreatic tumor formed of papillary proliferations of mucin-producing epithelial cells that have some gastroenteric differentiation. According to the degree of epithelial dysplasia, the tumors are classified as adenoma, borderline tumor, or carcinoma. A tumor with an invasive component is a papillary-mucinous carcinoma; cystic duct dilatation due to excessive secretion of mucin characterizes the ductectatic mucin-hypersecreting variant. Intraductal papillary-mucinous tumors are also referred to as *intraductal papilloma* (108,113), *papillary adenoma* (127), *villous adenoma* (132,140), *diffuse intraductal papillary adenocarcinoma* (97,101), *diffuse villous carcinoma of the duct of Wirsung* (110), *carcinoma in situ of the pancreas* (137), *diffuse papillomatosis, carcinoma in situ* (103,130), *multiple primitive endoluminal tumors of the main pancreatic duct* (109), *intraductal mucin-hypersecreting neoplasm* (131), *ductectatic type of pancreatic ductal carcinoma* (107), *mucinous ductal ectasia* (98), *mucin-producing tumor (or carcinoma)* (129, 142), and *mucus-hypersecreting tumor* (106).

**General Considerations.** Early case reports and recent studies from France (98,99, 109), Japan (112,129), and other countries (101, 122,135) have shown the existence of a group of pancreatic neoplasms that are characterized by their primarily intraductal papillomatous growth pattern, with or without marked mucin secretion. These lesions have been given a plethora of names (see above) depending on whether they have been described by endoscopic gastroenterologists, radiologists, surgeons, or pathologists. This has led to much confusion concerning the nature and biology of these lesions. Some interpreted the lesions as reactive changes of the duct system and accordingly described them as atypical papillary hyperplasias (104,128,136), others regarded the lesions as precursors of the usual ductal adenocarcinoma (101,119,137), and still others considered the lesions a variant of the mucinous cystic tumors (112,115,124). It appears, therefore, that this is a heterogeneous group of lesions. However, our own experience with these tumors (122,131,135) and careful review of the world literature has led us to believe that these neoplasms, although heterogeneous in regard to their epithelial differentiation, form a tumor group that is morphologically and biologically distinct from ductal adenocarcinoma, mucinous cystic tumor, and ductal papillary hyperplasia.

*Classification.* Like mucinous cystic tumors, intraductal papillary-mucinous tumors may have a spectrum of epithelial dysplasia from almost benign looking epithelium (mild dysplasia) through moderate to severe dysplasia and carcinoma in situ changes (106,135). As there are also frankly invasive tumors (118,135,142), the existence of an adenoma-carcinoma sequence is likely. Although there are no data as yet on the risk of malignancy for an individual intraductal papillary-mucinous tumor, it seems that this risk increases with the degree of tumor dysplasia. We therefore classify intraductal papillary-mucinous neoplasms according to the grade of dysplasia into adenoma, tumor of borderline malignant potential, and intraductal carcinoma (109); the already frankly invasive lesion should be called papillary-mucinous carcinoma.

**General Features.** This is an uncommon tumor of the pancreas, accounting for approximately 1 percent of all exocrine pancreatic tumors (100,121). To date some 150 cases have been published in the English-speaking literature; 106 cases are included in 11 studies of at least three cases each (98,106,107,112,116a,122,126,130,131, 135,142). Two thirds of the patients are men. The peak age for both sexes occurs in the sixth decade (range, 30 to 87 years; mean, 62 years) (98, 106,107,118,122,126,131,142). The tumor occurs in all races (118,122,130,142), but the largest number of cases have been accumulated in Japan.

The etiology of the tumor is not known. Yamada et al. (142) noted that most patients in their series were smokers.

**Clinical Features.** Most patients have pancreatitis-like manifestations: epigastric discomfort, episodes of heavy pain, and hyperamylasemia, often for many years (98,111,116a,122,131). Eventually about half of these patients develop pancreatic insufficiency with diabetes, steatorrhea, or both. Symptoms of acute pancreatitis are especially observed in patients with mucin-hypersecreting tumors and are due to temporary complete occlusion of the main duct by viscous mucin. Symptoms of chronic pancreatitis with pancreatic insufficiency are due to permanent occlusion of the main duct in the head of the pancreas, either by papillary proliferations or by large amounts of viscous mucin which cannot be washed off by normal pancreatic secretion. If the papillary tumor involves the ampulla (105,122,137) or if sticky mucin within the ampulla compresses the common bile duct, jaundice may develop. Symptoms are absent (or partly absent) in those patients whose lesions only involve the tail section of the main duct.

In some patients serum CEA and CA19-9 may be moderately elevated (126), but usually the serum levels of these tumor markers are within normal limits. Ultrasonography and CT may detect a polypoid lesion (or lesions) in the main pancreatic duct or reveal a diffuse or segmental cystic ectasia of the main duct (112,126). In addition, there may be grape-like cystic dilatations of the branch ducts (or one of the branch ducts), particularly in the uncinate process (112). Angiography is usually noncontributory. Endoscopic retrograde pancreatography shows diffuse dilatation of the main pancreatic duct with filling defects caused by either papillary tumors or mucin plugs (98,126,131). In patients with mucin-hypersecreting tumors a widely open ampulla of Vater filled with mucoid material is often observed. Aspirated secretions or mucin from the main dilated duct may contain high levels of CEA and CA19-9 (98).

**Gross Findings.** Sixty to 80 percent of the tumors occur in the head of the pancreas (98,106, 107,118,122,126,130,131,142). On external inspection the pancreas appears to be thickened, somewhat nodular, and hard in consistency. The cut surface shows a dilated main pancreatic duct with a diameter ranging from 1 to 8 cm. The ectatic pancreatic duct may contain solitary or multiple sessile tumors or sticky mucinous material (fig. 4-30). In more than half of the cases the only change in the main duct or a few of the secondary ducts is an extreme dilatation due to plugs of sticky mucin.

The average size of the tumors in the main duct is 2 to 4 cm. They are soft and friable and tan to grey-white. In a few cases, the entire main pancreatic duct is studded with tumor tissue (figs. 4-30, 4-31) which may also involve the ampulla of Vater and the minor papilla where the tumor protrudes into the duodenum (101,105,122,130, 137). Some tumors in the head of the pancreas may produce fistulas into the duodenum (107, 142). Marchal et al. (117) described a patient with biliary papillomatosis which involved the ampulla of Vater and the adjacent main pancreatic duct. Morohoshi et al. (123) reported on a patient with congenital biliary dilation (choledochal cyst) and an anomalous arrangement of the pancreatobiliary duct system in association with papillary cholecystic tumors and intraductal papillary-mucinous tumors in the head of the pancreas.

Extreme intraductal mucin accumulation in the absence of a grossly visible tumor characterizes the ductectatic mucin-hypersecreting variant of intraductal papillary mucinous tumor (fig. 4-30). This variant occurs predominantly in the head of the pancreas (fig. 4-32) and only occasionally in the tail (fig. 4-29) or in one or a few secondary (branch) ducts in the uncinate process. The inner surface of the dilated mucin-filled ducts is smooth but may have tiny papillary excrescences.

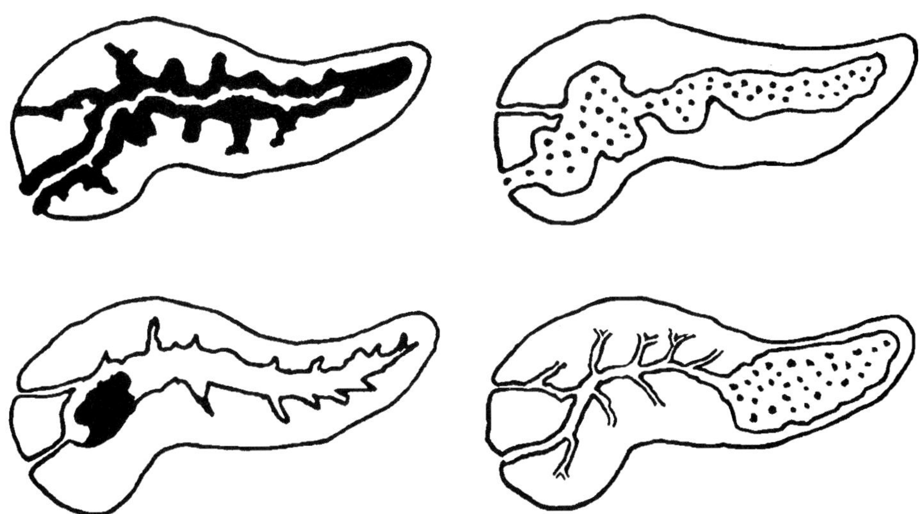

Figure 4-30
INTRADUCTAL PAPILLARY-MUCINOUS TUMOR
This drawing shows the four prototypes of intraductal papillary-mucinous tumor. Upper left, diffuse papillary tumor growth within the entire pancreatic duct system. Lower left, focal papillary growth in the main pancreatic duct. Upper right, diffuse involvement of the entire pancreatic duct system by a mucin hypersecreting tumor. Lower right, focal involvement of the pancreatic duct system by a mucin hypersecreting tumor.

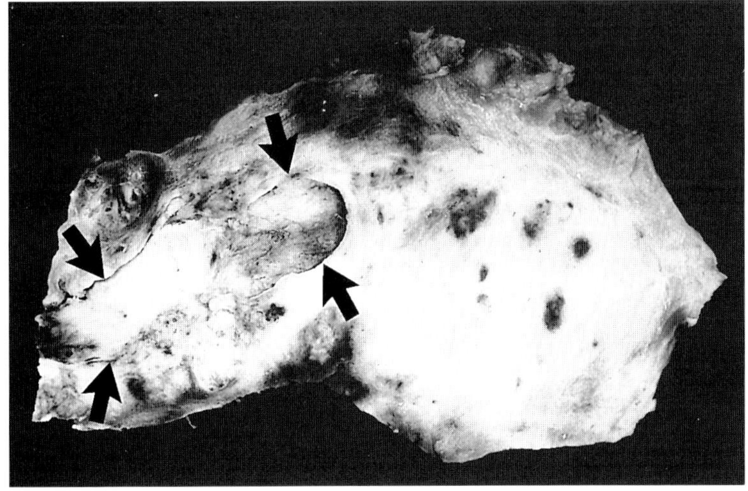

Figure 4-31
INTRADUCTAL PAPILLARY-MUCINOUS TUMOR
This left-sided pancreatectomy specimen shows a markedly dilated main pancreatic duct filled with tumor tissue (arrows). The surrounding pancreatic tissue is severely fibrotic.

The pancreatic tissue surrounding a dilated main pancreatic duct that is occluded by a papillary tumor or sticky mucin is severely fibrotic (fig. 4-31). Invasive tumors are barely recognized by gross inspection. The surface and the cut section of the pancreas usually have the same appearance as in noninvasive tumors (113,127,138); occasionally, the periductal parenchyma may appear somewhat gelatinous.

**Microscopic Findings.** The involved duct segments are lined by atypical mucin-producing columnar epithelium which forms papillary proliferations. When intraductal tumors are grossly visible, the duct lumen is often entirely filled by small or large papillae. Large polypoid papillae have multiple branches and a fibrovascular stalk (fig. 4-33). Small papillae are seen in ductectatic mucin-hypersecreting tumors (fig. 4-34), and parts

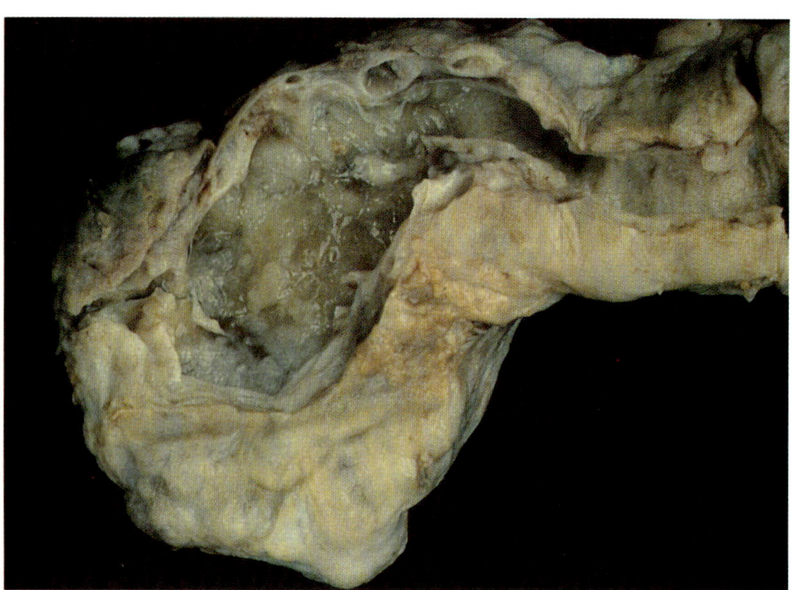

Figure 4-32
INTRADUCTAL PAPILLARY-MUCINOUS TUMOR

The head of the pancreas shows a markedly dilated pancreatic duct which is filled with sticky mucin. Due to the occlusion of the duct by mucin, the upstream part of the main duct is also dilated. This lesion was originally misinterpreted as mucinous cystic tumor. (Fig. 7.4 from Klöppel G. Nonendocrine tumors. In: Klöppel G, Heitz PU, eds. Pancreatic pathology. Edinburgh: Churchill Livingstone, 1984.)

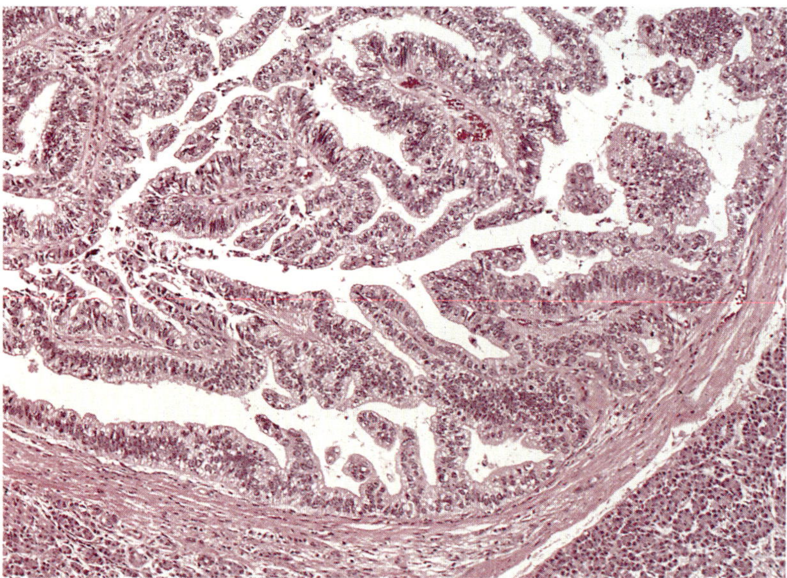

Figure 4-33
INTRADUCTAL PAPILLARY-MUCINOUS TUMOR

Cross section through the main pancreatic duct which is filled with epithelial papillary proliferations.

of the neoplastic epithelium may be even desquamated so that the duct wall appears denuded. The columnar tumor cells stain with nondiastase digestible PAS (fig. 4-35) and Alcian blue (pH 2.7 and pH 1.0) suggesting the production and secretion of acidic mucin, variable proportions of sulfomucins and sialomucins, and neutral mucin (142). In some cases, goblet-like cells are found admixed with columnar cells as well as scattered argyrophilic cells (118,122). In a few cases, a conspicuous oncocytic differentiation may be observed (Klimstra D, personal communication, 1996).

As in mucinous cystic tumors, differentiation of the neoplastic epithelium may vary from case to case and within the same tumor; all gradations, from almost benign-appearing epithelium to carcinoma in situ changes, may be encountered. Since severely dysplastic lesions are often focal, extensive tissue sampling (if possible the whole lesion) is mandatory in each case. Classification of intraductal papillary-mucinous tumor as adenoma, borderline lesion, or carcinoma is based on the most severe grade of epithelial dysplasia found in the neoplasm (135).

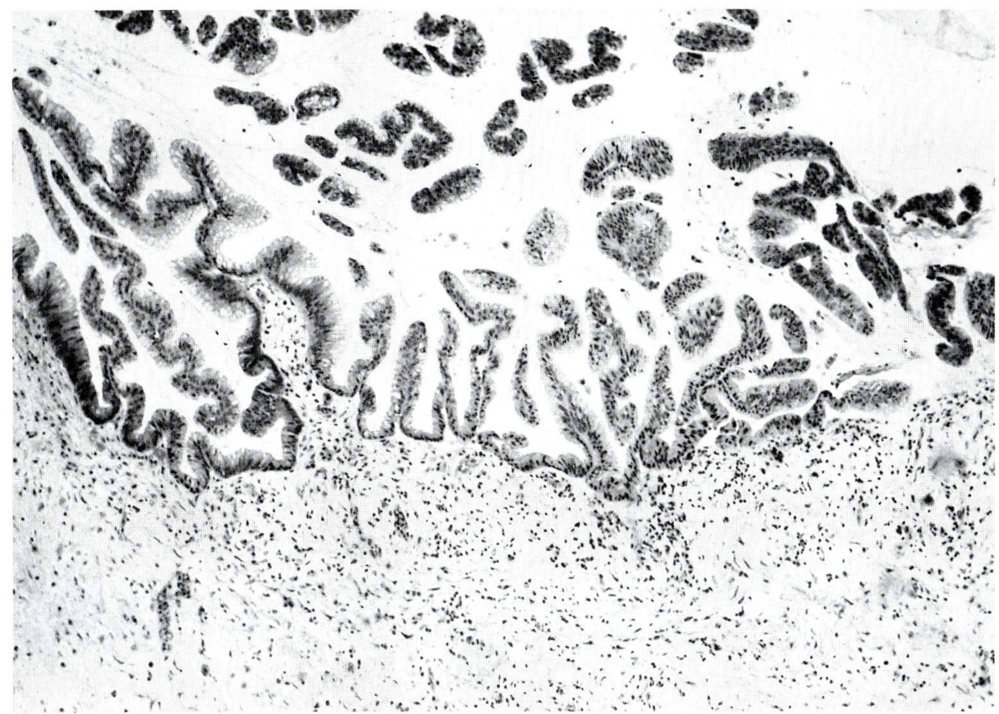

Figure 4-34
INTRADUCTAL PAPILLARY-MUCINOUS TUMOR
The wall of the main pancreatic duct is lined by tall columnar mucin-producing epithelium which forms varying sized papillae. The tips of the papillae are sectioned tangentially and appear therefore to be free floating in mucin.

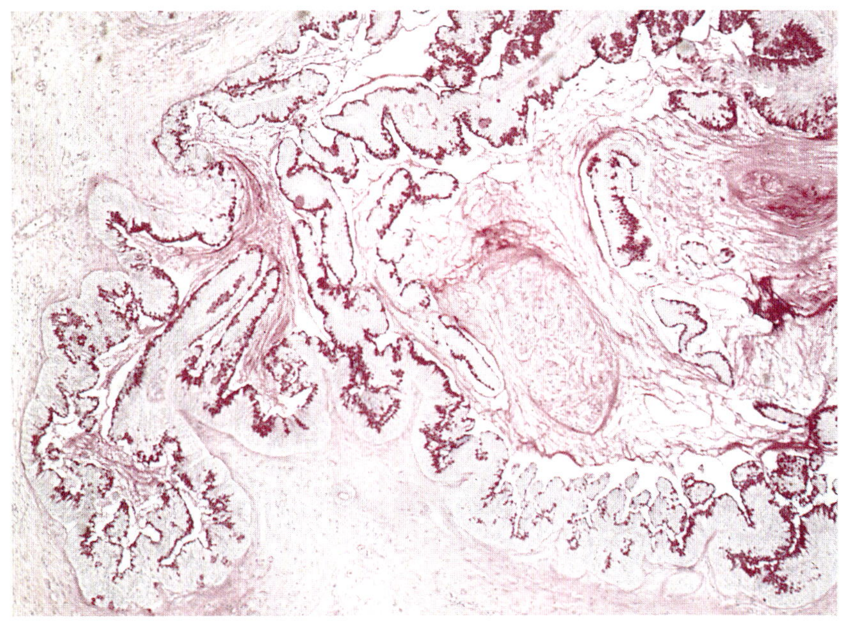

Figure 4-35
INTRADUCTAL PAPILLARY-MUCINOUS TUMOR
The PAS stain of the mucin-producing tumor epithelium reveals the extension of the neoplastic epithelium into a secondary duct.

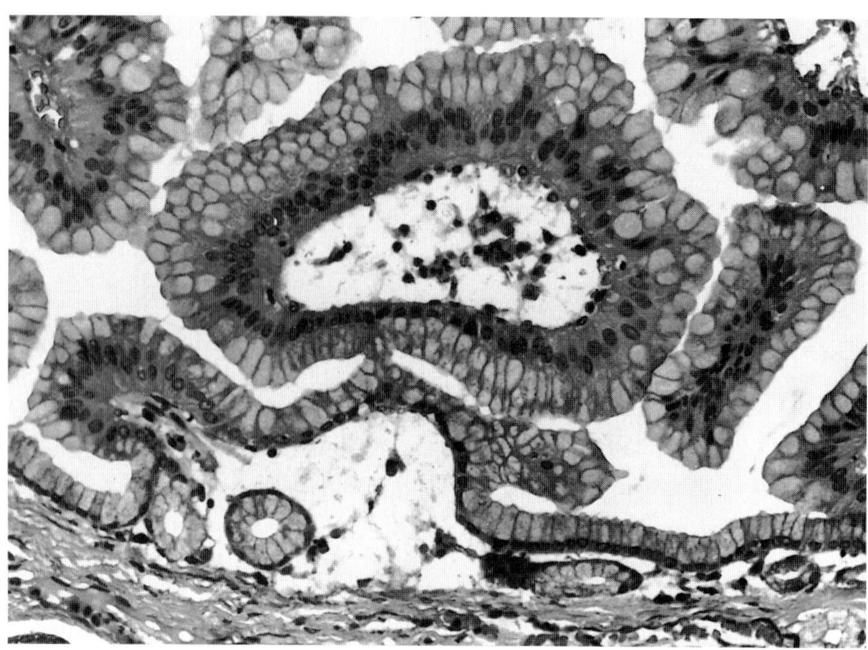

Figure 4-36
INTRADUCTAL PAPILLARY-MUCINOUS ADENOMA

Mild dysplasia is illustrated. The wall of the duct is lined by tall columnar epithelium which forms plump papillae. The epithelial cells show apical mucin accumulation, minimal pleomorphism, and regular oval nuclei. Note the goblet-like appearance of some columnar cells.

*Adenomas* have only mild dysplasia: all papillae are well formed and have a fibrovascular stalk. There may also be some small glands in the stroma underlying some polypoid growth. Papillae and glands are lined by tall columnar cells containing abundant mucin in their apical portion and a round to oval nucleus of slightly increased size in the basal portion (fig. 4-36). The nuclei are usually not hyperchromatic and contain one or two inconspicuous nucleoli. Due to the abundance of mucin-containing cytoplasm, the nuclear/cytoplasmic ratio is often lower than in normal ductal cells. Mitoses are almost absent.

*Tumors of borderline malignant potential* have mild or moderate dysplasia: the tumor cells form more irregular and elongated papillae with small fibrovascular stalks (fig. 4-37, top). The cells are still columnar and show nuclear polarization, but their mucin content is variable. The nuclei are often irregular in size, slightly hyperchromatic, and elongated (fig. 4-37, bottom). Occasionally they may contain a conspicuous nucleolus. Focally, there is nuclear crowding and stratification. The nuclear/cytoplasmic ratio is greater than with mild dysplasia. Mitoses are frequent.

*Intraductal carcinomas* have severe dysplasia-carcinoma in situ changes which may be diffusely or focally developed. In these tumors, the papillae are crowded and display irregular branching and budding (fig. 4-38A,B). They are not supported by fibrovascular tissue stalks. In addition, intraluminal bridging may form a cribriform pattern. Small areas of focal necrosis may occur. The cells contain no or minimal mucin, but have distinctly enlarged and irregularly shaped nuclei with a conspicuous nucleolus. Nuclear stratification is striking and many nuclei approach the cell surface. Mitoses are common (fig. 4-38C). Tumors predominantly composed of severely dysplastic elements are also described as in situ carcinoma of the pancreas (105,137).

In borderline tumors and intraductal carcinomas, and less frequently in adenomas, the neoplastic epithelium typically extends into secondary ducts or extends from a secondary duct (if this was the place of origin) to the main pancreatic duct, but remains confined within the duct system (fig. 4-39). In areas where intraductal tumor extension is difficult to distinguish from invasion by neoplastic ductal structures, serial sectioning of the tissue may become necessary: intraductal tumor branches respect the lobular distribution of normal ducts and resemble ductal hyperplasia, whereas invasive ductular structures are irregular in shape and distribution (fig. 4-40, left).

*Papillary-mucinous carcinoma* is characterized by carcinomatous invasion of the pancreatic parenchyma, either focal or diffuse, in association

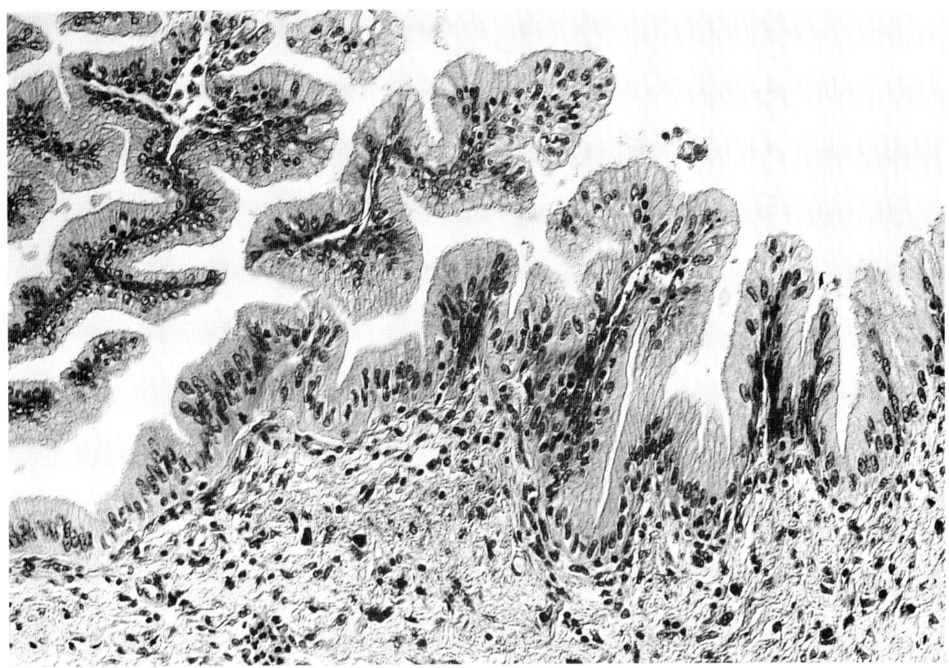

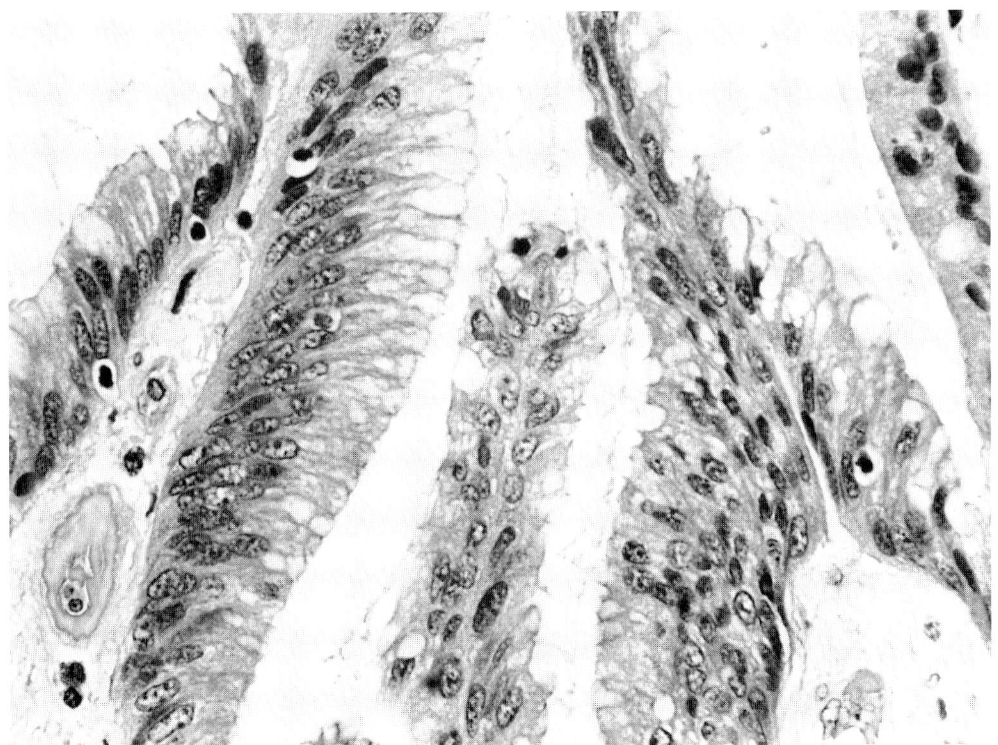

Figure 4-37

INTRADUCTAL PAPILLARY-MUCINOUS TUMOR, BORDERLINE

Top: Moderate dysplasia is seen. The wall of the duct is lined by columnar epithelium which forms irregularly shaped papillae with small fibrovascular stalks. The epithelium shows focal cellular stratification and nuclear crowding.

Bottom: The moderate dysplasia of the lining epithelium of the papillae is characterized by nuclear enlargement, stratification, and crowding.

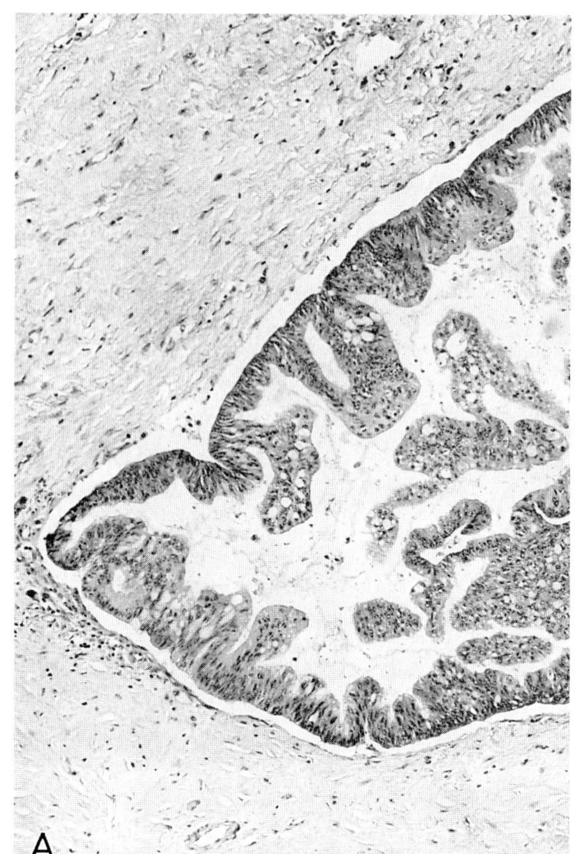


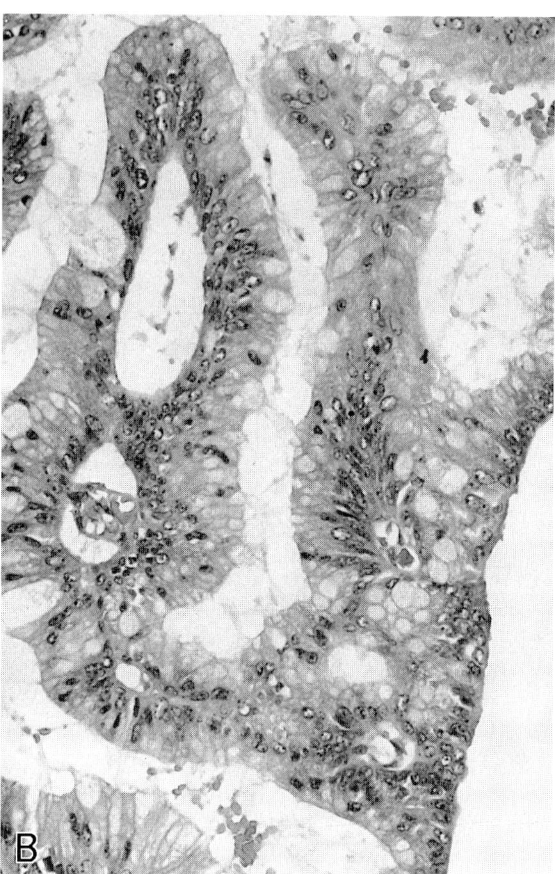


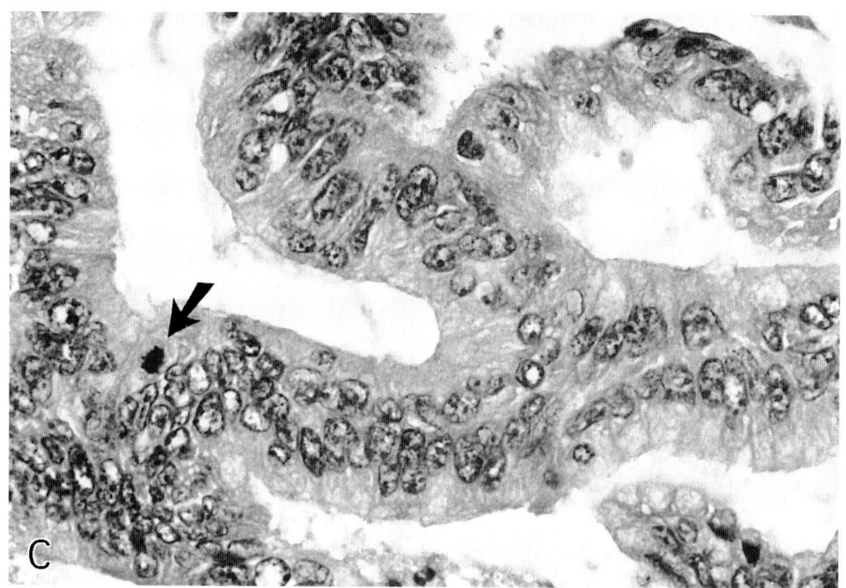


Figure 4-38
INTRADUCTAL PAPILLARY-MUCINOUS CARCINOMA

A: The severely atypical epithelium forms irregular projections without any tissue stalk.
B: The atypical epithelium shows branching and bridging.
C: The cells have varying sized nuclei, some of which show thick nucleoli and mitoses (arrow).

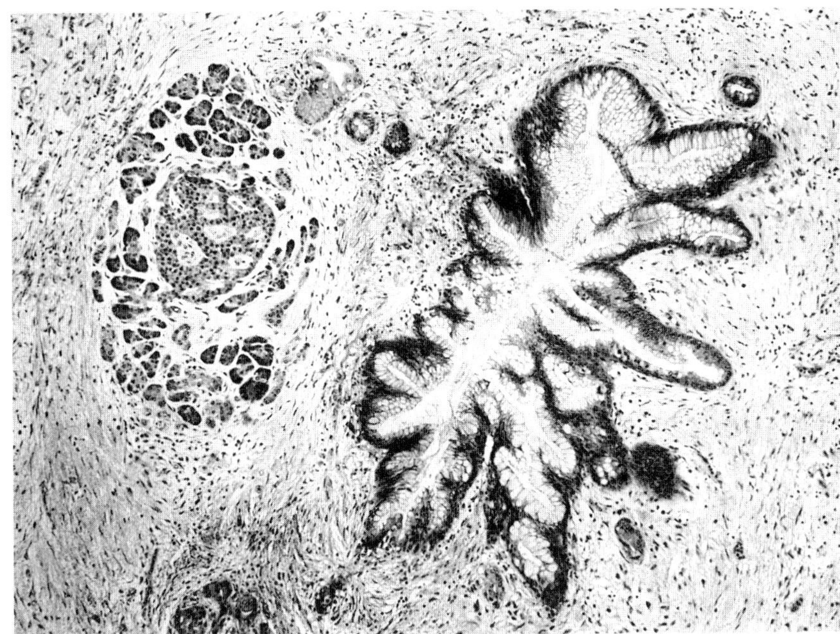

Figure 4-39
INTRADUCTAL PAPILLARY-MUCINOUS TUMOR

Cross section through a secondary duct lined by neoplastic columnar epithelium. The surrounding tissue displays chronic obstructive pancreatitis with a remnant of a lobulus containing an islet.

with an intraductal papillary-mucinous borderline tumor or carcinoma (fig. 4-40). The type of the infiltrating carcinoma either corresponds to the usual ductal adenocarcinoma (fig. 4-40, left) or, more frequently, to its mucinous noncystic variant (fig. 4-40, right) (135,142). In the latter type, there is muconodular infiltration around the dilated ducts, with pools of mucin surrounded by fibrous tissue and containing free-floating tumor cells and glands (142).

The pancreatic tissue surrounding the dilated duct system lacks any ovarian-type stroma but has the fibroatrophic changes of obstructive chronic pancreatitis. The normal acinar parenchyma is replaced by sclerotic tissue containing aggregates of variously sized islets, ducts, and usually also some mononuclear inflammatory cells (fig. 4-39). Calcifications have not been described in the literature and we have seen only one case with calcifications within and around tumor-involved ducts.

**Immunohistochemical Findings.** These tumors are positive for M1, a gastric type mucin marker, and M3SI, a small intestine goblet cell marker (134,135). They also stain for CEA, which labels the apical surface of well-differentiated columnar tumor cells (fig. 4-41) and the cytoplasm in cells with severe atypia. The cells may also stain for CA19-9 and B72.3 (122,131). DuPan-2, which is expressed in most ductal adenocarcinomas, is only seen in a few cases (135). The expression of the p53 protein seems to be restricted to tumors with moderate or severe dysplasia, while c-*erb*-B2 appears in all lesions, regardless of the degree of dysplasia (135). Endocrine cells (serotonin, somatostatin, and others) can occasionally be identified (125).

**Ultrastructural Findings.** Electron microscopy demonstrates tall columnar cells resembling pancreatic duct cells resting on the basal membrane. At their apical surface, they have well-developed microvilli and the cytoplasm usually contains multiple mucin granules (up to 300 nm in size) (122). Occasionally, the nuclei may be cleaved and show pseudonuclear inclusions.

**New Techniques.** Recently, five studies appeared which examined the incidence of point mutations at codon 12 in the K-*ras* gene in intraductal papillary-mucinous tumors (116,133, 135,139,144). The results of these studies showed point mutations in about 44 percent of 36 tumors. The point mutations were found not only in areas of severe dysplasia but also in those of mild dysplasia.

**Differential Diagnosis.** The major problem is the differentiation of intraductal papillary-mucinous tumor from mucinous cystic tumor, ductal adenocarcinoma, or ductal papillary hyperplasia. There is usually no difficulty in distinguishing intraductal neoplasms from other pancreatic

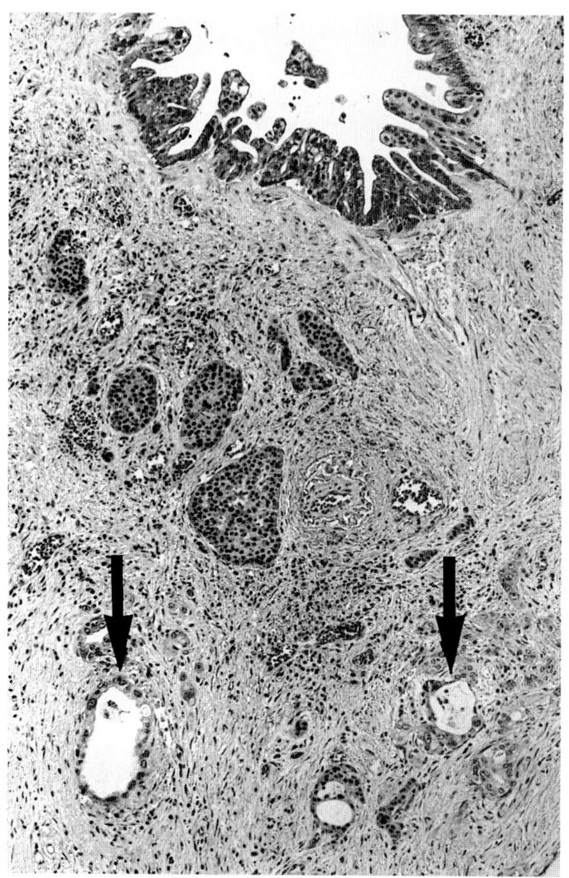

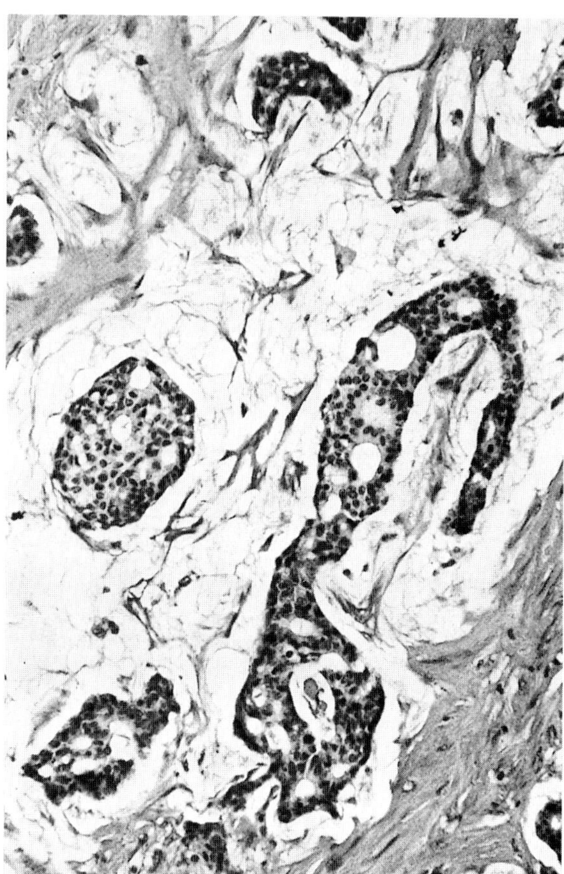

Figure 4-40
PAPILLARY MUCINOUS CARCINOMA

Left: The upper part of this illustration shows a secondary duct lined by severely dysplastic epithelium. The surrounding pancreatic tissue is fibrotic and contains only some islets. In the lower part of the illustration, there are atypical ductal structures (arrows) characterizing the invasive component of this tumor.

Right: Invasive component of another papillary mucinous carcinoma showing the features of a mucinous noncystic carcinoma.

tumors such as serous microcystic adenoma, solid-cystic tumor, acinar cell cystadenocarcinoma, cystic endocrine tumor, and non-neoplastic cysts. The distinction of intraductal papillary-mucinous tumor from chronic pancreatitis is more a clinical than morphologic problem.

*Mucinous Cystic Tumors.* These have almost the same cytologic features as intraductal papillary-mucinous tumors, however, they occur predominantly in women between 40 and 60 years of age, they are usually localized in the tail of the pancreas, patients present with nonspecific upper abdominal complaints and not with pancreatitis-like symptoms, and there is a large, often unilocular cyst with characteristic ovarian-type stroma and without involvement of the duct system. A cystic tumor that excretes massive amounts of mucin through the papillae or forms fistulae into the bile duct most likely represents an intraductal papillary-mucinous tumor rather than a mucinous cystic tumor (102,115,143).

*Ductal Adenocarcinoma.* Because of its poor prognosis, the common ductal adenocarcinoma has to be clearly distinguished from intraductal papillary-mucinous tumor. Usually this is not difficult because of the grossly obvious solid and invasive tumor growth of the former. There may be a problem distinguishing invasive papillary-mucinous carcinoma from ductal adenocarcinomas with intraductal spread; however, even in these cases the invasive component of ductal carcinoma outnumbers by far the intraductal component, while the reverse is true for the papillary-mucinous carcinoma.

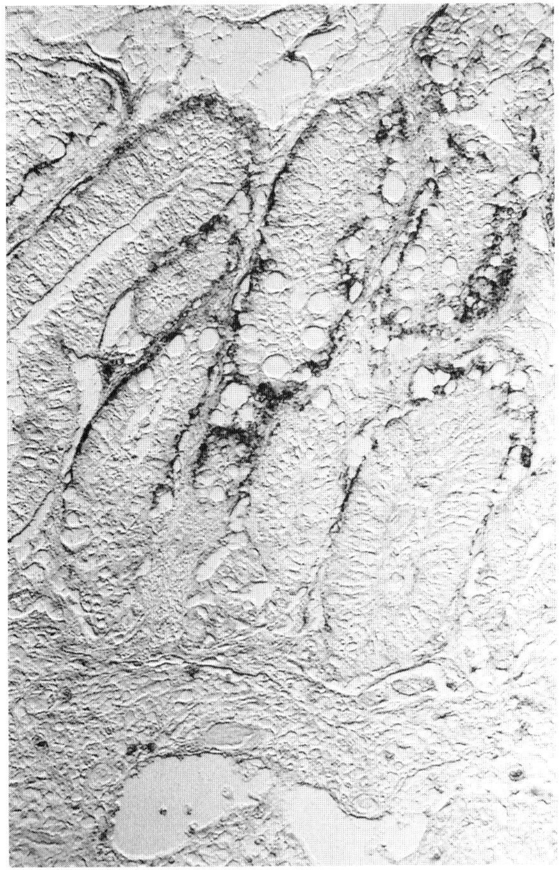

Figure 4-41
INTRADUCTAL PAPILLARY-MUCINOUS TUMOR

Neoplastic papillae showing apical immunoreactivity for CEA. (Fig. 7 from Rickaert F, Cremer M, Deviere J, et al. Intraductal mucin-hypersecreting neoplasms of the pancreas. A clinicopathologic study of eight patients. Gastroenterology 1991;101:512–9.)

*Ductal Papillary Hyperplasia.* The non-neoplastic pancreatic duct change known as ductal papillary hyperplasia has similar cytologic and histologic features to intraductal papillary-mucinous tumor. However, ductal papillary hyperplasia is a microscopically small lesion that usually occurs in secondary ducts and does not give rise to macroscopic changes or clinical symptoms (114).

*Chronic Pancreatitis.* This is characterized by uneven scarring of the pancreas parenchyma. The duct system, and particularly the main pancreatic duct, is irregularly distorted as well as strictured and contains, in advanced cases, calculi (calcified protein plugs). Often there is also an extrapancreatic pseudocyst. Microscopic ductal papillary hyperplasias may occur, but are never significant enough to represent the dominant lesion in the scarred pancreas.

**Frozen Section Diagnosis and Cytology.** Features seen on frozen section are a markedly dilated pancreatic duct system filled with papillary proliferations of well-differentiated or focal severely atypical columnar cells and an advanced chronic obstructive pancreatitis surrounding the ducts. In cases with mucin hypersecretion, the pancreatic duct system is filled with sticky mucin and the papillary pboliferations may be minimal or even absent.

Endoscopically obtained biopsies and cytologic examination of aspirated material from the pancreatic duct may show monomorphic populationc of large columnar cells with a benign appearance. In addition, there may also be groups of cells with loss of nuclear polarity and distinct nucleoli in enlarged nuclei, indicating malignancy.

**Spread, Metastasis, and Recurrence.** The invasive carcinomatous component follows the same pathways of local invasion (i.e., interstitial tissue, perineural sheaths, lymphatic channels, and parapancreatic fatty tissue), as does usual ductal adenocarcinoma. There may also be carcinomatous invasion of the bile duct and duodenum. The first distant metastases are in the regional parapancreatic lymph nodes (118, 135,142). In advanced cases there are usually peritoneal carcinomatosis and liver metastases (116a,118,135,138). Tumors may recur after incomplete local resection (130). We saw a borderline tumor that recurred 5 years after initial resection, without an invasive component.

**Treatment.** Because of the malignant potential of most intraductal papillary-mucinous tumors and their effects on the function of the pancreas, they should be completely resected. However, this is only possible in tumors limited to the head or body-tail of the pancreas in which intraoperative frozen section examination reveals no further spread of the tumor along the main pancreatic duct beyond the resection line. Difficulties arise when patients are too old for surgery or the tumor appears to involve the entire pancreatic duct from the ampulla to the tip of the tail. In the latter case, a total pancreatectomy has to be performed to ensure the removal of all potentially invasive tumor tissue (110,116a). Such an aggressive approach, however, has to be carefully weighed against the risk of the operation and the problems arising with resultant endocrine and exocrine pancreatic insufficiency. As most tumors are slow-growing neoplasms with a favorable prognosis (122,131), a conservative symptomatic approach should be considered in the above mentioned difficult situations.

**Prognosis.** Only 10 to 20 percent of intraductal papillary-mucinous tumors are invasive and the general prognosis is therefore good. Complete removal of the tumor cures most patients (116a,122,126,131,141) and survival periods of up to 10 years have been reported (97,131). Incomplete resection leads to recurrence (130). The prognosis of invasive intraductal papillary-mucinous carcinoma depends on the extent of invasion at the time of resection: patients with completely resected carcinomas in which the carcinomatous invasion is limited to the pancreas probably have a much better prognosis than those whose tumors invaded the parapancreatic region and lymph nodes. However, no studies are available confirming this assumption. In the few patients with follow-up after resection of a papillary-mucinous carcinoma, survival ranged from 6 to 63 months (116a,118,135,138) indicating that the prognosis probably depends on a number of different, not yet established, factors.

## DUCTAL ADENOCARCINOMA

**Definition.** This is a malignant epithelial tumor composed of mucin-producing glandular structures that show evidence of ductal differentiation. These tumors have also been referred to as *duct cell adenocarcinoma* or *duct cell carcinoma* of the pancreas; other terms include *pancreatic adenocarcinoma of ductal type* or, as often found in oncology or surgical textbooks, *exocrine pancreatic carcinoma* or simply *pancreatic cancer.*

**General Features.** Ductal adenocarcinoma and its variants (mucinous noncystic carcinoma, signet-ring cell carcinoma, adenosquamous carcinoma, and undifferentiated carcinoma) are by far the most common tumor types in the pancreas. They comprise 85 to 90 percent of all pancreatic tumors (173,218). In developed countries the annual age-adjusted incidence rates (world standard population) range from 8.0 to 12.0 per 100,000 males and from 4.5 to 7.0 per 100,000 females (186,234). Incidence rates from most third world countries range from 1.0 to 2.5 per 100,000 people. Incidence and mortality rates are almost identical, since survival rates for pancreatic carcinoma are extremely low. All studies on the incidence and mortality rates of pancreatic carcinoma have shown a steady increase between 1930 and 1980. Since 1980, however, the incidence rates have leveled off (164, 190). In the United States, pancreatic carcinoma is the fifth leading cause of cancer death, second only to cancer of the colon among neoplasms of the digestive system. The incidence rate at autopsy is approximately 2 percent (218).

Ductal adenocarcinoma is characteristically a tumor of elderly individuals: approximately 80 percent of cases occur in patients between the ages 60 and 80; patients below the age of 40 years are rare (208,214,229,302). The diagnosis of ductal adenocarcinoma of the pancreas should therefore be suspect in a young patient. However, exceptions occur: in a series of 243 ductal adenocarcinomas (including variants), 10 (4 percent) were found in patients younger than 40 years, the youngest being 17 years old (176).

Pancreatic adenocarcinoma occurs more frequently in men than in women, with a ratio varying between 2.0 to 1.0 and 1.1 to 1.0. American black patients of either sex have incidence rates 1.5 to 2.0 times those of white patients (234). This high rate is not paralleled in African populations.

There is no clear relationship to socioeconomic status in patients with pancreatic carcinoma. Concerning geographic differences it appears that, in general, pancreatic cancer rates are higher in the well-developed than in lesser developed countries.

To date, few clues to the etiopathogenesis of pancreatic carcinomas have emerged from epidemiologic studies. Factors that have been analyzed include past gastric surgery; pancreatitis; diabetes mellitus; allergic disease; tonsillectomy; chemical exposure; radiation exposure; use of tobacco, alcohol, coffee, and tea; and diet. Elevated risk of pancreatic carcinoma has been particularly ascribed to previous partial gastrectomy (242,265), pancreatitis (154,158,236), diabetes mellitus (207,212,250), beta-naphtylamine and benzidine exposure (245), smoking (166, 243,311), and increased intake of alcohol (163, 178), coffee (237,242), and dietary fat (178,190, 203) and meat (185,242). While the data on diabetes (237,242), occupational or radiation exposures (190,242), and alcohol (188) and coffee (242) intake have been inconsistent with regard to a significant elevation of risk for pancreatic carcinoma, the findings concerning gastric surgery, smoking, and diet prove to be more consistent. The question of whether chronic pancreatitis is a risk factor for pancreatic carcinoma has long been debated (149,190), but now seems to have received an answer from a multicentric trial performed by an international study group (240) which found that patients with chronic pancreatitis have a small but significantly increased risk for developing pancreatic cancer. An increased incidence (up to 6 percent) is particularly seen in patients with hereditary pancreatitis, an autosomal dominant disorder (193). Protective effects against the development of pancreatic carcinoma have been ascribed to allergic diseases (242), tonsillectomy (190), and high intake of fresh fruits and vegetables (185,190,203).

Thus far, no single factor or carcinogen has been implicated in pancreatic carcinogenesis in humans. Carcinogens, however, may well play a role, since experimental administration of certain chemical substances induce pancreatic tumors. The most potent carcinogens are nitrosoamine derivatives (N-nitroso-bis-hydroxy-propylamine and N-nitroso-bis-oxypropylamine), which induce ductular adenocarcinomas in Syrian golden hamsters (276), and azaserine, which induces acinar cell tumors in rats (239). Interestingly, mutations of the K-*ras* oncogene in codons 12 and 13 have been reported to occur at high frequency and at an early stage in hamster tumors, which morphologically resemble human ductal adenocarcinoma. In rat acinar tumors, in contrast, no such mutations were found (197). Recently, pancreatic tumors were also described in transgenic mice in which the gene encoding the SV40 L-antigen was placed under the control of rat elastase/enhancer (268). In addition to acinar cell carcinomas these mice developed insulinomas and D-cell hyperplasias (159). In transgenic mice in which c-*myc* expression was targeted to pancreatic acinar cells, tumors with ductal phenotype occurred, particularly in areas of stromal proliferation (197). Cell lines with a duct-like phenotype were also found to develop from a transplanted acinar cell carcinoma of the rat pancreas (274). Spontaneous pancreatic carcinomas in domestic animals are rare and do not help elucidate the etiology of pancreatic carcinoma.

Familial occurrence of pancreatic carcinoma is rare (189), but pancreatic cancer is among the malignancies observed in so-called cancer families (181,241). They have also been described in association with Peutz-Jeghers syndrome (161).

**Clinical Features.** The first, as yet nonspecific, symptoms associated with carcinoma of the head of the pancreas are gradually increasing abdominal pain (usually in the epigastrium with penetration to the back) and unexplained weight loss, seen in at least half of patients (150,246). Painless jaundice is a less frequent early sign (10 to 20 percent), but is found in more than half of the patients by the time of diagnosis. Rarer manifestations are pancreatitis (192), migratory thrombophlebitis (230), hypoglycemia (177), hypercalcemia (253), and endocarditis (251). Diabetes (fasting blood glucose level of more than 120 mg/dl) is present in 70 percent of the patients: 50 percent have a diabetes history of less than 2 years and 20 percent of more than 2 years (207). Diabetes of less than 2 years duration is characterized by insulin resistance and high islet amyloid polypeptide serum levels, which probably develop as a consequence of the pancreatic carcinoma (272). Patients with tumors in the body and tail of the pancreas present with symptoms related to liver metastasis or invasion of the peritoneal cavity (ascites).

Currently, the most important tests for establishing the diagnosis of pancreatic carcinoma are ultrasonography and CT, with or without guided percutaneous fine-needle biopsy, endoscopic retrograde cholangiography (ERCP), endoscopic ultrasonography, and tumor marker determinations (CA19-9 >37 U/ml, DuPan 2 ≥ 300 U/ml, CEA >3 ng/ml, Span1 >30 U/ml) (213). The sensitivity and specificity of any of these tests alone ranges from 55 to 95 percent. By applying combinations of these tests accuracy rates of more than 95 percent have been reported (see New Techniques). Magnetic resonance imaging has not yet proven its specific value in the diagnosis of pancreatic cancer, but endoscopic ultrasonography can contribute to the staging of the disease.

Recently, the detection of mutated K-*ras* oncogene in pancreatic juice or blood of patents with proven ductal adenocarcinoma of the pancreas has been described (227,291).

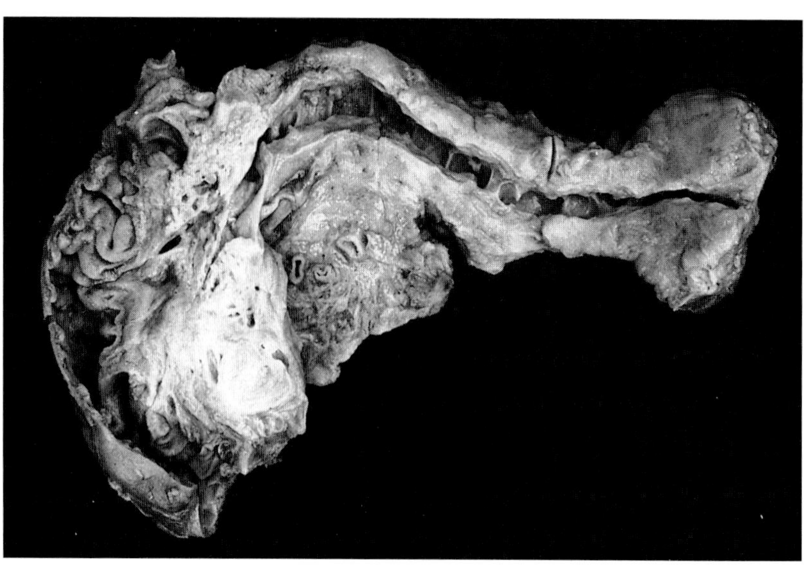

Figure 4-42
DUCTAL ADENOCARCINOMA
Autopsy specimen of the pancreas showing complete obstruction of the main pancreatic duct by a solid tumor in the head of the pancreas. The obstruction caused extreme prestenotic duct dilation with haustration and atrophy of the parenchyma. (Fig. 7-26 from Klöppel G. Pancreatic, nonendocrine tumors. In: Klöppel G, Heitz PU, eds. Pancreatic pathology. Edinburgh: Churchill Livingstone, 1984:79–113.)

**Gross Findings.** In autopsy series, 60 to 70 percent of pancreatic ductal adenocarcinomas are localized to the head of the gland (fig. 4-42), 5 to 10 percent to the body, 10 to 15 percent to the tail, and 10 to 15 percent to a combination of sites. In surgical series, 80 to 90 percent of the tumors are in the head of the pancreas; 50 percent in the upper half of the head close to the intrapancreatic part of the common bile duct (fig. 4-43A); the remainder in the area behind the ampulla of Vater or, rarely, in the uncinate process (fig. 4-43C) (217). The higher frequency of carcinomas in the pancreatic head in surgical series compared to autopsy series is due to their earlier detection and therefore better resectability than carcinomas in the body and tail of the pancreas. Occasionally, heterotopic pancreatic tissue gives rise to a carcinoma (151,191,293).

In surgical series, carcinomas of the head of the pancreas range from 1.5 to 10 cm, with a mean of 2.5 to 3.5 cm. Carcinomas of the body/tail average between 5 and 7 cm. Tumors with a diameter less than 2 cm are infrequent (198). In autopsy series, mean tumor size ranges from 4 to 8 cm both for tumors of the head and of the body/tail (169,231,248,249,256).

Grossly, typical ductal adenocarcinoma presents as a firm mass with ill-defined margins (fig. 4-43B). On cut surface the tumor is yellow to white and merges imperceptibly with the surrounding pancreatic tissue. Hemorrhage and necrosis are uncommon, but microcystic areas may occur. Small tumors with diameters less than 2 cm may be difficult to recognize grossly and sometimes are only identified by focal induration of the parenchyma.

Carcinomas of the head of the pancreas, with the exception of those arising in the uncinate process, have an intimate anatomic relationship with the distal common bile duct and the main pancreatic duct (fig. 4-44). By invasion of the walls of these ducts and periductal growth they produce duct stenosis and eventually total obstruction; this leads to dilatation of both duct systems upstream of the stenosis. The obstructed bile duct segment is usually about 1 cm long and lies 1 to 2 cm proximal to the ampulla of Vater. Although this stenosis is often incomplete, it results in extreme dilatation of the proximal bile duct with resultant jaundice. Complete obstruction of the main pancreatic duct leads to extreme prestenotic duct dilatation with duct haustration and fibrous atrophy of the parenchyma (fig. 4-42). These pancreatic changes are called obstructive chronic pancreatitis (see Tumor-Like Lesions). Depending on their localization within the head of the pancreas, the tumors may involve the ampulla and the duodenal wall (fig. 4-44), causing ulceration in advanced cases. Extrapancreatic extension of the tumor into the retroperitoneal tissue at the time of diagnosis is the rule. This leads to invasion of the mesenteric nerves and vessels. In advanced tumors, the peritoneum, stomach, and gallbladder may also be involved.

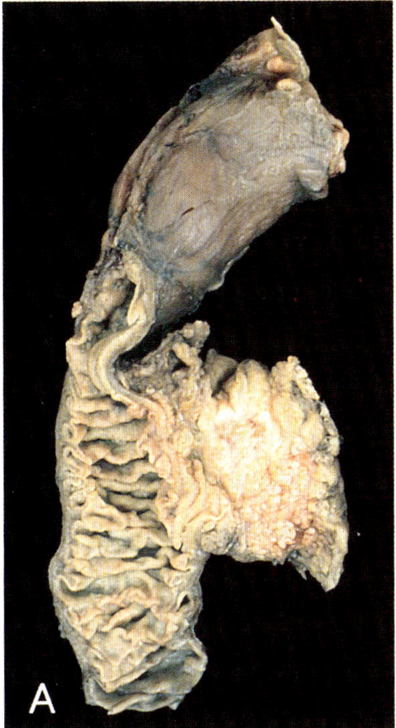


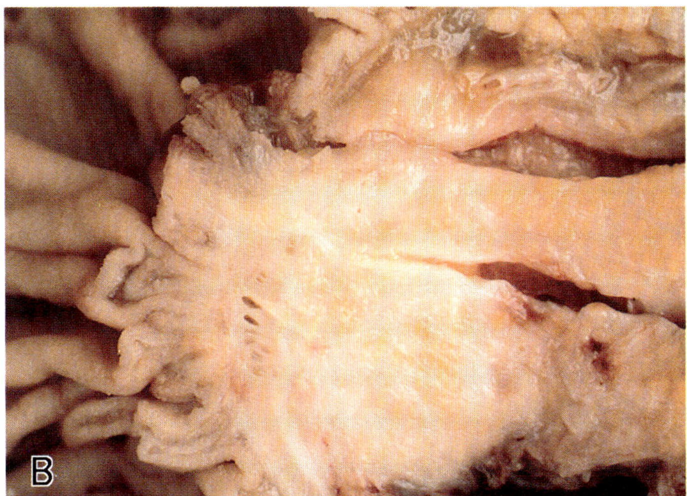


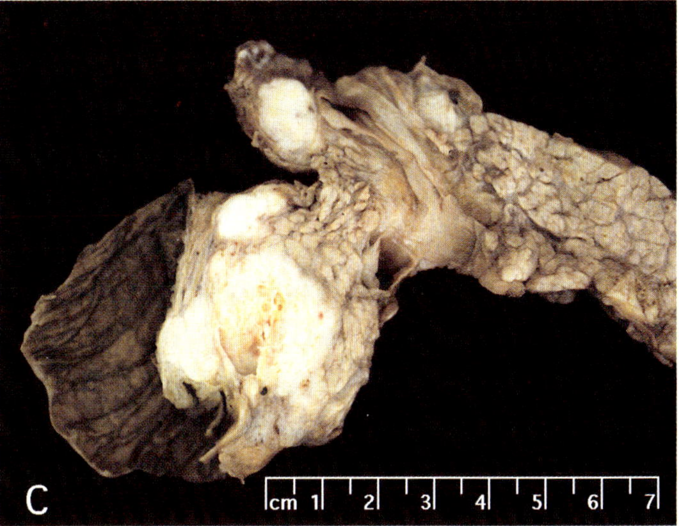


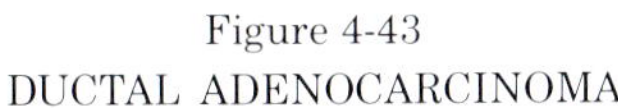

Figure 4-43
DUCTAL ADENOCARCINOMA

A: Whipple resection specimen showing a small ductal adenocarcinoma in the upper half of the head of the pancreas.

B: Whipple resection specimen showing a ductal adenocarcinoma with invasion of the ampulla and the duodenal wall, obstructing the common bile duct as well as the pancreatic duct. Note the ill-defined tumor demarcation.

C: Autopsy specimen showing a tumor mainly located in the uncinate process of the head of the pancreas. The tumor caused no jaundice.

Carcinomas in the body or tail of the pancreas are identical in color and consistency to those arising in the head. They obstruct the main pancreatic duct but, of course, do not involve the common bile duct (fig. 4-45). Extrapancreatic extension first involves the retroperitoneal tissue between pancreas, spleen, stomach, and left adrenal gland and later also the peritoneum, with subsequent peritoneal carcinomatosis. The adjacent organs most often invaded are the spleen, the left adrenal gland, and the stomach.

**Microscopic Findings.** Most ductal adenocarcinomas are moderately to well-differentiated tumors. They elicit a desmoplastic stromal reaction which accounts for their firm consistency. Well-differentiated carcinomas consist of large duct-like structures combined with medium-sized neoplastic glands, while the moderately differentiated carcinomas have a mixture of medium-sized duct-like structures with tubular neoplastic glands of various sizes and shape. A few carcinomas are poorly differentiated. They are composed of relatively small and irregularly formed neoplastic glands which show little resemblance to pancreatic ducts and often induce only a slight stromal reaction. Small variations in the degree of differentiation within the same neoplasm are frequent, but well-differentiated

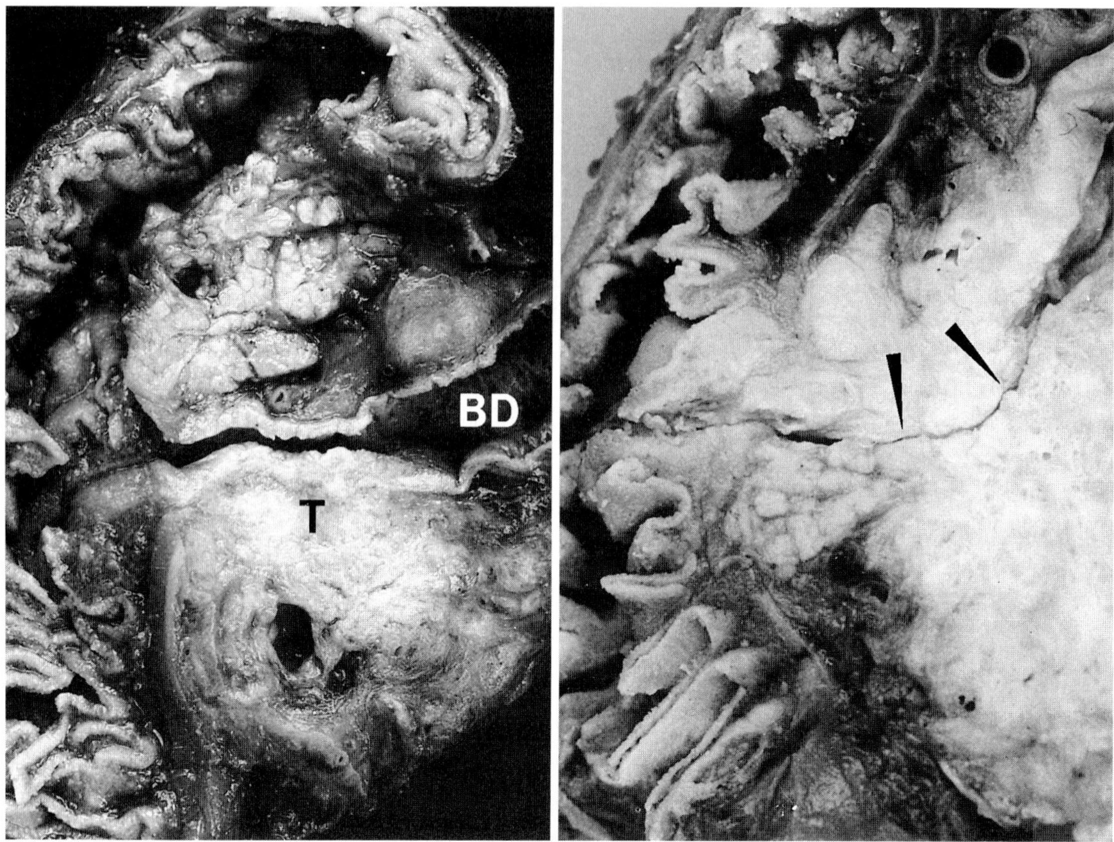


Figure 4-44
DUCTAL ADENOCARCINOMA

Whipple resection specimens showing ill-demarcated tumors in the head of the pancreas.

Left: This tumor (T) has a maximum diameter of 3 cm and obstructs the bile duct (BD).

Right: This advanced tumor invades the papilla of Vater and occludes the bile duct (arrowheads). (Fig. 3 from Klöppel G, Maillet B. Classification and staging of pancreatic nonendocrine tumors. Radiol Clin N Am 1989;27:105–19.)

tumors with foci of poor differentiation are uncommon. Adenocarcinomas in which the duct-like and tubular structures are outnumbered by other components, such as intensive mucin production, signet-ring cells, squamoid or squamous elements, or undifferentiated cell patterns, are considered variants of ductal adenocarcinoma and discussed below.

In well-differentiated carcinomas, the central tumor region has large, and occasionally even microcystic, duct-like structures and some medium-sized and tubular neoplastic glands, which are irregularly arranged within a desmoplastic stroma (fig. 4-46). A few non-neoplastic ducts as well as remnants of acini and individual islets may be found between the neoplastic glands (fig. 4-47). Sometimes the neoplastic duct-like glands are so well differentiated that they are difficult to distinguish from non-neoplastic ducts (fig. 4-47). However, their arrangement typically disregards the normal lobular architecture of the gland, while the distribution of non-neoplastic ducts usually follows a lobular pattern. Moreover, the mucin-containing neoplastic glands may be ruptured or incompletely formed, a feature that is also missing in normal ducts. Apart from a tubular architecture, the neoplastic glands may have cribriform patterns (fig. 4-48, left) or small papillary projections (without a distinct fibrovascular stalk), particularly in large duct-like structures (fig. 4-48, right). The mucin-producing tumor cells tend to be columnar, have an eosinophilic and occasionally pale or clear cytoplasm (fig. 4-49), and are usually larger than those of non-neoplastic ducts. They contain large round to ovoid nuclei which may

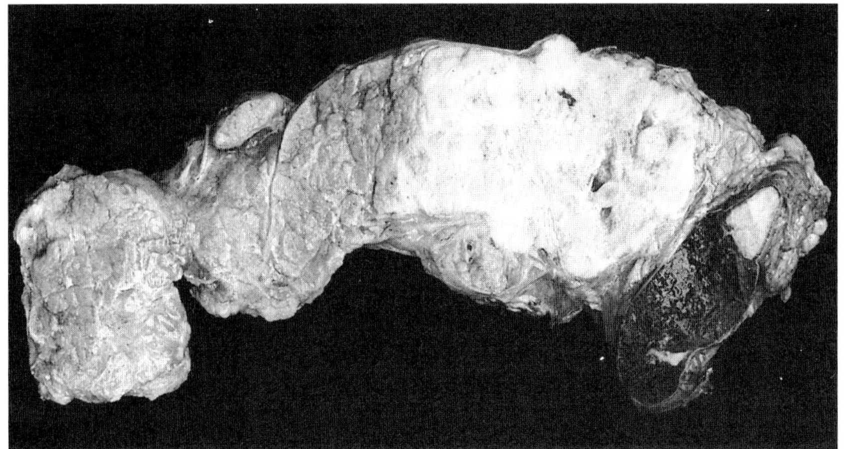

Figure 4-45
DUCTAL ADENOCARCINOMA
Autopsy specimen of the pancreas showing a large solid tumor in the tail. The attached spleen exhibits a small anemic infarct. (Fig. 11B from Klöppel G. Pathology of pancreatic nonendocrine tumors. In: Go VL, Gardner JD, Brooks FP, Lebenthal E, Di Magno EP, Scheele GA, eds. The pancreas: biology, pathobiology and disease, 2nd ed. New York: Raven Press, 1993:871–97.)

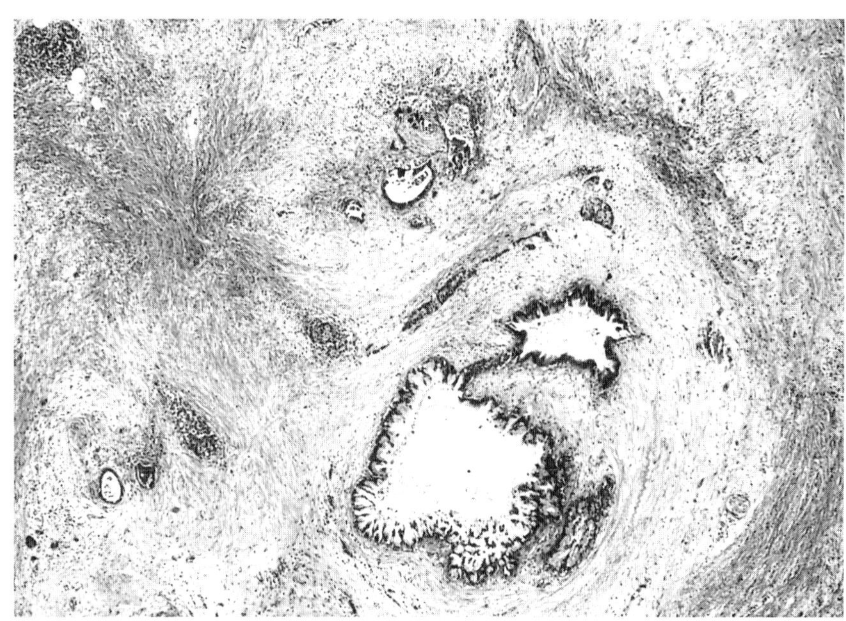

Figure 4-46
DUCTAL ADENOCARCINOMA, WELL-DIFFERENTIATED
Large duct-like neoplastic structures and some smaller neoplastic glands embedded in dense fibrous stroma.

vary in size, with sharp nuclear membranes and distinct nucleoli that are not found in normal duct cells (fig. 4-50). Moreover, although the tumor cell nuclei tend to be situated at the base of the cell, they always show some loss of polarity. The mitotic activity is low. Extension into the adjoining pancreatic tissue occurs mainly via the interlobular septa where the infiltrating duct-like tumor glands also elicit a marked desmoplastic stromal response (fig. 4-51, top). Particularly in these areas, the tumor glands may be misinterpreted as hyperplastic ducts as seen in chronic pancreatitis. A helpful criterion for the differentiation between neoplastic duct-like structures and non-neoplastic ducts is the immunoreactivity of neoplastic glands for CEA (fig. 4-51, bottom) (see also Immunohistochemical Findings). Another route of intrapancreatic extension is as an in situ component via large ducts (fig. 4-52). In rare cases, the tumor may even spread along the main pancreatic duct into tumor-free tissue distant from the main tumor mass (222).

Moderately differentiated carcinomas, which have predominantly medium-sized duct-like and tubular structures of various shape, completely replace the acinar tissue (fig. 4-53). The neoplastic glands are embedded in desmoplastic stroma and form irregular patterns. Large duct-like structures are infrequent, while incompletely formed glands are common. Compared with

Figure 4-47
DUCTAL ADENOCARCINOMA, WELL-DIFFERENTIATED

This tumor shows atypical duct-like structures (arrows) and a carcinoma in situ lesion (asterisk) embedded in sclerotic tissue containing remnants of acini and normal ducts. The inset shows neoplastic epithelium adjacent to epithelium of a non-neoplastic duct.

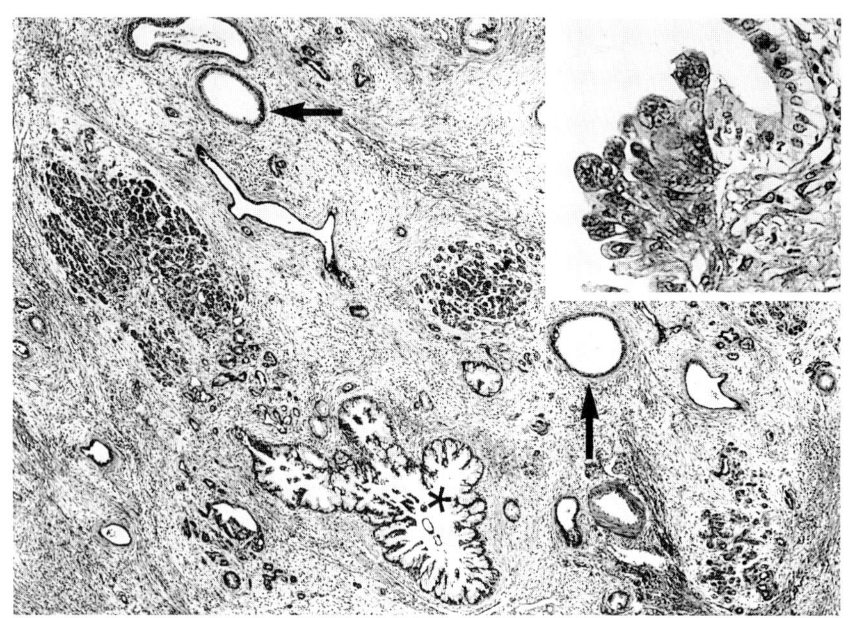

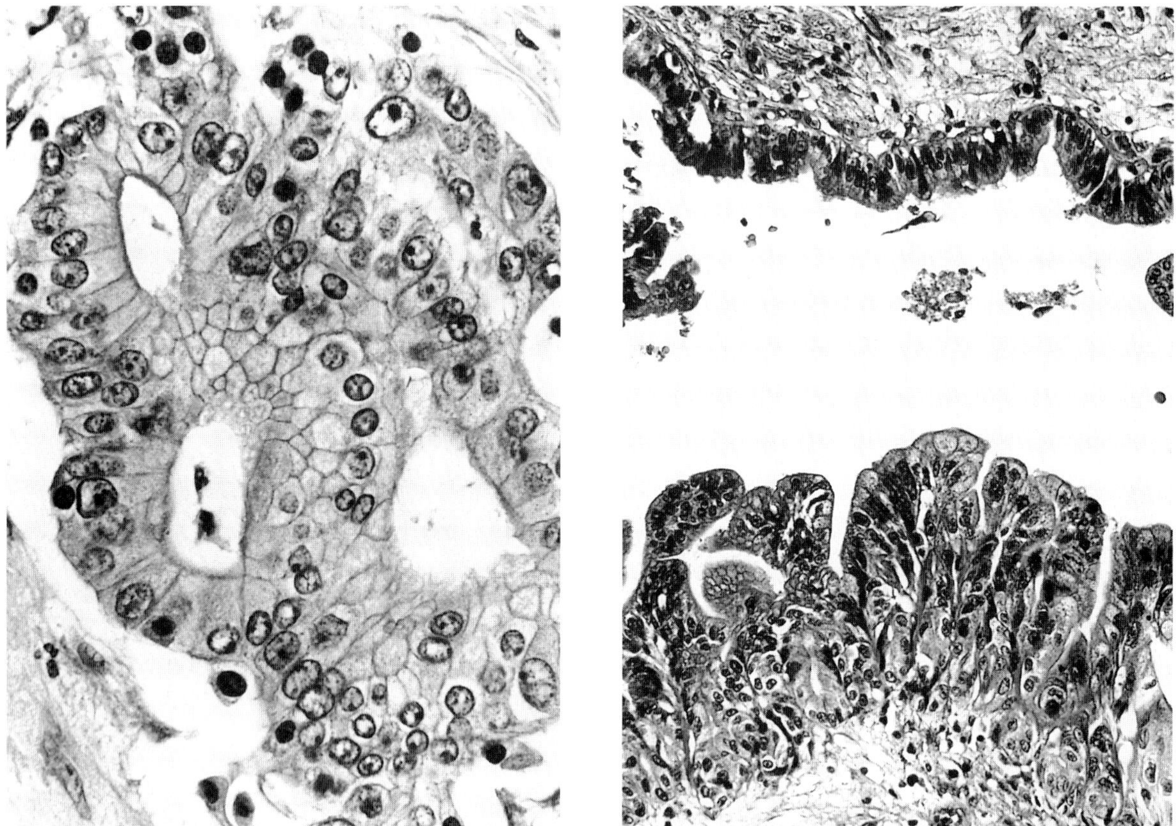

Figure 4-48
DUCTAL ADENOCARCINOMA, WELL-DIFFERENTIATED

Left: The tumor gland shows a cribriform structure.
Right: Part of a large duct-like structure containing papillary projections without a distinct fibrovascular stalk.

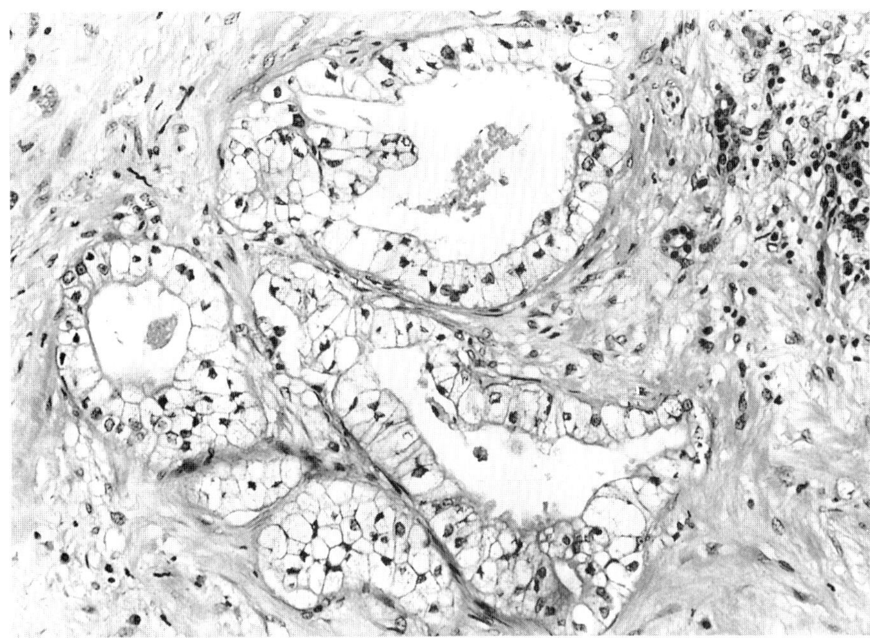

Figure 4-49
DUCTAL
ADENOCARCINOMA,
WELL-DIFFERENTIATED

This tumor shows glands lined by cells with a clear cytoplasm and an occasionally condensed hyperchromatic nucleus.

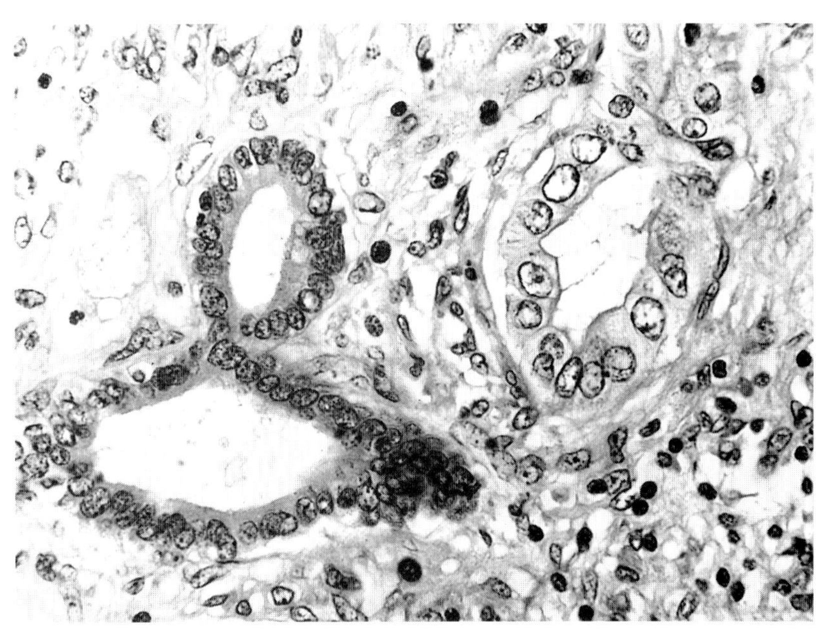

Figure 4-50
DUCTAL ADENOCARCINOMA,
WELL-DIFFERENTIATED

The illustration compares a neoplastic gland (right) with a normal duct (left). Note the big, round to ovoid nuclei which vary in size and have a sharp nuclear membrane. Some of them also display a distinct nucleolus which is absent in the nonneoplastic duct cell nuclei.

well-differentiated carcinoma there is a much greater degree of cellular atypia (fig. 4-54). The tumor cell nuclei vary greatly in size, chromatin distribution, and appearance of nucleoli. Mitotic figures are frequent. The cytoplasm is usually slightly eosinophilic, but clear cells may also occur. Mucin production appears to be decreased and intraductal in situ components are less frequently seen than in well-differentiated carcinomas. Foci of poor and irregular glandular differentiation may be found at the margins of carcinomas (fig. 4-55), particularly where they invade the peripancreatic tissue.

Poorly differentiated carcinomas consist of a mixture of densely packed, small, irregular glands as well as solid tumor cell sheets and nests (fig. 4-56), which entirely replace the acinar tissue. Large duct-like structures and intraductal tumor components are lacking, but small foci (comprising per definition less than 20

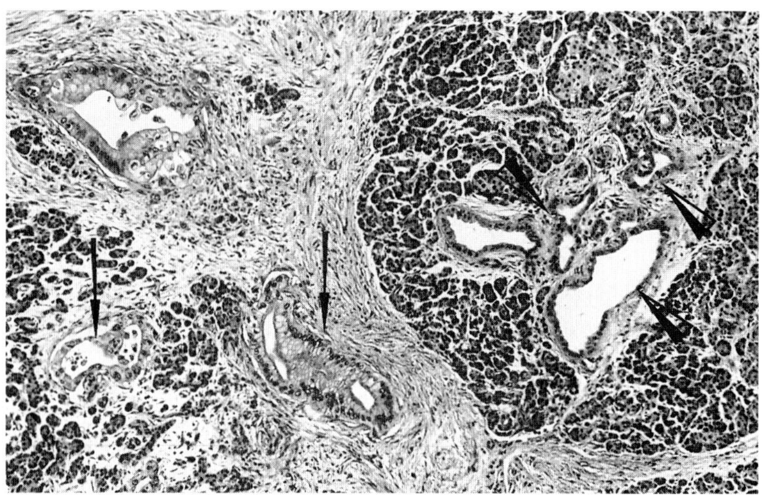

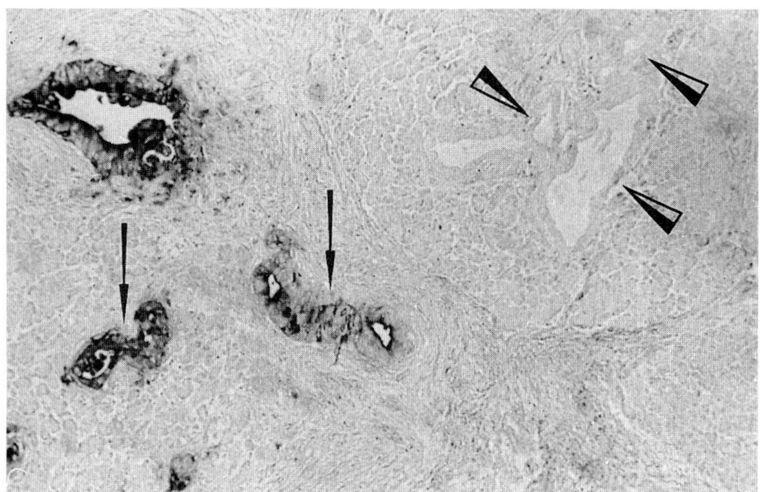

Figure 4-51
DUCTAL ADENOCARCINOMA,
WELL-DIFFERENTIATED

Top: Tumor invasion into the adjoining pancreatic tissue via the interlobular septa where the infiltrating duct-like tumor glands (arrows) elicit a marked desmoplastic stromal response.

Bottom: Immunostaining for CEA labels the neoplastic glands (arrows), but not the normal ducts (arrowheads).

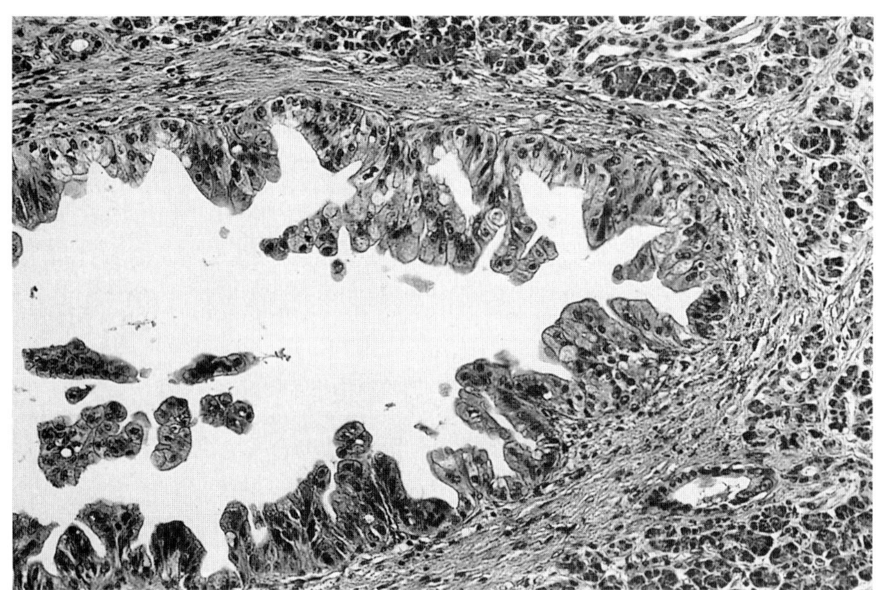

Figure 4-52
DUCTAL
ADENOCARCINOMA,
WELL-DIFFERENTIATED

This illustration shows intraductal tumor spread by severely atypical epithelium. The lesion is equivalent to a carcinoma in situ component.

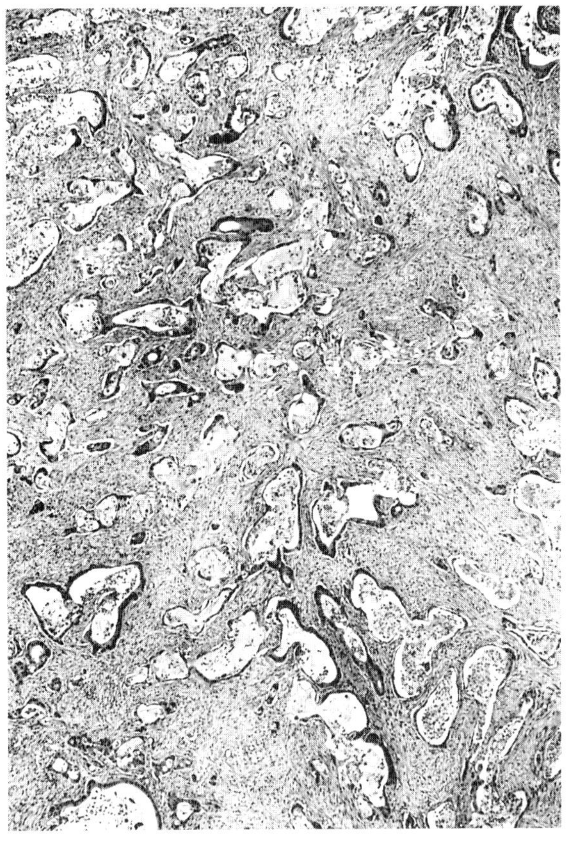

Figure 4-53
DUCTAL ADENOCARCINOMA,
MODERATELY DIFFERENTIATED

Low-power view of a tumor composed of medium-sized duct-like and tubular structures of various shapes and arrangements.

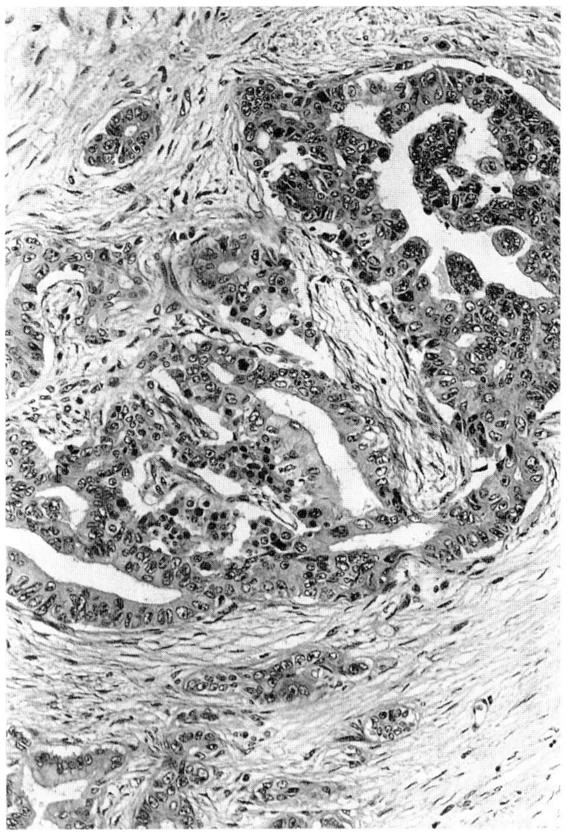

Figure 4-54
DUCTAL ADENOCARCINOMA,
MODERATELY DIFFERENTIATED

Atypical duct-like structures and small tubular complexes with a cribriform pattern.

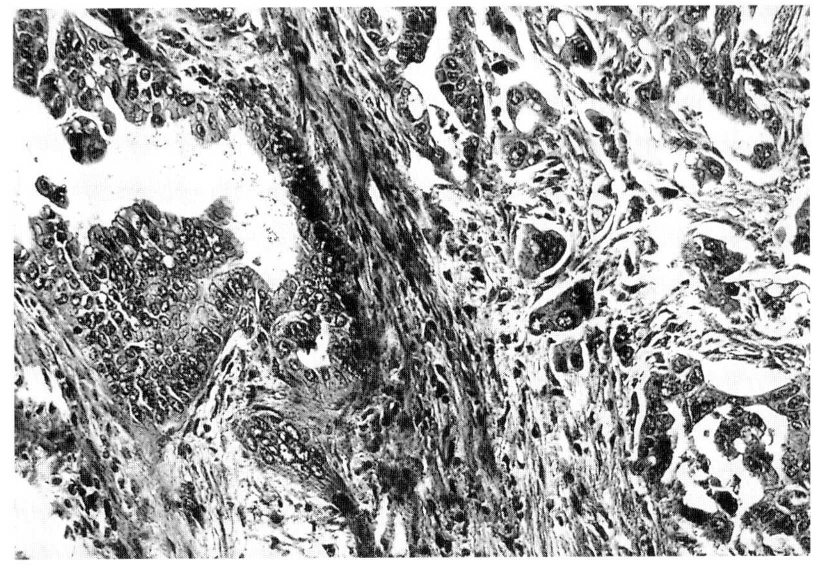

Figure 4-55
DUCTAL ADENOCARCINOMA

The illustration shows a focus of a duct-like tumor structure adjacent to poorly differentiated tumor glands.

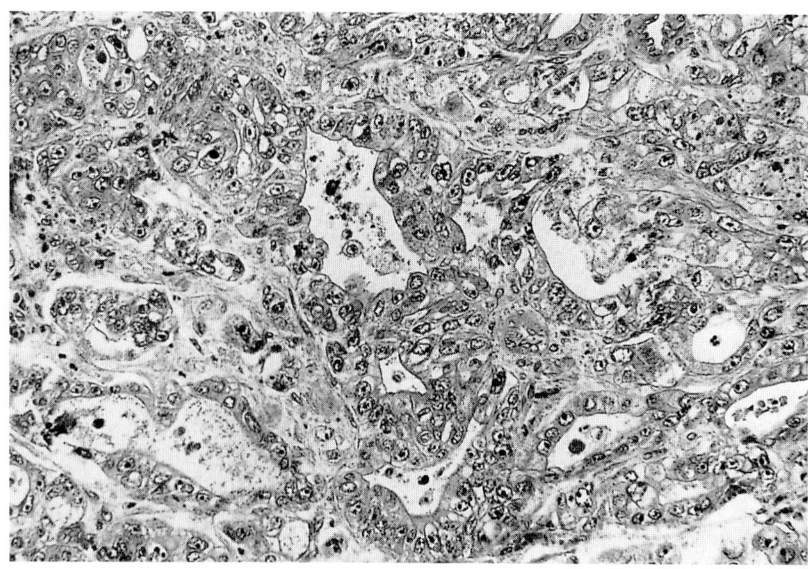

Figure 4-56
DUCTAL ADENOCARCINOMA, POORLY DIFFERENTIATED
The tumor is composed of irregularly shaped glands formed by severely atypical cells.

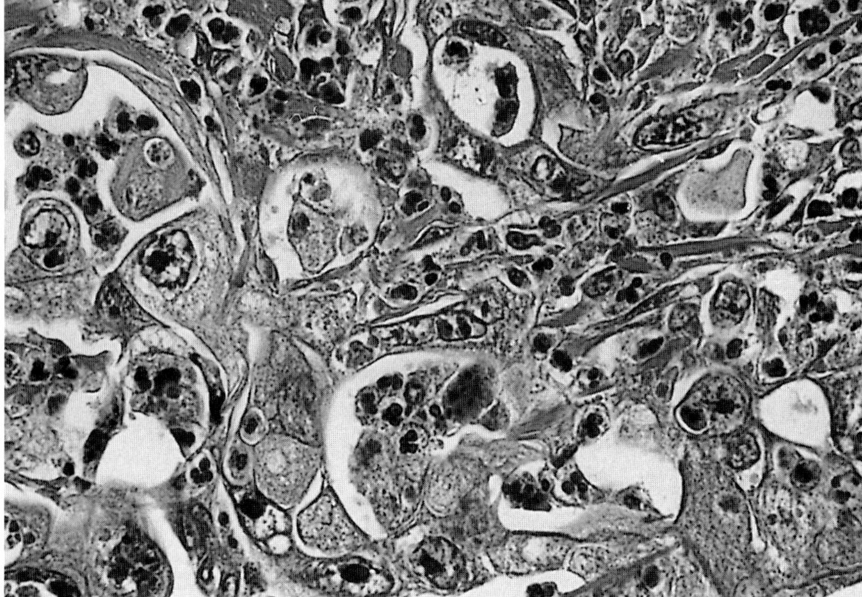

Figure 4-57
DUCTAL ADENOCARCINOMA, POORLY DIFFERENTIATED
Many tumor cells contain big bizarre nuclei with large conspicuous nucleoli.

percent of the tumor tissue) of squamoid differentiation or anaplasia may occur. Usually there is little stromal reaction, but a scattering of inflammatory cells and foci of necrosis and hemorrhage may be present. The neoplastic cells display marked atypia and, in general, little mucin production, although single cells may display mucin-filled intracytoplasmic vacuoles. Some tumor cells, particularly those forming solid clusters, contain large and occasionally bizarre nuclei (fig. 4-57). The mitotic activity is high (fig. 4-58). At the advancing edge of the tumor, the gland and the peripancreatic tissue are invaded by small tumor cell clusters.

Multifocal tumor development in grossly normal-appearing pancreatic tissue distant to a macroscopic tumor in the head of the pancreas has been reported in 15 to 40 percent of cases. In our own study of 37 total pancreatectomy specimens from tumors in the head of the gland no multifocal cancer developed but there was continuous intraductal tumor growth beyond the usual Whipple resection line in 3 (8 percent) cases (see Spread, Metastasis, and Recurrence).

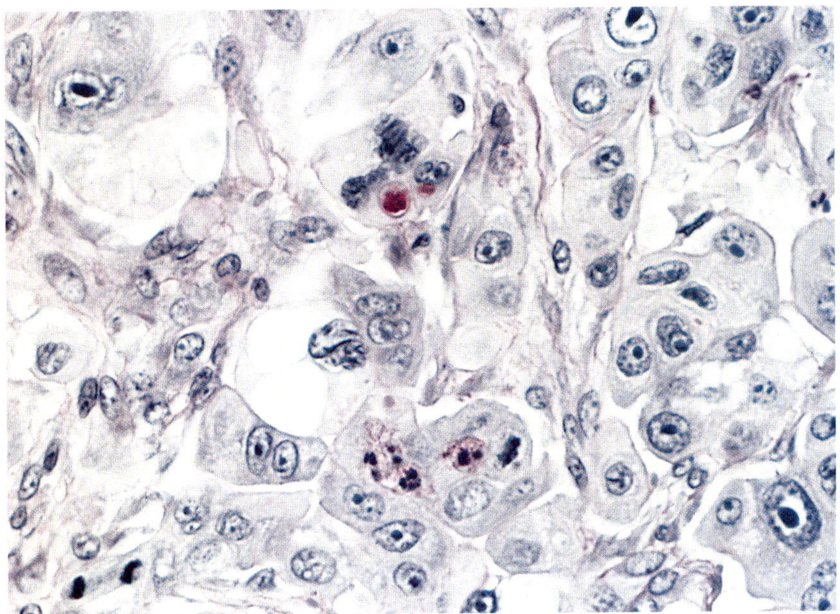

Figure 4-58
DUCTAL ADENOCARCINOMA, POORLY DIFFERENTIATED
Only single tumor cells show intracytoplasmic PAS positivity.

The pancreatic ducts outside the tumor may show ductal papillary hyperplasia with mucinous cell hypertrophy (see Tumor-Like Lesions, Duct Changes). This is more common in patients with a pancreatic carcinoma than in those without a tumor (172,219,228). It may be found anywhere in the non-neoplastic tissue. The ductal cells involved in papillary hyperplasia have a benign appearance or may display some minor degree of atypia. Severe epithelial atypia with irregular budding and bridging, equivalent to severe ductal dysplasia-carcinoma in situ, may be found in the vicinity of the tumors in 8 to 29 percent of the cases (222). Similar duct changes have also been described remote from the macroscopic tumor, but in our experience this is rare. Squamous metaplasia, another duct change, occurs as frequently as in chronic pancreatitis (219).

All ductal adenocarcinomas are associated with more or less developed fibrosclerotic and inflammatory changes in the adjoining non-neoplastic pancreas. These changes are due to carcinomatous duct obstruction (obstructive chronic pancreatitis). In cases of complete occlusion of the main duct, there is marked upstream dilatation of the duct and almost complete fibrotic atrophy of the parenchyma. In contrast to chronic pancreatitis due to alcoholism, intraductal calcifications are, as a rule, absent (see Tumor-Like Lesions, Chronic Pancreatitis).

The pancreatic islets usually disappear within moderately and poorly differentiated tumors. In well-differentiated tumors, islets may be found entrapped in tumor tissue where they are intimately admixed with tumor glands. In addition, scattered neuroendocrine cells occur attached to or intermingled between neoplastic columnar cells (see Immunohistochemical Findings). Only in exceptional cases do the endocrine cells constitute a second cell component of the ductal carcinoma (see Mixed Ductal-Endocrine Carcinoma).

**Microscopic Grading.** Apart from distinguishing well, moderately, and poorly differentiated carcinomas, some grading systems determine the grade of malignancy in ductal adenocarcinomas of the pancreas. Miller et al. (249) graded pancreatic tumors using the system of Broder, which distinguishes four grades cellular atypia: high-grade carcinomas were larger and the frequency of venous thrombosis and metastasis was higher than in low-grade tumors. Mannell et al. (246) reported a correlation between shorter patient survival and pancreatic carcinomas with high cellular atypia (Broder's grades 3 and 4).

We developed another grading system which is based on the combined assessment of the histologic and cytologic features of the tumor as well as its mitotic activity (Table 4-1) (221). If there is intratumor heterogeneity (i.e., a variation in the degree of differentiation and mitotic

Table 4-1

**HISTOLOGIC GRADING OF PANCREATIC DUCTAL ADENOCARCINOMA**

| Tumor Grade | Glandular Differentiation | Mucin Production | Mitoses (per 10 HPF) | Nuclear Atypia |
|---|---|---|---|---|
| 1 | Well-differentiated duct-like glands | Intensive | <5 | Little polmorphism, polar arrangement |
| 2 | Moderately differentiated duct-like and tubular glands | Irregular | 6-10 | Moderate polymorphism |
| 3 | Poorly differentiated glands, muco-epidermoid and pleomorphic structures | Abortive | >10 | Marked polymorphism and increased nuclear size |

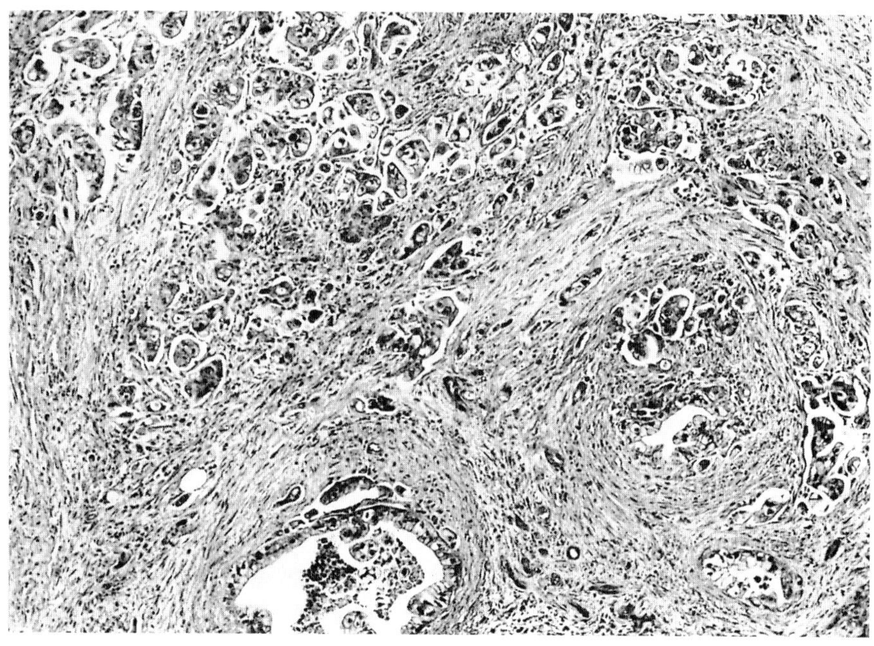

Figure 4-59
DUCTAL ADENOCARCINOMA

This tumor shows marked variation in differentiation. Duct-like glands (bottom) are seen adjacent to undifferentiated clusters of severely atypical cells.

activity) (fig. 4-59), which in our experience is seen in approximately 30 percent of cases, a higher grade is assigned. This rule also applies if only a minor component (less than half of the tumor) is of lower grade. Using this system, we found a correlation between grade and survival time and established grade as an independent prognostic variable (221,223). Recently it was shown that prognosis may also be predicted when only the mitotic index of ductal adenocarcinoma is considered (238).

**Histochemical and Immunohistochemical Findings.** The diagnostic utility of all histochemical and immunohistochemical markers so far available is limited because none of these markers is able to unequivocally distinguish ductal adenocarcinoma of the pancreas from extrapancreatic mucin-producing adenocarcinoma, a distinction of importance in cases of liver metastasis from an unknown primary. However, some markers help separate ductal adenocarcinoma from nonduct-type tumors of the pancreas or non-neoplastic duct changes such as ductal papillary hyperplasia.

Histochemically, ductal adenocarcinomas mainly stain for sulfated (acid) mucins (positive for high-iron diamine) but focal staining occurs for neutral mucins (positive for Alcian blue pH 2.5 and periodic acid–Schiff after pretreatment with diastase) (285). Among lectins, the strongest binding, mainly at the cell surface of the neoplastic epithelium, is observed with peanut lectin (220).

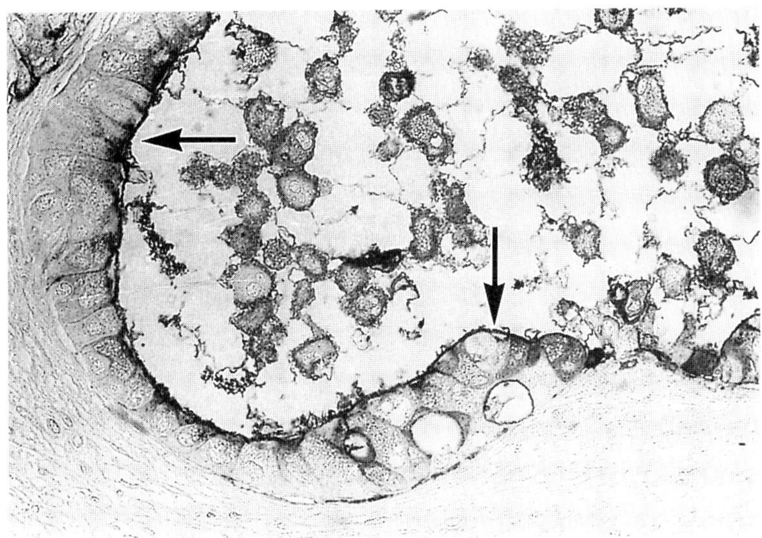

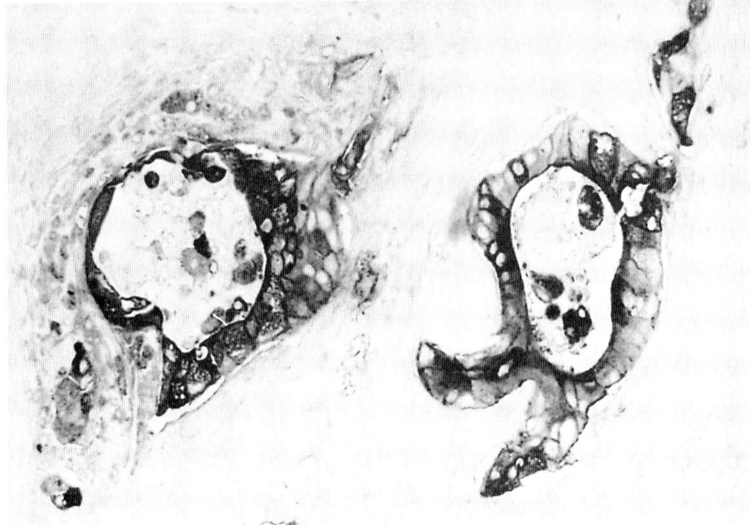

Figure 4-60
DUCTAL ADENOCARCINOMA

Top: Well-differentiated adenocarcinoma with apical immunostaining for CEA (arrows).

Bottom: Moderately differentiated adenocarcinoma with apical cytoplasmic immunostaining for CEA.

Immunohistochemically, the best known markers for ductal adenocarcinoma are M1, CEA, CA19-9, DuPan 2, Span1, CA125, and TAG72 (see Table 3-1) (157,285,292,295,304). As already mentioned, their use as tissue markers for pancreatic carcinoma is limited by their lack of tumor and tissue specificity, and even a combination of positive markers does not increase this specificity. The serologic expression of CEA, CA19-9, and DuPan 2, however, may be a useful diagnostic adjunct for pancreatic carcinoma (see Clinical Features).

*M1.* The M1 mucin antibody characterizes the mucin produced in foveolar cells of the stomach. It is expressed in 95 percent of ductal adenocarcinomas (285). Ductal papillary hyperplasia and neoplastic duct-like structures cannot be distinguished by use of this antibody.

*CEA.* Nearly all ductal adenocarcinomas stain for CEA, even if monospecific antibodies against CEA that do not recognize other members of the CEA family such as NCA55, NCA95, and BGP are used (157,302). The strongest staining, of the luminal contents, luminal borders, and cytoplasm, is found in well-differentiated tumors (figs. 4-51, 4-60, top); staining is usually weak and focal in poorly differentiated tumors (fig. 4-60, bottom) and absent in the normal pancreas and in chronic pancreatitis, except for an occasional ductal papillary hyperplasia that may show discrete labeling of the

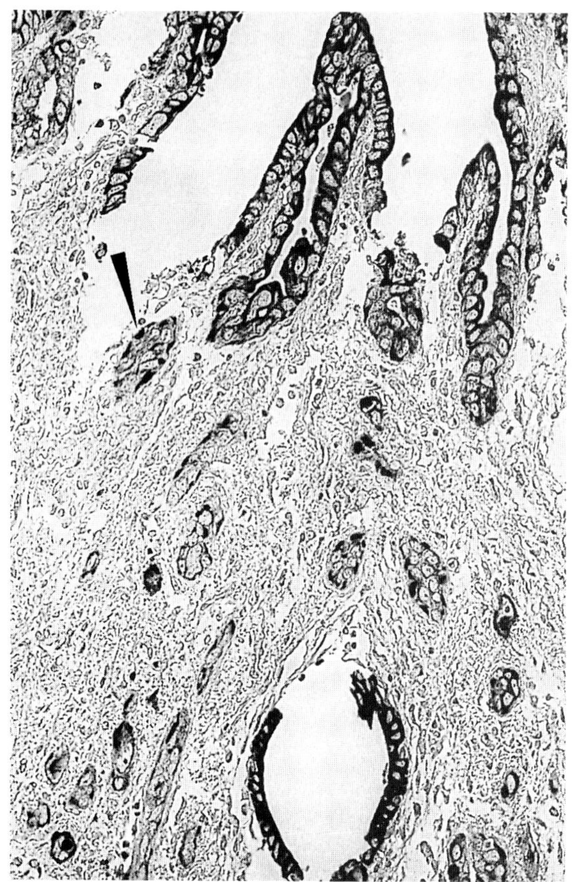

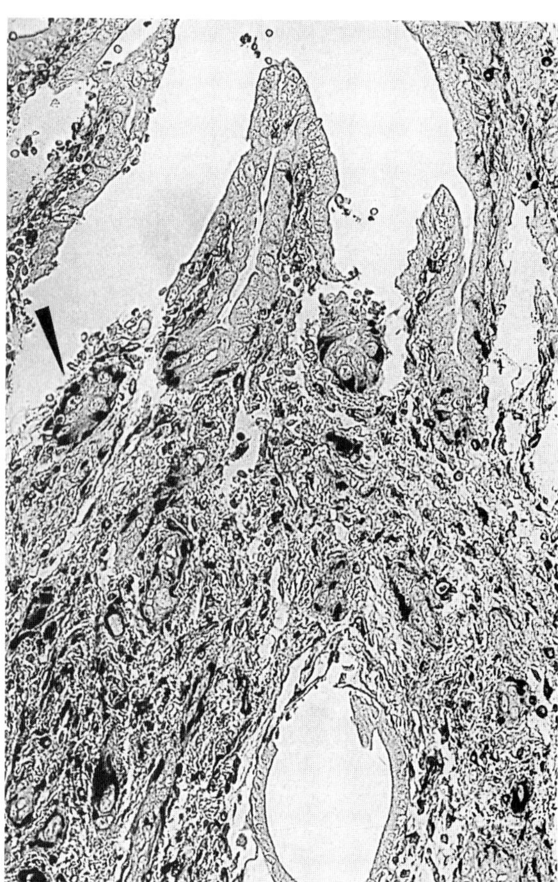

Figure 4-61
DUCTAL ADENOCARCINOMA
This tumor shows keratin (left) as well as vimentin (right) expression in a number of tumor cells (arrowheads).

luminal borders (157). CEA is negative in serous cystadenoma, acinar cell carcinoma, pancreatoblastoma, and endocrine tumors.

*CA19-9.* This marker is expressed in more than 80 percent of ductal adenocarcinomas. Immunoreactivity is predominantly found in the luminal contents and along the luminal borders. It also stains the epithelium of normal pancreatic ducts, particularly in chronic pancreatitis (152,257,295), and the tumor cells of some serous cystadenomas and acinar cell carcinomas.

*DuPan 2 and Span1.* These markers are expressed in about 90 percent of ductal adenocarcinomas. Their patterns of immunoreactivity and specificity are comparable to those of CA19-9 (292,295).

*CA125 and TAG72.* Both markers show a cytoplasmic pattern of staining and are expressed in more than 50 percent and 80 percent of the tumors, respectively. Their patterns of immunoreactivity and specificity are also comparable to those of CA19-9.

*Cytokeratins.* Normal pancreatic and biliary ductal cells as well as pancreatic centroacinar cells express the cytokeratins 7, 8, 18, 19, and occasionally 4 (269,284). Acinar cells contain only keratins 8 and 18, and islet cells 8, 18, and occasionally 19. Ductal adenocarcinomas express the same cytokeratins, 7, 8, 18, and 19, as does normal duct epithelium (269). More than 50 percent of the tumors also express cytokeratin 4 (284). As the usual keratin pattern of colon carcinomas is 8, 18, and 19, it is possible to discriminate between ductal adenocarcinoma of the pancreas and colon carcinoma.

*Other Markers.* Ductal adenocarcinomas are usually negative for vimentin (284) and only occasionally coexpress vimentin and keratin (fig. 4-61) (215). With rare exceptions (184; see Mixed Ductal-Endocrine Carcinoma), they also fail to stain

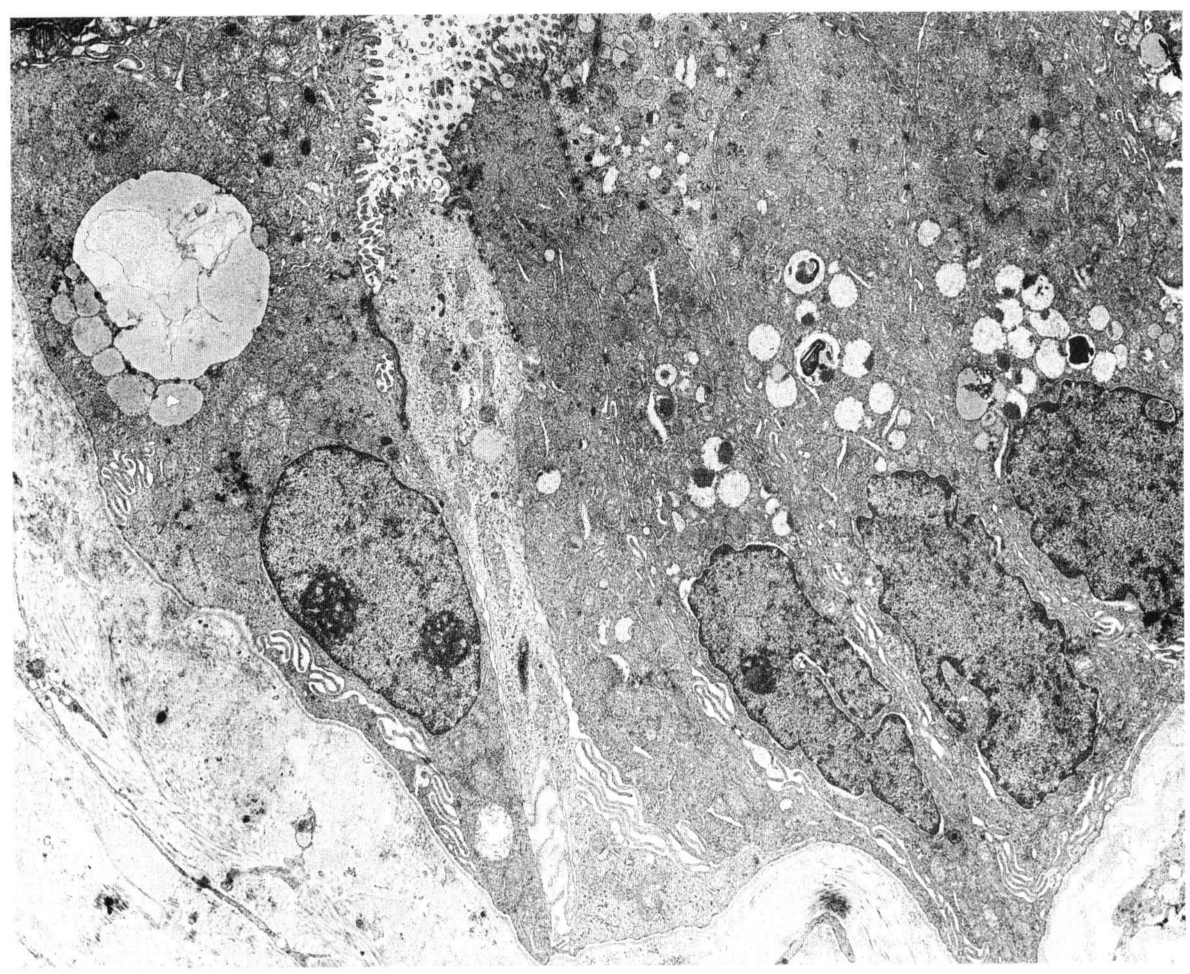

Figure 4-62
DUCTAL ADENOCARCINOMA, WELL-DIFFERENTIATED
Electron micrograph of a well-differentiated ductal adenocarcinoma. The luminal surface of the cells (top) shows many microvilli. In the apical part of the cells there are many large mucin granules with granular contents and sometimes a dense eccentric core. The cells reside on a well-developed basal membrane (X28,000).

with endocrine markers such as synaptophysin and the chromogranins, but may contain, particularly if well differentiated, some scattered (possibly non-neoplastic) endocrine cells in close association with neoplastic cells (160). They are generally negative for pancreatic enzymes such as trypsin, chymotrypsin, and lipase (201,257).

In summary, there is no immunohistochemical marker specific for ductal adenocarcinoma. However, antibodies specific for CEA, i.e., those not cross-reacting with other antigens of the CEA family, are good markers for distinguishing non-neoplastic duct changes from neoplastic ducts. Moreover, they help separate ductal adenocarcinoma from nonduct-type tumors such as acinar cell carcinoma and neuroendocrine tumor (see Table 3-1). Other useful markers are the different cytokeratins, since ductal adenocarcinomas always stain for cytokeratins 7, 8, 18, and 19, while 25 percent of the acinar cell carcinomas and almost all endocrine tumors do not stain for cytokeratin 7.

**Ultrastructural Findings.** On electron microscopy, the most frequently recognized cell types in ductal adenocarcinomas resemble pancreatic duct cells. The tumor cells are characterized by mucin granules in the apical cytoplasm (fig. 4-62), irregular microvilli on the luminal surface, and a more or less polarized arrangement of the differently sized nuclei (173,211,

285). The content of the mucin granules (size, 0.4 to 2.0 µm) varies from solid electron dense to filamentous and punctate; often there is a dense eccentric core. Some cells have features of gastric foveolar cells: granules with a punctate-cerebroid structure (285). In addition to mucin granules the cytoplasm usually contains numerous small vesicles. Well-differentiated carcinomas have strictly polarized cells, with their basal plasma membrane in contact with a well-differentiated basal lamina (fig. 4-62). Loss of tumor differentiation is characterized by loss of cell polarity, disappearance of a basal lamina, appearance of irregular luminal spaces, and loss of mucin granules (211).

**New Techniques.** Studies of the DNA content of ductal adenocarcinomas, using either image cytometry or flow cytometry, reveal "nondiploid" or aneuploid distributions in 15 to almost 100 percent of the cases (145,153,182,310). From these reports it appears that a nondiploid or aneuploid DNA content is associated with advanced tumor stage and shorter survival. A more precise prediction of the prognosis according to the DNA content is so far not possible.

The expression of argyrophilic nucleolar organizer regions (AgNORs) has been studied in 33 ductal adenocarcinomas (266). It was found that patients with tumors with low AgNOR counts per cell (less than 3.25) have a better prognosis 2 and 3 years after surgery than those with tumors with a high AgNOR count. AgNOR positivity was not related to the stage of the tumor. Immunohistochemical examination of the proliferating cell nuclear antigen (PCNA) in percutaneous biopsies from patients suspected of having pancreatic carcinoma revealed that PCNA labeling is significantly higher in ductal adenocarcinoma tissue than in chronic pancreatitis tissue (232).

Recently, several studies using immunocytochemical and hybridization techniques have shown that ductal adenocarcinomas frequently overexpress some growth factors and their receptors, and commonly contain certain activated oncogenes and inactivated tumor suppressor genes. Pancreatic carcinomas overexpress the epidermal growth factor receptor, overexpress the c-*erb*-B2 proto-oncogene, produce large quantities of transforming growth factor alpha, and have an exceptionally high point mutation rate (75 to 90 percent) at codon 12 of the K-*ras* gene (149,197,271,279,282,287,312). In addition, a mutated p53 suppressor gene and nuclear expression of the p53 protein occur in 40 to 60 percent of the cases (155,280). To date no clear prognostic relevance has been established for any of the above mentioned changes. In particular, there is as yet no correlation between K-*ras* and p53 mutations and survival, tumor grade, or stage (155,194, 259). For the differential diagnosis it is of interest that K-*ras* codon 12 mutations are either absent from or only rarely present in pancreatic acinar cell carcinomas (201,271), solid-pseudopapillary tumors (271), or endocrine tumors (271). K-*ras* point mutations were demonstrated in non-neoplastic pancreatic duct lesions such as ductal papillary hyperplasia (313), although this has not been confirmed by others (233,290). Finally, the rate of K-*ras* mutations in ampullary carcinomas and bile duct carcinomas, tumors that are histologically and immunocytochemically indistinguishable from ductal adenocarcinoma of the pancreas, does not exceed 20 percent (258,281).

Cytogenetic analyses have identified gene rearrangements or losses particularly in chromosomes 1p, 1q, 6q, 12p, 16q, and 17p. Allelic losses were common for chromosomes 17p and 18q, the sites of the p53 and *DCC* gene loci, respectively, but mutations of the *APC* gene were not found (286). Although the number of chromosomal examinations that have so far been performed is small, it appears that ductal adenocarcinoma lacks any diagnostic chromosomal change.

**Differential Diagnosis.** The major differential diagnosis of ductal adenocarcinoma is chronic pancreatitis (see Diagnosis of Pancreatic Carcinoma). The tumors that have to be differentiated from ductal adenocarcinoma include pancreatic neoplasms with a less grave prognosis: ampullary carcinoma, intraductal papillary-mucinous tumor, acinar cell carcinoma, endocrine tumor, solid-pseudopapillary tumor, and pancreatoblastoma.

*Chronic Pancreatitis.* Clinically, patients younger than 40 years are more likely to have chronic pancreatitis than carcinoma. The opposite is true for patients older than 50 years, particularly if they present with painless jaundice of relatively short duration. On gross inspection, most carcinomas present as ill-defined and firm masses in the head of the pancreas. However, this feature may be simulated by chronic pancreatitis because of its common focal accentuation (fig. 4-63). On the cut surface at the level of the common bile duct, the situation usually becomes much clearer, since many tumors produce a severe stenosis or complete obstruction of the common bile duct and the main pancreatic duct, thereby producing a marked upstream dilatation of both duct systems. Moreover, the stenosis of the bile duct is related to an ill-defined mass in the adjoining parenchyma. In chronic pancreatitis, the common bile duct may also be stenotic but this stenosis is never complete and is usually tubular (fig. 4-63). The pancreatic duct exhibits strictures and saccular dilatations and may contain calculi. The parenchyma reveals an irregular fibrosis: small scars alternate with areas displaying a still preserved lobular parenchyma. In addition, there may be pseudocysts, usually at the margin of the gland. Microscopically, the neoplastic duct-like structures and glands are embedded in fibrous tissue and may therefore simulate the ductal and ductular proliferations found in chronic pancreatitis. However, in contrast to chronic pancreatitis in which the remaining small ducts, even in cases with severe fibrosis, are still arranged in a lobular pattern, the tumor glands are unevenly distributed in the fibrotic tissue (fig. 4-64). In addition, they may have an abnormal shape, variable mucin content, ruptured epithelium, and incomplete or absent basal membranes when immunostained for laminin. If the biopsy sample comes from the periphery of the tumor, the tumor glands may show perineural invasion and frank infiltration of fatty tissue (fig. 4-65), findings not seen in chronic pancreatitis. At times, the close association of endocrine cell clusters with nerves may simulate perineural tumor invasion (156). However, the solid arrangement and monomorphic appearance of the endocrine cells distinguish them from the gland-forming cells of a ductal adenocarcinoma. Another source of misinterpretation are the tiny accessory ducts found around the common bile duct or in the duodenal wall. They are arranged in a lobular pattern and lack the disorganization of neoplastic glands. Cytologically, the cells of the neoplastic ducts have relatively large nuclei with conspicuous nucleoli and an occasional mitosis. In chronic pancreatitis, the ducts are lined with cells that have a uniform nucleus without a distinct nucleolus. Immunohistochemically, nonneoplastic ducts usually do not stain for CEA using monospecific monoclonal antisera that does not recognize nonspecific cross-reacting antigens (figs. 4-51, 4-66). In ductal adenocarcinoma, most neoplastic ducts are labeled by CEA. Since chronic inflammation secondary to duct obstruction is always found in the periphery of ductal adenocarcinoma, tissues from peripheral areas may only show chronic pancreatitis. A diagnosis of chronic pancreatitis in a small biopsy from the surface of a pancreas therefore does not exclude a carcinoma, since that may only be present in a sample from the deeper part of the suspicious tissue.

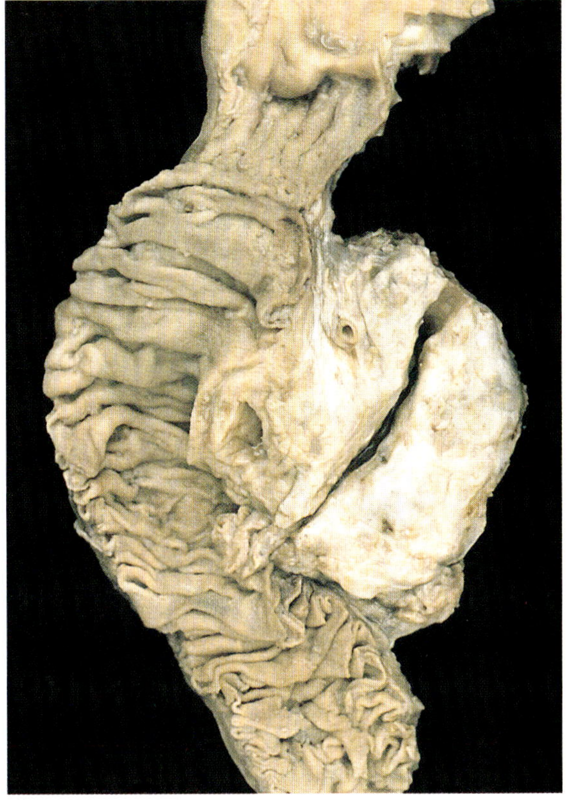

Figure 4-63
CHRONIC PANCREATITIS
Whipple resection specimen from a patient with chronic pancreatitis. The cut surface shows tubular stenosis of the common bile duct. Differentiation from a ductal adenocarcinoma is hardly possible on the basis of the gross appearance of this inflammatory lesion.

*Ampullary Carcinoma.* Distinguishing ductal adenocarcinoma of the pancreas from adenocarcinoma of the ampulla of Vater is not possible on

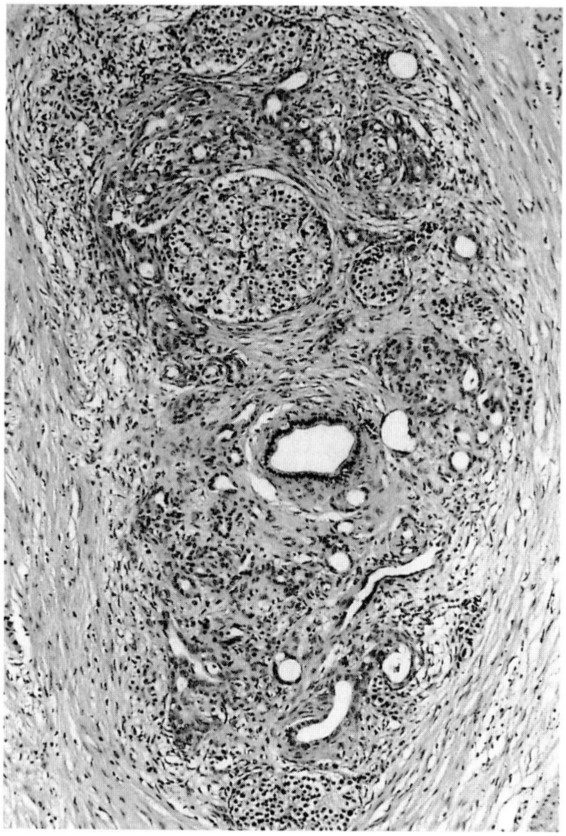

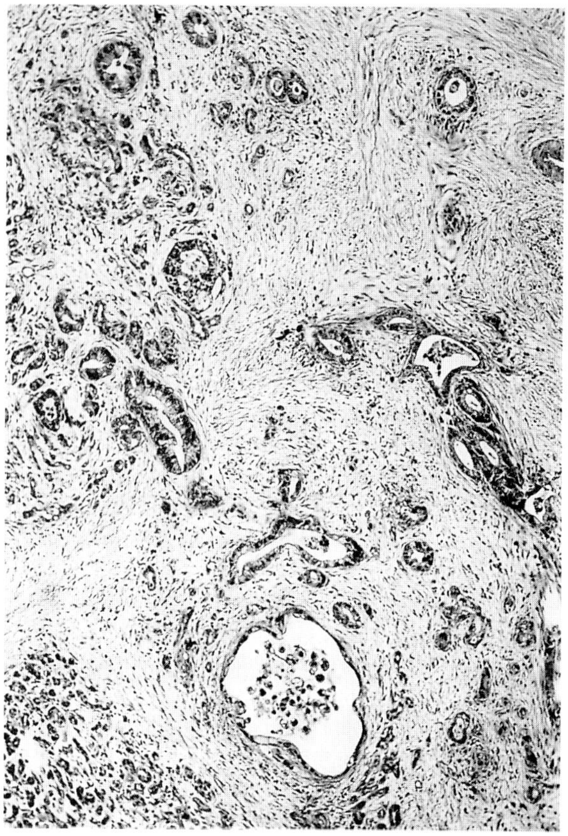

Figure 4-64
DUCTAL ADENOCARCINOMA: DIFFERENTIAL DIAGNOSIS WITH CHRONIC PANCREATITIS

Left: The illustration shows chronic pancreatitis with remnants of acini, islets, and ducts. These structures are still distributed in a lobular pattern.

Right: This illustration shows a ductal adenocarcinoma characterized by its unevenly distributed tumoral glands.

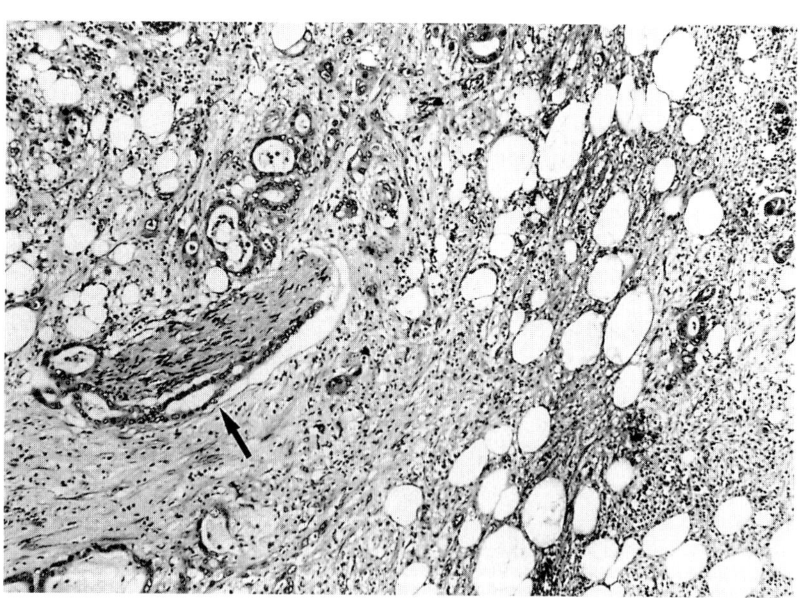

Figure 4-65
DUCTAL ADENOCARCINOMA WITH PERINEURAL INVASION

The neoplastic glands show perineural invasion (arrow) as well as invasion of fatty tissue.

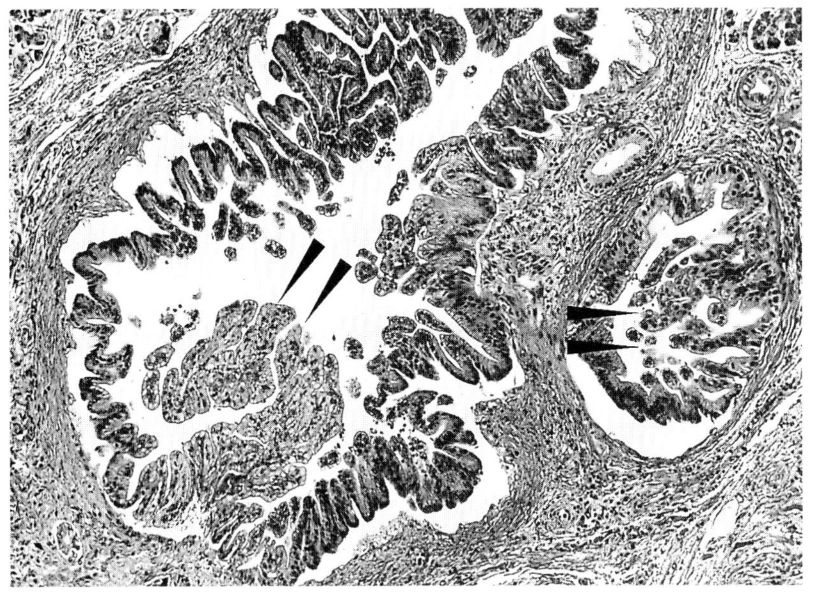

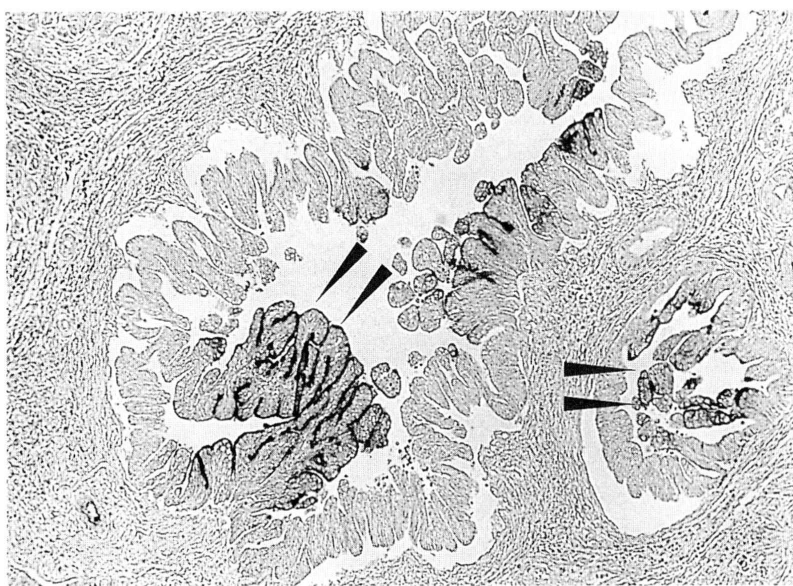

Figure 4-66
DUCTAL ADENOCARCINOMA:
INTRADUCTAL TUMOR SPREAD

Top: Intraductal foci of well-differentiated ductal adenocarcinoma (arrowheads).

Bottom: Immunostaining for CEA reveals the neoplastic cells (arrowheads).

histologic or immunohistochemical grounds, because both tumors share the same microscopic features. The only way to distinguish between the two is by careful assessment of the macroscopic and microscopic localization of the lesion. The same is true for carcinomas of the intrapancreatic segment of the common bile duct (fig. 4-67). However, if such tumors are advanced, even careful macroscopic evaluation may not differentiate adenocarcinomas of the distal bile duct from those of the head of the pancreas. This raises the question of whether the predilection of pancreatic carcinomas for the head of the gland is in part due to the fact that a considerable number of head carcinomas originate from the preampullary part of the common bile duct. Periampullary carcinomas of duodenal origin that invade the pancreas may be recognized by tubulopapillary glands lined predominantly by cells with an intestinal phenotype.

*Other Tumors.* Differentiation of ductal adenocarcinoma from intraductal papillary-mucinous tumor, acinar cell carcinoma, neuroendocrine tumor, solid-cystic tumor, and pancreatoblastoma

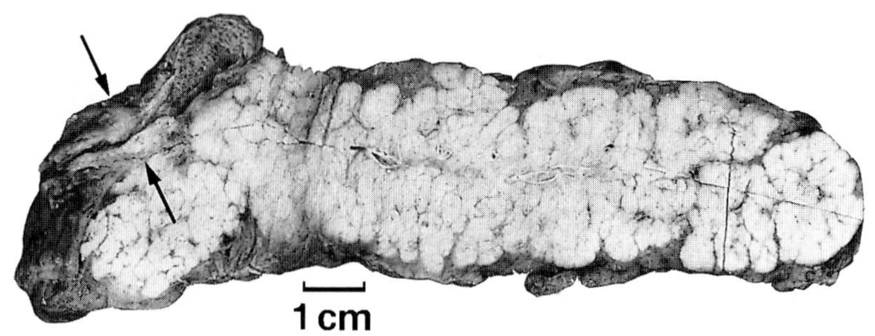


Figure 4-67
DUCTAL ADENOCARCINOMA:
DIFFERENTIAL DIAGNOSIS

Autopsy specimen of the pancreas showing a carcinoma (arrows) in the distal preampullary part of the common bile duct. There is no tumor infiltration of the adjacent pancreatic tissue.

relies on the distinctive histologic pattern, the immunohistochemical marker constellation (see Table 3-2), and the biology of the respective tumors. In intraductal papillary-mucinous tumors the proliferation of neoplastic duct cells is confined to the duct system, and even in those tumors that already show frank invasion by tumor glands, the bulk of neoplastic tissue still lies within the ducts. Patients with intraductal papillary-mucinous tumors often present with a long history of a pancreatitis-like syndrome. Acinar cell carcinomas show a conspicuous acinar structure or a solid endocrine-like pattern. They stain for pancreatic enzymes and are usually negative for CEA (201,257). Endocrine tumors exhibit solid, trabecular and microglandular structures, with occasional true glandular formations, but do not produce mucin. They stain for neuroendocrine markers and usually one or more pancreatic hormones. Entrapped non-neoplastic ductular structures in endocrine tumors are not evidence of true ductal differentiation. Endocrine tumors occur at all ages and can be associated with distinct syndromes; patient survival is much longer than in ductal adenocarcinoma, even for malignant tumors. Solid pseudopapillary tumors consist of monomorphic cells arranged in a solid or pseudopapillary pattern with large areas of hemorrhage (224). The large, well-demarcated tumors stain focally for alpha-1-antitrypsin, occur predominantly in young women, and are usually benign. Pancreatoblastomas are rare tumors of children and display acinar cell differentiation with scattered squamoid nests.

*Metastases.* Distinguishing between liver metastases from pancreatic ductal adenocarcinoma and those from other mucin-producing adenocarcinomas is impossible on histologic grounds alone. The only hint may be that metastases from pancreatic carcinomas often display small glands embedded in marked desmoplastic stroma accompanied by cholestasis, features also found in bile duct carcinomas. Ductal adenocarcinomas may be distinguished from most gastrointestinal carcinomas by their cytokeratin pattern: they express cytokeratins 7, 8, 18, and 19, while the latter tumors express only cytokeratins 8, 18, and 19 (269). As ductal adenocarcinomas also express CEA, CA19-9, and other tumor markers as do mucin-producing adenocarcinomas of gastrointestinal, biliary, or pulmonary origin, these antigens are not suitable for their differentiation. Metastases from carcinomas of the pancreas to the ovary or lung may simulate primary mucinous tumor of the ovary (314), or primary lung adenocarcinoma, respectively (165).

**Frozen Section Diagnosis.** Correct frozen section diagnosis is critical for intraoperative diagnosis and therapy. Frozen section evaluation identifies suspicious lesions in the pancreas and detects remaining tumor tissue at the resection margins after tumor removal. Frozen section analysis is important in differentiating ductal adenocarcinoma and chronic pancreatitis. The criteria for distinguishing the two diseases have already been discussed in the section on differential diagnosis. Helpful morphologic criteria for ductal adenocarcinoma, as defined by Hyland et al. (204), are nuclear size variation equal to or greater than 4 to 1, incomplete glandular lumens, and disorganized duct distribution. Another unequivocal feature of malignancy is perineural invasion. Frozen sections from a pancreatic resection margin should be searched for perineural and lymphatic invasion of the attached peripancreatic fatty tissue and the cytologic features of all papillary duct changes carefully evaluated. Papillary projections of the duct epithelium without a fibrous core and with distinct cellular atypia indicate intraductal tumor spread. Cross sections from the distal common bile duct should also be screened for perineural and lymphatic invasion in the surrounding fatty tissue. The small accessory glands in the wall of the bile duct, which are arranged in groups, should not be misinterpreted as malignant glands.

**Cytologic Findings.** Cytologic assessment of pancreatic lesions is critical for preoperative and intraoperative diagnosis and therapy. The success of this method not only depends on the experience of the cytopathologist but also on the experience of the clinician who must accurately localize and biopsy the lesion. Sometimes even multiple biopsies are required before a correct diagnosis is possible. Cytologic material may be obtained by two different approaches: percutaneous fine-needle biopsy (FNB) aspirates guided by computerized tomography or ultrasonography, and pancreatic juice cytology obtained during an endoscopic retrograde cholangio-pancreatography. The sensitivity of percutaneous FNB is between 70 and 90 percent (147,252), while that of cytologic examination of pure pancreatic juice is 76 percent (261). Cytologic samples from ductal adenocarcinomas typically contain tightly packed small or large clusters of neoplastic cells which are characterized by their irregular and enlarged nuclei, distinct nuclear membranes, and prominent nucleoli (147,216); mitoses are occasional. The cytoplasm of the malignant cells is usually scanty. Sometimes the neoplastic cells are grouped in small loose sheets which show palisading of nuclei. Marked cellular pleomorphism, lack of cohesion of the cells, and abundant necrotic debris indicate a poorly differentiated tumor. Frequently, there are groups of benign ductal cells with some irregularity in size. These cells are differentiated from malignant cells by their appearance in monolayered sheets, their distinct cell borders, uniform nuclei, and a preserved nuclear/cytoplasmic ratio. Cytologic specimens may further contain acinar and stromal cells. Acinar cells contain, within abundant granular cytoplasm, uniform round nuclei with finely stippled chromatin and small inconspicuous nucleoli. Other cells that may be observed are endothelial cells and inflammatory cells. In pancreatic juice samples obtained by endoscopic cannulation the exfoliated cells may be distinctly degenerated if the specimens still contain contrast medium. This can create problems of interpretation and falsify the results (261).

**Spread, Metastasis, and Recurrence.** Ductal adenocarcinoma of the pancreas infiltrates peripancreatic retroperitoneal fatty tissue early in the course of the disease. It invades perineural sheaths (fig. 4-65), lymphatic channels, and eventually the peritoneum and mesenteric blood vessels. Carcinomas of the pancreatic head also spread by direct invasion into the wall of the duodenum. They metastasize most commonly to the lymph nodes of the superior head and posterior pancreaticoduodenal groups (173). The anterior pancreaticoduodenal and the inferior head lymph nodes as well as lymph nodes around the celiac trunk and the aorta are less frequently involved. Lymph nodes in the pancreatic body, which may be affected in advanced cases, are not removed in a standard Whipple procedure (175). Carcinomas of the body and tail directly extend through the retroperitoneal tissue to the stomach, spleen, peritoneum, colon, and left adrenal gland. They metastasize especially to the superior body and head lymph nodes and may also spread via lymphatic channels to pleura and lung (see fig. 1-9). Distant metastases occur primarily in the liver and peritoneum (247). Other metastatic sites, in approximate order of frequency, are: lung, bone, kidney, brain, and skin (umbilicus). Ovarian metastases are rare, but may simulate a primary mucinous tumor (314). In about 10 to 15 percent of autopsies there are no distant metastases (Table 4-2) (225,248).

Despite surgery, most patients with pancreatic carcinoma die of tumor recurrence within 1 to 2 years. The origin of the recurrent tumor appears to be, in descending order of frequency, microscopic tumor cell nests remaining in the retroperitoneal spaces behind the head of the pancreas and the large mesenteric vessels; metastases to local lymph nodes or liver; and tumor remaining in the rest of the gland in the case of a Whipple resection (223). Results of a postmortem examination of patients who died of recurrent tumor after "curative" resection for pancreatic carcinoma showed local retroperitoneal recurrence in 80 percent, hepatic metastasis in 66 percent, peritoneal dissemination in 53 percent, and lymph

Table 4-2

**METASTATIC SPREAD (INCLUDING DIRECT INVASION) IN 164 PATIENTS WITH CARCINOMA OF THE PANCREAS***

| Site of Metastasis | Number of Carcinomas by Site: Head (n=106) | Body/ Tail (n=34) | Head, Body, and Tail (n=24) |
|---|---|---|---|
| Regional lymph nodes | 85 | 34 | 24 |
| Juxtaregional lymph nodes | 52 | 25 | 18 |
| Liver | 80 | 28 | 21 |
| Stomach | 15 | 7 | 13 |
| Peritoneum | 23 | 17 | 11 |
| Lungs | 28 | 8 | 7 |
| Pleura | 29 | 13 | 6 |
| Pericardium | 3 | 2 | 1 |
| Colon | 3 | 4 | 4 |
| Spleen | 6 | 11 | 4 |
| Adrenal glands | 15 | 9 | 5 |
| Bones | 13 | 5 | 3 |
| Kidneys | 9 | 7 | 6 |
| Skin | 1 | 1 | 2 |
| No metastases | 15 | 1 | — |

*From reference 73.

Table 4-3

**UICC STAGE CLASSIFICATION (1987)**

PRIMARY TUMOR (T)
TX Primary tumor cannot be assessed
T0 No evidence of primary tumor
T1 Tumor limited to the pancreas
T1a: Tumor 2 cm or less in greatest dimension
T1b: Tumor more than 2 cm in greatest dimension
T2 Tumor extends directly to the duodenum, bile duct, or peripancreatic tissues
T3 Tumor extends directly to the stomach, spleen, colon, or adjacent large vessels

REGIONAL LYMPH NODES (N)
NX Regional lymph nodes cannot be assessed
N0 No regional lymph node metastasis
N1 Regional lymph node metastasis

DISTANT METASTASIS (M)
MX Presence of distant metastasis cannot be assessed
M0 No distant metastasis
M1 Distant metastasis

STAGE GROUPING *

| | | | |
|---|---|---|---|
| Stage I | T1 | N0 | M0 |
| | T2 | N0 | M0 |
| Stage II | T3 | N0 | M0 |
| Stage III | Any T | N1 | M0 |
| Stage IV | Any T | Any N | M1 |

*It is recommended to subdivide stage I into stage Ia encompassing T1 N0 M0, and stage Ib encompassing T2 N0 M0. In addition, information should be provided about the absence (R0 - no residual tumor detected) or the presence (R1 - microscopic residual tumor; R2 - macroscopic residual tumor) of residual tumor after resection.

node recurrence in 47 percent (210). Recurrence in the remainder of the gland has been attributed to intrapancreatic multifocal cancer (299, 307,308), a high incidence of multicentricity (15 to 40 percent [222]), or continuous cancer development (73.5 percent [262]). In our experience, tumor recurrence in the pancreatic remnant after a Whipple resection seems to be less than expected from the incidence rates for multicentricity; the high frequency of multicentricity given in the literature may be overestimated. Ishikawa (206) saw no residual cancer in the pancreatic remnant at autopsy if the Whipple resection specimen was free of cancer at the cut margin.

**Staging.** In the 1970s, several staging systems for pancreatic carcinomas were in use (174,200,225). By 1977, they were replaced by the revised Union Internationale Contre Cancer (UICC) staging system based on the size and extent of the primary tumor (T), the status of regional lymph nodes (N), and the presence of metastatic disease (M) (199). This TNM staging system is presented in Table 4-3. A more complex staging classification was proposed by the Japan Pancreas Society in 1987 (Table 4-4). The UICC classification considers lymph node metastasis the most important prognostic factor, whereas the Japanese classification primarily relies on the prognostic value of tumor size and local spread. Thus, in the UICC classification, all tumors without lymph node involvement are included in stages I and II, regardless of whether they are limited to the pancreas (T1) or extend to the peripancreatic tissues (T2) and adjacent organs (such as the stomach or the large vessels; T3). In the Japanese

Table 4-4

**JAPANESE STAGE CLASSIFICATION (1987)**

| | | | | | |
|---|---|---|---|---|---|
| Stage I | $T_1$ (0–2 cm) | $N_0$ | $S_0$ | $Rp_0$ | $V_0$ |
| Stage II | $T_2$ (2.1–4.0 cm) | $N_1$ | $S_1$ | $Rp_1$ | $V_1$ |
| Stage III | $T_3$ (4.1–6.0 cm) | $N_2$ | $S_2$ | $Rp_2$ | $V_2$ |
| Stage IV | $T_4$ (>6.1 cm) | $N_3$ | $S_3$ | $Rp_3$ | $V_3$ |

Distant metastasis including hepatic metastasis or peritoneal dissemination is allocated to stage IV.
T: size of tumor; N: lymph node metastasis; N0: No lymph node involvement; N1: involvement of primary group of lymph nodes (situated closely to the tumor); N2: involvement of secondary group of lymph nodes between N1 and N3; N3: involvement of tertiary group of lymph nodes regarded as juxtaregional lymph nodes; S: serosal invasion; Rp: retroperitoneal invasion; V: invasion of portal venous systems; S0, Rp0, V0: absence of invasion; S1, Rp1, V1: suspected invasion; S2, Rp2, V2: definite invasion; S3, Rp3, V3: severe invasion.

classification, on the other hand, stage I includes only tumors up to 2 cm in size without retroperitoneal invasion, while tumors above 2 cm or with suspected retroperitoneal invasion already belong to stage II (303).

**Treatment.** Surgical resection is the most effective treatment of ductal adenocarcinoma, but only 10 to 20 percent of the tumors are amenable to so called curative resection because at the time of diagnosis the tumor is so widespread that total removal is impossible. Tumors of the head of the pancreas are usually resected by a Whipple operation (rarely, by a total pancreatectomy), currently often combined with a radical lymphadenectomy, while tumors in the body and tail are treated with distal pancreatectomy. In recent years the mortality rate of these operations has been reduced from 10 to 20 percent to 2 to 6 percent (187,298,301).

Unresectable carcinomas are treated with palliative bypass operations. Response to chemotherapy with 5-fluorouracil occurs in at most 10 percent of patients (162,270). Radiotherapy alone is largely ineffective (309).

**Prognosis.** Ductal adenocarcinoma is fatal in most cases (51). The mean survival time of the untreated patient is 3 months, while the mean survival time after radical resection varies from 10 to 20 months (171,180,187,298). The 5-year survival rate of patients treated by resection remains disappointing (3.5 percent) (195), although in selected and stage-stratified series survival figures of 25 percent (298) or even 37 percent (301) have been reported. In the individual patient prognosis is related to tumor site, size, stage, and grade.

*Site.* At the time of diagnosis carcinomas of the body or the tail of the pancreas are usually more advanced than those of the head, because body-tail tumors may spread insidiously into extrapancreatic tissue and metastasize readily before detection (174).

*Size.* The survival time is longer in patients with tumors confined to the pancreas and less than 3 cm in diameter (17 to 29 months) than in patients with tumors of greater size and/or regional lymph node involvement (6 to 15 months) (174). There seems to be no further improvement of prognosis in patients with tumors less than 2 cm in diameter (223), because even in these "small carcinomas," which comprise approximately 10 percent of all resected tumors (198), involvement of the peripancreatic tissue and regional lymph nodes is observed in 40 to 75 percent of cases (198,244,260,301). Resected carcinomas smaller than 2 cm, limited to the pancreas, and without lymph node metastases (early pancreatic carcinoma) are rare (less than 5 percent of patients) (198).

*Stage.* Patients with tumors confined to the pancreas (T1 according to UICC classification) and no residual tumor following resection (R0) have the most favorable prognosis of all patients undergoing surgical resection (187,254,298,301, 303). This implies that local spread to peripancreatic tissues, i.e., retroperitoneal invasion with or without involvement of the portal venous system, is the most important prognostic feature. Tumors that involve one or two peripancreatic lymph nodes seem to have the same prognosis as tumors involving no lymph nodes (187,217,246, 298,301,303). For the few patients displaying favorable prognostic features, i.e., small tumor confined to the pancreas without or with limited (single) lymph node involvement, postoperative cumulative 5-year survival rates of 26 to 46 percent (187,298,301) with a mean survival time of about 38 months (187, 303) have been reported.

*Grade.* Although the stage of pancreatic carcinoma at the time of diagnosis predicts, in great part, the patient's prognosis, it appears that histologic grade may also play a role as prognostic parameter. Based on the criteria of the grading system summarized in Table 4-1, it was found that G1 tumors showed generally a lower stage at the time of surgery than G2 and G3 carcinomas. Moreover, the median postoperative survival times correlated significantly with tumor grade (221), mitotic index (238), and severe cellular atypia (246). As grading systems are, to a large extent, subjective, reproducibility may be low. It is thus not surprising that there are also studies that found no relationship between grade and survival in pancreatic carcinomas (310).

*Other Factors.* Nuclear parameters, such as median nuclear size, nuclear area, and nuclear perimeter, have been shown to help evaluate prognosis for ductal adenocarcinoma (183,221). Recent studies on the DNA content of ductal adenocarcinoma revealed associations with tumor stage, tumor grade, and, although only minimally, with survival (145,153,182,310). Other unfavorable prognostic factors include presenting symptoms such as steatorrhea and back pain, while age, sex, and past medical history showed no influence on survival (246).

## DUCTAL ADENOCARCINOMA VARIANTS

Mucinous noncystic adenocarcinoma, signet-ring cell carcinoma, adenosquamous carcinoma, and undifferentiated (anaplastic) carcinoma are considered variants of ductal adenocarcinoma because most of these carcinomas, even if poorly differentiated, contain some foci of neoplastic glands with ductal differentiation (169,173,218). Also biologically, these tumors (with the exception of the signet-ring cell tumor) do not differ significantly from ductal adenocarcinoma. Although some of the osteoclast-like giant cell tumors may also contain neoplastic ducts, they are not considered variants of ductal adenocarcinoma; they probably constitute a heterogeneous group in which some show epithelial and others mesenchymal differentiation.

### Mucinous Noncystic Adenocarcinoma

This uncommon tumor (relative frequency, 1 to 3 percent [218]) is characterized by abundant extracellular mucin production (more than 50 percent of the tumor consists of mucin), which results in a gelatinous cut surface (fig. 4-68). It has therefore also been called *colloid carcinoma.* The tumors may be very large and are usually well demarcated. The development of pseudomyxoma peritonei has been described (168). Similar to ductal adenocarcinoma, they occur predominantly in the head of the pancreas; sex distribution and median age are also similar. It is of interest that the invasive component of some intraductal papillary-mucinous tumors resembles mucinous noncystic carcinoma.

Microscopically, mucinous adenocarcinomas show large pools of mucin which are partially lined by well-differentiated cuboidal cells (fig. 4-69). The mucin lakes usually contain clumps or strands of tumor cells. Some floating cells may be of signet-ring cell type. These carcinomas should not be confused with mucinous cystic tumors; the latter have a much better prognosis (see Mucinous Cystic Tumor).

### Signet-Ring Cell Carcinoma

The extremely rare signet-ring cell carcinoma is composed almost exclusively of cells filled with mucin. We found only one reported in the literature (297) and have had one case of our own (fig. 4-70). Apart from signet-ring cells, the carcinoma may show a small portion of poorly differentiated glands. Immunohistochemically, the signet-ring cells stain intensely for CEA. The tumors exhibit a markedly infiltrative spread and may involve almost the entire pancreas, resulting in diffuse enlargement of the gland. Our patient survived only 3 months. Signet-ring cell carcinomas of the stomach infiltrating the pancreas are indistinguishable from those arising primarily in the pancreas.

### Adenosquamous Carcinoma

This rare tumor (relative frequency, 3 to 4 percent [205,218]) is characterized by variable proportions of mucin-producing glandular elements and squamous components (figs. 4-71, 4-72). The squamous components should account for at least 30 percent of the tumor tissue as seen on the sections. In gross appearance, male to female ratio, and localization, adenosquamous carcinoma resembles usual ductal adenocarcinoma (173,218). It has also been called *mucoepidermoid carcinoma* and *adenoacanthoma.*

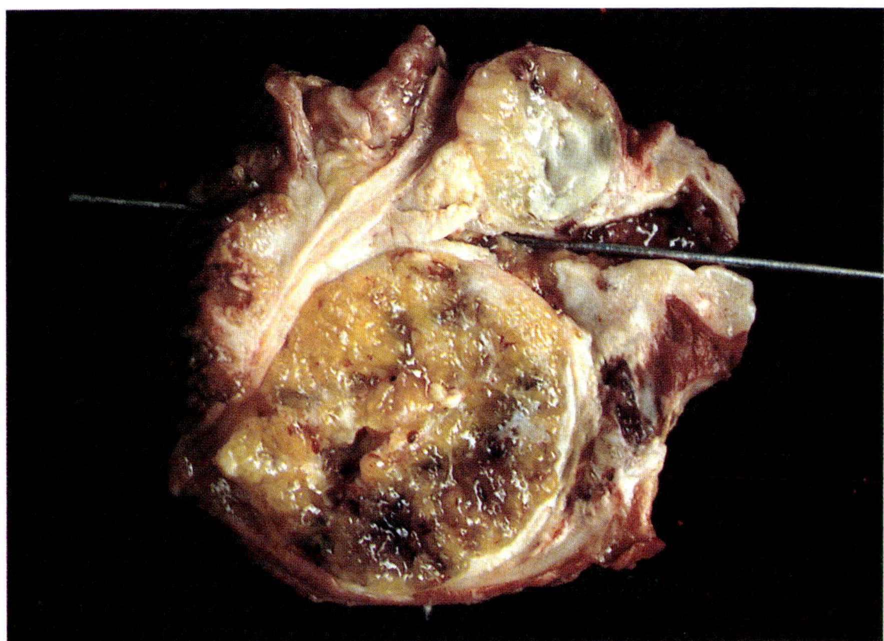

Figure 4-68
MUCINOUS NONCYSTIC ADENOCARCINOMA

The Whipple resection specimen shows a well-demarcated tumor in the head of the pancreas with a nodular pattern and a gelatinous cut surface. The probe indicates the pancreatic duct which runs into the minor papilla.

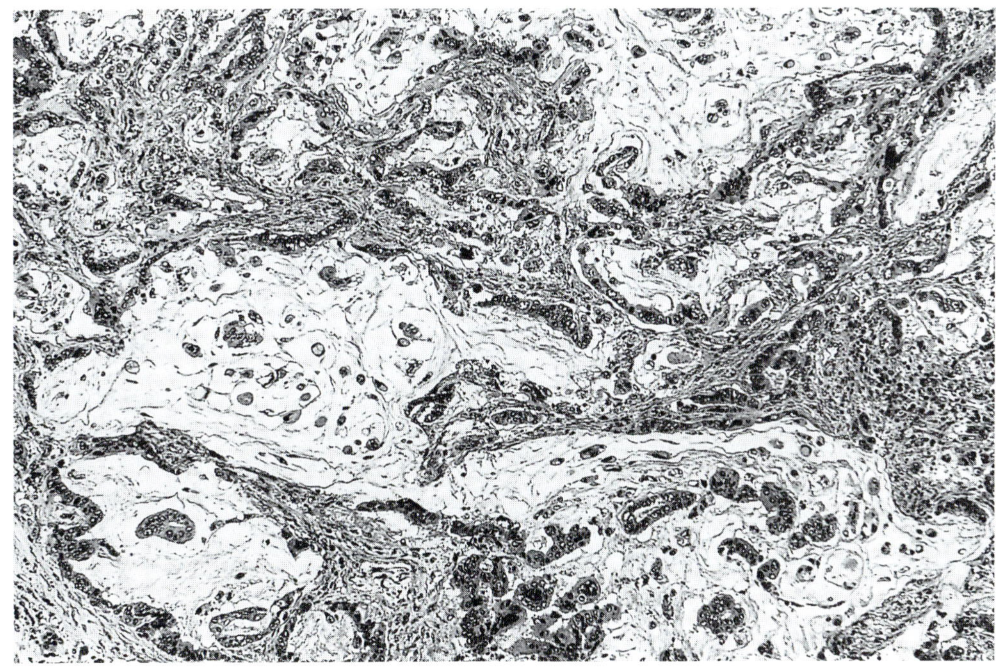

Figure 4-69
MUCINOUS NONCYSTIC ADENOCARCINOMA

This tumor shows large pools of mucin partly lined by neoplastic epithelium. Remnants of glandular tumor structures are free floating within mucin.

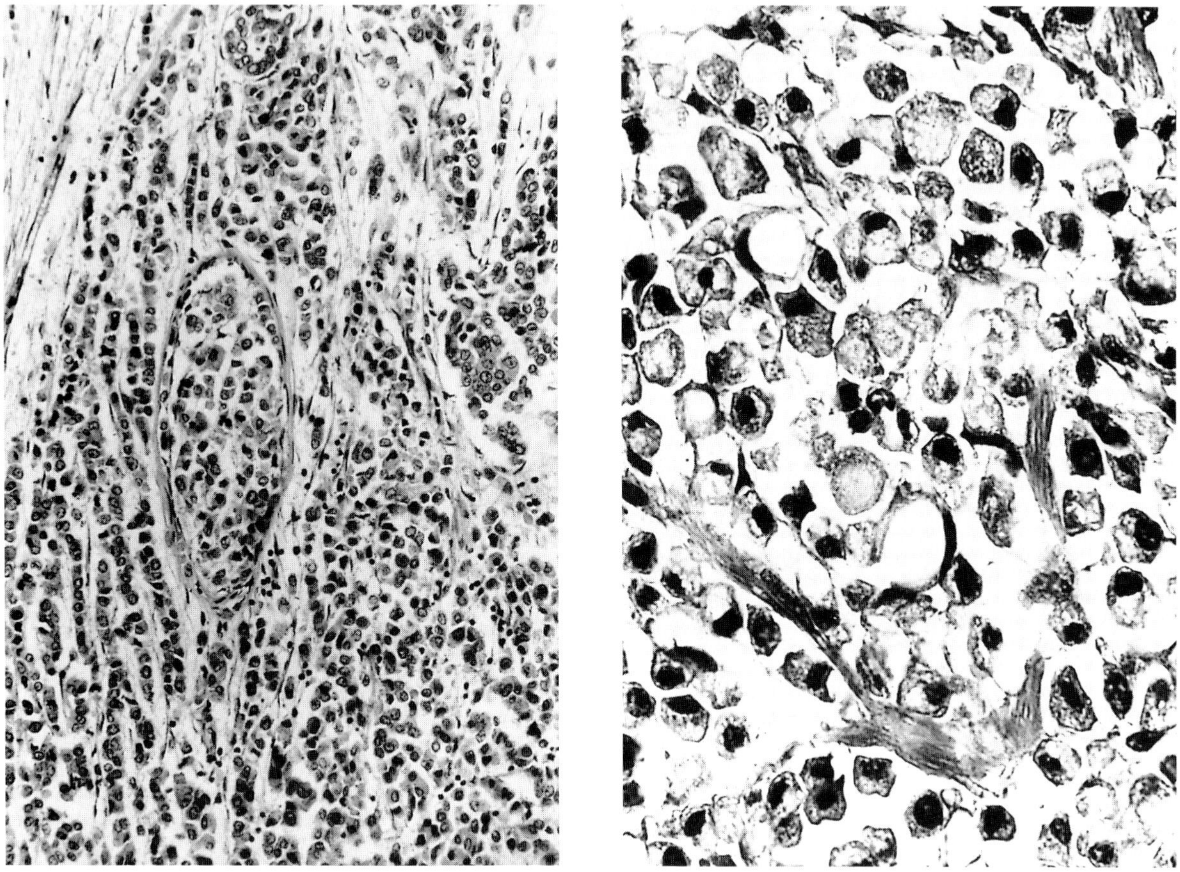

Figure 4-70
SIGNET-RING CELL CARCINOMA

Left: This tumor consists of strands of relatively small tumor cells with many signet-ring cells admixed. Right: Collection of typical signet-ring cells.

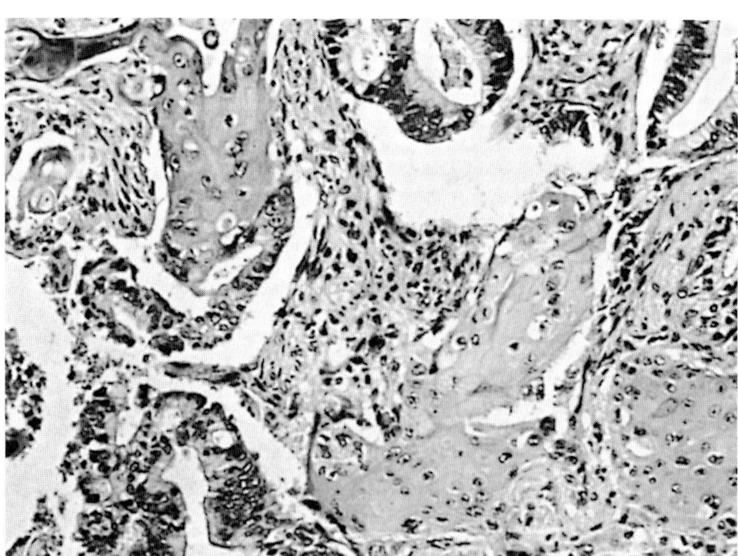

Figure 4-71
ADENOSQUAMOUS CARCINOMA

Mixture of adenocarcinoma and squamous carcinoma. (Fig. 159 from Fascicle 19, Second Series.)

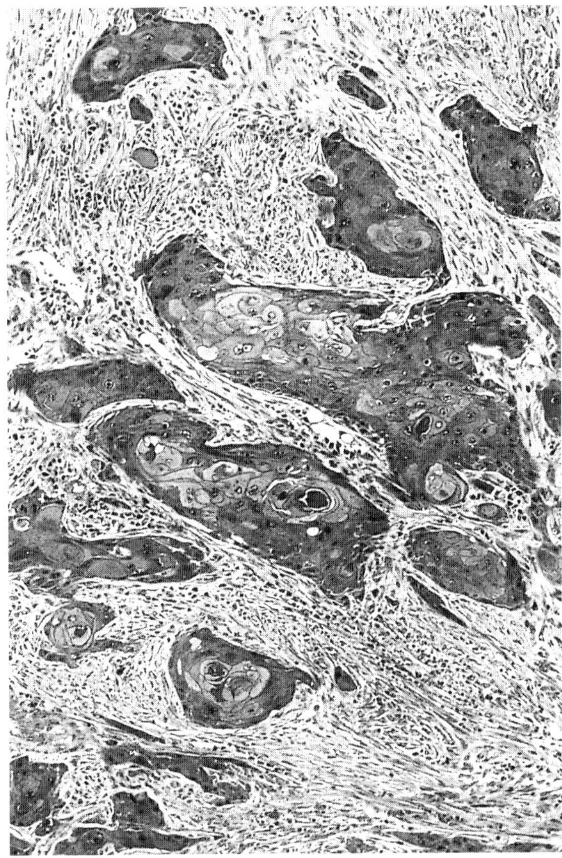

Figure 4-72
ADENOSQUAMOUS CARCINOMA
This tumor exhibits areas with pure squamous differentiation.

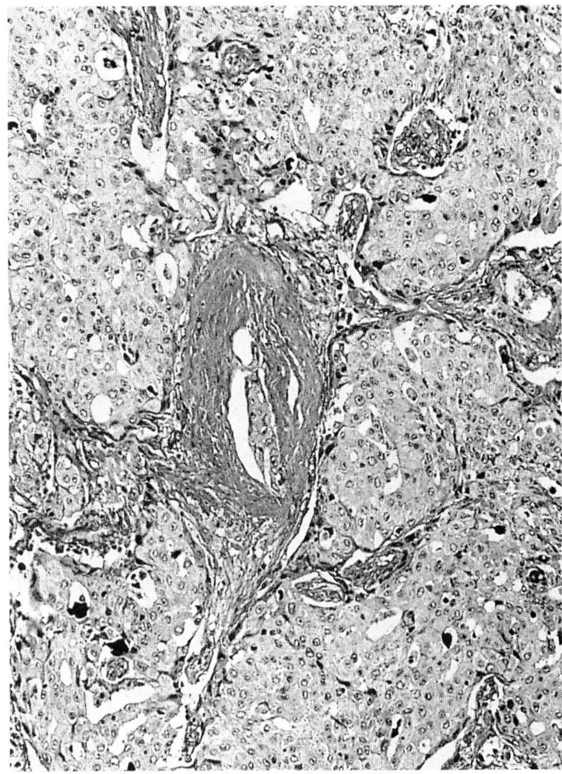

Figure 4-73
ADENOSQUAMOUS CARCINOMA
This tumor displays areas with an intimate intermingling of glandular and squamoid components, forming a mucoepidermoid pattern.

Microscopically, variably differentiated ductal structures are admixed with solid squamoid cell complexes or typical squamous elements (fig. 4-72). The squamous components are arranged in solid sheets with intercellular bridges. If well differentiated, they may contain keratohyaline granules and occasional squamous pearls. The glandular component, which produces mucin, is usually moderately or poorly differentiated. In areas with an intimate intermingling of glandular and squamoid components the tumor displays a mucoepidermoid pattern (fig. 4-73). The existence of pure squamous cell carcinomas has been doubted, since extensive sampling of tissue from carcinomas with squamous patterns usually reveals some foci of tumor glands (205). In metastases, the adenocarcinoma component is usually the only pattern present. Immunohistochemically, the tumor cells are positive for cytokeratins and CEA. While CEA is present predominantly in the duct-like elements, the squamous components stain for cytokeratin 13, in addition to cytokeratins 7, 8, 18, and 19 (fig. 4-74). Electron microscopically, intracytoplasmic aggregates of tonofibrils with desmosomal attachments have been described in the squamous cells (173,267).

## Undifferentiated (Anaplastic) Carcinoma

Most of these uncommon tumors (relative frequency, 2 to 7 percent) are composed of large undifferentiated cells showing extreme anaplasia; a few tumors predominantly have a spindle cell pattern (146,173,179,218,288,300). Other terms for this tumor include *giant cell carcinoma, pleomorphic large cell carcinoma,* and *sarcomatoid carcinoma.*

In age and sex distribution undifferentiated carcinoma is similar to ductal adenocarcinoma.

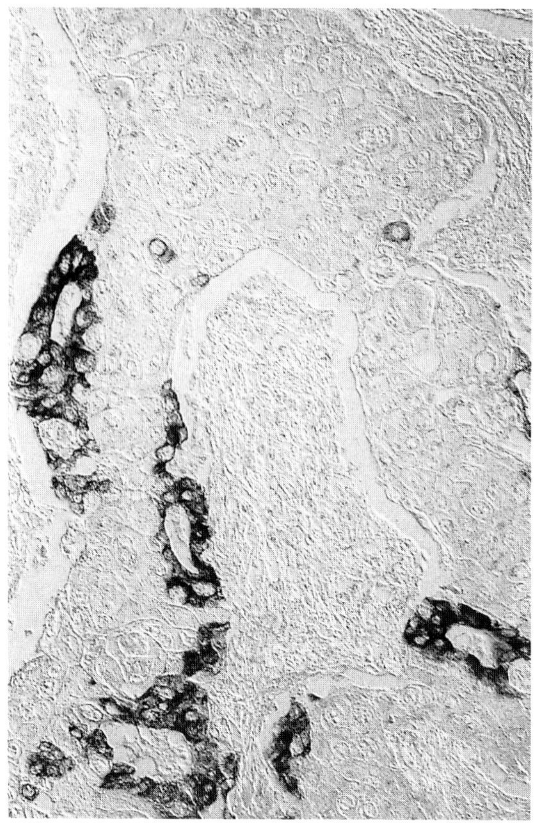
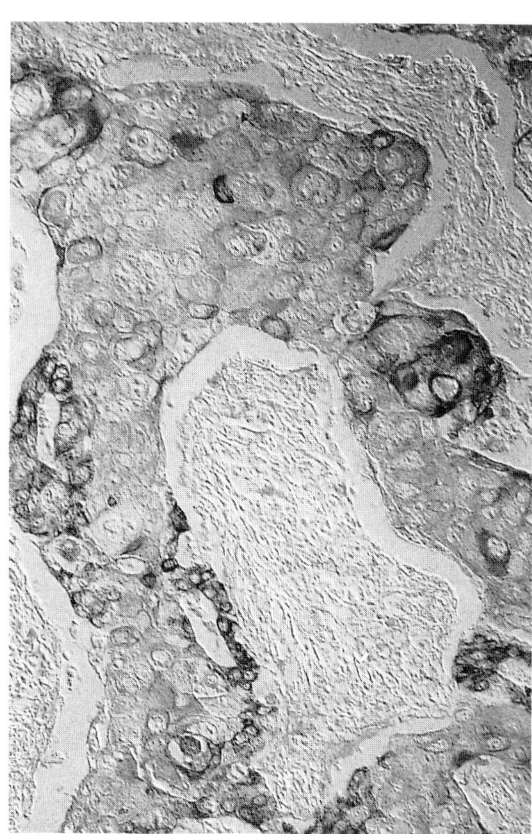

Figure 4-74
ADENOSQUAMOUS CARCINOMA
Left: Immunostaining for the keratin marker CAM5.2 reveals cytokeratins 8 and 18 in the glandular components (Nomarski optic).
Right: Immunostaining for cytokeratin 13 labels the squamoid components (Nomarski optic).

The tumors arise, however, somewhat more frequently in the body and tail than in the head of the pancreas. They present as large masses (range, 3 to 15 cm; average, 6 cm) of soft consistency, usually displaying necrosis and hemorrhage (fig. 4-75). At the time of diagnosis many patients already have widespread metastatic disease. The prognosis is extremely poor.

Microscopically, some tumors display a pleomorphic large cell pattern and others exhibit a spindle cell pattern. The pleomorphic large cell pattern is characterized by mononucleated or multinucleated giant cells growing in poorly cohesive, sarcomatoid formations, supported by scanty fibrous tissue (fig. 4-76). The cells have large, often bizarre nuclei and an eosinophilic cytoplasm. Occasionally, there is engulfment of red blood cells or other tumor cells ("cell cannibalism") (fig. 4-77). Tumors consisting predominantly of spindle cells (fig. 4-78) may also contain areas of squamoid differentiation (179). High mitotic rates as well as perineural, lymphatic, and blood vessel invasion are found in almost all cases of undifferentiated carcinoma. Although the pleomorphic pattern simulates a sarcoma, particularly malignant fibrous histiocytoma, anaplastic carcinomas appear to derive from duct cells, because foci of glandular differentiation are found in almost all of these tumors after extensive sampling (fig. 4-79). The epithelial nature of the pleomorphic cells is revealed by immunohistochemical demonstration of cytokeratins (fig. 4-80). The keratin-positive cells may also coexpress vimentin. CEA, which decorates the glandular components, is absent from the pleomorphic elements (fig. 4-81). Electron microscopy reveals microvilli and mucin granules in some of the tumors (173). Undifferentiated

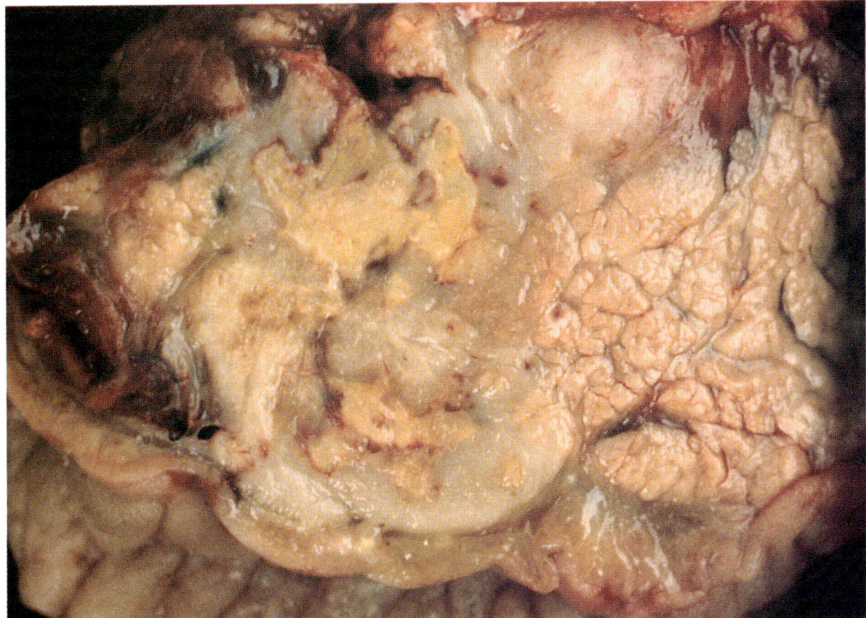

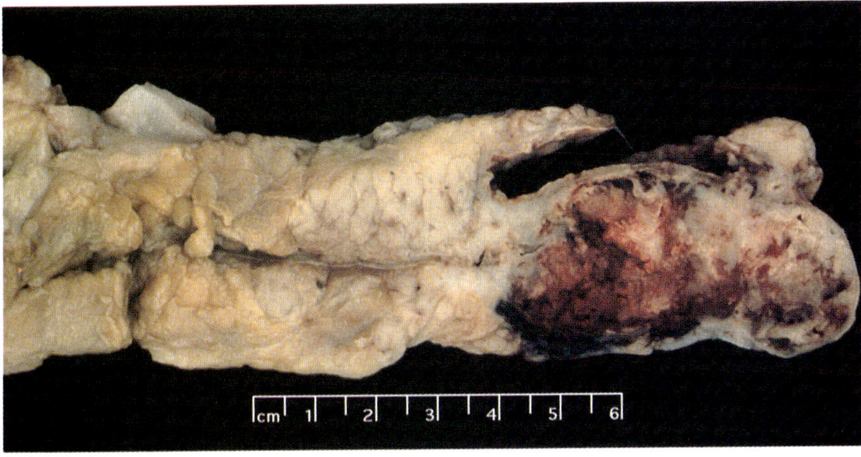


Figure 4-75
UNDIFFERENTIATED CARCINOMA

Top: The Whipple resection specimen shows an ill-demarcated tumor in the head of the pancreas with large areas of central necrosis (yellow areas).

Bottom: Tumor mass in the tail of the pancreas with extensive hemorrhagic necrosis.

carcinomas with a neoplastic mesenchymal component (carcinosarcoma) have so far not been described. Anaplastic pancreatic tumors containing osteoclast-like giant cells (278) are dealt with in a separate chapter.

Undifferentiated carcinomas have to be distinguished from metastases from amelanotic melanoma (S-100 positivity), pleomorphic rhabdomyosarcoma (desmin and/or actin positivity), pleomorphic sarcomas (vimentin positivity in the absence of cytokeratin positivity), and choriocarcinoma (human choriogonadotropin beta positivity). Distinction from a metastasis from large cell lung carcinoma may be very difficult or even impossible.

## Mixed Ductal-Endocrine Carcinoma

Mixed ductal-endocrine carcinoma of the pancreas is a malignant epithelial neoplasm in which the ductal and endocrine cells are intimately admixed in the primary tumor as well as in its metastases, and the endocrine cells comprise at least one third to half of the tumor tissue (235). The ductal differentiation is defined by mucin production and the presence of a duct type marker such as CEA. The endocrine cells are characterized by the presence of general endocrine markers and hormonal products (see chapter on Normal Histology for a discussion of markers). The existence of these tumors suggests that

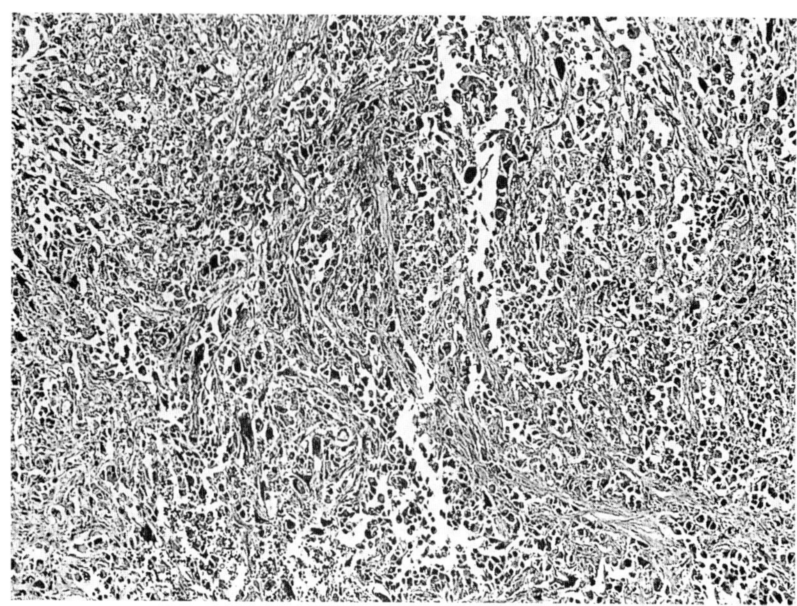

Figure 4-76
UNDIFFERENTIATED (ANAPLASTIC) CARCINOMA

Microscopically, undifferentiated (anaplastic) carcinoma with a pleomorphic large cell pattern exhibits mononucleated or multinucleated giant cells growing in poorly cohesive, sarcomatoid formations and supported by scanty fibrous tissue.

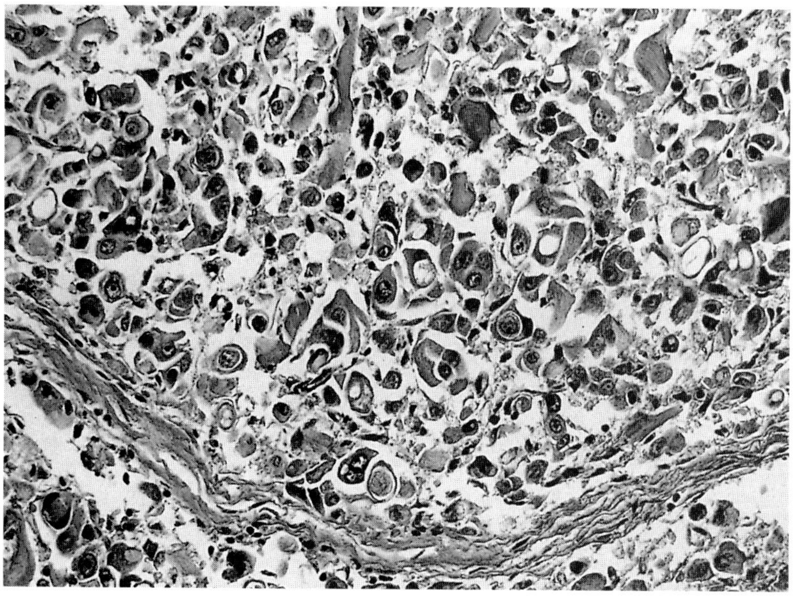

Figure 4-77
UNDIFFERENTIATED (ANAPLASTIC) CARCINOMA

The tumor cells show occasional engulfment of red blood cells or other tumor cells (cell cannibalism).

neoplastic cells of the pancreas may, in principle, have the potential for dual (ductal and endocrine) differentiation, reflecting the common embryologic origin of the two components of the pancreas. Biologically, mixed carcinoma behaves like usual ductal adenocarcinoma. Acinar cell carcinomas (201,283,305), pancreatoblastoma (202) with some endocrine and ductal elements, and endocrine tumors with ductal components (264,277,296) are not discussed here because their behavior is dictated by the acinar and endocrine elements.

Mixed ductal-endocrine carcinoma is also referred to as *mixed carcinoid-adenocarcinoma, mucinous carcinoid tumor* (173), or simply *mixed exocrine-endocrine tumor* (184). However, as the term mixed exocrine-endocrine carcinoma in principle comprises all tumors with a dual exocrine and endocrine differentiation and thus also includes tumors with acinar and endocrine elements, it is more accurate to designate a carcinoma showing ductal as well as endocrine differentiation as mixed ductal-endocrine carcinoma.

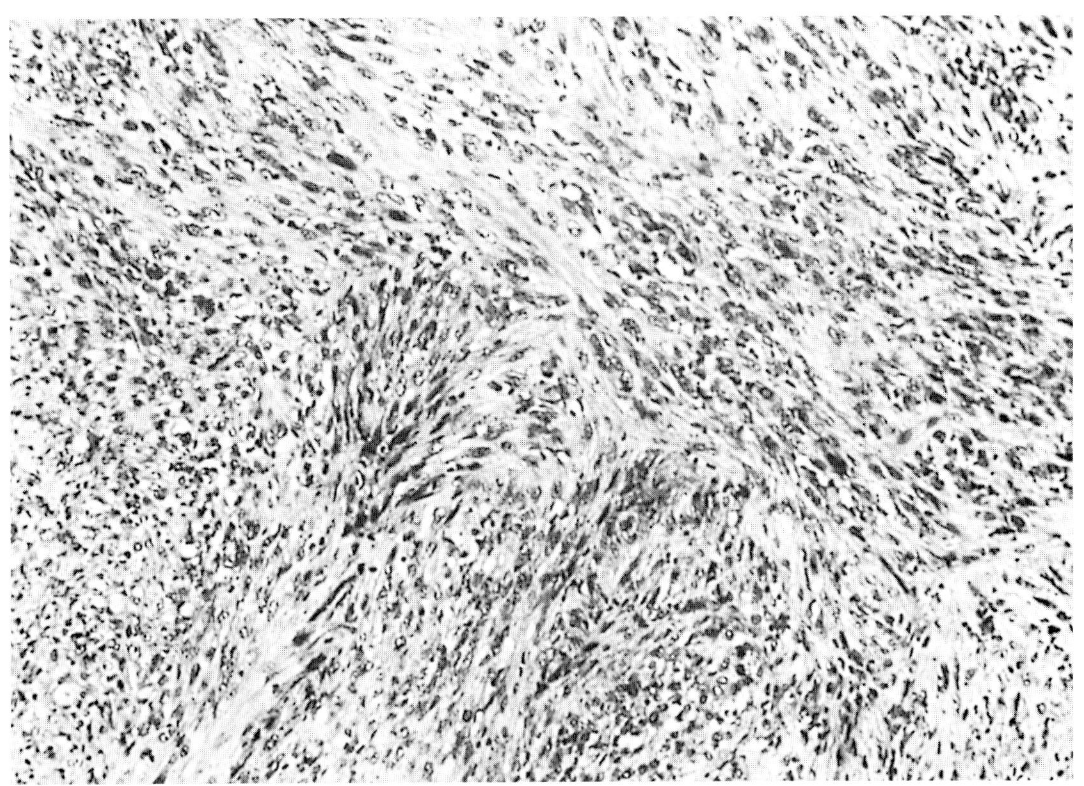

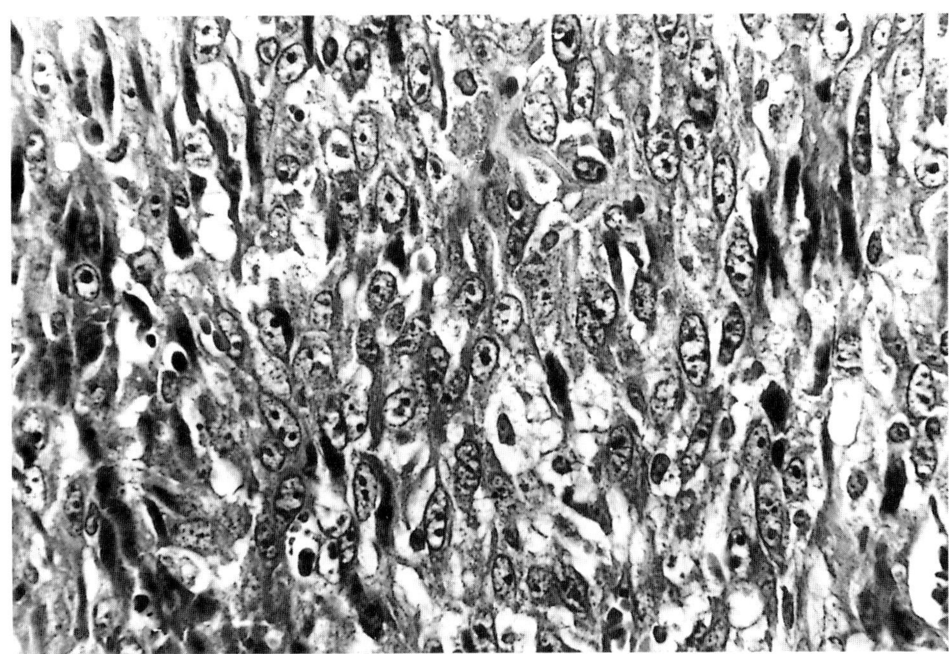

Figure 4-78
UNDIFFERENTIATED (ANAPLASTIC) CARCINOMA

Top: Spindle cell sarcomatoid features, present in this area, were noted in about 50 percent of the tissue of this neoplasm. The rest was adenosquamous carcinoma. (Fig. 164 from Fascicle 19, Second Series.)

Bottom: This tumor consists predominantly of spindle cells.

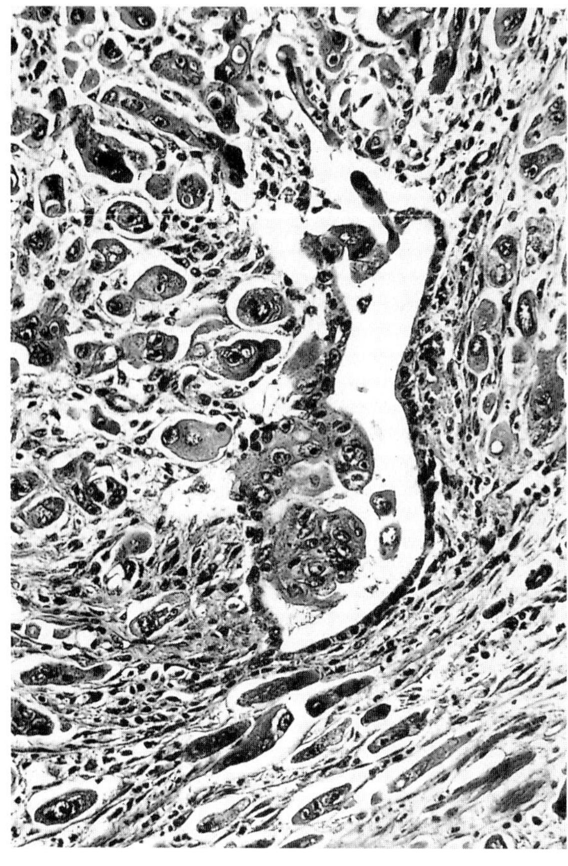

Figure 4-79
UNDIFFERENTIATED (ANAPLASTIC) CARCINOMA
This tumor shows a focus of glandular differentiation within a sarcomatoid pattern.

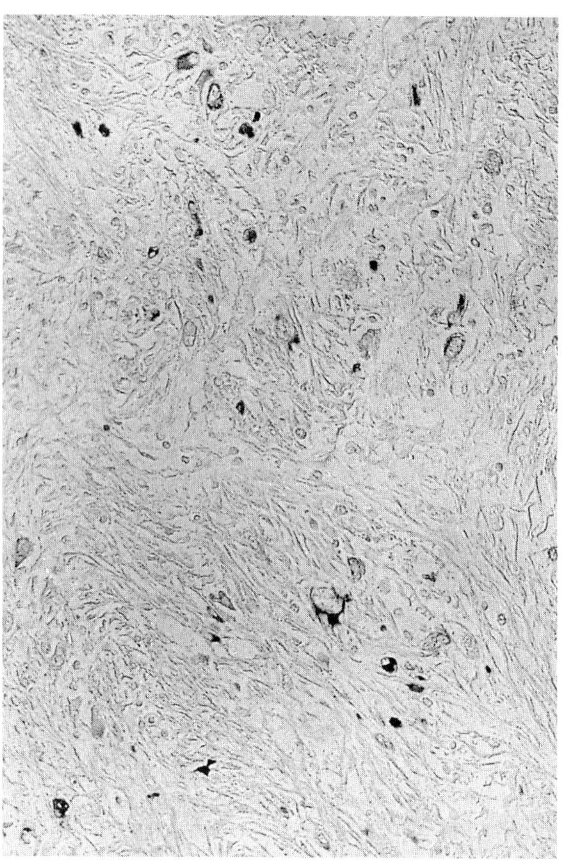

Figure 4-80
UNDIFFEBENTIATED (ANAPLASTIC) CARCINOMA
Immunostaining for cytokeratin reveals the epithelial nature of the pleomorphic tumor cells.

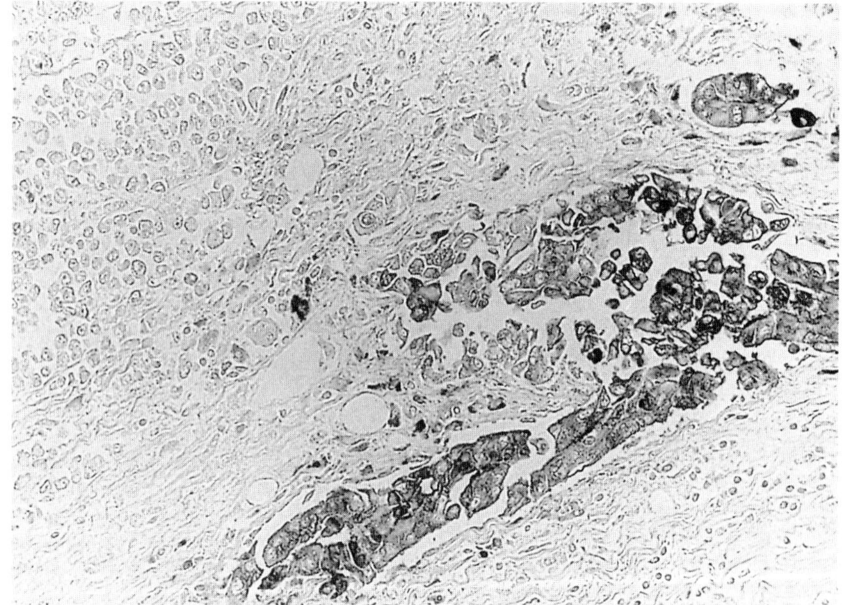

Figure 4-81
UNDIFFERENTIATED (ANAPLASTIC) CARCINOMA
Tumor with positive immunostaining for CEA in the glandular components of the tumor. Pleomorphic cells remain unstained.

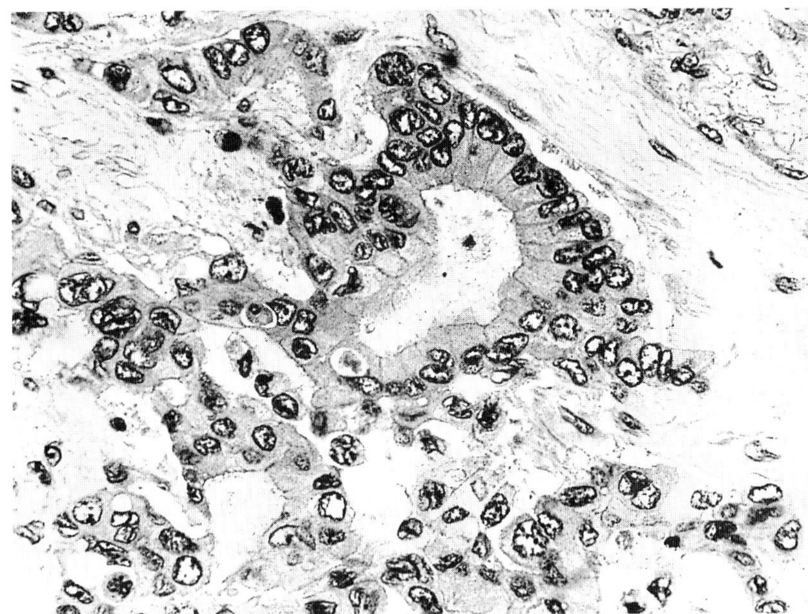

Figure 4-82
MIXED DUCTAL-ENDOCRINE CARCINOMA
This tumor shows features of a rather poorly differentiated adenocarcinoma. (Figures 4-82 and 4-83 are from the same patient.)

Tumors that are composed of two topographically separate components (i.e., collision tumors) are by definition not included in the mixed ductal-endocrine category.

Mixed ductal-endocrine carcinomas are exceptionally rare in the pancreas: only two examples, reported by Eusebi et al. (184) and Sessa et al. (285) appear to fulfill the criteria given above. In both patients, who were 65 and 62 years old, the tumors formed solid masses to the head of the pancreas and metastasized to the liver. Microscopically, moderately differentiated ductal adenocarcinoma structures were found intimately intermingled with more solid areas. Using histochemistry, immunohistochemistry, and electron microscopy, mucin-producing and neuroendocrine cells were demonstrated in the primary tumor as well as the metastases. An interesting feature in Eusebi's case (included in the series studied by Chejfec et al. [167]) was the presence of single tumor cells displaying both neuroendocrine granules as well as mucinous vesicles. Cells with dual differentiation are called amphicrine cells. Amphicrine cells displaying mucin as well as hormone production were present in a case of metastasizing mixed carcinoma of the pancreas that was observed in Brussels (275). The patient, an 84-year-old woman, presented with obstructive jaundice because of a tumor in the head of the pancreas. Histologically, this tumor was composed of poorly differentiated glands and more solid cell clusters supported by a dense stroma (figs. 4-82, 4-83). The tumor was not associated with an endocrine syndrome, but produced and secreted somatostatin. Recently, a pancreatic exocrine carcinoma producing ACTH was reported (196). However, from the morphologic description and illustration it is difficult to tell whether this tumor fulfills all the criteria of a mixed ductal-endocrine carcinoma.

Mixed ductal-endocrine carcinomas should be separated from ductal adenocarcinomas with scattered endocrine cells associated with neoplastic glands. Scattered endocrine cells have been reported in 40 to 80 percent of ductal adenocarcinomas (160,170,184,226,272,289). They seem to be particularly frequent in well-differentiated tumors where they are either lined up along the base of the neoplastic ductal structures or lie between the neoplastic columnar cells (fig. 4-84). Immunohistochemically, all four islet hormones as well as amylin (IAPP), serotonin, and occasionally gastrin have been identified in these cells. In the dorsal head region of the pancreas, which is rich in pancreatic polypeptide (PP) cells, most of the tumor-associated endocrine cells produce PP (fig. 4-85) (160). Scattered endocrine cells in ductal adenocarcinomas might be neoplastic considering their close association

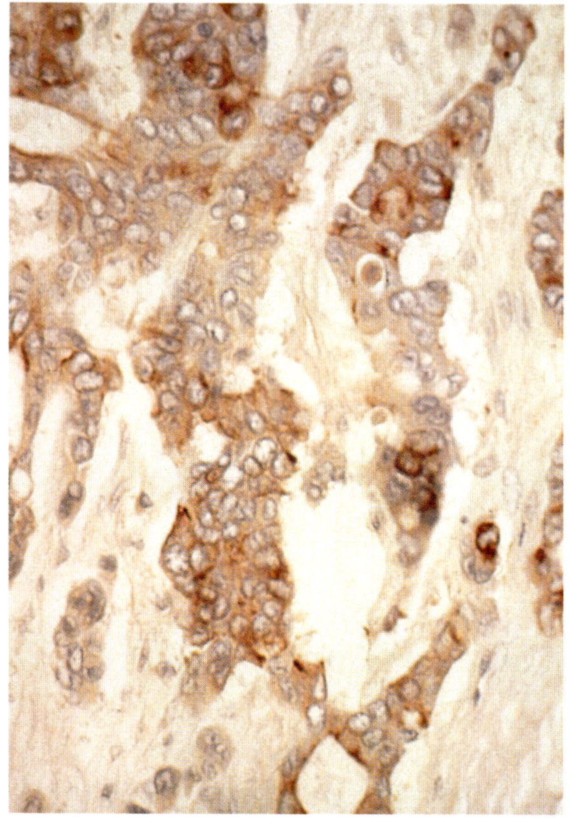

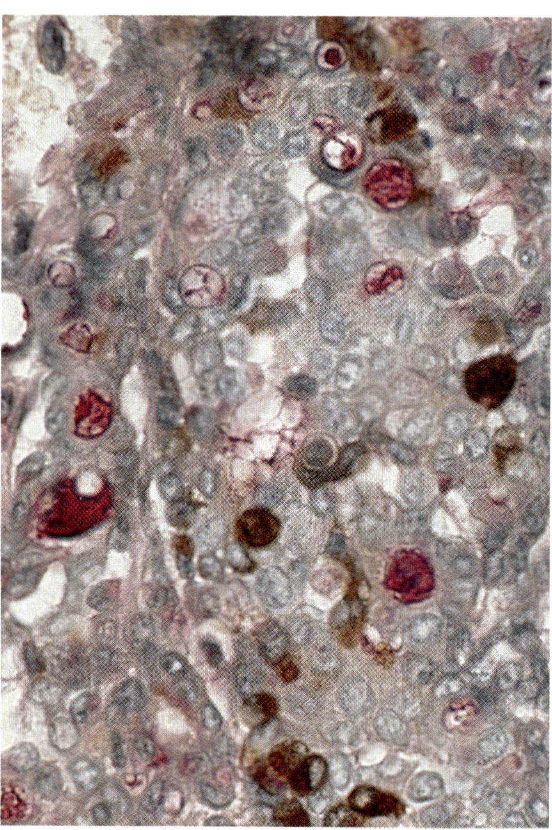

Figure 4-83
MIXED DUCTAL-ENDOCRINE CARCINOMA

Left: Immunostaining reveals numerous unevenly distributed somatostatin-positive tumor cells.
Right: Immunostaining for somatostatin (brown) combined with PAS diastase-resistent staining (purple) reveals the intimate admixture of hormone- and mucin-producing tumor cells.

with neoplastic glands. Usually, however, the metastases from such tumors lack the endocrine cell population seen in the primary tumor. At least in part, these cells may represent non-neoplastic rather than true neoplastic endocrine cells. It may be possible that growth and arrangement of endocrine cells in the vicinity of tumor cells may be influenced by factors released by the neoplastic cells.

## Other Rare Carcinomas

Other very rare carcinomas of probable ductal phenotype include *clear cell carcinoma* and *ciliated cell carcinoma*. Clear cell carcinomas resembling renal cell carcinoma have been described by Cubilla and Fitzgerald (173) and Kanai et al. (209). The glycogen-rich cells are arranged in nests and sheets. A few of these cells also contain mucin. Foci of mucin-producing cells are useful in distinguishing these tumors from metastatic carcinoma from kidney, adrenal gland, or liver (294). A clear cell change is occasional in ductal adenocarcinomas or anaplastic carcinomas (306).

Ciliated cell carcinomas have been described by Sommers and Meissner (288) and Morinaga et al. (255). Microscopically, these tumors show the pattern of a ductal adenocarcinoma, but contain many ciliated cells, as demonstrated by electron microscopy in Morinaga's case.

Carcinomas distinguished by a microglandular pattern as described by Cubilla and Fitzgerald (173) most likely do not represent a separate entity but today may be classified with the use of immunohistochemical markers either as acinar cell carcinoma or endocrine tumor. Oncocytic carcinoma and choriocarcinoma are discussed in the chapter on Miscellaneous Carcinomas.

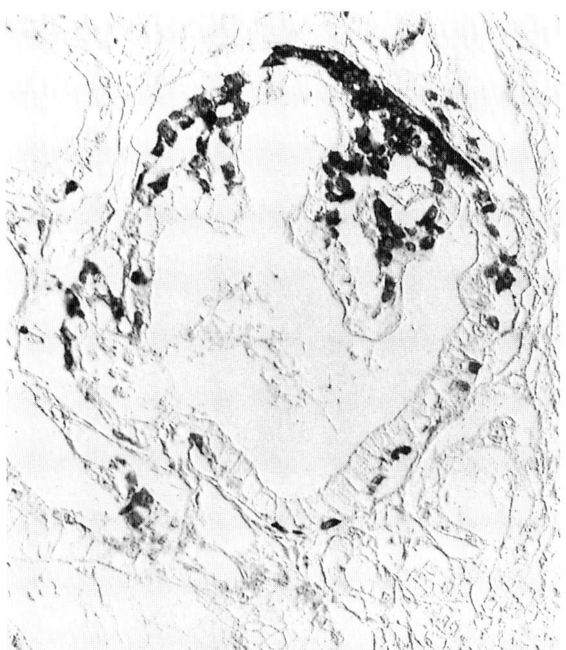

Figure 4-84
DUCTAL ADENOCARCINOMA WITH ASSOCIATED ENDOCRINE CELLS
Well-differentiated adenocarcinoma with endocrine cells immunostained for synaptophysin. The endocrine cells are either lined up along the base of the neoplastic ductal structures or lie between the neoplastic columnar cells (Nomarski optic).

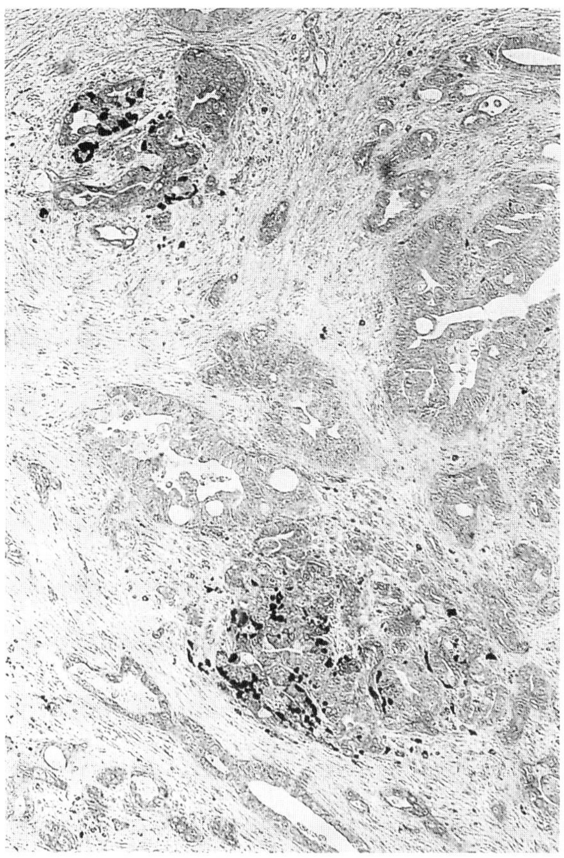

Figure 4-85
DUCTAL ADENOCARCINOMA WITH ASSOCIATED ENDOCRINE CELLS
Ductal adenocarcinoma occurring in the pancreatic polypeptide (PP)-rich head region of the pancreas shows abundant tumor-associated endocrine cells that immunostain for PP.

## OSTEOCLAST-LIKE GIANT CELL TUMOR

**Definition.** This tumor is composed of proliferating undifferentiated epithelial or mesenchymal cells admixed with non-neoplastic osteoclast-like giant cells. Thebe may be a ductal adenocarcinoma component and an association with a mucinous cystic tumor.

**General Features.** This rare tumor closely resembles giant cell tumor of bone and has also been observed in many other organs. In the pancreas at least 21 cases have so far been described in detail (317,322). Mean patient age is 60 years but there is a wide age range from 32 to 82 years. Women are more frequently affected than men. The main symptoms are abdominal pain, weight loss, jaundice, and a palpable mass.

**Gross Findings.** Most tumors occur in the head of the pancreas, and present as relatively large (greatest diameter, 5 to 8 cm) masses with a rubbery firm consistency and a lobulated whitish yellow and focally necrotic cut surface. Gross invasion into adjacent organs is common, but metastatic spread is found in only 50 percent of patients at the time of diagnosis.

**Microscopic Findings.** The tumors are composed of two cell populations: a neoplastic and a non-neoplastic population. The neoplastic cells are spindle shaped to ovoid and vary in size. The cytoplasm is faintly eosinophilic and contains a large, irregularly shaped, hyperchromatic nucleus with a distinct nucleolus. Mitotic activity is high and atypical mitotic figures are frequent. Intermixed with these proliferating cells are non-neoplastic, multinucleated (more than 20 uniformly small nuclei), osteoclast-like giant cells (fig. 4-86). These cells show no mitotic activity. In addition, there may be foci of osteoid formation (fig. 4-87) and entrapped normal ducts.

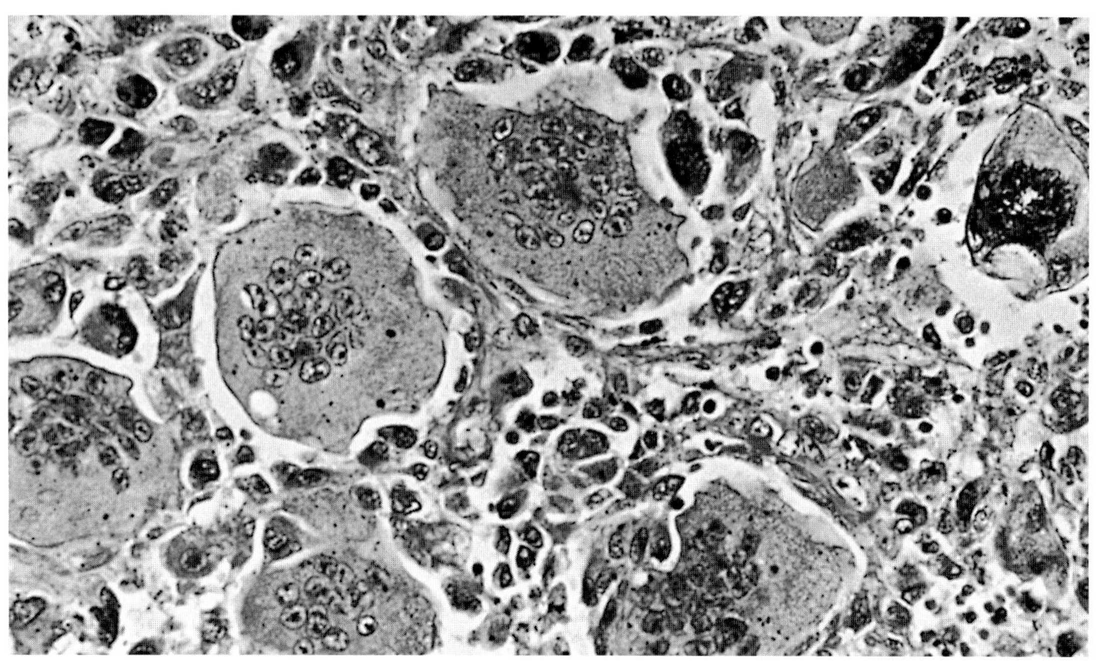

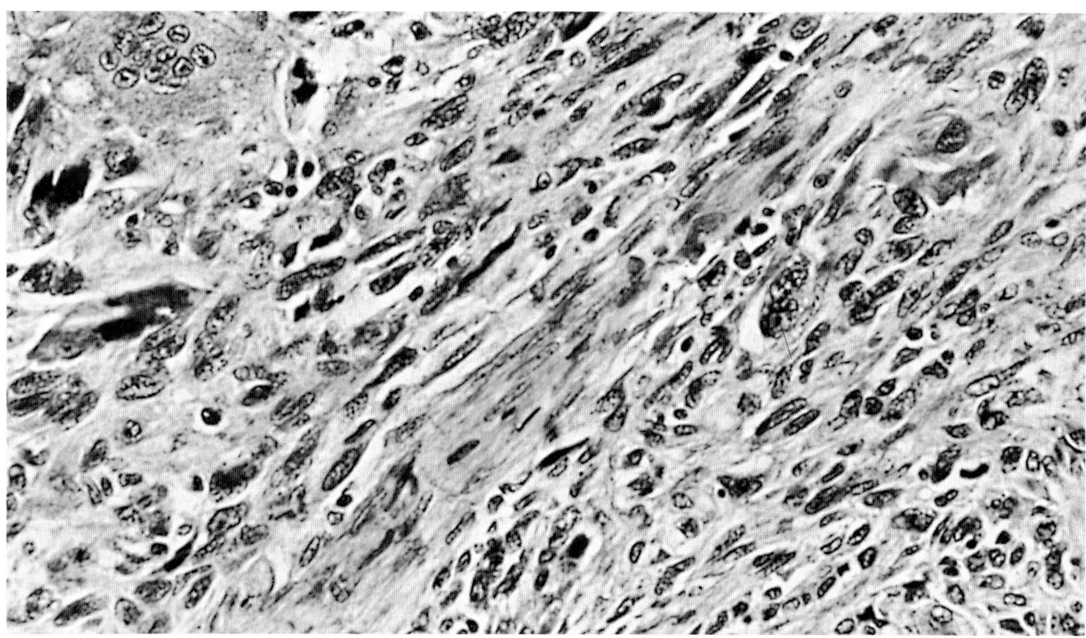

Figure 4-86
OSTEOCLAST-LIKE GIANT CELL TUMOR

Top: Osteoclast-like giant cells and bizarre tumor giant cells are mixed with a few spindle and smaller pleomorphic cells. The osteoclast-like cells are relatively uniformly nucleated, and each nucleus has little chromatin and one small distinct nucleolus. (Fig. 152 from Fascicle 19, Second Series.)

Bottom: Elongated spindle cells vary from those with small cell nuclei and relatively little chromatin to cells containing much chromatin. An osteoclast-like giant cell can be seen in the upper left corner. (Fig. 153 from Fascicle 19, Second Series.)

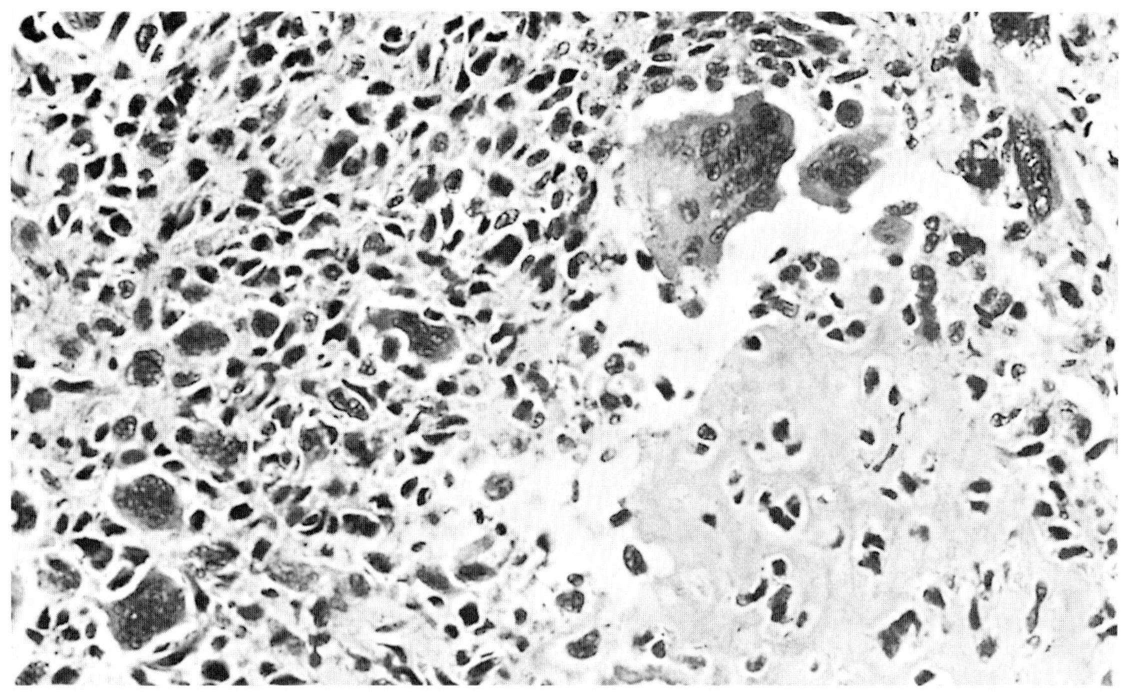

Figure 4-87
OSTEOCLAST-LIKE GIANT CELL TUMOR
Osteoid formation (lower right) with a few osteoclast-like giant cells. Dispersed throughout most of the tissue on the left side are many small, pleomorphic, mononucleated cells. (Fig. 154 from Fascicle 19, Second Series.)

Some tumors also contain areas of ductal adenocarcinoma (fig. 4-88) (316,318,321,326), while others lack neoplastic glands (324,325). Goldberg et al. (319) observed hyperplasia and epithelial atypia in the main pancreatic duct adjacent to the tumor. The osteoclast-like giant cell tumors reported by Mentes and Posen (320, 323) and the one observed by us (Zamboni G. et al., unpublished observation, 1996) were present in the wall of a mucinous cystadenocarcinoma.

**Immunohistologic and Ultrastructural Findings.** Conflicting opinions exist with respect to tumor origin. Originally it was thought to be of epithelial origin (324). This assumption was based on electron microscopic findings, such as presence of microvilli, desmosomes, and zymogen-like granules, and was later corroborated by immunohistochemical data showing positivity for keratin in the mononuclear tumor cells (322) and occasionally also in the osteoclast-like giant cells (315). However, there are also a number of reports on the demonstration of vimentin (in the absence of keratin and ultrastructural features of epithelial cells) in the mononuclear polygonal cells and the osteoclast-like cells (317, 319,321,325). Osteoclast-like cells stain for a macrophage marker (EBM11) and leukocyte common antigen (fig. 4-89), but not for HLA-DR and lysozyme. This antigenic profile suggests that osteoclast-like giant cell tumors are of mesenchymal origin. Suster (325) therefore uses the term *malignant fibrous histiocytoma (giant cell type)* of the pancreas for these tumors. The same authors, after reviewing the literature, also discuss the possibility that osteoclast-like giant cell tumors may show a spectrum of cell differentiation that includes epithelial features at one end and nonepithelial features at the other end.

**Prognosis.** Early reports on this tumor suggest that the prognosis is more favorable than for usual ductal adenocarcinoma (316). Whether this applies to all osteoclast-like giant cell tumors is so far not known. In one of the most recent reports, survival for 11 patients was 12 months (317). However, survival up to 15 years has also been reported (317).

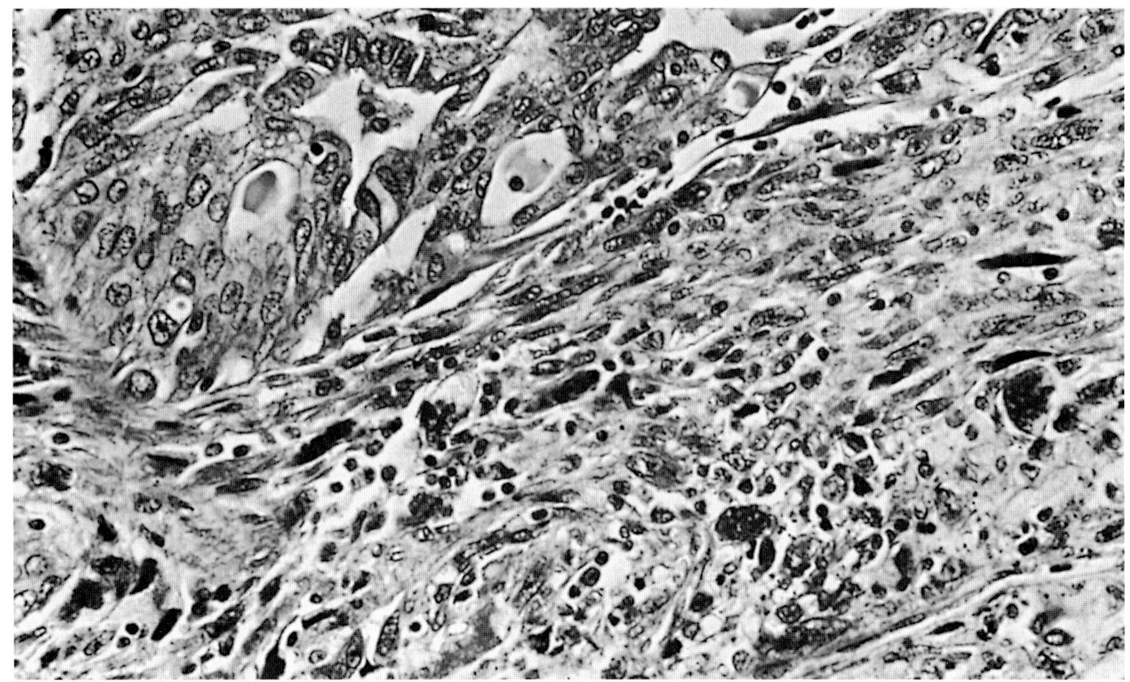

Figure 4-88
OSTEOCLAST-LIKE GIANT CELL TUMOR

Rare small focus of adenocarcinoma in one of the sections of a giant cell tumor of osteoclastoid type. (Fig. 155 from Fascicle 19, Second Series.)

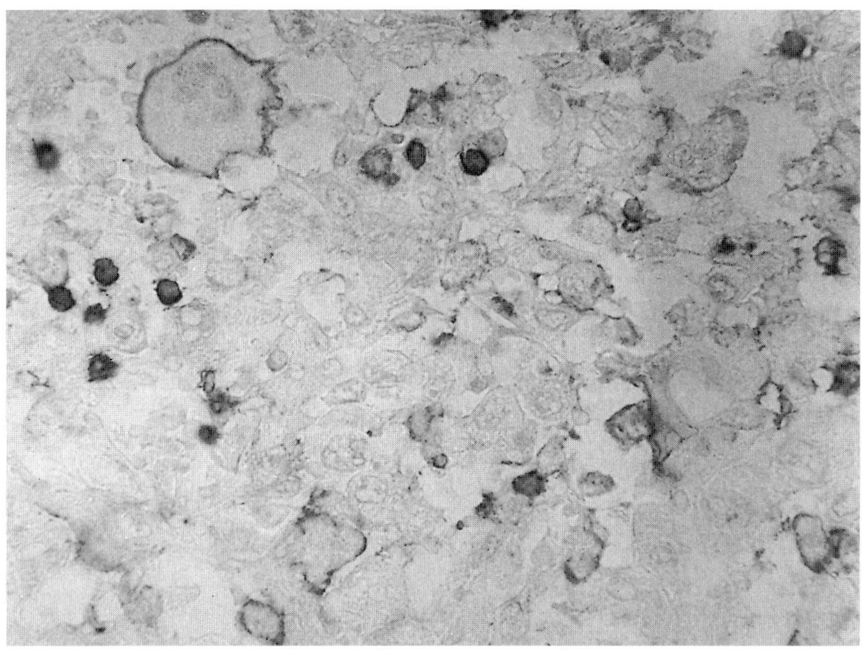

Figure 4-89
OSTEOCLAST-LIKE GIANT CELL TUMOR

Immunostaining for leukocyte common antigen (LCA) labels the cell membranes of osteoclast-like giant cells. In addition, there is cytoplasmic labeling of non-neoplastic macrophages and lymphocytes between nonlabeled tumor cells.

## ACINAR CELL CARCINOMA

**Definition.** This is an epithelial tumor showing evidence of acinar cell differentiation and an occasional endocrine cell component. In approximately 15 percent of patients, the tumor produces a syndrome characterized by polyarthralgia, extrapancreatic fat necrosis, and eosinophilia (355,369,380). These tumors have also been referred to as *acinic cell carcinoma* and *acinous cell carcinoma* of the pancreas.

**General Features.** Acinar cell carcinoma is an uncommon tumor, accounting for 1 to 2 percent of all exocrine pancreatic tumors (333,335,368). The incidence figures of 13 percent and 10.5 percent reported by Miller et al. (366) and Webb (395), respectively, are most likely too high because of the imprecise histologic criteria applied at that time and the lack of histochemical and immunohistochemical diagnostic confirmation.

The tumor is more frequent in males than females (ratio, 2 to 1) (345,355). Patients range in age from 3 to 90 years (360,369). If the few acinar cell carcinomas described in children and adolescents (age range, 3 to 16 years; mean, 8 years) (340,345,355,360,365,374,396) are not considered, the mean age of adult patients in the two largest series reported by Klimstra (355) and Hoorens (345) is 62 years (range, 40 to 81 years) and 55 years (range, 28 to 78 years), respectively. There seems to be no racial predominance.

The etiology of the tumor is not known. Experimentally, it can be produced in rats treated with azaserine or 4-hydroxyaminoquinolone-1-oxide (362,383). The rat pancreatic acinar cell line AR42J, one of the most widely used cell culture systems for studies of pancreatic acinar cells, is derived from a chemically induced pancreatic acinar cell carcinoma. Recently, it has been shown that this cell line combines exocrine and endocrine properties (381). Acinar cell neoplasms also develop in mice made transgenic for the activated human c-H-*ras* oncogene and SV40 tumor antigen targeted to the elastase-1 promoter/enhancer gene (377). Pancreatic neoplasms with mixed acinar and ductal features have been produced in c-*myc*-expressing transgenic mice (382).

**Clinical Features.** Patients usually present with symptoms related either to metastasis or local expansion. These symptoms are nonspecific and include abdominal pain, loss of appetite and weight, nausea, and vomiting. Jaundice is rare. Five of 7 cases reported by Cubilla and Fitzgerald (335) presented as metastases from an occult primary.

More than 30 patients have presented with a syndrome characterized by polyarthralgia-polyarthritis and disseminated (mainly subcutaneous) fat necrosis (327–331,339,342,345,348,350,355, 364,375,378,380,384,385,387,391,394,397). Some also had peripheral eosinophilia and fever (331, 380). In Klimstra's series (355), 16 percent of the patients were affected by the syndrome, while in our own series only 1 of 22 patients was affected. In most of the recently reported cases, the syndrome is associated with high serum lipase and trypsin production by the tumor (348,394), while a rise in serum alpha-amylase is rare (339,348). It is therefore likely that disseminated fat necrosis and polyarthralgia are caused by the enzymatic activity of lipase and possibly other enzymes as well. However, in a few cases there was an increase of serum lipase (as well as amylase and elastase-1) without concomitant symptoms (334,349). Two acinar cell carcinomas were associated with a myeloma-like cast nephropathy (367,379), and thrombotic endocarditis was reported in three patients (395).

Markedly elevated serum alpha-fetoprotein (AFP) levels were detected in five patients (352, 371,373). The serum levels of other tumor markers such as CEA and CA19-9 were, with a few exceptions (347,349), normal.

Ultrasonography reveals a midrange echogenic mass, with some low echogenic areas suggesting necrosis (378). A sharply demarcated mass with irregular low-density areas may be also demonstrated by CT (361).

**Gross Findings.** In adults, the tumors are well-circumscribed nodular masses with a soft consistency, evenly distributed throughout the pancreas. The cut surface reveals large, yellowish brown to red nodules, separated by fine fibrous strands and often showing necrotic foci (fig. 4-90). Occasionally the tumor has a cystic appearance (see Variants). There is no clear preferential localization, but the head appears somewhat more affected than the other parts of the pancreas. The tumors range from 2 to 30 cm (mean, 10 cm) in diameter (345,355,369). Four tumors were attached to the pancreas (345,355). Some tumors invade the surrounding tissues (duodenum, stomach, peritoneum). In children,

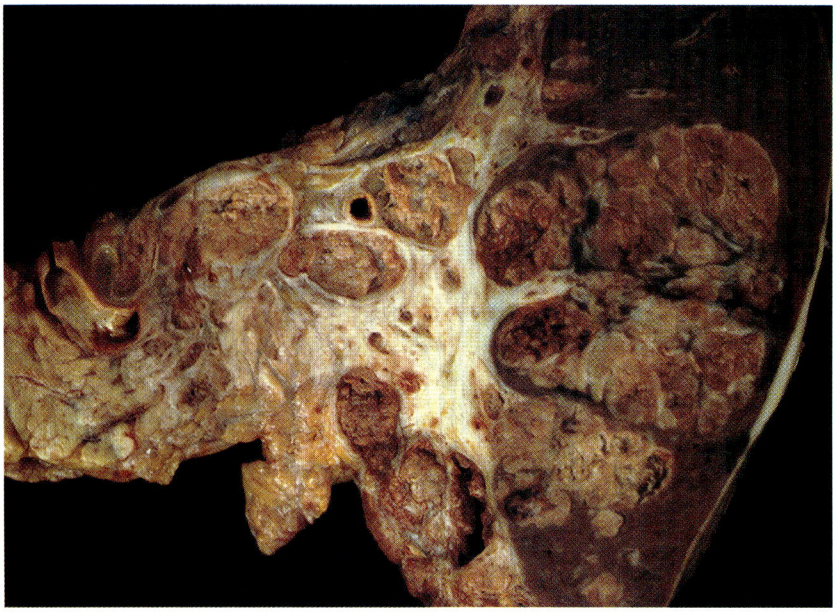

Figure 4-90
ACINAR CELL CARCINOMA
Cut surface of an acinar cell carcinoma displays large yellowish brown to red nodules, separated by fibrous strands and frequently showing necrotic foci.

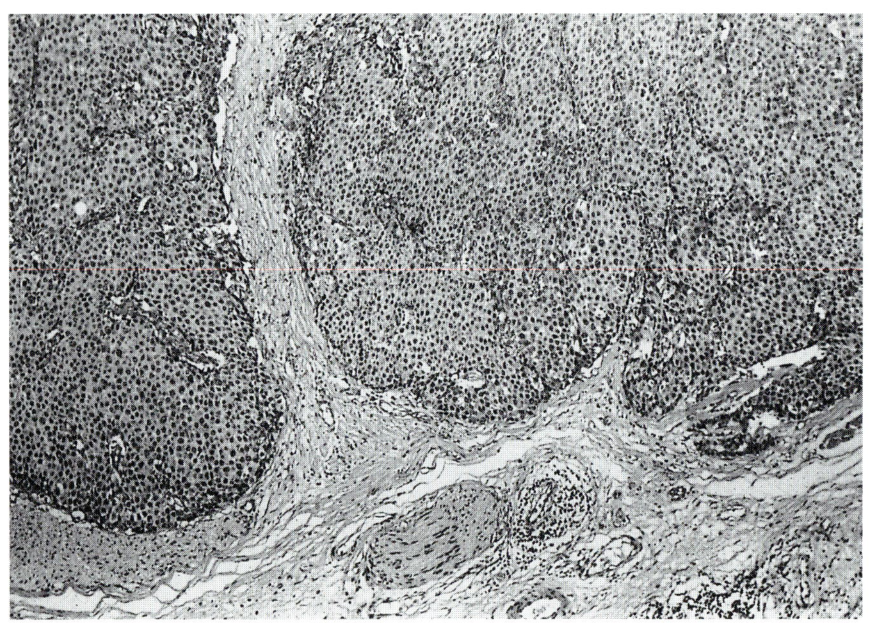

Figure 4-91
ACINAR CELL CARCINOMA
At low magnification the markedly cellular tumor tissue shows gross lobulation by broad fibrous strands. Within the large tumor lobules there is only scant stroma.

the gross appearance of the tumor is similar to that of pancreatoblastomas (355,360,365,374).

**Microscopic Findings.** In adults, features common to most tumors are a gross lobulation of markedly cellular neoplastic tissue by fibrous strands; scanty stroma within the large tumor lobules (fig. 4-91); broad nodular tumor invasion into adjacent pancreatic tissue, the spleen, the mesentery, or the duodenum; and frequent vascular invasion.

In most tumors, acinar areas alternate with trabecular and solid formations (fig. 4-92). The uniform tumor cells are rich in granular cytoplasm and are faintly positive with diastase-resistent PAS. The nuclei are irregular in size, but are usually locally polarized in the cytoplasm (fig. 4-93). Generally, there is more than 1 mitosis per 10 high-power fields. Mucin stains are negative.

A few tumors have a purely acinar pattern, reminiscent of normal pancreatic acinar tissue

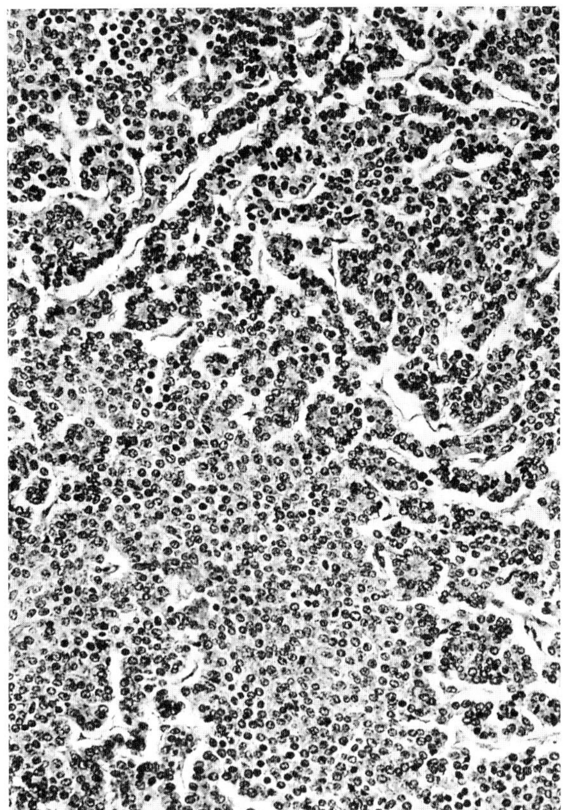

Figure 4-92
ACINAR CELL CARCINOMA
This tumor shows a mixed pattern, with acinar areas alternating with trabecular and solid formations.

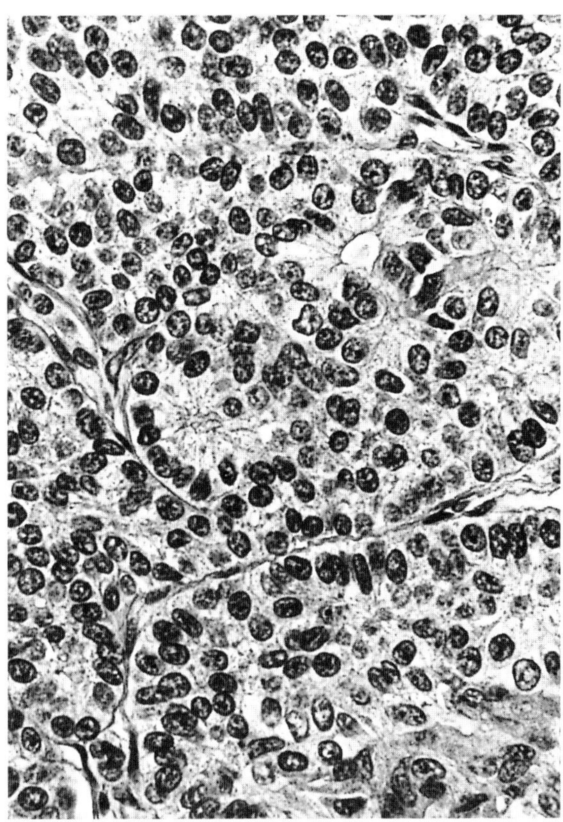

Figure 4-93
ACINAR CELL CARCINOMA
The nuclei are somewhat irregular in size. In acinar formations they show a polarized arrangement.

(fig. 4-94). The tumor cells have round nuclei of uniform size within abundant eosinophilic cytoplasm; the cytoplasm is finely granular and PAS-positive in its apical portion (fig. 4-95, top). Some tumors have areas with dilated acini that form "microglandular" structures (fig. 4-95, bottom), occasionally containing secretory material. The mitotic activity is generally low (less than 1 mitosis in 10 high-power fields).

Some tumors have a solid pattern, reminiscent of low-grade endocrine tumors (fig. 4-92). Usually there are necrotic areas. The small round cells have scanty cytoplasm and contain vesicular, irregular nuclei with distinct nucleoli (fig. 4-96). There are often more than 5 mitoses per 10 high-power fields.

The acinar tumors that have been described in children (340,355,360,365,374,396) are characterized by well-differentiated acinar tissue, a solid growth pattern, or both (see Differential Diagnosis).

**Histochemical and Immunohistochemical Findings.** The most useful markers for acinar cell carcinoma of the pancreas are pancreatic enzymes. The butyrate esterase stain, which detects lipase activity histochemically, is positive in 75 percent of cases (355). Immunohistochemically, all tumors stain strongly for at least one of the following pancreatic enzymes: trypsin, lipase, chymotrypsin, and phospholipase A2 (figs. 4-97, 4-98) (345,355,369). Pancreatic stone protein, another marker for zymogen granules (353), is also expressed in almost all tumors (345). In Hoorens' series (345), none of the tumors stained with antisera against alpha-amylase, while in Klimstra's study (355) one third of the tumors did. In one case report, the tumor stained for elastase-1 but not for amylase (349). Enzyme staining is localized in the apical portion of most cells arranged in an acinar pattern, while it is focal and usually restricted to single cells in tumors with solid patterns.

Figure 4-94
ACINAR CELL CARCINOMA
This tumor shows a pure acinar pattern, reminiscent of normal pancreatic acinar tissue.

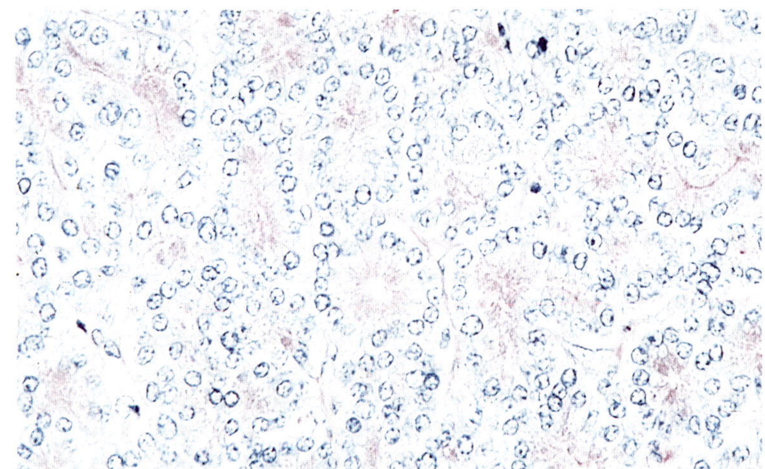

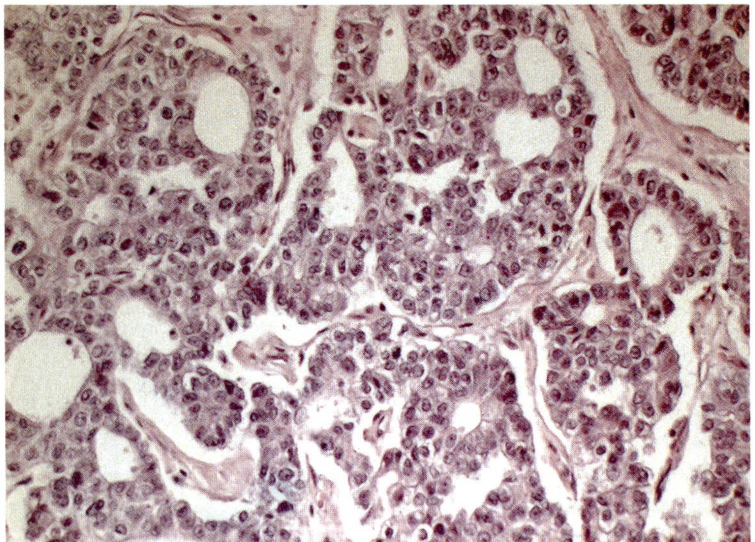

Figure 4-95
ACINAR CELL CARCINOMA
Top: The tumor cells have abundant cytoplasm, which is finely granular and PAS positive in its apical portion.
Bottom: This area shows dilated acini forming "microglandular" structures.

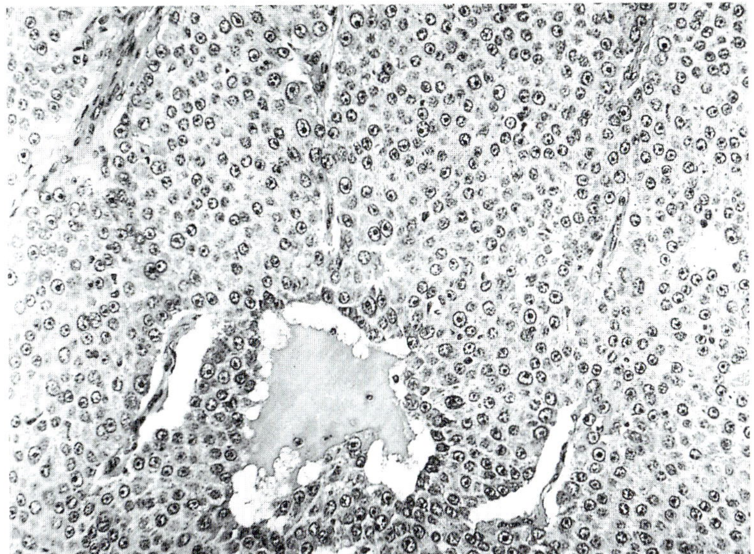

Figure 4-96
ACINAR CELL CARCINOMA
This tumor shows round cells with scant cytoplasm, slightly irregular nuclei, and distinct nucleoli.

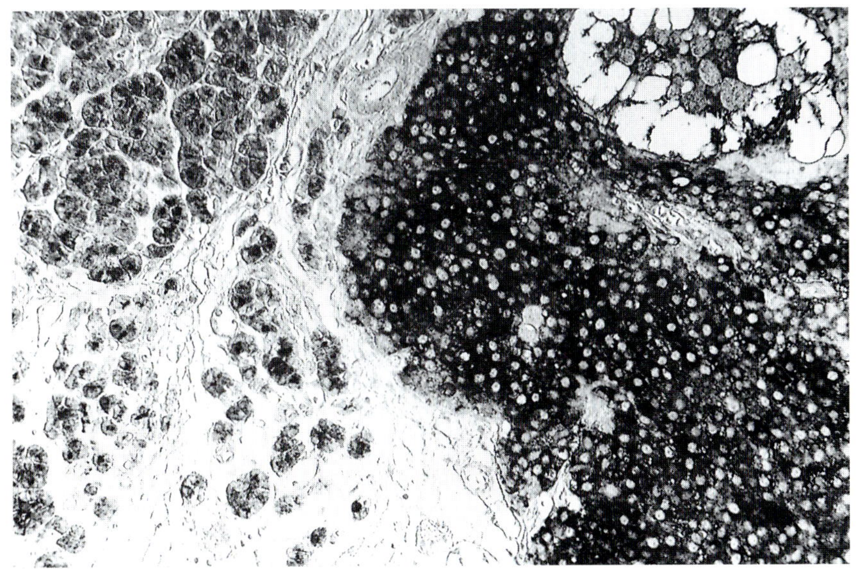

Figure 4-97
ACINAR CELL CARCINOMA
This tumor shows intense immunostaining for trypsin. Note the trypsin positivity of the normal acinar tissue (left) adjacent to the tumor (right).

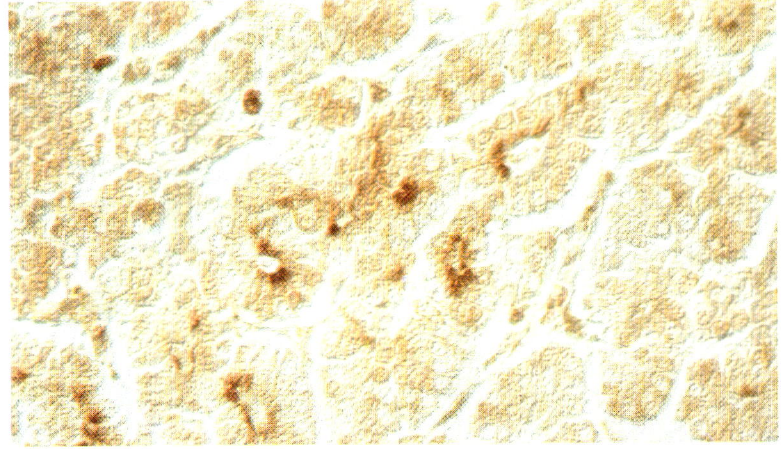

Figure 4-98
ACINAR CELL CARCINOMA
Immunostaining for trypsin labels the apical portion of the tumor cells.

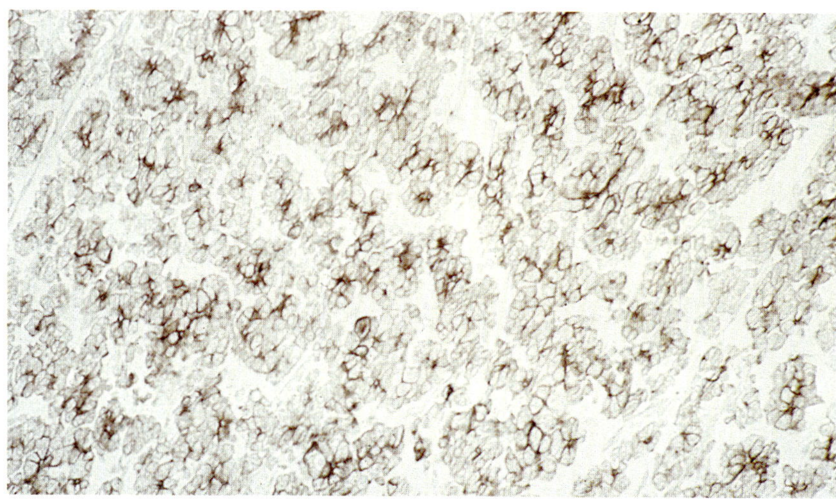

Figure 4-99
ACINAR CELL CARCINOMA
Immunostaining for CAM5.2 (cytokeratins 8 and 18) labels all tumor cells.

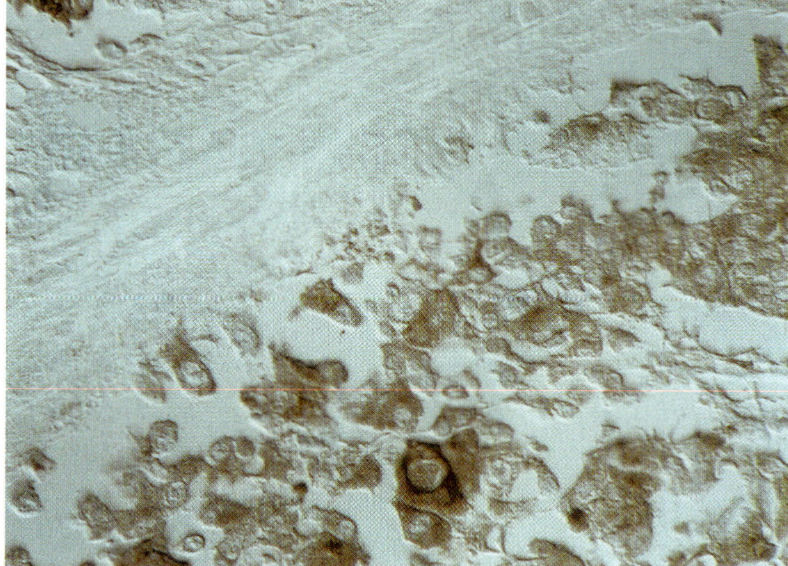

Figure 4-100
ACINAR CELL CARCINOMA
Immunostaining for synaptophysin labels some tumor cells.

Keratin is present in all tumors when the marker CAM5.2 for cytokeratins 8 and 18 is used (fig. 4-99) (345); while three fourths of tumors stain with the keratin marker AE1/AE3 (355). Alpha-1-antitrypsin is diffusely expressed in most tumors. CA19.9 and B72.3 (TAG72) are positive in one third of tumors, most of which have a mixed or solid pattern (345). Rarely, tumors stain for CEA or alpha-fetoprotein (AFP) (345,352,355,371,373). No reaction is found with the mucin marker M1 (345).

Endocrine cells staining for synaptophysin and chromogranin A are found in up to one fourth of tumors (fig. 4-100) (345,355). Usually they occur in tumors with a solid pattern, where they are scattered throughout the tissue. In a few of these tumors, the endocrine cells stain also for somatostatin and glucagon. When one tumor with a large number of scattered endocrine cells was double stained for synaptophysin and trypsin, most stained cells showed only one reaction product, but occasional single cells coexpressed synaptophysin and trypsin (345). Screening for mutant p53 overexpression has been negative in all 19 tumors tested (345).

**Ultrastructural Findings.** The tumor cells often form acinar-like complexes. The cells contain large electron-dense granules, abundant rough endoplasmic reticulum, well-developed Golgi complexes, some mitochondria, and a few

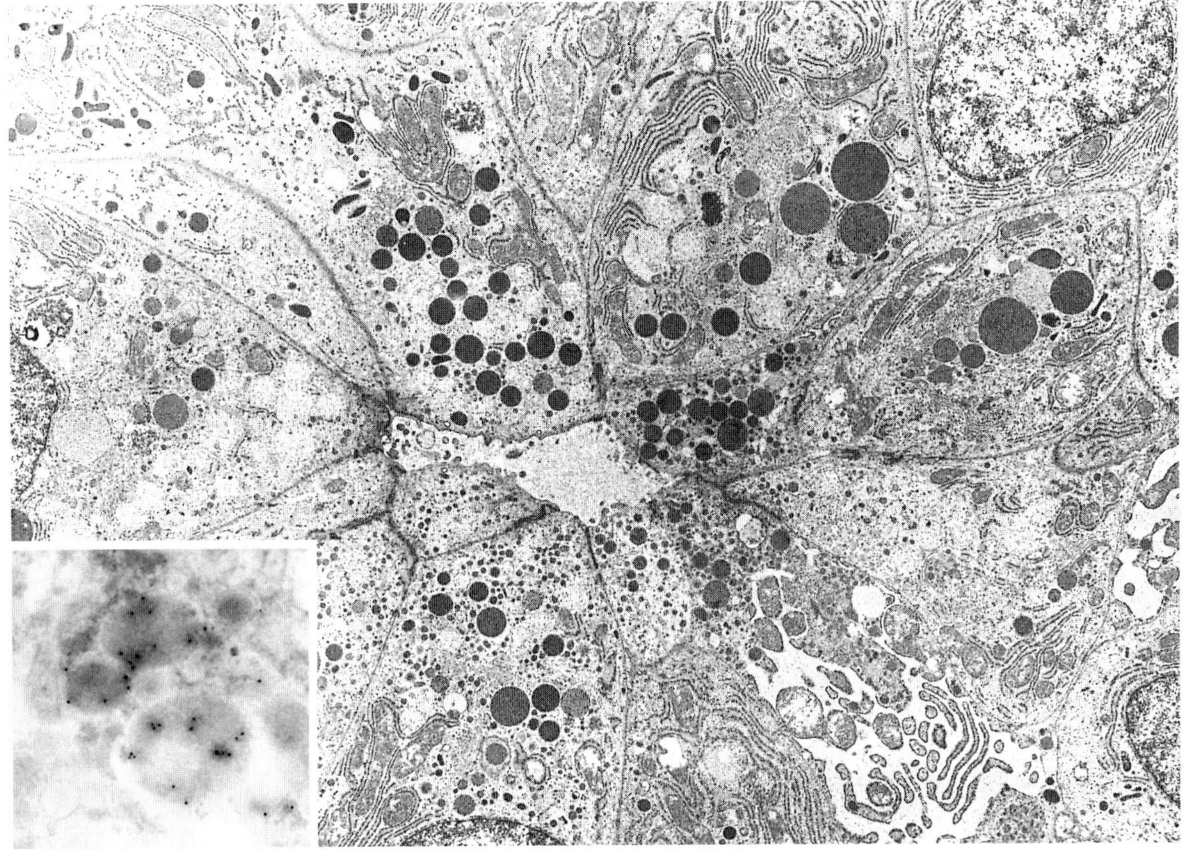

Figure 4-101
ACINAR CELL CARCINOMA

Electron micrograph showing dense zymogen granules of varying sizes (ranging from 200 to 700 nm) in the apical portion of the tumor cells. In addition, the cytoplasm contains abundant rough endoplasmic reticulum and well-developed Golgi complexes (X6340). The inset shows immunogold labeling for trypsin in zymogen granules (X12,000). (Fig. 7 from Hoorens A, Lemoine NR, McLellan E, et al. Pancreatic acinar cell carcinoma: an analysis of cell lineage markers, p53 expression, and Ki-ras mutation. Am J Pathol 1993;143:685–98.)

lysosomes (fig. 4-101) (332,335,336,343,345,346, 355,369). Small microvilli are found at the apical surface. The rather uniform electron-dense granules (mean diameter, 400 to 500 nm; range, 170 to 1800 nm) (392), which are commonly oriented towards the luminal space, are round and lack a halo between their homogenous dark-staining contents and the granule membrane (fig. 4-101). Their appearance is consistent with that of normal pancreatic zymogen granules, i.e., uniformly electron-dense granules with a tightly fitting membrane. However, the size of the neoplastic zymogen granules may vary considerably, both within a tumor and from tumor to tumor: of five tumors reported by Tucker (392), at least one had zymogen granules in the size range of those of endocrine tumors (75 to 350 nm). Sometimes, pleomorphic granules (fig. 4-102) and inclusion bodies with fibrillary internal structures, resembling the zymogen granules of the fetal pancreas, occur (355,392). The zymogen nature of the granules is demonstrated by positive immunogold labeling of trypsin (345). Occasionally, single cells with endocrine secretory granules may be identified (392). Cells with neurosecretory granules admixed with typical acinar cells have been described in two tumors, subsequently called acinar-endocrine cell tumor (386) and pancreatic carcinoma with duct, endocrine, and acinar differentiation (393); they most likely represent acinar cell carcinomas with an endocrine component.

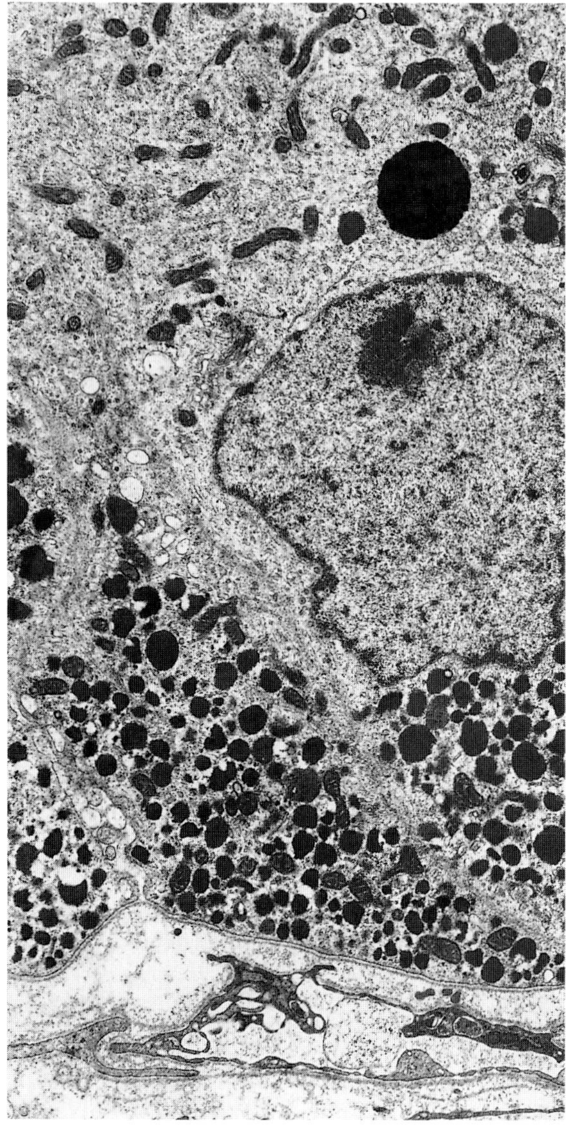

Figure 4-102
ACINAR CELL CARCINOMA

This electron micrograph shows tumor cells with many pleomorphic and rather small zymogen granules (mean diameter 400 to 500 nm; range 200 to 1000 nm), commonly oriented towards the luminal space. They are round and lack a halo between their homogeneous dark-staining contents and the granule membrane (X6340).

**New Techniques.** DNA from formalin-fixed tumor specimens from 16 patients with acinar cell carcinoma was amplified and screened for the presence of a mutation at codon 12 of the K-*ras* oncogene. Only one tumor had this mutation (345). This low frequency of K-*ras* mutation contrasts sharply with the high K-*ras* mutation rates found in ductal adenocarcinomas (see Ductal Adenocarcinoma).

**Differential Diagnosis.** The differential diagnosis of acinar cell carcinoma includes endocrine tumors, solid-pseudopapillary tumor, pancreatoblastoma, ductal adenocarcinoma, mucinous cystic tumor, acinar cell adenoma, and so-called focal acinar cell transformation (atypical acinar cell nodule). The tumors described as microglandular carcinomas by Cubilla and Fitzgerald (335) are probably acinar cell carcinomas.

*Endocrine Tumors.* It is important to distinguish acinar cell carcinomas from endocrine tumors of the pancreas (islet cell tumors) because of the better prognosis of the latter. While it is not difficult to separate well-differentiated acinar cell carcinomas from well-differentiated endocrine tumors, acinar cell carcinomas with a solid and partly trabecular pattern may be confused with low-grade endocrine tumors. Histologic criteria in favor of an endocrine tumor are absence of foci of acinar differentiation, greater regularity in the arrangement of nuclei in solid areas, absence of intracellular PAS-positivity, dense and unevenly distributed fibrous stroma, and usually a more distinct demarcation from the surrounding normal tissues. Immunohistochemical criteria include diffuse staining for endocrine markers such as synaptophysin and often chromogranin A, and the absence of pancreatic enzymes such as trypsin or lipase (345, 369). Diagnostic ultrastructural criteria are the presence of typical endocrine granules (i.e., granules with a small halo between an electron-dense core and a distinct granule membrane), usually in the size range of 100 to 200 nm in almost all cells, and the absence of acinar configurations of tumor cells that have large zymogen granules (300 to 1000 nm).

*Solid-Pseudopapillary Tumors.* These differ from acinar cell carcinomas by their almost exclusive occurrence in young women, favorable prognosis, cystic-hemorrhagic gross presentation, solid and pseudopapillary histologic pattern, distinct fibrovascular and myxoid stroma, and monomorphic appearance of cells which often have clear cytoplasm. Immunohistochemically, they show strong focal positivity for alpha-1-antitrypsin and diffuse positivity for neuron-specific enolase and vimentin, but are negative for synaptophysin and chromogranin. They are usually negative for keratin markers such as CAM5.2. In our recent study of solid-pseudopapillary tumors no pancreatic enzymes could be detected (369), although positive reactions have been reported by others (see Solid-Pseudopapillary Tumor).

*Pancreatoblastoma.* This tumor has the acinar pattern of acinar cell carcinoma, but in addition displays the squamoid corpuscles lacking in acinar tumors. Moreover, pancreatoblastomas may have a neoplastic stromal component which is absent from acinar cell carcinomas. The rare acinar cell carcinomas that have been described in children (340,351,355,360,365,370,374,396) are difficult to distinguish from pancreatoblastoma because they are similar both grossly and in growth behavior. These tumors may actually represent pancreatoblastomas with well-developed acinar differentiation but minimal or even absent squamoid and mesenchymal differentiation. Further studies are needed to clarify this issue. It is noteworthy that a few pancreatoblastomas have also been described in adults (344,357).

*Ductal Adenocarcinoma.* This tumor is easily separated from acinar cell carcinoma. Grossly, ductal adenocarcinomas are firm, ill-demarcated tumors which occur predominantly in the head of the pancreas. They have duct-like glands and small tubular structures composed of cuboidal cells that stain for mucin and are embedded in fibrous stroma. Immunohistochemically, they are almost all positive for M1, CEA, and CA19-9, and are usually negative for pancreatic enzymes and pancreatic stone protein (345,369). Ultrastructurally, ductal carcinoma cells have mucin granules and lack zymogen granules.

*Acinar Cell Adenomas.* These have been reported in few patients (338,360,390,395). Because of their rarity and the absence of clear criteria separating them from acinar cell carcinomas, it has to be questioned whether acinar cell adenomas really exist or only represent acinar cell carcinomas of low-grade malignancy. The only acinar cell tumor that we observed incidentally at autopsy was a well-demarcated pancreatic tumor without metastasis but with gross invasion of the splenic vein (358,369). We and others (355) therefore suggest that acinar cell adenoma be diagnosed with greatest caution and restricted to those cases without morphologic indications of malignancy after at least 5 years of follow-up.

*Focal Acinar Cell Transformation.* Synonyms for this include focal eosinophilic degeneration of acinar cells (388), focal acinar cell dysplasia (354, 363), atypical acinar cell lesions (390), atypical acinar cell nodules (359,387), and hyperplastic acinar cell nodule (376). This is a non-neoplastic change in the pancreas characterized by irregular but sharply outlined acinar cell clusters measuring 300 to 3000 mm in greatest dimension. The cytoplasm of the cells often shows homogeneous eosinophilia or loss of basophilia, but it may also be vacuolated (372). Ultrastructurally, a marked dilatation of the rough endoplasmic reticulum is seen (359). Mitoses are infrequent and inflammatory changes are absent. The reported incidence of focal eosinophilic degeneration of acinar cells ranges from 1.2 to 43.5 percent (354,363,376,388). So far most studies have failed to identify any clear association between focal acinar cell transformation (which is most likely a degenerative lesion) and acinar cell carcinoma (see also Tumor-Like Lesions, Acinar Changes).

*Microglandular Carcinoma.* This lesion was described by Cubilla and Fitzgerald (335) as a histologic tumor entity of the pancreas. However, these authors questioned whether this tumor is a truly distinct entity because cases examined by electron microscopy seemed to contain neuroendocrine-type granules. Recent studies based on immunohistochemical stains were not able to confirm the concept of a microglandular carcinoma of the pancreas as an entity, but rather suggest that pancreatic tumors with a microglandular pattern represent either neuroendocrine tumors or acinar cell carcinomas (358,368,369).

**Frozen Section Diagnosis and Cytology.** A correct frozen section diagnosis of acinar cell carcinoma is supported by the endocrine-like pattern of the tumor which, nevertheless, shows discrete acinar formations. However, it is almost impossible to differentiate between an acinar cell carcinoma with a predominantly solid pattern and a low-grade endocrine tumor on a frozen section.

In fine-needle aspiration specimens, the diagnosis is based on the presence of numerous cell clusters forming acinar structures (349). The tumor cells are monomorphous, have a granular cytoplasm, and contain an eccentrically located nucleus with finely granular chromatin and a distinct nucleolus.

**Spread, Metastasis, and Recurrence.** More than half of the patients with acinar cell carcinoma present with metastases at the time of diagnosis, which usually affect the regional lymph nodes or the liver (335,343). Extra-abdominal metastases are rare and are seen only in advanced cases (345,367,369,395). The tumors may spread locally to involve the duodenum, stomach, and peritoneum.

**Prognosis and Treatment.** The overall 1-, 3-, and 5-year survival rates for treated and untreated patients in Klimstra's study (355) were 57, 26, and 5.9 percent, respectively. Cubilla and Fitzgerald (335) reported 1- and 5-year survivals of 14 and 0 percent, respectively. The reported mean survival periods are 5 (395), 18 (355), and 42 months (345). Patients without metastatic disease at diagnosis seem to survive longer than those with metastases (14.2 versus 21.6 months [355]). Patients treated by resection have a longer life expectancy than those without surgical intervention (22.6 versus 6 months [355]). Patients younger than 60 years had a significantly better prognosis in Klimstra's study (355) than those over 60 years (13.4 versus 25.6 months). Of the pathologic parameters examined, only tumor size of less than 10 cm seems to influence survival, while histologic subtype and mitotic rate have no prognostic impact (355). The longest reported survivors lived 66 months (355) and 90 months (345) before dying of tumor.

Radiation and chemotherapy are given mostly for palliative purposes. Good response to chemotherapy was recently reported in a few patients with liver metastases, who received combinations of 5-fluorouracil, streptozotocin, methotrexate, doxorubicin, and cisplatin (348,355,394). In a patient with lipase secretion and subcutaneous fat necrosis, treatment with a somatostatin analogue resulted in symptomatic improvement (337).

## ACINAR CELL CARCINOMA VARIANTS

### Acinar Cell Cystadenocarcinoma

This rare variant presents as a large, encapsulated, multicystic lesion with tumor diameters up to 25 cm (332,345,389). The cut surface shows multiple, watery, fluid-filled cysts ranging in size from a few millimeters to several centimeters (fig. 4-103). There may be also some solid areas.

The tumors are composed of acinar and microglandular complexes as well as microcysts and macrocysts (fig. 4-104). The cells lining the cysts are cylindrical or cuboidal. In large cysts the epithelium tend to be flattened. The cytoplasm as well as the cyst content is faintly diastase-resistent PAS positive and may be focally calcified. The immunohistochemical and ultrastructural features are the same as those in the usual acinar cell carcinoma.

The main entities in the differential diagnosis are mucinous cystic tumor and serous cystadenoma because grossly these tumors may have a similar appearance. Histologically, however, acinar cell differentiation is easy to recognize (332,345,389).

The prognoses of acinar cell cystadenocarcinoma and usual acinar cell carcinoma are the same.

### Mixed Acinar-Endocrine Carcinoma

To date, mixed acinar-endocrine carcinoma has not been clearly defined; a number of reports have described acinar cell carcinomas under the terms mixed acinar-endocrine tumor (356), mixed exocrine-endocrine tumor (341), acinar-endocrine cell tumor (393), and pancreatic carcinoma with duct, endocrine, and acinar differentiation (386). In all these studies, endocrine cells, in addition to acinar and occasionally duct-like cells, were demonstrated by immunohistology or electron microscopy. The endocrine cells constituted a significant proportion of the tumor tissue, although exact figures were not given. However, since endocrine cells were found in approximately 40 percent of cases in two large series of acinar cell carcinomas (345,355), it is clear that the presence of endocrine cells in these tumors is not an exceptional event. It is difficult to distinguish acinar cell carcinoma with "scattered" endocrine cells and mixed acinar-endocrine carcinoma. Analogous to mixed ductal-endocrine carcinoma (see Ductal Adenocarcinoma Variants), we propose that for a tumor to be called mixed acinar-endocrine carcinoma at least one third to half of the entire cell population be comprised of endocrine (or acinar) cells (356). Moreover, the two cell populations should be intimately mixed with each other. Mixed acinar-endocrine carcinomas may also exhibit cells with amphicrine features (i.e., presence of endocrine and acinar cell characteristics).

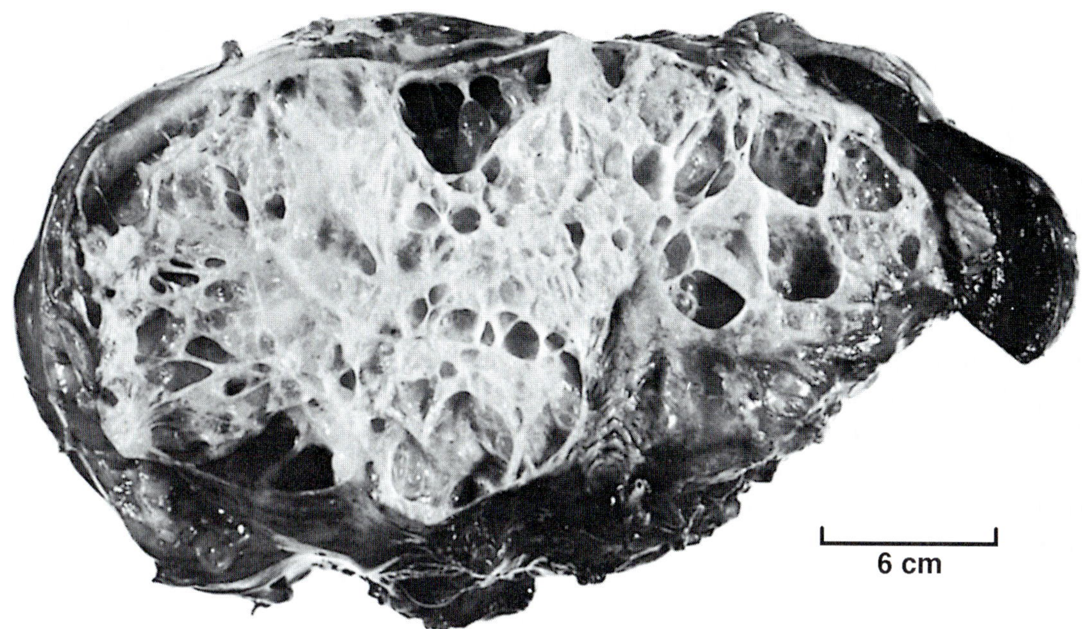


Figure 4-103
ACINAR CELL CYSTADENOCARCINOMA

Multiloculated, 7,000 g cystic neoplasm involving the body and tail of the pancreas. The thick fibrous capsule surrounds a mass with a multiloculated appearance. Cysts contain serous watery fluid and vary in size from pinpoint to 7 cm in diameter. They are lined by a smooth, white, glistening surface. No normal pancreatic tissue was identified grossly in the specimen. The neoplasm was attached to, but did not invade, the spleen (upper right corner). Small nodules on the peritoneum were composed of microcysts containing a thin fluid similar to that of the primary tumor. (Fig. 219 from Fascicle 19, Second Series.)

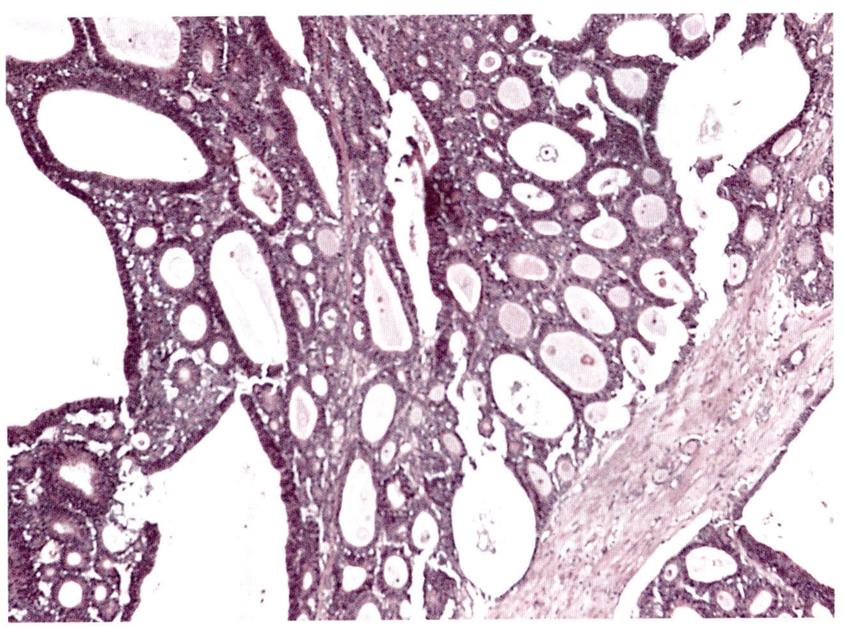

Figure 4-104
ACINAR CELL CARCINOMA

This area of a cystic acinar cell carcinoma is composed of numerous microcysts of varying size.

Since currently there is no clearly defined mixed acinar-endocrine carcinoma entity, it is not possible to determine prognosis. However, it may be anticipated that the prognosis of patients with such tumors does not differ from that of the usual acinar cell carcinoma.

## PANCREATOBLASTOMA

**Definition.** This malignant tumor is composed of epithelial tissue with acinar differentiation, squamoid cell nests, and occasional endocrine cells. Some tumors have a pronounced mesenchymal component. The tumor usually occurs in infants, but has also been reported in adults (408,432). It is referred to as *pancreaticoblastoma and infantile type carcinoma of the pancreas* (402,405).

**General Features.** Although pancreatoblastoma is an extremely rare tumor, it is the most common pancreatic neoplasm in childhood. Since the first report by Becker in 1957 (398), only 33 patients with this tumor have been described (Table 4-5). Cubilla and Fitzgerald's (402) pancreatic tumor series (645 cases) included only 1 patient (0.2 percent) with pancreatoblastoma.

Pancreatoblastoma is more frequent in males than females, with a ratio of 2 to 1. The patient age at presentation ranges from a few hours after birth to 9 years (mean, 4 years). Recently, seven cases in adults, aged 19 to 56 years, have been described (408,420,432). The tumor is more common in Asians (about two thirds of patients) than in Caucasians (Table 4-5).

Pancreatoblastomas were described in three newborns with the Beckwith-Wiedemann syndrome (403,421,433) which, apart from visceromegaly and islet hyperplasia, is known for its high rate of associated blastic tumors.

**Clinical Features.** Patients usually present with an abdominal mass and either no symptoms, or with nonspecific complaints including epigastric pain (40 percent), loss of appetite and weight (20 percent), and diarrhea and vomiting. Jaundice occurs in less than 15 percent of patients.

Elevated serum alpha-fetoprotein (AFP) levels are reported in one fourth to one third of patients (400,412,416,417,425,430). Other tumor markers such as CEA, CA19-9, and DuPan 2 are not helpful in the diagnosis of this tumor.

Ultrasonography and CT reveal a well-demarcated, solid and often multilobulated tumor in the upper abdomen, which may show low echogenic areas, central attenuations, and displacement of adjacent organs (400,406,434,438).

**Gross Findings.** These large, solitary tumors have no preferential location in the pancreas (Table 4-5). They may replace the entire pancreas or be only attached to it (400,410,411,414).

The tumor presents as a soft solid mass, usually surrounded by a fibrous capsule (fig. 4-105). Tumors range from 7 to 18 cm (Table 4-5). The cut section shows yellow-tan areas with incomplete lobulation, which may contain some small pseudocystic or hemorrhagic foci (fig. 4-106). True cysts do not occur.

In advanced stages, the tumor is no longer demarcated, but invades the pancreas and may also involve the parapancreatic retroperitoneal tissue and adjacent organs. Metastases occur in regional lymph nodes, liver, and lung.

**Microscopic Findings.** The usually encapsulated tumors are characterized by lobules and nests of relatively uniform cells separated by dense fibrous stroma. The cells grow in acinar, glandular, or more solid patterns which blend with scattered squamoid cell nests (or stratified cell cords) (fig. 4-107). In the acinar and glandular areas the cells are columnar or cuboidal; have a slightly eosinophilic, finely granular cytoplasm; and contain a round to oval nucleus situated at the basal pole. PAS stain reveals fine cytoplasmic granularity resistant to diastase digestion; Alcian blue stain is negative. The squamoid cell nests and cords ("squamoid corpuscles") are composed of polygonal tumor cells with basophilic or clear cytoplasm which may contain a few tiny PAS-positive granules. Occasionally the squamoid nests show central keratinization (402,410). Foci of necrosis may be present. Mitoses are usually rare, but may be frequent in some tumors. The fibrous stroma separating the epithelial areas may contain some tubular structures.

Rarely, pancreatoblastomas have, in addition to lobular epithelial areas, a conspicuous mesenchymal component including chondroid and osteoid tissues (fig. 4-108) (399,402,420).

The fibrous capsule may be infiltrated by epithelial tumor cells. Moreover, frank invasion of the duodenal wall, the stomach wall, and the peritoneum may occur (402,405,422). Vascular invasion is rare.

Table 4-5

**LITERATURE SURVEY OF PANCREATOBLASTOMA (1957–1994)**

| Case | Author | No./ Sex | Race* | Site/Size (cm)‡ | Clinical Features (Serum AFP [ng/ml]) | Metastasis (Invasion) | Follow-Up/ (Time period) |
|---|---|---|---|---|---|---|---|
| 1 | Becker (1957) | 1/M | C | H/7 | abdominal pain, hematemesis, melena | none | died (3y) |
| 2 | Moynan (1964) | 5/F | ? | H/2.5 | vomiting, fever, epigastric mass | liver, lung | died (9d) |
| 3 | Fonkalsrud (1966) | 3/M | C | H/ egg-size | anorexia, diarrhea | colon | healthy (5y) |
| 4 | Frabel (1971) | 4/M | C | H/15 | abdominal mass | (mesenteric vein, colon) | died (7d) |
| 5 | Tsukimoto (1973) | 4/F | J | H/6x5x5 | jaundice, nausea, vomiting, abdominal pain, anorexia | liver | died (30d) |
| 6 | Kakudo (1976) | 3/F | J | T 15x5x5 | anorexia, weight loss, abdominal pain | none | died (2y) |
| 7 | Horie (1977) | 4/M | J | H/11x9x8.5 | abdominal mass, diarrhea abdominal pain, fever | none | healthy (16y) |
| 8 | Horie (1977) | 5/M | J | H/7x6x4 | abdominal mass | none | healthy (2y) |
| 9 | Benjamin (1980) | 7/M | C | H/10 | epigastric mass, weight loss | none | healthy (10m) |
| 10 | Cho** (1980) | 4/M | K | T/11x9x8 | ? | ? | died (22m) |
| 11 | Jung** (1982) | 4/M | K | H/10x8x7 | ? | ? | ? |
| 12 | Imamura (1984) | 5/F | J | BT/13x8x6 | abdominal mass (8780) | none | died (15m) |
| 13 | Shimizu (1984) | 6/M | J | B/14x9.5x6 | abdominal mass | liver | died (in op.) |
| 14 | Cubilla (1984) | 3/M | P | H/4x3x2 | abdominal mass, jaundice | lung | died (1y) |
| 15 | Buchino (1984) | 4/M | C | B/11x8.5x8 | abdominal pain and girth (7176) | none | healthy (29m) |
| 16 | Ko** (1984) | 3/F | K | B/5x4x4 | ? | ? | ? |
| 17 | Ichijima (1984) | 6/F | J | T/8x5x4 | abdominal mass | none | healthy (10y) |
| 18 | Ohaki (1985) | 6/M | J | T/7 | diarrhea, jaundice, general fatigue (800) | liver, lung (portal vein) | died (3y) |
| 19 | Huh** (1986) | 7/M | K | H/5x5x4 | ? | liver | healthy (22m) |
| 20 | Iseki (1986) | 8/M | J | T/18x9.5x8.5 | abdominal mass and pain, diarrhea (98.3) | (spleen) | healthy (2y) |
| 21 | Koh (1986) | neonate/M | I | T/7.5 | Beckwith-Wiedemann syndrome, nephroblastoma (2y, after resect.) | none | healthy (4y) |
| 22 | Potts (1986) | neonate/M | ? | T/7 | Beckwith-Wiedemann syndrome | none | healthy (10m) |
| 23 | Palosaari (1986) | 37/M | C | H/8 | abdominal mass and pain, weight loss | liver | recurrence (15m) |
| 24 | Sasaki (1987) | 2/F | J | T/10x10 | abdominal mass (700) | lymph node | healthy (6m) |
| 25 | Tsukamoto** (1987) | 7M | J | HBT/? | ? | liver | died (13m) |
| 26 | Takemiya** (1987) | 3/F | J | T/17x13x8 | ? | ? | died (9m) |
| 27 | Fukuda** (1987) | 4/M | J | B/12x10x9 | ? | ? | healthy (3y) |
| 28 | Drut (1988) | neonate/M | ? | B/10 | Beckwith-Wiedemann syndrome | none | died (10d) |
| 29 | Morohoshi (1989) | 7/F | J | HB/6x5 | diarrhea, vomiting, abdominal mass (10,000) | liver, lung | died (10m) |
| 30 | Sakaida (1992) | 4/M | J | T/12.5x11x6 | abdominal mass (112) | ? | healthy |
| 31 | Sakaida (1992) | 6/F | J | H/5x4x4 | jaundice | liver | healthy |
| 32 | Shinagawa† (1992) | 30/F | J | H/5x3 | jaundice, epigastric discomfort (350) | none | healthy (6m) |
| 33 | Hoorens (1994) | 39/F | C | T/13 | abdominal mass | none | healthy (30m) |

*Race: C = Caucasian, J = Japanese, Ch = Chinese, K = Korean, P = Peruvian, I = Indian.
**According to reference 412.
†Personal contact.
‡H = head; T = tail; B = body; BT = body-tail.

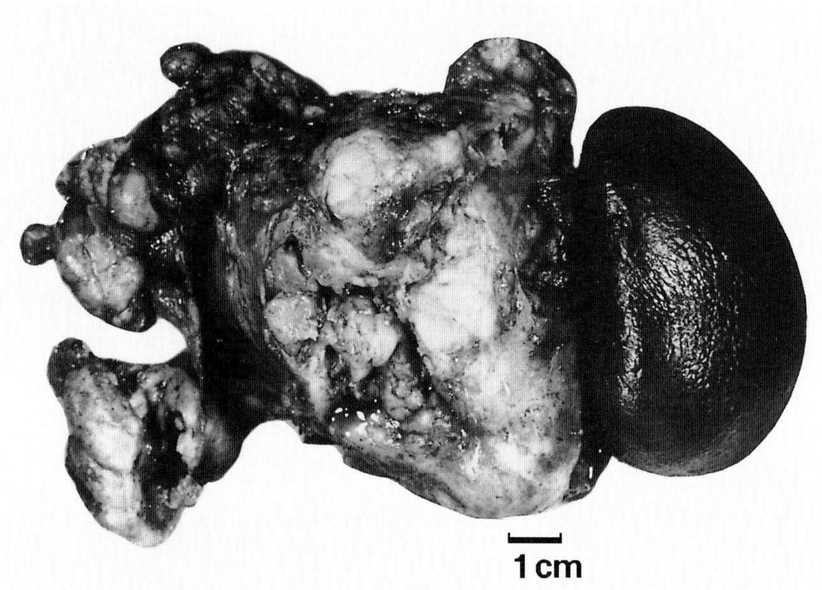


Figure 4-105
PANCREATOBLASTOMA
This large tumor presented as a soft, solid, well-demarcated mass in the tail of the pancreas. (Fig. 1 from Hoorens A, Gebhard F, Kraft K, Lemoine NR, Klöppel G. Pancreatoblastoma in an adult: its separation from acinar cell carcinoma. Virchows Arch 1994;424:485–90.)

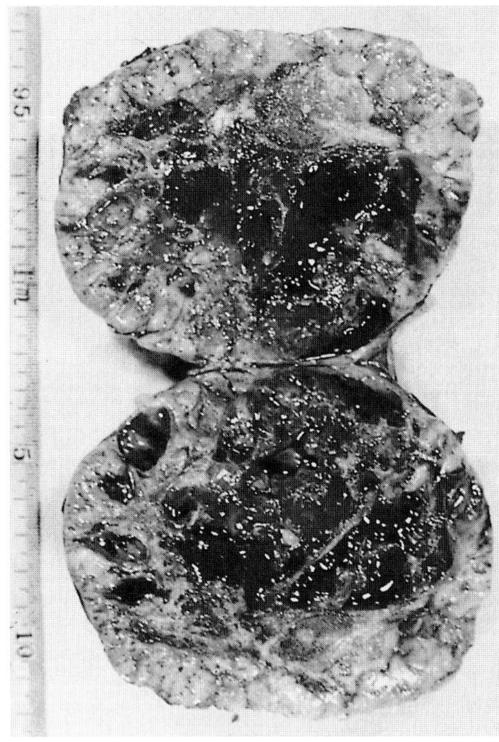

Figure 4-106
PANCREATOBLASTOMA
The cut surface of this well-demarcated tumor shows lobulation and hemorrhagic necrosis. (Fig. 7.41 from Klöppel G. Pancreatic, non-endocrine tumours. In: Klöppel G, Heitz PU, eds. Pancreatic pathology, Edinburgh: Churchill Livingstone, 1984:79–113.)

**Immunohistochemical Findings.** The tumor cells arranged in an acinar or solid pattern are positive for the keratin marker CAM5.2 and usually also for lipase, trypsin, chymotrypsin, and alpha-1-antitrypsin, but not alpha-amylase (408,424). The squamoid corpuscles do not stain for CAM5.2 (fig. 4-109) and are not immunoreactive for pancreatic enzymes or endocrine markers (401,408,420,438). The nature of these cell clusters is, therefore, unclear. Some tumors are positive for AFP (400,415,416,425,428,429), CEA (400,425), or CA19-9 (425).

A few pancreatoblastomas contain subpopulations of endocrine cells that stain with the Grimelius reaction or antisera against neuron-specific enolase, synaptophysin, chromogranin A, and pancreatic hormones, particularly somatostatin (400,402,415,435,438). Endocrine cells are scattered among the other epithelial cells, but may occasionally form nests similar to endocrine islets (401).

**Ultrastructural Findings.** The tumor cells forming acinar structures have microvilli on the luminal surface and are connected by desmosomes. Their cytoplasm contains large electron-dense zymogen-like granules, 300 to 700 nm in diameter; well-developed Golgi complexes; and abundant rough endoplasmic reticulum (399,400, 412,414,415,417,418,438). In addition, individual cells have endocrine-type granules measuring from 100 to 200 nm in diameter (438). Tumor

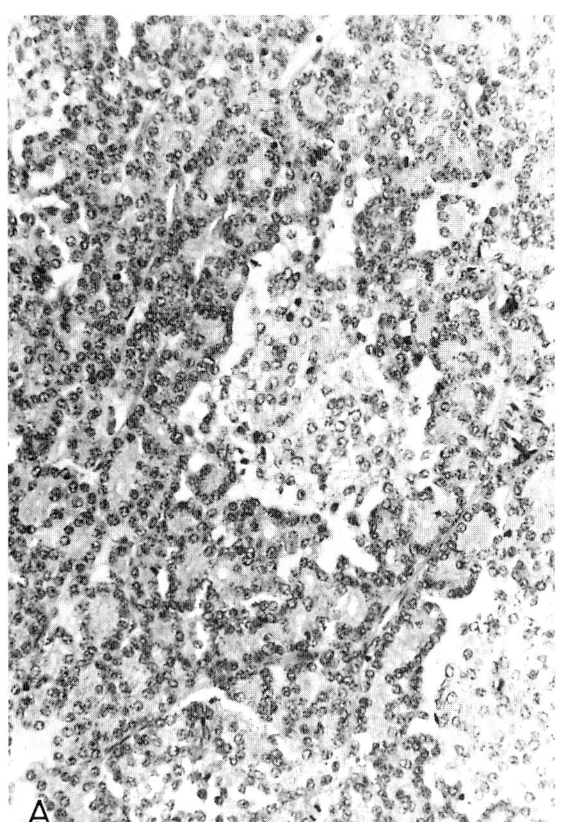


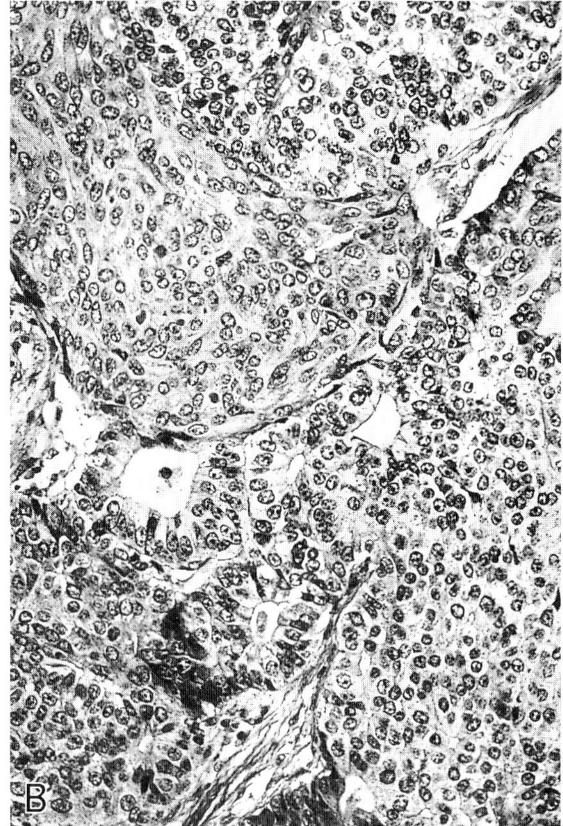


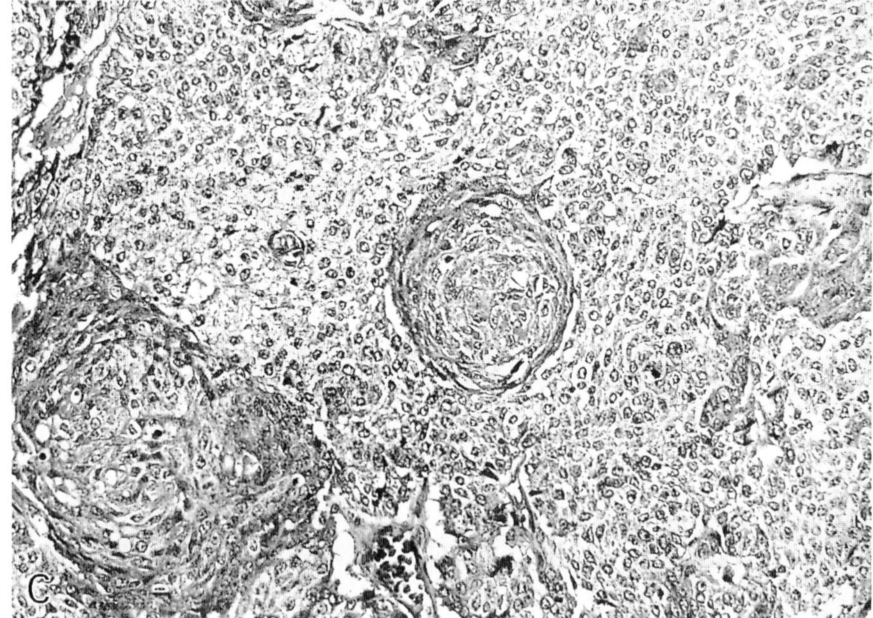


Figure 4-107
PANCREATOBLASTOMA

A: The tumor cells grow in an acinar pattern and include groups of cells with pale cytoplasm ("squamoid corpuscles").
B: This tumor shows a mixed solid-glandular pattern.
C: Solid tumor tissue with scattered squamoid corpuscles.

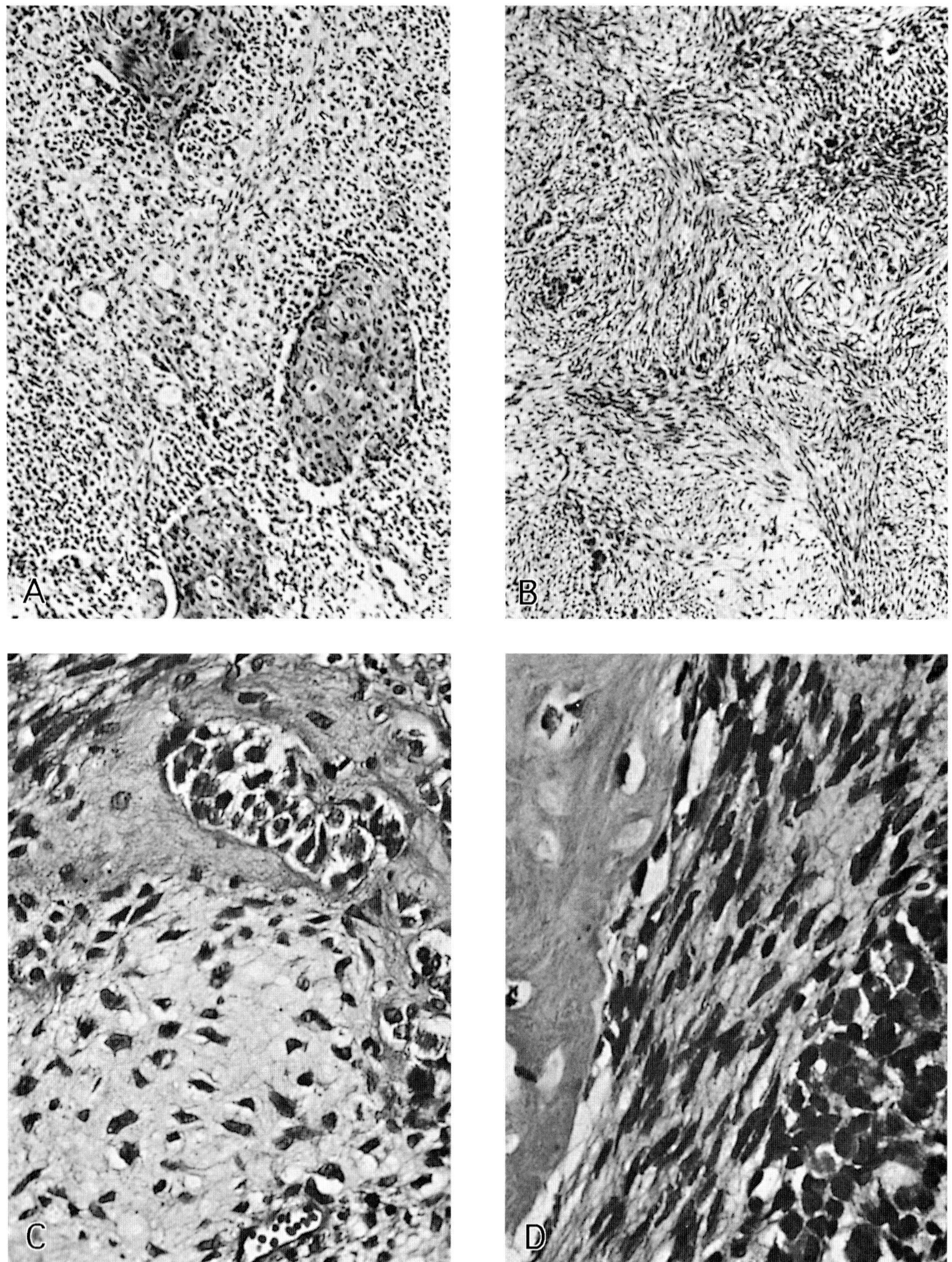


Figure 4-108
PANCREATOBLASTOMA

A: Nests of squamous or epidermoid tissue in a background of small, diffusely infiltrating cells.
B: Spindle cells with sarcomatoid features.
C: Chondroid tissue surrounded by spindle cells.
D: Spindle cells (center), epithelial cells (right), and osteoid (left)
(Figs. 198–201 from Fascicle 19, Second Series.)

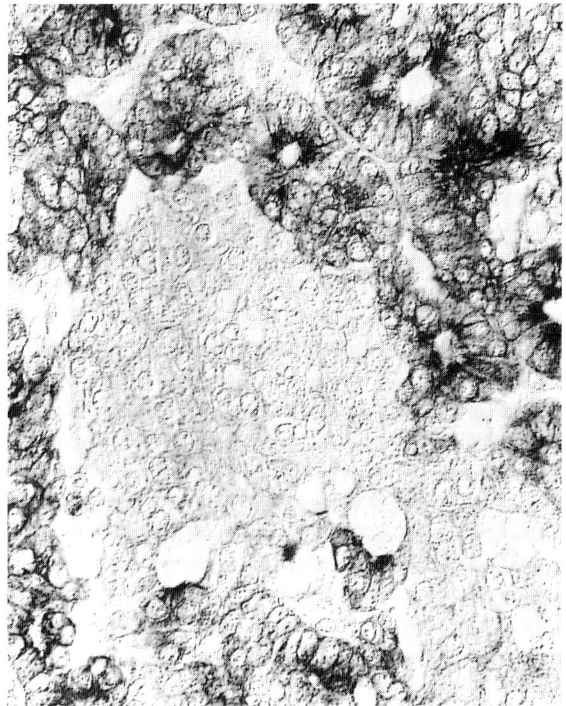

Figure 4-109
PANCREATOBLASTOMA
Immunostaining for the cytokeratin marker CAM5.2 shows positive tumor cells arranged in an acinar pattern. The squamoid corpuscles fail to stain for this keratin marker (Nomarski optic).

cells containing both the larger zymogen-type granules and the smaller neuroendocrine-like granules have been described (400,410,438).

**Differential Diagnosis.** The differential diagnosis of pancreatoblastoma includes acinar cell carcinoma, endocrine tumor, and solid-pseudopapillary tumor.

*Acinar Cell Carcinoma.* Pancreatoblastomas with a prevailing acinar pattern and occurring in adults may be difficult to separate from acinar cell carcinoma. The only criterion which distinguishes the latter tumor is the absence of squamoid nests. The acinar cell carcinomas (407,419,422,423,431, 440) and acinar cell adenomas (422) that have been described in children appear to differ biologically from respective tumors in adults (see Acinar Cell Carcinoma [109,419,420]). These tumors could, therefore, represent pancreatoblastomas in which squamoid differentiation is minimal or absent.

*Endocrine Tumor.* Pancreatoblastomas with a solid pattern and no evidence of acinar formation are histologically difficult to differentiate from endocrine tumors. Immunohistochemically, however, the latter neoplasms are diffusely positive for synaptophysin and usually also chromogranin A, while the few endocrine cells, which may be present in pancreatoblastomas, are found scattered between the other tumor cells. Moreover, endocrine tumors lack the AFP positivity occasionally observed in pancreatoblastomas.

*Solid-Pseudopapillary Tumor.* Solid-pseudopapillary tumors also occur in childhood. However, they are easily recognized by their predilection for females (not younger than 9 years) and their distinct histologic pattern characterized by solid areas alternating with pseudopapillary structures and degenerative pseudocystic lesions (424). Immunohistologically, they display a strong focal positivity for alpha-1-antitrypsin and a diffuse positivity for neuron-specific enolase and vimentin, features missing in pancreatoblastomas.

**Frozen Section Diagnosis and Cytology.** Clues to a correct frozen section diagnosis include the organoid and acinar features and the demonstration of squamoid nests in a cellular tumor. Cytologically, there may be tight clusters of small epithelial cells in acinar groupings admixed with stromal fragments consisting of bland-appearing spindle-shaped cells. The epithelial cells have granular cytoplasm and round nuclei with finely granular chromatin (437).

**Spread, Metastasis, and Recurrence.** Local invasion at presentation by pancreatoblastoma usually involves the duodenum, stomach, transverse colon, portal vein, and peritoneum. Metastases to the regional lymph nodes or liver are rare at diagnosis and only appear after the tumor has recurred locally.

**Prognosis and Treatment.** There is no doubt about the malignant potential of pancreatoblastoma because the tumor can invade adjacent organs and vessels and is capable of regional and distant metastases. The relevance of the mitotic rate or other microscopic features to the malignant potential of the tumor has yet to be investigated. Postoperative prognosis is fairly good in patients in whom the tumor is discovered prior to metastasis. About two thirds of patients are well 1 year after resection, and one fourth are alive and tumor free after 5 years. The longest follow-up after surgery is 28 years (410). Pancreatoblastomas are responsive to radiotherapy and chemotherapy (406,418,420).

## SOLID-PSEUDOPAPILLARY TUMOR

**Definition.** This benign or low-grade malignant epithelial tumor occurs predominantly in young women and is composed of monomorphous cells variably expressing epithelial, mesenchymal, and endocrine markers. These tumors have also been referred to as *solid-cystic tumor, papillary-cystic tumor,* and *solid and papillary epithelial neoplasms.*

**General Considerations.** *Terminology.* The term solid-cystic tumor was proposed because of the tumor's gross features (460); the designations papillary-cystic (443) and solid and papillary tumor, in contrast, mainly relate to the most obvious histologic features (448). In the early literature, the tumors were also described as "papillary tumor of the pancreas—benign or malignant" (451), "papillary epithelial neoplasm of pancreas in a child" (453), or "adenocarcinoma of the pancreas in childhood" (441,483). Since these terms do not exactly reflect what is observed either at the macroscopic or microscopic level, we propose the name solid-pseudopapillary tumor. This term correctly encompasses the two most conspicuous histologic features encountered in these tumors, the solid areas and the pseudopapillary regions.

*Classification.* Follow-up of a large number of cases has shown that the majority of solid-pseudopapillary tumors are benign. Only a small number recur or develop metastases after resection. But even in the metastasizing cases the tumors are slow growing and are therefore best designated as low-grade malignancies. Criteria that distinguish tumors that may become malignant from those that will probably remain benign are angioinvasion, perineural invasion, and deep invasion of the surrounding pancreatic parenchyma. If these features are present, we classify the neoplasm as solid-pseudopapillary carcinoma; if these features are lacking, the tumor is considered a neoplasm with borderline malignant potential. The reason for placing these tumors in the borderline category is that even tumors without the above mentioned histologic criteria of malignancy may give rise to metastases.

*Origin.* Almost all reports on solid-pseudopapillary tumors discuss their origin in detail. This indicates that there is not much known about it. We therefore restrict our considerations on the origin of these neoplasms to a minimum. The fact that solid-pseudopapillary tumors may express epithelial as well as mesenchymal markers and occasionally also seem to show exocrine and endocrine features suggest an origin from an omnipotent cell, i.e., a stem cell. Such a cell may be from the ductular-centroacinar cell compartment which, during embryogenesis, is thought to give rise to exocrine and endocrine cells. However, it must be emphasized that the presumed omnipotent nature of the tumor cells is not quite obvious from the structure and behavior of these cells. They neither have the features of a highly proliferative blastic cell nor show evidence of clear-cut terminal differentiation to either an acinar or endocrine cell. In addition, their strongly sex-linked occurrence is not in keeping with an origin from a stem cell. We believe that there is little evidence to date in support of an origin of solid-pseudopapillary tumors from a stem cell. Molecular biology studies may clarify this situation.

**General Features.** The tumor is uncommon, but has been recognized with increasing frequency in recent years (460,465,466,470,473, 482). It accounts for approximately 1 to 2 percent of all exocrine pancreatic tumors (448,458,469). The tumor occurs predominantly in adolescent girls and young women (age range, 8 to 67 years; mean, 35 years) (460,465,466,473,481,482). It is rare in men (age range, 25 to 72 years; mean, 35 years) (459,467,473,481,484,486). The tumor occurs in all races (461,474).

The etiology of the tumor is not known. Its unique sex and age distribution point to genetic and hormonal factors in the pathogenesis. However, so far no association with endocrine disturbances and, in particular, disorders with overproduction of estrogen or progesterone, have been reported. Moreover, few women developed a tumor after long-term use of contraceptives (448,449,479).

The impressive degenerative changes of the tumor, which are particularly a feature of large lesions, probably result from a vasculature that consists predominantly of poorly supported small vessels (474).

**Clinical Features.** The tumors are either found incidentally on routine physical examination or they cause abdominal discomfort and pain (473), occasionally after abdominal trauma (459, 476,478). Jaundice is rare (475), even in tumors that originate from the head of the pancreas, and

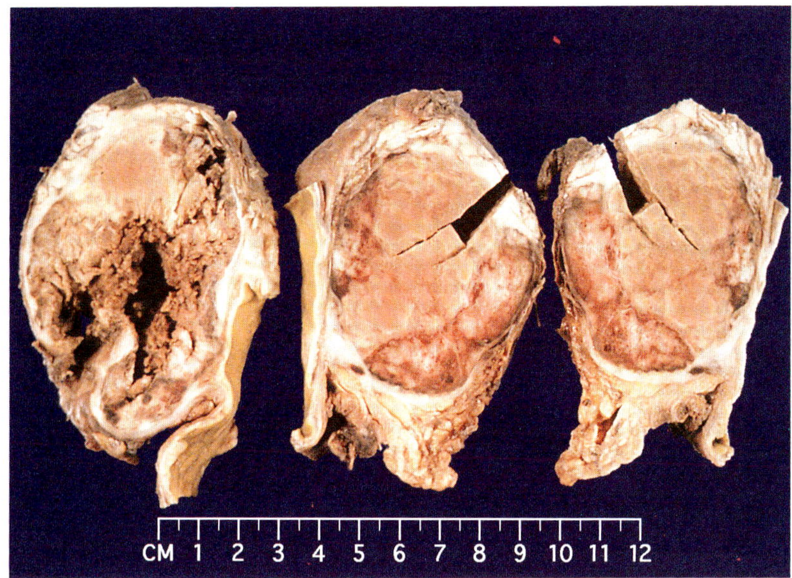


Figure 4-110
SOLID-PSEUDOPAPILLARY TUMOR
Whipple resection specimen showing a large, round, well-demarcated mass in the head of the pancreas. The tumor is partly necrotic and cystic. (Courtesy of Dr. Andreas Schulz, Giessen, Germany.)

there is no associated functional endocrine syndrome. All known tumor markers are normal.

Ultrasonography and CT reveal a sharply demarcated, variably solid and cystic mass without any internal septation (446,452). On angiography the tumors are usually hypovascular or mildly hypervascular lesions that displace surrounding vessels (452,490).

**Gross Findings.** The tumors occur evenly distributed in the pancreas (470,473). They present as large, round, solitary masses (size range, 3 to 18 cm; average, 8 to 10 cm) that are usually so well demarcated from the remaining pancreas that they can be easily removed (fig. 4-110). So far only one patient had two synchronous tumors in the head and tail (475). Invasion of adjacent organs (duodenal wall, spleen, or transverse colon) or the portal vein is rare (fig. 4-111) (472, 479–481). The cut surface of the encapsulated and often fluctuant tumors reveals lobulated, light brown solid areas admixed with zones of hemorrhage and necrosis as well as cystic spaces filled with necrotic debris (fig. 4-110). Occasionally, the hemorrhagic-cystic changes involve almost the entire tumor tissue so that the tumor may be mistaken for a pseudocyst (fig. 4-112). The capsule, but also the inner portion of the mass, may contain calcifications (473). A few tumors were attached to the pancreas or were in extrapancreatic locations (454,457,459).

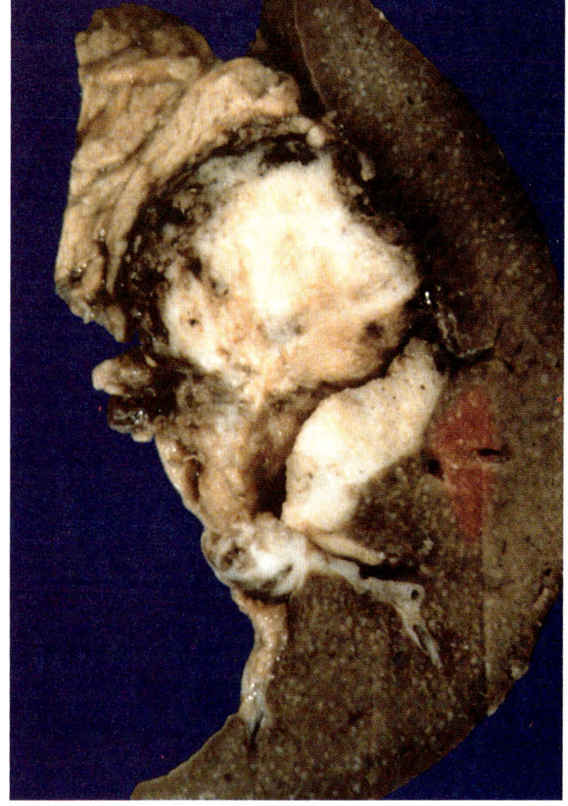

Figure 4-111
SOLID-PSEUDOPAPILLARY TUMOR
Left-sided resection specimen of the pancreas showing a tumor invading the spleen. This tumor gave rise to liver metastases. (Courtesy of Dr. Manfred Stolte, Bayreuth, Germany.)

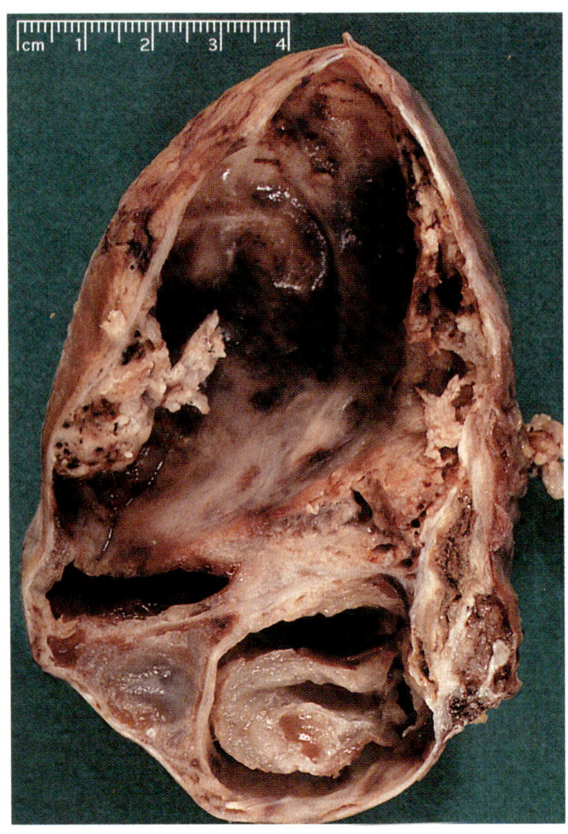


Figure 4-112
SOLID-PSEUDOPAPILLARY TUMOR
The cut surface of this tumor reveals a uniloculated cyst. Only the capsule shows some solid tissue areas. (Courtesy of Dr. Helmut Lüchtrath, Koblenz, Germany.)

**Microscopic Findings.** In small tumors all tumor tissue is preserved. In large tumors the preserved tissue is usually found in the tumor periphery under the fibrous capsule. This tissue exhibits a solid monomorphous pattern with variable sclerosis (fig. 4-113), and more centrally, a pseudopapillary pattern (fig. 4-114). These components often gradually merge into each other. In both patterns the uniform polygonal cells are arranged around delicate and often hyalinized fibrovascular stalks. Tumor cells that are radially arranged around the minute fibrovascular stalks may resemble rosettes or ducts (fig. 4-115). In the solid parts disseminated aggregates of tumor cells with foamy cytoplasm (fig. 4-116) or cholesterol crystals surrounded by foreign body cells may be found (fig. 4-117). The spaces between the pseudopapillary structures are filled with red blood cells. The hyalinized connective tissue strands may contain foci of calcification and even ossification (467).

The tumor cells have either an eosinophilic or clear vacuolar cytoplasm (fig. 4-113, right). Occasionally they contain eosinophilic, diastase-resistant, PAS-positive globules of varying size; these also occur outside the cells (fig. 4-115, left). Glycogen or mucin cannot be demonstrated. The round to oval nuclei have finely dispersed chromatin and are often grooved or indented (fig. 4-115, right). Mitoses are usually rare, but in a few instances may be prominent (473). Occasionally there is vessel invasion (488). The tumor tissue is usually well demarcated from the normal pancreas, although a separating layer of connective tissue may be missing (fig. 4-118, top). Occasionally, however, the tumor invades surrounding pancreatic parenchyma (467,473).

*Criteria of Malignancy.* Although criteria of malignancy have not yet been clearly established, we believe that unequivocal perineural invasion or angioinvasion, with or without deep invasion into the surrounding tissue (fig. 4-118, bottom), indicates malignant behavior. Nishihara et al. (473) compared the histologic features of 3 metastasizing and 19 nonmetastasizing solid-pseudopapillary tumors. They found that venous invasion, degree of nuclear atypia, mitotic rate, and prominence of necrobiotic cell nests (cells with pyknotic nuclei and eosinophilic cytoplasm) were helpful histologic parameters for predicting malignancy. It must be emphasized that even in the absence of all the above criteria malignant behavior cannot be excluded. It is therefore necessary to classify all benign-appearing solid-pseudopapillary tumors as borderline lesions.

**Histochemical and Immunohistochemical Findings.** The tumor cells do not stain with PAS (except for the PAS-positive globules) or Alcian blue (pH 2.5). Grimelius-positive cells may occur. The most useful markers are alpha-1-antitrypsin, alpha-1-antichymotrypsin, neuron-specific enolase (NSE), and vimentin (447,459,460,465, 470,473,491). The cellular positivity for alpha-1-antitrypsin and alpha-1-antichymotrypsin is always intense but involves only small cell clusters or single cells, a finding that characterizes this tumor (fig. 4-119). Alpha-1-antitrypsin also stains the PAS-positive globules. Positivity for NSE (fig. 4-120) and vimentin, in contrast, is

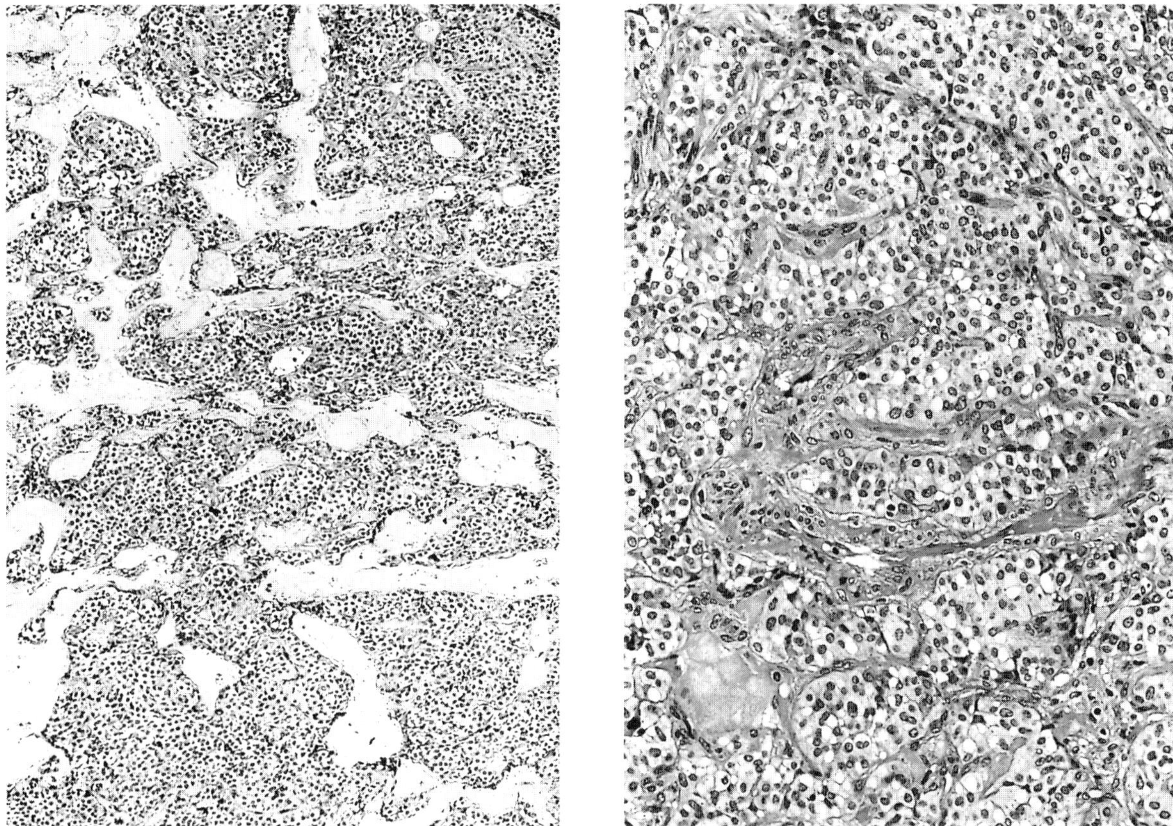

Figure 4-113
SOLID-PSEUDOPAPILLARY TUMOR

Left: The tumor tissue shows a solid monomorphous pattern with variable sclerosis.

Right: Higher magnification of the tumor tissue reveals the monomorphous character of the cell population. Some of the cells are vacuolated.

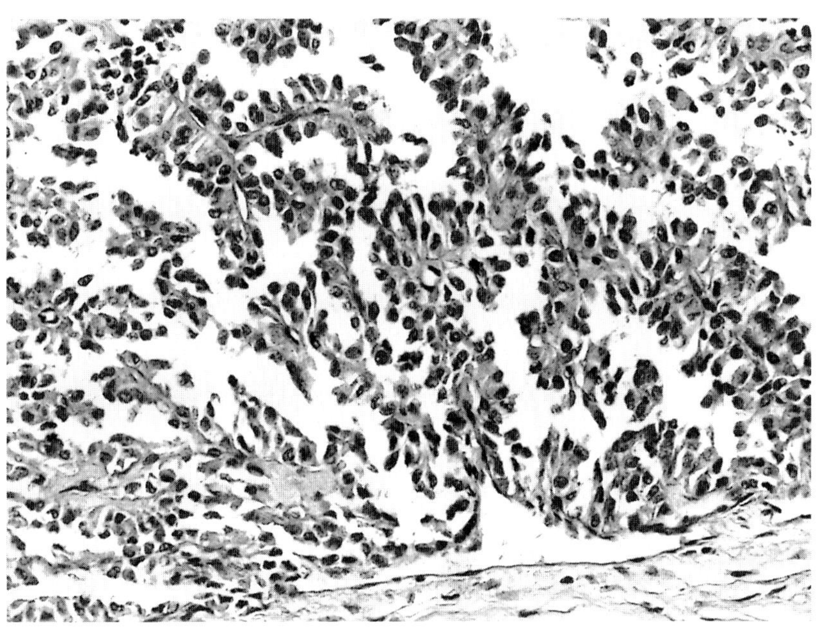

Figure 4-114
SOLID-PSEUDOPAPILLARY TUMOR

This area of the tumor displays a pseudopapillary pattern with cystic degeneration.

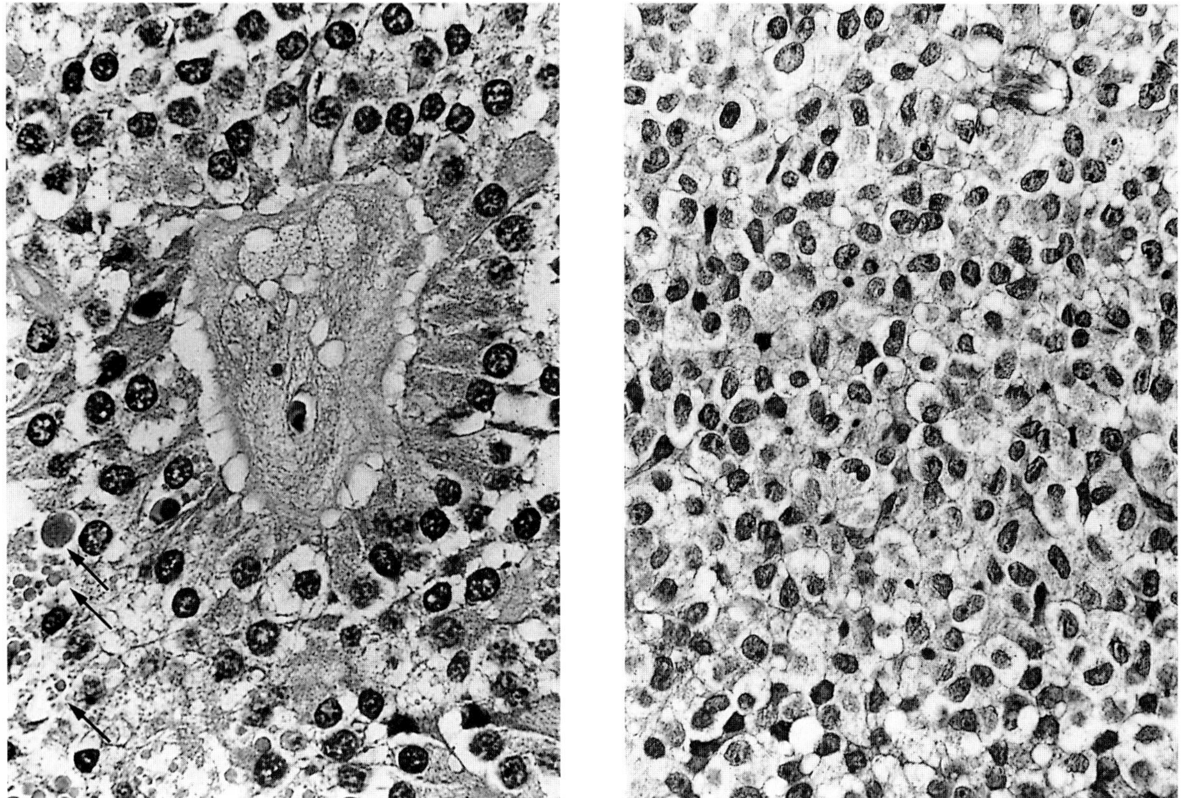

Figure 4-115
SOLID-PSEUDOPAPILLARY TUMOR

Left: Tumor cells are radially arranged around a delicate and somewhat hyalinized fibrovascular stalk. Arrows point to small hyaline globules within and between the cells.

Right: The nuclei of the monomorphic tumor cells lack a conspicuous nucleolus but show indentations.

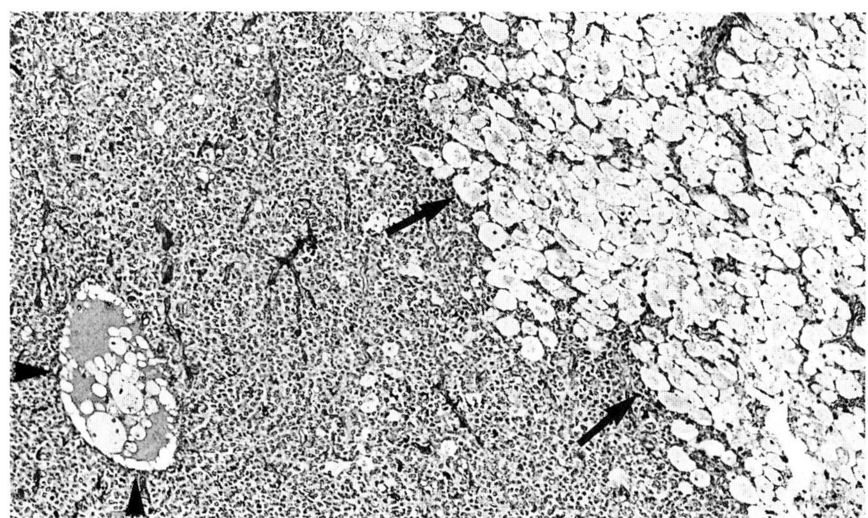

Figure 4-116
SOLID-PSEUDOPAPILLARY TUMOR

In the solid part of the tumor there is an aggregate of large tumor cells with foamy cytoplasm (arrows). Arrowheads point to a small cyst filled with eosinophilic fluid and some foam cells.

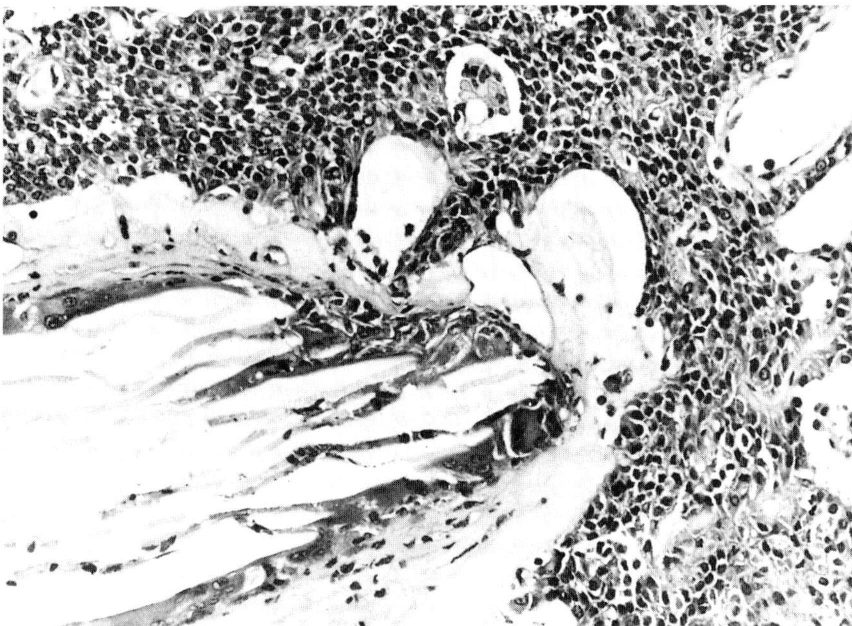

Figure 4-117
SOLID-PSEUDOPAPILLARY TUMOR
The tumor tissue includes cholesterol crystals surrounded by foreign body cells.

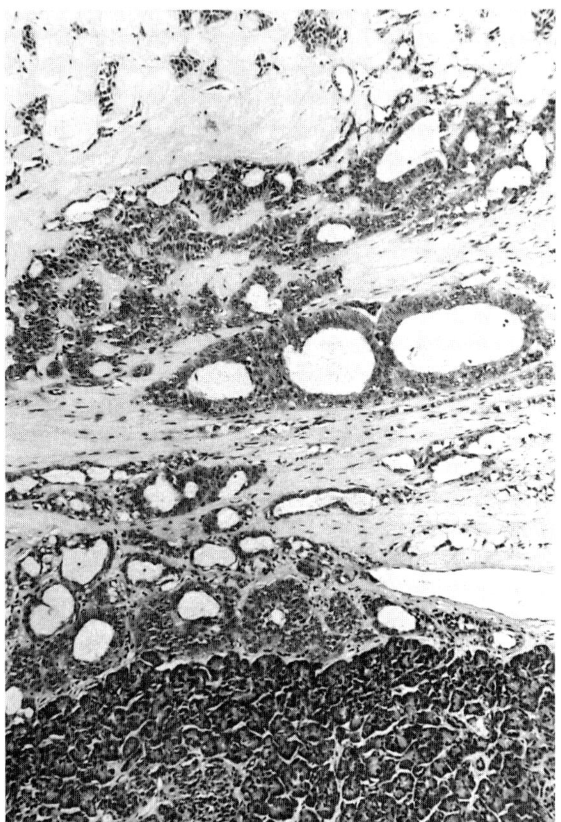

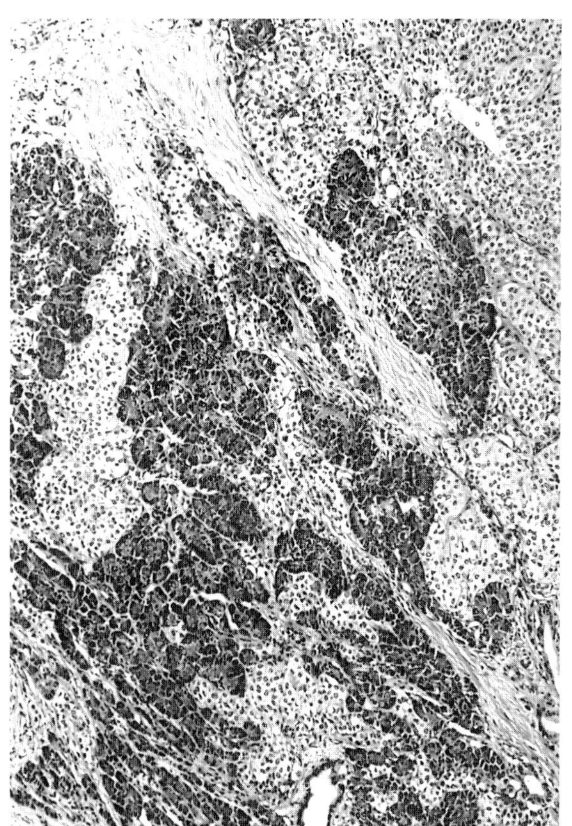

Figure 4-118
SOLID-PSEUDOPAPILLARY TUMOR
Left: The tumor tissue (top) is sharply demarcated from the adjoining pancreatic parenchyma (bottom), but lacks a clear capsule. Right: Margin of a malignant tumor with deep invasion into the adjacent pancreatic tissue.

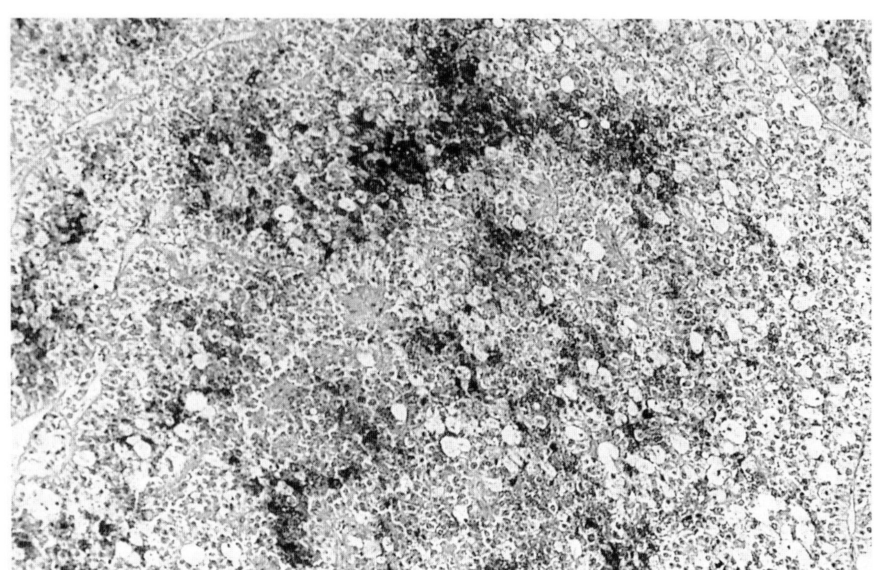

Figure 4-119
SOLID-PSEUDOPAPILLARY TUMOR
Tumor tissue with intense focal immunostaining for alpha-1-antitrypsin.

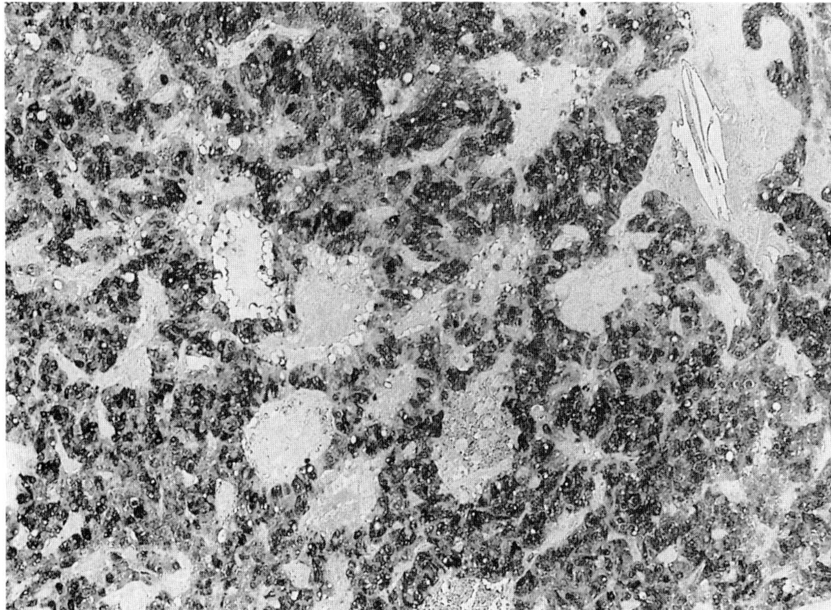

Figure 4-120
SOLID-PSEUDOPAPILLARY TUMOR
Tumor tissue with diffuse immunostaining for NSE.

usually diffuse. Inconsistent results have been reported for epithelial markers, neuroendocrine markers, pancreatic enzymes, islet cell hormones, and other antigens such as CEA or CA19-9. Most reports record negative results for synaptophysin and chromogranin A as well as for CEA, CA19-9, and AFP. A few tumors stain for S-100 protein or cytokeratin markers (459,468,473). Immunoreactivity for trypsin, chymotrypsin, amylase, and phospholipase A2 has been reported by some authors (442,465,466,468,472,482), but has not been confirmed by others (454,459,470). Similarly, focal positivity for glucagon, somatostatin, and insulin has been described in some tumors (468, 471,485,489), but not in others (459,463–465, 470,473,482). Estrogen and progesterone receptors have been demonstrated by biochemical assays in four solid-pseudopapillary tumors (445, 463,487). Immunohistologically, most studies fail to detect nuclear estrogen receptors (445, 468,487), while progesterone receptors were recently demonstrated in eight tumors (492).

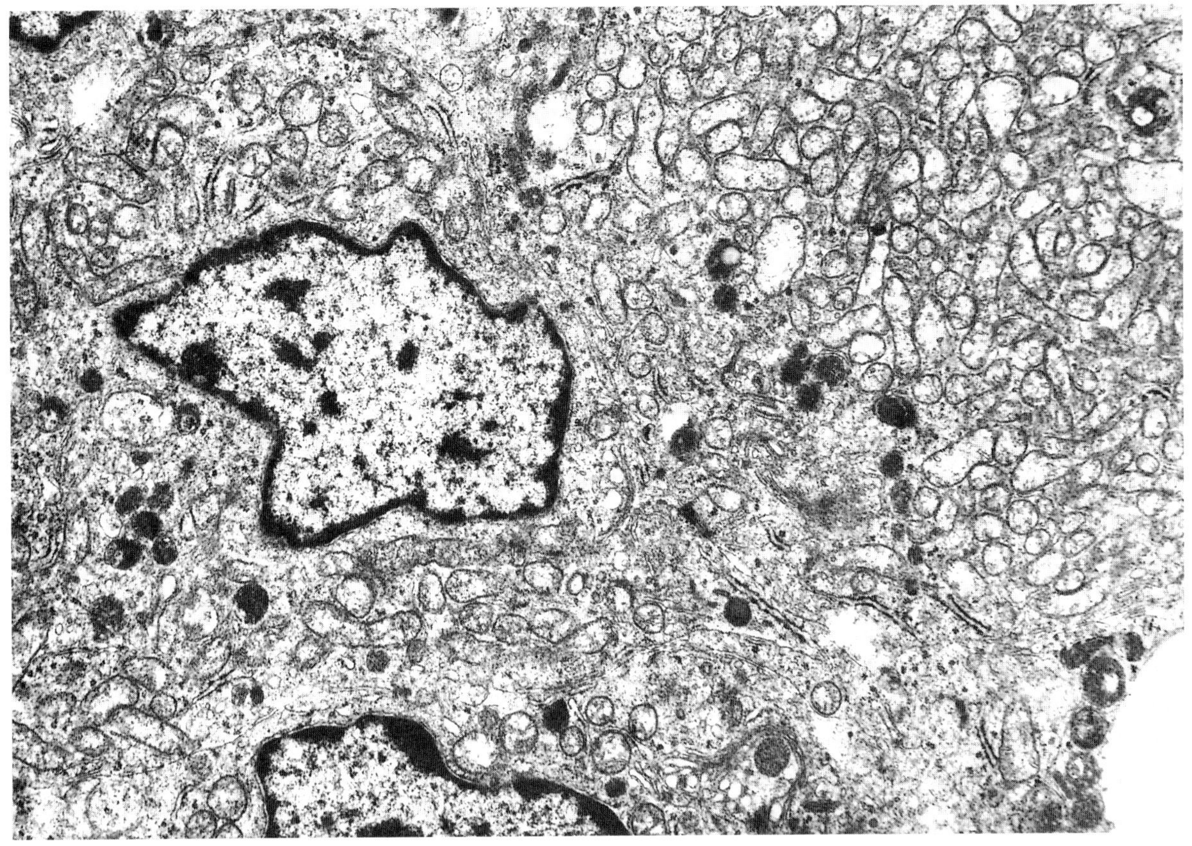

Figure 4-121
SOLID-PSEUDOPAPILLARY TUMOR
This electron micrograph shows tumor cells with an abundant cytoplasm containing multiple mitochondria and a few dense bodies. The nuclei have a polygonal shape. (Courtesy of Dr. H.D. John, Mainz, Germany.)

**Ultrastructural Findings.** The tumor cells have round or markedly indented nuclei which contain a small single nucleolus and a narrow rim of marginated heterochromatin. The cytoplasm is abundant and rich in mitochondria (fig. 4-121). The rough endoplasmic reticulum is sparse to moderate, with occasionally prominent Golgi complexes. Stacks of annulate lamellae may also be noted. Some tumor cells have a vacuolated clear cytoplasm. Most conspicuous are tumor cells containing large, osmiophilic, zymogen-like granules of variable sizes (500 to 3000 nm). The contents of these granules often disintegrate and form multilamellated vesicles and lipid droplets (fig. 4-122) (460,464,468,491). The exact nature of these granules, which are randomly distributed in the cytoplasm, is not known, but they probably represent deposits of alpha-1-antitrypsin. Neurosecretory granules have been described in a few tumors (455,456,471,480,486, 489). Intermediate cell junctions are rarely observed and microvilli are lacking, but small intercellular spaces are frequent.

**New Techniques.** Morphometric analyses differentiate solid-pseudopapillary tumors from well-differentiated ductal adenocarcinoma by lower mean nuclear volume and mitotic index, but not by silver-stained AgNOR counts (455).

DNA flow cytometric analysis of two solid-pseudopapillary tumors showed a diploid range of DNA content, with an additional aneuploid population in one of the tumors (455). In another study diploid DNA was found in eight non-metastasizing solid-pseudopapillary tumors and aneuploid DNA in one metastasizing tumor (473). The malignant solid-pseudopapillary tumors reported by Cappellari et al. (444) had an aneuploid DNA histogram.

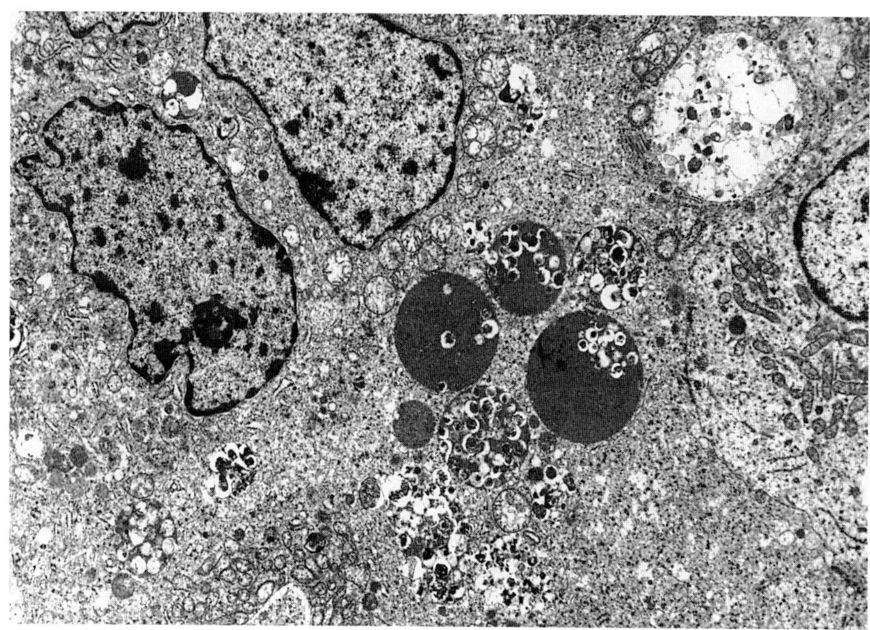

Figure 4-122
SOLID-PSEUDOPAPILLARY TUMOR

Electron micrograph showing large osmiophilic, zymogen-like granules of variable sizes. Often, there is disintegration of the granule content, thereby forming multilamellated vesicles. (Courtesy of Dr. H.D. John, Mainz, Germany.

**Differential Diagnosis.** The differential diagnosis of solid-pseudopapillary tumor includes endocrine tumor, acinar cell carcinoma, pancreatoblastoma, ductal adenocarcinoma, and cystic tumors.

*Endocrine Tumor.* It is important to distinguish solid-pseudopapillary tumors from endocrine tumors because of the better prognosis of the former. Histologically, the solid areas of solid-pseudopapillary tumors resemble endocrine tumor tissue because of their monomorphous cell pattern. However, endocrine tumors usually lack the widespread hemorrhagic-degenerative changes and pseudopapillary pattern seen in most solid-pseudopapillary tumors. Immunohistochemical criteria in favor of solid-pseudopapillary tumor include strong focal positivity for alpha-1-antitrypsin, diffuse immunoreactivity for vimentin, and negativity for endocrine markers such as synaptophysin and usually chromogranin A. Neuron-specific enolase is positive in both tumors. Electron microscopically, endocrine tumors lack the large zymogen-like granules and abundance of mitochondria seen in many solid-pseudopapillary tumors. Moreover, their nuclei are usually round and not indented.

*Acinar Cell Carcinoma.* These tumors occur more often in men than in women. In contrast to solid-pseudopapillary tumors they are not well demarcated and have a nodular cut surface; in the case of an acinar cystadenocarcinoma, the cut surface is multicystic. Microscopically, they lack pseudopapillary changes and instead have an acinar or trabecular pattern. If they are solid, they are rich in mitoses. Immunohistochemically, they express pancreatic enzymes such as trypsin or lipase and lack a strong focal positivity for alpha-1-antitrypsin. They also stain consistently with cytokeratin markers, a feature rarely observed in solid-pseudopapillary tumors.

*Pancreatoblastoma.* When solid-pseudopapillary tumors occur in children under 10 years of age they have to be distinguished from pancreatoblastoma. Although pancreatoblastomas may also show necrotic changes, they lack the delicate fibrovascular tissue stalks and pseudopapillary pattern. Moreover, pancreatoblastomas, as acinar cell carcinomas, usually display epithelial cells arranged in an acinar pattern. These cells are consistently positive for pancreatic enzymes and negative for vimentin.

*Ductal Adenocarcinoma.* This is easily separated from solid-pseudopapillary tumor by gross appearance, histologic pattern, and sex and age distribution. Cystic tumors of the pancreas, in contrast to solid-pseudopapillary tumor, are composed of true cystic structures lined by epithelial cells, either expressing mucin (mucinous cystic tumor) or glycogen (serous cystadenoma).

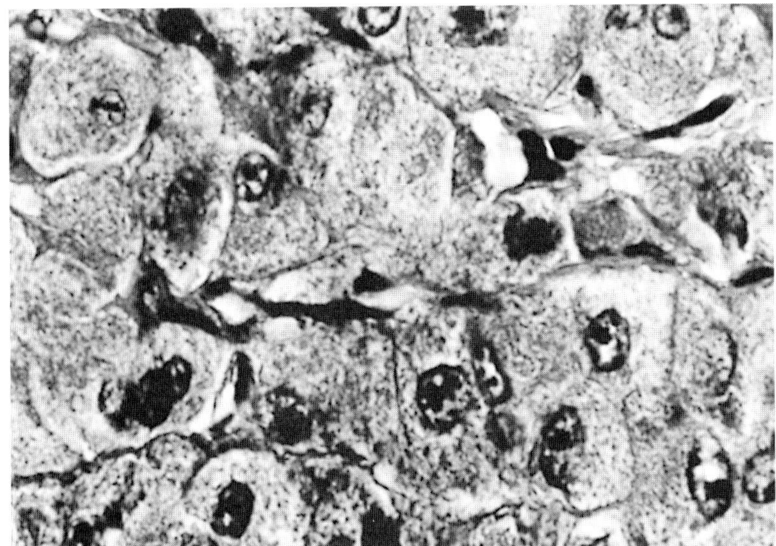

Figure 4-123
ONCOCYTIC CARCINOMA
Large cells with abundant, finely granular, eosinophilic cytoplasm. There is irregularity in size and shape of nuclei, which have prominent nucleoli. (Fig. 232 from Fascicle 19, Second Series.)

**Frozen Section Diagnosis and Cytology.** On frozen section, a heterogeneous pattern with endocrine-like parts alternating with zones of pseudopapillary architecture and hemorrhagic degeneration is seen. Fine-needle aspiration cytology is characterized by pronounced cellularity, a bland, uniform nuclear appearance with even chromatin distribution, the presence of occasional cells with foamy cytoplasm, and perivascular papillary clustering of tumor cells (444,450,486,488).

**Spread, Metastasis, and Recurrence.** There are only a few reports of metastasizing solid-pseudopapillary tumor (for review see 466 and 473). Of 18 patients reported, the tumor metastasized to the regional lymph nodes in 4, the peritoneum and greater omentum in 5, the liver in 11, and the subcutis in 1 (446,473). The metastatic deposits in the liver are usually solitary lesions which grossly resemble the primary tumors in the pancreas. Multiple liver metastases are rare (444, 481,493). Local tumor recurrence has been observed 3 to 10 years after tumor resection (481).

**Prognosis and Treatment.** In general, the prognosis is very good: after complete tumor removal more than 95 percent of patients are cured. Even in patients whose tumors spread locally, recurred (448,451,462), or metastasized (444,466,477) long disease-free periods have been recorded after initial diagnosis and resection. Only a few patients have died of a metastasizing solid-pseudopapillary tumor (466,474).

## MISCELLANEOUS CARCINOMAS

### Oncocytic Carcinoma

Oncocytic carcinomas that appear to be of nonendocrine origin have been reported by Huntrakoon (498), Chen and Baithun (495), Nozawa et al. (499), Bondeson et al. (494), and Sironi et al. (500,501). The tumor cells were large with abundant finely granular eosinophilic material (fig. 4-123). Electron microscopically, they were packed with mitochondria, but devoid of zymogen or neuroendocrine granules (fig. 4-124). Immunohistochemical examinations were not performed.

### Choriocarcinoma

A case of pancreatic choriocarcinoma which presented as an inflammatory cyst was reported by Childs et al. (496). This widely metastasized tumor was large and occurred in the body of the pancreas. The tumor produced and secreted the beta-subunit of human chorionic gonadotropin.

### Nonmucinous, Glycogen-Poor Cystadenocarcinoma

This tumor presented in the head of the pancreas as a large encapsulated and bosselated mass, measuring 19 cm in greatest diameter (497). It consisted of numerous tiny and some larger cysts with watery contents. Metastases were found in lymph nodes, liver, adrenal gland, lung, and bone marrow. Microscopically, large parts of the tumor were similar to serous

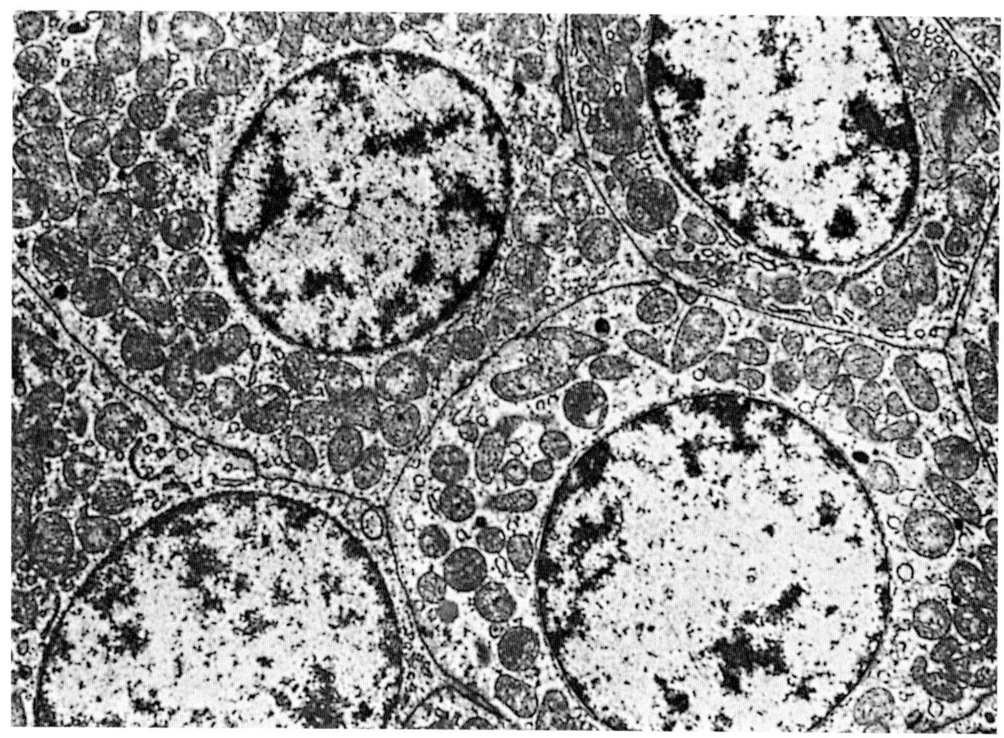

Figure 4-124
ONCOCYTIC CARCINOMA
Tumor in the tail of the pancreas. Four cells with abundant mitochondria in the cytoplasm are shown. The cytoplasm of all cells are packed with mitochondria. Few glands were present in other areas. (Fig. 233 from Fascicle 19, Second Series.)

microcystic adenoma. In some areas, however, the cysts were tiny and lined by a distinctly atypical pseudostratified columnar epithelium. This type of epithelium was also found in the metastases. The tumor cells were negative for mucins. Immunohistochemically, they stained for CEA and focally for neuron-specific enolase and synaptophysin, but not for chromogranin A. Ultrastructurally, some cells showed oncocytic changes and contained many lipid droplets.

## MATURE TERATOMA

**Definition.** This is a benign extragonadal germ cell tumor with mature tissues derived from all three germinal layers. It has been referred to as *dermoid cyst of the pancreas* (502,503).

So far 12 teratomas have been described in the pancreas (503). Eight of these 12 patients were younger than 27 years. In almost all patients the tumors were palpable and often also painful.

**Gross and Histologic Findings.** The tumors may occur anywhere within the pancreas or may be attached to it (502–504). They are usually large (8 to 12 cm) and consist of unilocular or multilocular cysts filled with thick yellowish sebaceous material. Histologically, the cyst is lined by a single layer of ciliated epithelium or stratified squamous epithelium. The wall contains dermal appendages (sebaceous glands and hair follicles) and sometimes other tissues, such as teeth, cartilage, bone, and glia. In the outer layer of the wall there are usually small pancreatic ducts. Foci of immature tissue have not yet been observed in pancreatic teratomas.

**Differential Diagnosis.** The differential diagnosis includes all other cystic lesions of the pancreas, which however can be easily excluded on histologic grounds. The only difficulty may be in differentiating a dermoid cyst from a so called lymphoepithelial cyst (see Tumor-Like Lesions), because both are lined by squamous epithelium. The lymphoepithelial cyst lacks epidermal appendages and instead has a subepithelial layer of lymphoid tissue.

## REFERENCES

### Serous Cystadenoma


1. Alpert LC, Truong LD, Bossart MI, Spjut HJ. Microcystic adenoma (serous cystadenoma) of the pancreas. A study of 14 cases with immunohistochemical and electron microscopic correlation. Am J Surg Pathol 1988;12:251–63.
2. Amir G, Hurvitz H, Neeman Z, Rosenmann E. Neonatal cytomegalovirus infection with pancreatic cystadenoma and nephrotic syndrome. Pediatr Pathol 1986;6:393–401.
3. Becker WF, Welsh RA, Pratt HS. Cystadenoma and cystadenocarcinoma of the pancreas. Ann Surg 1965;161:845–63.
4. Beerman MH, Fromkes JJ, Carey LC, Thomas FB. Pancreatic cystadenoma in Von Hippel-Lindau disease: an unusual cause of pancreatic and common bile duct obstruction. J Clin Gastroenterol 1982;4:537–40.
5. Bickler S, Wile AG, Melicharek M, Recher L. Pancreatic involvement in Hippel-Lindau disease. West J Med 1984;140:280–2.
6. Bogomoletz WV, Adnet JJ, Widgren S, Stavrou M, McLaughlin JE. Cystadenoma of the pancreas: a histological, histochemical and ultrastructural study of seven cases. Histopathology 1980;4:309–20.
7. Chang CH, Perrin EV, Hertzler J, Brough AJ. Cystadenoma of the pancreas with cytomegalovirus infection in a female infant. Arch Pathol Lab Med 1980;104:7–8.
8. Chen J, Baithun SI. Morphological study of 391 cases of exocrine pancreatic tumors with special reference to the classification of exocrine pancreatic carcinoma. J Pathol 1985;146:17–29.
9. Compagno J, Oertel JE. Microcystic adenoma of the pancreas (glycogen-rich cystadenomas): a clinicopathologic study of 34 cases. Am J Clin Pathol 1978;69:289–98.
10. Corbally MT, McAnena OJ, Urmacher C, Herman B, Shiu MH. Pancreatic cystadenoma. A clinicopathologic study. Arch Surg 1989;124:1271–4.
11. Doll DC, List AF, Yarbro JW. Evans' syndrome associated with microcystic adenoma of the pancreas. Cancer 1987;59:1366–8.
12. Egawa N, Maillet B, Schröder S, Mukai K, Klöppel G. Serous oligocystic and ill-demarcated adenoma of the pancreas: a variant of serous cystic adenoma. Virchows Arch 1994;424:13–7.
13. Friedman AC, Lichtenstein JE, Dachman AH. Cystic neoplasms of the pancreas. Radiological-pathological correlation. Radiology 1983;149:45–50.
14. Gundersen AE, Janis JF. Pancreatic cystadenoma in childhood. Report of a case. J Pediatr Surg 1969;4:478–81.
15. Helpap B, Vogel J. Immunohistochemical studies on cystic pancreatic neoplasms. Pathol Res Pract 1989;84:39–45.
16. Hodgkinson DJ, ReMine WH, Weiland LH. Pancreatic cystadenoma. A clinicopathologic study of 45 cases. Arch Surg 1978;113:512–9.
17. Horton WA, Wong V, Eldridge R. Von Hippel-Lindau disease: clinical and pathological manifestations in nine families with 50 affected members. Arch Int Med 1976;136:769–77.
18. Itai Y, Ohhashi K, Furui S, et al. Microcystic adenoma of the pancreas: spectrum of computed tomographic findings. J Comput Assist Tomogr 1988;12:797–803.
19. Kamei K, Funabiki T, Ochiai M, Amano H, Kasahara M, Sakamoto T. Multifocal pancreatic serous cystadenoma with atypical cells and focal perineural invasion. Int J Pancreatol 1991;10:161–72.
20. Kim YI, Seo JW, Suh JS, Lee KU, Choe KJ. Microcystic adenomas of the pancreas. Report of three cases with two of multicentric origin. Am J Clin Pathol 1990;94:150–6.
21. Laitio M, Lev R, Orlic D. The developing human fetal pancreas: an ultrastructural and histochemical study with special reference to exocrine cells. J Anat 1974;117:619–34.
22. Lewandrowski K, Warshaw A, Compton C. Macrocystic serous cystadenoma of the pancreas: a morphologic variant differing from microcystic adenoma. Hum Pathol 1992;23:871–5.
23. Lo JW, Fung CH, Yonan TN, Martinez N. Cystadenoma of the pancreas. An ultrastructural study. Cancer 1977;39:2470–4.
24. Mathieu D, Guigui B, Valette PJ, et al. Pancreatic cystic neoplasms. Radiol Clin North Am 1989;27:163–76.
25. Montag AG, Fossati N, Michelassi F. Pancreatic microcystic adenoma coexistent with pancreatic ductal carcinoma. A report of two cases. Am J Surg Pathol 1990;14:352–5.
26. Morohoshi T, Held G, Klöppel G. Exocrine pancreatic tumours and their histological classification. A study based on 167 autopsy and 97 surgical cases. Histopathology 1983;7:645–61.
27. Neumann HP, Dinkel E, Brambs HJ, et al. Pancreatic lesions in the Hippel-Lindau syndrome. Gastroenterology 1991;101:465–71.
28. Nyongo A, Huntrakoon M. Microcystic adenoma of the pancreas with myoepithelial cells. A hitherto undescribed morphologic feature. Am J Clin Pathol 1985;84:114–20.
29. Osborn M, van Lessen G, Weber K, Klöppel G, Altmannsberger M. Differential diagnosis of gastrointestinal carcinomas by using monoclonal antibodies specific for individual keratin polypeptides. Lab Invest 1986;55:497–504.
30. Pyke CM, van Heerden JA, Colby TV, Sarr MG, Weaver AL. The spectrum of serous cystadenoma of the pancreas. Clinical, pathologic, and surgical aspects. Ann Surg 1992;215:132–9.
31. Schüssler MH, Skoudy A, Ramaekers F, Real FX. Intermediate filaments as differentiation markers of normal pancreas and pancreas cancer. Am J Pathol 1992;140:559–68.
32. Seifert G. Cystic, traumatic and vascular lesions. In: Klöppel G, Heitz PH, eds. Pancreatic pathology. Edinburgh: Churchill Livingstone, 1984:73–7.
33. Shorten SD, Hart WR, Petras RE. Microcystic adenomas (serous cystadenomas) of pancreas. A clinicopathologic investigation of eight cases with immunohistochemical and ultrastructural studies. Am J Surg Pathol 1986;10:365–72.

34. Warfel KA, Faught PR, Hull MT. Pancreatic cystadenoma in an infant: ultrastructural study. Pediatr Pathol 1988;8:559–65.
35. Warshaw AL, Compton CC, Lewandrowsky K, Cardenosa G, Mueller PR. Cystic tumors of the pancreas. New clinical, radiologic, and pathologic observations in 67 patients. Ann Surg 1990;212:432–45.
36. Yamaguchi K, Enjoji M. Cystic neoplasms of the pancreas. Gastroenterology 1987;92:1934–43.
37. Young NA, Villani MA, Khoury P, Naryshkin S. Differential diagnosis of cystic neoplasms of the pancreas by fine-needle aspiration. Arch Pathol Lab Med 1991;115:571–7.

**Serous Cystadenocarcinoma**

38. Friedman HD. Nonmucinous, glycogen-poor cystadenocarcinoma of the pancreas. Arch Pathol Lab Med 1990;114:888–91.
39. George DH, Murphy F, Michalski R, Ulmer BG. Serous cystadenocarcinoma of the pancreas: a new entity? Am J Surg Pathol 1989;13:61–6.
40. Kamei K, Funabiki T, Ochiai M, Amano H, Kasahara M, Sakamoto T. Multifocal pancreatic serous cystadenoma with atypical cells and focal perineural invasion. Int J Pancreatol 1991;10:161–72.
41. Yoshimi N, Sugie S, Tanaka T, et al. A rare case of serous cystadenocarcinoma of the pancreas. Cancer 1992;69:2449–53.

**Mucinous Cystic Tumor**

42. Akwari OE, Tucker A, Seigler HF, Itani KM. Hepatobiliary cystadenoma with mesenchymal stroma. Ann Surg 1990;211:18–27.
43. Albores-Saavedra J, Angeles-Angeles A, Nadji M, Henson DE, Alvarez L. Mucinous cystadenocarcinoma of the pancreas. Morphologic and immunocytochemical observations. Am J Surg Pathol 1987;11:11–20.
44. Albores-Saavedra J, Nadji M, Henson DE, Angeles-Angeles A. Entero-endocrine cell differentiation in carcinomas of the gallbladder and mucinous cystadenocarcinomas of the pancreas. Path Res Pract 1988;183:169–75.
45. Bätge B, Bosslet K, Sedlacek HH, Kern HF, Klöppel G. Monoclonal antibodies against CEA-related components discriminate between pancreatic duct type carcinomas and nonneoplastic duct lesions as well as nonduct type neoplasias. Virchows Arch [A] 1986;408:361–74.
46. Becker WF, Welsh RA, Pratt HS. Cystadenoma and cystadenocarcinoma of the pancreas. Ann Surg 1965;161:845–63.
47. Bogomoletz WV, Adnet JJ, Widgren S, Stavrou M, McLaughlin JE. Cystadenoma of the pancreas: a histological, histochemical and ultrastructural study of seven cases. Histopathology 1980;4:309–20.
48. Campbell JA, Cruickshank AH. Cystadenoma and cystadenocarcinoma of the pancreas. J Clin Pathol 1962;15:432–7.
49. Chen J, Baithun SI, Ramsay MA. Histogenesis of pancreatic carcinomas: a study based on 248 cases. J Pathol 1985;146:65–76.
50. Compagno J, Oertel JE. Mucinous cystic neoplasms of the pancreas with overt and latent malignancy (cystadenocarcinoma and cystadenoma). A clinicopathologic study of 41 cases. Am J Clin Pathol 1978;69:573–80.
51. Corbally MT, McAnena OJ, Urmacher C, Herman B, Shiu M. Pancreatic cystadenoma. A clinicopathologic study. Arch Surg 1989;124:1271–4.
52. Cross MR. Mucinous cystadenoma of the pancreas. Endoscopy as an aid to diagnosis. Gastroenterology 1980;79:944–7.
53. Cullen PK, ReMine WH, Dahlin DC. A clinicopathological study of cystadenocarcinoma of the pancreas. Surg Gynecol Obstet 1963;117:189–95.
54. Czernobilsky B, Dgani R, Roth LM. Ovarian mucinous cystadenocarcinoma with mural nodule of carcinomatous derivation. Cancer 1983;51:141–8.
55. Didolkar MS, Holyoke ED. Cystadenoma of the pancreas. Surg Gynecol Obstet 1975;140:925–8.
56. El Nakadi B, Greuse M, Debaize JP, Salhadin A. Nouvelle complication des néoplasies kystiques du pancréas: la fistule cysto-duodénale. Acta Chir Belg 1992;92:52–4.
57. Fetissof F, Dubois MP, Legue E, deCalan L, Jobard P. Tumeurs mucineuses retropertitonéales et pancréatiques. Etude immunohistochimique. Ann Pathol 1985;5:53–7.
58. Friedman AC, Lichtenstein JE, Dachman AH. Cystic neoplasms of the pancreas. Radiological-pathological correlation. Radiology 1983;149:45–50.
59. Helpap B, Vogel J. Immunohistochemical studies on cystic pancreatic neoplasms. Pathol Res Pract 1989;184:39–45.
60. Herrera L, Glassman CI, Komins JI. Mucinous cystic neoplasm of the pancreas demonstrated by ultrasound and endoscopic retrograde pancreatography. Am J Gastroenterology 1980;73:512–5.
61. Hodgkinson DJ, ReMine WH, Weiland LH. A clinicopathologic study of 21 cases of pancreatic cystadenocarcinoma. Ann Surg 1978;188:679–84.
62. Hodgkinson DJ, ReMine WH, Weiland LH. Pancreatic cystadenoma. A clinicopathologic study of 45 cases. Arch Surg 1978;13:512–9.
63. Ishak KG, Willis GW, Cummins SD, Bullock AA. Biliary cystadenoma and cystadenocarcinoma: report of 14 cases and review of the literature. Cancer 1977;38:322–38.
64. Itai Y, Moss AA, Ohtomo K. Computed tomography of cystadenoma and cystadenocarcinoma of the pancreas. Radiology 1982;145:419–25.
65. Ito Y, Blackstone MO, Frank PH, Skinner DB. Mucinous biliary obstruction associated with a cystic adenocarcinoma of the pancreas. Gastroenterology 1977;73:1410–2.
66. Laucirica R, Schwartz MR, Ramzy I. Fine needle aspiration of pancreatic cystic epithelial neoplasms. Acta Cytol 1992;36:881–6.
67. Lichtenstein L. Papillary cystadenocarcinoma of pancreas. Case report, with notes on classification of malignant cystic tumors of pancreas. Am J Cancer 1934;21:542–53.

68. Margolis RM, Jang N. Zollinger-Ellison syndrome associated with pancreatic cystadenocarcinoma. N Engl J Med 1984;311:1380–1.
69. Mathieu D, Guigui B, Valette PJ, et al. Pancreatic cystic neoplasms. Radiol Clin North Am 1989;27:163–76.
70. Morinaga S, Ohyama R, Koizumi J. Low-grade mucinous cystadeno-carcinoma in the spleen. Am J Surg Pathol 1992;16:903–8.
71. Morohoshi T, Held G, Klöppel G. Exocrine pancreatic tumours and their histological classification. A study based on 167 autopsy and 97 surgical cases. Histopathology 1983;7:645–61.
72. Nishida K, Shiga K, Kato K, et al. Two cases of pancreatic cystadenocarcinoma with elevated CA 19-9 levels in the cystic fluid in comparison with two cases of pancreatic cystadenoma. Hepatogastroenterology 1989;36:442–5.
73. Posen JA. Giant cell tumor of the pancreas of the osteoclastic type associated with a mucous secreting cystadenocarcinoma. Hum Pathol 1981;12:944–7.
74. Prat J, Scully RE. Ovarian mucinous tumors with sarcoma-like mural nodules: a report of seven cases. Cancer 1979;44:1332–44.
75. Probstein JG, Blumenthal HT. Progressive malignant degeneration of a cystadenoma of the pancreas. Arch Surg 1960;81:683–9.
76. Rego JA, Ruvira LV, Garcia AA, Freijanes PS, Penaranda JM, Soto JM. Pancreatic mucinous cystadenocarcinoma with pseudosarcomatous mural nodules. A report of a case with immunohistochemical study. Cancer 1991;67:494–8.
77. ReMine SG, Frey D, Rossi RL, Munson JL, Braasch JW. Cystic neoplasms of the pancreas. Arch Surg 1987;122:443–6.
78. Santini D, Bazzocchi F, Ricci M, Mazzoleni G, Campione O, Marrano D. Mucinous cystic tumour of the pancreas. A histological and histochemical study. Pathol Res Pract 1988;183:767–70.
79. Schwerk WB. Ultrasonically guided percutaneous puncture and analysis of aspirated material of cystic pancreatic lesions. Digestion 1981;21:184–92.
80. Seifert G. Cystic, traumatic and vascular lesions. In: Klöppel G, Heitz PH, eds. Pancreatic pathology. Edinburgh: Churchill Livingstone, 1984;73–7.
81. Sessa F, Bonato M, Frigerio B, et al. Ductal cancers of the pancreas frequently express markers of gastrointestinal epithelial cells. Gastroenterology 1990;98:1655–65.
82. Smith E, Matzen P. Mucus-producing tumors with mucinous biliary obstruction causing jaundice: diagnosed and treated endoscopically. Am J Gastroenterol 1985;80:287–9.
83. Stahlschmidt M, Schäfer A, Schmitt-Köppler A. Zystadenom in heterotopen Pankreasgewebe. Leber Magen Darm 1974;4:247–50.
84. Tatsuta M, Iishi H, Ichii M, et al. Values of carcinoembryonic antigen, elastase 1, and carbohydrate antigen determinant in aspirated pancreatic cystic fluid in the diagnosis of cysts of the pancreas. Cancer 1986;57:1836–9.
85. Tenti P, Aguzzi A, Riva C, et al. Ovarian mucinous tumors frequently express markers of gastric, intestinal, and pancreatobiliary epithelial cells. Cancer 1992;69:2131–42.
86. Tsujimura T, Kawano K, Taniguchi M, Yoshikawa K, Tsukaguchi I. Malignant fibrous histiocytoma coexistent with mucinous cystadenoma of the pancreas. Cancer 1992;70:2792–6.
87. von Segesser L, Rohner A. Pancreatic cystadenoma and cystadenocarcinoma. Br J Surg 1984;71:449–51.
88. Warren KW, Hardy KJ. Cystadenocarcinoma of the pancreas. Surg Gynecol Obstet 1968;127:734–6.
89. Warshaw AL, Compton CC, Lewandrowski K, Cardenosa G, Mueller PR. Cystic tumors of the pancreas. New clinical, radiologic, and pathologic observations in 67 patients. Ann Surg 1990;212:432–45.
90. Warshaw AL, Rutledge PL. Cystic tumors mistaken for pancreatic pseudocysts. Ann Surg 1987;205:393–8.
91. Wheeler DA, Edmondson HA. Cystadenoma with mesenchymal stroma (CMS) in the liver and bile ducts. A clinicopathologic study of 17 cases, 4 with malignant change. Cancer 1985;56:1434–45.
92. Yamada M, Kozuka S, Yamao K, Nakazawa S, Naitoh Y, Tsukamoto Y. Mucin-producing tumor of the pancreas. Cancer 1991:68;159–68.
93. Yamaguchi K, Enjoji M. Cystic neoplasms of the pancreas. Gastroenterology 1987;92:1934–43.
94. Young NA, Villani MA, Khoury P, Naryshkin S. Differential diagnosis of cystic neoplasms of the pancreas by fine-needle aspiration. Arch Pathol Lab Med 1991; 115:571–7.
95. Yu HC, Shetty J. Mucinous cystic neoplasm of the pancreas with high carcinoembryonic antigen. Arch Pathol Lab Med 1985;109:375–7.
96. Zamboni G, Bonetti F, Castelli P, et al. Mucinous cystic tumor of the pancreas recurring after 11 years as cystadenocarcinoma with foci of choriocarcinoma and osteoclast-like giant cell tumor. Surg Pathol 1994;5:253–62.

**Intraductal Papillary-Mucinous Tumor**

97. Armstrong O, Charleux H. Adénocarcinome papillaire intracanalaire du pancréas. Un cas et revue de la littérature. Presse Méd 1983;12:1763–5.
98. Bastid C, Bebnard JP, Sarlec H, Payan MJ, Sahel J. Mucinous ductal ectasia of the pancreas: a premalignant disease and a cause of obstructive pancreatitis. Pancreas 1991;6:15–22.
99. Caroli J, Hadchouel P, Mercadier M, Lageron A. Papillome bénin du canal de Wirsung? Diagnostic par cathétérisme rétrograde. Med Chir Dig 1975;4:163–6.
100. Chen J, Baithun SI, Ramsay MA. Histogenesis of pancreatic carcinomas: a study based on 248 cases. J Pathol 1985;146:65–76.
101. Conley CR, Scheithauer BW, van Heerden JA, Weiland LH. Diffuse intraductal papillary adenocarcinoma of the pancreas. Ann Surg 1987;205:246–9.
102. Cross MR. Mucinous cystadenoma of the pancreas. Endoscopy as an aid to diagnosis. Gastroenterology 1980;79:944–7.
103. Cubilla AL, Fitzgerald PJ. Tumors of the exocrine pancreas. Atlas of Tumor Pathology, 2nd Series, Fascicle 19. Washington, D.C.: Armed Forces Institute of Pathology, 1984.
104. Ferrari BT, O'Halloran RL, Longmire WP, Lewin KJ. Atypical papillary hyperplasia of the pancreatic duct mimicking obstructing pancreatic carcinoma. N Engl J Med 1979;301:531–2.

105. Fitzgerald PJ, Cubilla AL. Exocrine pancreas. In: Henson DE, Albores-Saavedra J, Vuitch F, eds. The pathology of incipient neoplasia. Philadelphia: WB Saunders, 1986:217–31.
106. Furukawa T, Takahashi T, Kobari M, Matsuno S. The mucus-hypersecreting tumor of the pancreas. Development and extension visualized by three-dimensional computerized mapping. Cancer 1992;70:1505–13.
107. Furuta K, Watanabe H, Ikeda S. Differences between solid and duct-ectatic types of pancreatic ductal carcinomas. Cancer 1992;69:1327–33.
108. Haban G. Papillomatose und Carcinom des Gangsystems der Bauchspeicheldrüse. Virchows Arch [A] 1936;297:207–20.
109. Halphen M, Hoang C, Hautefeuille P, et al. Tumeurs intra-canalaires primitives multiples du canal de Wirsung: démonstration d'une filiation entre tumeurs bénignes et malignes. Gastroenterol Clin Biol 1988;12:163–8.
110. Hivet M, Maisel A, Horiot A, Conte J. Carcinome villeux diffus du canal de Wirsung. Pancréatectomie totale. Med Chir Dig 1975;4:159–62.
111. Itai Y, Kokubo T, Atomi Y, Kuroda A, Haraguchi Y, Terano A. Mucin-hypersecreting carcinoma of the pancreas. Radiology 1987;165:51–5.
112. Itai Y, Ohhashi K, Nagai H, et al. Ductectatic mucinous cystadenoma and cystadenocarcinoma of the pancreas. Radiology 1986;161:697–700.
113. Klöppel G. Pancreatic non-endocrine tumours. In: Klöppel G, Heitz PU, eds. Pancreatic pathology. Edinburgh: Churchill Livingstone, 1984:79–113.
114. Klöppel G, Bommer G, Rückert K, Seifert G. Intraductal proliferation in the pancreas and its relationship to human and experimental carcinogenesis. Virchows Arch [A] 1980;387:221–33.
115. Kohler B, Köhler G, Riemann JF. Pancreoscopic diagnosis of intraductal cystadenoma of the pancreas. Dig Dis Sci 1990;35:382–4.
116. Lemoine NR, Jain S, Hughes CM, et al. Ki-ras oncogene activation in preinvasive pancreatic cancer. Gastroenterology 1992;102:203–36.
116a. Loftus EV, Olivares-Pakzad BA, Batts KP, Adkins MC, Stephens DH, Sarr MG, DiMagno EP. Intraductal papillary-mucinous tumors of the pancreas: clinicopathologic features, outcome, and nomenclature. Gastroenterology 1996;110:1909–18.
117. Marchal G, Vernette M, Roustan J, Henry G. Papillomatose biliaire cancérisée avec atteinte de l'ampoule de Vater et du canal de Wirsung. Hépatectomie gauche élargie et duodéno-pancréatectomie en un temps. J Chir (Paris) 1974;107:555–78.
118. Milchgrub S, Campuzano M, Casillas J, Albores-Saavedra J. Intraductal carcinoma of the pancreas. Cancer 1992;69:651–6.
119. Mizumoto K, Inagaki T, Koizumi M, et al. Early pancreatic duct adenocarcinoma. Hum Pathol 1988; 19:242–4.
120. Mizumoto K, Tsutsumi M, Kitazawa S, et al. Intraductal carcinoma in a surgically resected pancreas with chronic pancreatitis. Int J Pancreatology 1990;7:279–85.
121. Morohoshi T, Held G, Klöppel G. Exocrine pancreatic tumours and their histological classification. A study based on 167 autopsy and 97 surgical cases. Histopathology 1983;7:645–61.
122. Morohoshi T, Kanda M, Asanuma K, Klöppel G. Intraductal papillary neoplasms of the pancreas. A clinicopathologic study of six patients. Cancer 1989;64:1329–35.
123. Moroshoshi T, Kunimura T, Kanda M, et al. Multiple carcinomata associated with anomalous arrangement of the biliary and pancreatic duct system. A report of two cases with a literature survey. Acta Pathol Jpn 1990;40:755–63.
124. Nicki NJ, Lawson JM, Cotton PB. Mucinous pancreatic tumors: ERCP findings. Gastrointest Endosc 1991; 37:133–8.
125. Nishihara K, Fukuda T, Tsuneyoshi M, Kominami T, Maeda S, Saku M. Intraductal papillary neoplasm of the pancreas. Cancer 1993;72:689–96.
126. Obara T, Maguchi H, Saitoh Y, et al. Mucin-producing tumor of the pancreas: a unique clinical entity. Am J Gastroenterol 1991;86:1619–25.
127. Obara T, Saitoh Y, Maguchi H, et al. Papillary adenoma of the pancreas with excessive mucin secretion. Pancreas 1992;7:114–7.
128. Obara T, Saitoh Y, Maguchi H, et al. Multicentric development of pancreatic intraductal carcinoma through atypical papillary hyperplasia. Hum Pathol 1992;23:82–5.
129. Ohhashi K, Murakami F, Takekoshi T, et al. Four cases of "mucin-producing" cancer of the pancreas based on specific findings of the papilla of Vater [Japanese]. Prog Dig Endosc 1982;20:348.
130. Ponsot P, Molas G, Vilgrain V, Gayet B, Fékété F, Paolaggi JA. Adénomes, adénomatoses et adénocarcinomes pancréatiques intra-canalaires. Gastroenterol Clin Biol 1989;13:663–70.
131. Rickaert F, Cremer M, Devière J, et al. Intraductal mucin-hypersecreting neoplasms of the pancreas. A clinicopathologic study of eight patients. Gastroenterology 1991; 101:512–9.
132. Rogers PN, Seywright MM, Murray WR. Diffuse villous adenoma of the pancreatic duct. Pancreas 1987;2:727–30.
133. Satoh K, Sawai T, Shimosegawa T, et al. The point mutation of c-Ki-ras at codon 12 in carcinoma of the head region and in intraductal mucin-hypersecreting neoplasm of the pancreas. Int J Pancreatol 1993;2:135–43
134. Sessa F, Bonato M, Frigerio B, et al. Ductal cancers of the pancreas frequently express markers of gastrointestinal epithelial cells. Gastroenterology 1990;98:1655–65.
135. Sessa F, Solcia E, Capella C, et al. Intraductal papillary-mucinous tumors represent a distinct group of pancreatic neoplasms: an investigation of tumor cell differentiation and K-ras, p53 and c-erbB-2 abnormalities in 26 patients. Virchows Arch 1994;425:357–67.
136. Shimizu M, Itoh H, Okumura S, et al. Papillary hyperplasia of the pancreas. Hum Pathol 1989;20:806–7.
137. Smith RC, Kneale K, Goulston K. In situ carcinoma of the pancreas. Aust N Z J Surg 1986;56:369–73.
138. Stömmer P, Gebhardt C, Schultheiss KH. Adenocarcinoma of the pancreas with a predominant intraductal component: a special variety of ductal adenocarcinoma. Pancreas 1990;5:114–8.
139. Tada M, Omata M, Ohto M. Ras gene mutations in intraductal papillary neoplasms of the pancreas. Analysis in five cases. Cancer 1991;67:634–7.
140. Warshaw AL, Berry J, Gang DL. Villous adenoma of the duct of Wirsung. Dig Dis Sci 1987;32:1311–3.

141. Warshaw AL, Compton CC, Lewandrowski K, Cardenosa G, Mueller PR. Cystic tumors of the pancreas. New clinical, radiologic and pathologic observations in 67 patients. Ann Surg 1990;212:432–45.
142. Yamada M, Kozuka S, Yamao K, Nakazawa S, Naitoh Y, Tsukamoto Y. Mucin-producing tumor of the pancreas. Cancer 1991;68:159–68.
143. Yamaguchi K, Tanaka M. Mucin-hypersecreting tumor of the pancreas with mucin extrusion through an enlarged papilla. Am J Gastroenterol 1991;86:835–9.
144. Yanagisawa A, Kato Y, Ohtake K, et al. c-Ki-ras point mutations in ductectatic-type mucinous cystic neoplasms of the pancreas. Jpn J Cancer Res 1991;82:1057–60.

**Ductal Adenocarcinoma**

145. Alanen KA, Joensuu H, Klemi PJ, Nevalainen TJ. Clinical significance of nuclear DNA content in pancreatic carcinoma. J Pathol 1990;160:313–20.
146. Alguacil-Garcia A, Weiland LH. The histologic spectrum, prognosis and histogenesis of the sarcomatoid carcinoma of the pancreas. Cancer 1977;39:1181–9.
147. Al-Kaisi N, Siegler EE. Fine needle aspiration cytology of the pancreas. Acta Cytologica 1989;33:145–52.
148. Almoguera C, Shibata D, Forrester K, Martin J, Arnheim N, Perucho M. Most human carcinomas of the exocrine pancreas contain mutant c-K-ras genes. Cell 1988;53:549–54.
149. Ammann RW, Akovbiantz A, Largiader F, Schueler G. Course and outcome of chronic pancreatitis. Longitudinal study of a mixed medical-surgical series of 245 patients. Gastroenterology 1984;86:820–8.
150. Ansari A, Burch GE. A correlative study of proven carcinoma of the pancreas in 83 patients. Am J Gastroenterol 1968;50:456–75.
151. Arkin A, Weisberg SW. Carcinoma of the pancreas, a clinical and pathologic study of seventy-five cases. Gastroenterology 1949;13:118–26.
152. Atkinson BF, Ernst CS, Herlyn M, Steplewski Z, Sears HF, Koprowski H. Gastrointestinal cancer-associated antigen in immunoperoxidase assay. Cancer Res 1982;42:4820–3.
153. Baisch H, Klöppel G, Reinke B. DNA ploidy and cell-cycle analysis in pancreatic and ampullary carcinoma: flow cytometric study of formalin-fixed paraffin-embedded tissue. Virchows Arch [A] 1990;417:145–50.
154. Bartholomew LG, Gross JB, Comfort MW. Carcinoma of the pancreas associated with chronic relapsing pancreatitis. Gastroenterology 1958;35:473–81.
155. Barton CM, Staddon SL, Hughes CM, et al. Abnormalities of the p53 tumour suppressor gene in human pancreatic cancer. Br J Cancer 1992;64:1076–82.
156. Bartow SA, Mukai K, Rosai J. Pseudoneoplastic proliferation of endocrine cells in pancreatic fibrosis. Cancer 1981;47:2627–33.
157. Bätge B, Bosslet K, Sedlacek HH, Kern HF, Klöppel G. Monoclonal antibodies against CEA-related components discriminate between pancreatic duct type carcinomas and nonneoplastic duct lesions as well as nonduct type neoplasias. Virchows Arch [A] 1986;408:361–74.
158. Becker V. Carcinoma of the pancreas and chronic pancreatitis—a possible relationship [Editorial]. Acta Hepato-Gastroenterol 1978;25:257–9.
159. Bell RH, Memoli VA, Longnecker DS. Hyperplasia and tumors of the islets of Langerhans in mice bearing an elastase I-SV40 T-antigen fusion gene. Carcinogenesis 1990;11:1393–8.
160. Bommer G, Friedel U, Heitz PH, Klöppel G. Pancreatic PP cell distribution and hyperplasia: immunocytochemical morphology in the normal pancreas, chronic pancreatitis and pancreatic carcinoma. Virchows Arch [A] 1980;387:319–31.
161. Bowlby LS. Pancreatic adenocarcinoma in an adolescent male with Peutz-Jeghers syndrome. Hum Pathol 1986;17:97–9.
162. Bukowski RM, Fleming TR, Macdonald JS, Oishi N, Taylor SA, Baker LH. Evaluation of combination chemotherapy and phase II agents in pancreatic adenocarcinomas. Cancer 1993;71:322–5.
163. Burch GE, Ansari A. Chronic alcoholism and carcinoma of the pancreas. A correlative hypothesis. Arch Intern Med 1968;122:273–5.
164. Cancer facts and figures. New York, American Cancer Society, 1988.
165. Cassiere SG, McLain DA, Emory WB, Hatch HB. Metastatic carcinoma of the pancreas simulating primary bronchogenic carcinoma. Cancer 1980;46:2319–21.
166. Cederlöf R, Hrubec Z, Lorich U. The relation of smoking and some social covariables to mortality and cancer morbidity. Part I. Stockholm Dept. of Environmental Hygiene. The Karolinska Institute, 1974.
167. Chejfec G, Capella C, Solcia E, Jao W, Gould VE. Amphicrine cells, dysplasia, and neoplasias. Cancer 1985;56:2683–90.
168. Chejfec G, Rieker WJ, Jablokow VR, Gould VE. Pseudomyxoma peritonei associated with colloid carcinoma of the pancreas. Gastroenterology 1986;90:202–5.
169. Chen J, Baithun SI. Morphological study of 391 cases of exocrine pancreatic tumours with special reference to the classification of exocrine pancreatic carcinoma. J Pathol 1985;146:17–29.
170. Chen J, Baithun SI, Pollock DJ, Berry CL. Argyrophilic and hormone immunoreactive cells in normal and hyperplastic pancreatic ducts and exocrine pancreatic carcinoma. Virchows Arch [A] 1988;413:399–405.
171. Connolly MM, Dawson PJ, Michelassi F, Moossa AR, Lowenstein F. Survival in 1001 patients with carcinoma of the pancreas. Ann Surg 1987;206:366–73.
172. Cubilla AL, Fitzgerald PJ. Morphological lesions associated with human primary invasive nonendocrine pancreas cancer. Cancer Research 1976;36:2690–8.
173. Cubilla AL, Fitzgerald PJ. Tumors of the exocrine pancreas. Atlas of Tumor Pathology. 2nd Series, Fascicle 19. Washington, DC: Armed Forces Institute of Pathology, 1984:162.
174. Cubilla AL, Fitzgerald PJ, Fortner JG. Pancreas cancer—duct cell adenocarcinoma: survival in relation to site, size, stage and type of therapy. J Surg Oncology 1978;10:465–82.
175. Cubilla AL, Fortner J, Fitzgerald PJ. Lymph node involvement in carcinoma of the head of the pancreas area. Cancer 1978;41:880–7.
176. De Vuyst M, Rickaert F, De Roy G, Klöppel G. The spectrum of ductal adenocarcinomas and other tumors of the pancreas in patients younger than 40 years of age [Abstract]. Path Res Pract 1993;189:681.

177. Diaso RB, Eanes RZ, Chen ML, Madge GE, Mellette SJ. Adenocarcinoma of the pancreas associated with hypoglycemia: case report and review of the literature. Cancer 1979;43:2457–64.
178. Durbec JP, Chevillotte G, Bidart JM, Berthezene P, Sarles H. Diet, alcohol, tobacco and risk of cancer of the pancreas: a case-control study. Br J Cancer 1983;47:463–70.
179. Dworak O, Kessler H, Riedel C. Spindelzelliges karzinom des pankreas: ein fallbericht mit immunhistologischer untersuchung. Pathologe 1992;13:221–3.
180. Edis AJ, Kiernan PD, Taylor WF. Attempted curative resection of ductal carcinoma of the pancreas: review of the Mayo Clinic experience, 1951-75. Mayo Clin Proc 1980;55:531–6.
181. Ehrenthal D, Haeger L, Griffin T, Compton C. Familial pancreatic adenocarcinoma in three generations. A case report and a review of the literature. Cancer 1987;59:1661–4.
182. Eskelinen M, Lipponen P, Collan Y, Marin S, Alhava E, Nordling S. Relationship between DNA ploidy and survival in patients with exocrine pancreatic cancer. Pancreas 1991;6:90–5.
183. Eskelinen M, Lipponen P, Marin S, et al. Prognostic factors in human pancreatic cancer, with special reference to quantitative histology. Scand J Gastroenterol 1991;26:483–90.
184. Eusebi V, Capella C, Bondi A, Sessa F, Vezzadini P, Mancini AM. Endocrine-paracrine cells in pancreatic exocrine carcinomas. Histopathology 1981;5:599–613.
185. Falk RT, Pickle LW, Fontham ET, Correa P, Fraumeni JF. Life-style risk factors for pancreatic cancer in Louisiana: a case-control study. Am J Epidemiol 1988;128:324–36.
186. Fontham ET, Correa P. Epidemiology of pancreatic cancer. Surg Clin North Am 1989;69:551–67.
187. Gall FP, Kessler H, Hermanek P. Surgical treatment of ductal pancreatic carcinoma. Eur J Surg Oncol 1991;17:173–81.
188. Ghadirian P, Simard A, Baillargeon J. Tobacco, alcohol, and coffee and cancer of the pancreas. A population-based, case-control study in Quebec, Canada. Cancer 1991;67:2664–70.
189. Ghadirian P, Simard A, Baillargeon J, Perret C. Cancer of the pancreas in two brothers and one sister. Int J Pancreatol 1987;2:383–91.
190. Gold EB, Gordis L, Diener MD, et al. Diet and other risk factors for cancer of the pancreas. Cancer 1985;55:460–7.
191. Goldfarb WB, Bennett D, Monafo W. Carcinoma in heterotopic gastric pancreas. Ann Surg 1963;158:56–8.
192. Greenberg RE, Bank S, Stark B. Adenocarcinoma of the pancreas producing pancreatitis and pancreatic abscess. Pancreas 1990;5:108–13.
193. Gross JB. Hereditary pancreatitis. In: Go VL, Gardner JD, Brooks FP, Lebenthal E, DiMagno EP, Scheele GA, eds. The exocrine pancreas: biology, pathobiology and diseases. New York: Raven Press, 1986:829–39.
194. Grünewald K, Lyons J, Fröhlich A, et al. High frequency of Ki-ras codon 12 mutations in pancreatic adenocarcinomas. Int J Cancer 1989;43:1037–41.
195. Gudjonsson B. Cancer of the pancreas. 50 years of surgery. Cancer 1987;60:2284–303.
196. Gullo L, De Giorgio R, D'Errico A, Grigioni W, Parenti M, Corinaldesi R. Pancreatic exocrine carcinoma producing adrenocorticotropic hormone. Pancreas 1992;7:172–6.
197. Hall PA, Lemoine NR. Models of pancreatic cancer. In: Cancer surveys, Vol 16: The molecular pathology of cancer. Imperial Cancer Research Fund, 1993:135–55.
198. Hermanek P. Staging of exocrine pancreatic carcinoma. Eur J Surg Oncol 1991;17:167–72.
199. Hermanek P, Sobin LH, eds. UICC: TNM classification of malignant tumors, 4th ed. Berlin: Springer, 1987.
200. Hermreck AS, Thomas CH, Friesen SR. Importance of pathologic staging in the surgical management of adenocarcinoma of the exocrine pancreas. Am J Surg 1974;127:653–7.
201. Hoorens A, Lemoine NR, McLellan E, et al. Pancreatic acinar cell carcinoma. An analysis of cell lineage markers, p53 expression, and Ki-ras mutations. Am J Pathol 1993;143:685–98.
202. Horie A, Haratake J, Jimi A, Matsumoto M, Ishi N, Tsutsumi Y. Pancreatoblastoma in Japan, with differential diagnosis from papillary cystic tumor (ductuloacinar adenoma) of the pancreas. Acta Pathol Jpn 1987;37:47–63.
203. Howe GR, Jain M, Miller AB. Dietary factors and risk of pancreatic cancer: results of a Canadian population-based case-control study. Int J Cancer 1990;45:604–8.
204. Hyland C, Kheir SM, Kashlan MB. Frozen section diagnosis of pancreatic carcinoma: a prospective study of 64 biopsies. Am J Surg Pathol 1981;5:179–91.
205. Ishikawa O, Matsui Y, Aoki I, Iwanaga T, Terasawa T, Wada A. Adenosquamous carcinoma of the pancreas: a clinicopathologic study and report of three cases. Cancer 1980;46:1192–6.
206. Ishikawa O, Ohhigashi H, Imaoka S, et al. Clinicopathological study on the appropriate range of pancreatic resection to obtain operative curability of the pancreatic head cancer. J Jpn Surg Soc 1984;85:363–9.
207. Ishikawa O, Ohhigashi H, Wada A, et al. Morphologic characteristics of pancreatic carcinoma with diabetes mellitus. Cancer 1989;64:1107–12.
208. Ivy EJ, Sarr MG, Reiman HM. Nonendocrine cancer of the pancreas in patients under age forty years. Surgery 1990;108:481–7.
209. Kanai N, Nagaki S, Tanaka T. Clear cell carcinoma of the pancreas. Acta Pathol Jpn 1987;37:1521–6.
210. Kayahara M, Nagakawa T, Ueno K, Ohta T, Takeda T, Miyazaki I. An evaluation of radical resection for pancreatic cancer based on the mode of recurrence as determined by autopsy and diagnostic imaging. Cancer 1993;72:2118–23.
211. Kern HF, Röher HD, von Bülow M, Klöppel G. Fine structure of three major grades of malignancy of human pancreatic adenocarcinoma. Pancreas 1987;2:2–13.
212. Kessler II. Cancer mortality among diabetics. JNCI 1970;44:673–86.
213. Kiriyama S, Hayakawa T, Kondo T, et al. Usefulness of a new tumor marker, Span-1, for the diagnosis of pancreatic cancer. Cancer 1990;65:1557–61.
214. Kissane JM. Tumors of the exocrine pancreas in childhood. In: Humphrey GB, ed. Pancreas tumors in children, part 6. London: Martinus Nijhoff, 1982:99–129.
215. Klöppel G. Immunocytochemical tumour markers in neoplasms of the gut, pancreas, and liver. In: Klapdor R, ed. New tumour markers and their monoclonal antibodies. (4th Symposium on tumour markers, Hamburg) New York: Georg Thieme Verlag, 1987:303–14.

216. Klöppel G. Pancreatic biopsy. In: Klöppel G, Heitz PH, eds. Pancreatic pathology. New York: Churchill Livingstone, 1984:114–22.
217. Klöppel G. Pancreatic carcinoma: structural features and biological behaviour. In: Becker V, Hübner K, eds. The pancreas in connection with the epigastric unit. New York: Fischer, 1988:122–36.
218. Klöppel G. Pancreatic, non-endocrine tumours. In: Klöppel G, Heitz PH, eds. Pancreatic pathology. New York: Churchill Livingstone, 1984:79–113.
219. Klöppel G, Bommer G, Rückert K, Seifert G. Intraductal proliferation in the pancreas and its relationship to human and experimental carcinogenesis. Virchows Arch [A] 1980;387:221–33.
220. Klöppel G, Fitzgerald PJ. Pathology of non-endocrine pancreatic tumors. In: Go VL, Gardner JD, Brooks FP, Lebenthal E, DiMagno EP, Scheele GA, eds. The exocrine pancreas. New York: Raven Press, 1986:649–74.
221. Klöppel G, Lingenthal G, von Bülow M, Kern HF. Histological and fine structural features of pancreatic ductal adenocarcinomas in relation to growth and prognosis: studies in xenografted tumours and clinico-histopathological correlation in a series of 75 cases. Histopathology 1985;9:841–56.
222. Klöppel G, Lohse T, Bosslet K, Rückert K. Ductal adenocarcinoma of the head of the pancreas: incidence of tumor involvement beyond the Whipple resection line. Histological and immunocytochemical analysis of 37 total pancreatectomy specimens. Pancreas 1987;2:170–5.
223. Klöppel G, Maillet B. Classification and staging of pancreatic nonendocrine tumors. Radiol Clin North Am 1989;27:105–19.
224. Klöppel G, Morohoshi T, John HD, et al. Solid and cystic acinar cell tumor of the pancreas. Virchows Arch [A] 1981;392:171–83.
225. Klöppel G, Sosnowski J, Eichfuss HP, Rückert K, Klapdor R. Aktuelle Aspekte des Pankreaskarzinoms. Klinische und morphologische Analysen zur Diagnostik und Therapie. Dtsch Med Wschr 1979;104:1801–5.
226. Kodama T, Mori W. Morphological behavior of carcinoma of the pancreas. 2. Argyrophilic cells of Langerhans' islets in the carcinomatous tissues. Acta Pathol Jpn 1983;33:483–93.
227. Kondo H, Sugano K, Fukayama N, et al. Detection of point mutations in the K-ras oncogene at codon 12 in pure pancreatic juice for diagnosis of pancreatic carcinoma. Cancer 1994;73:1589–94.
228. Kozuka S, Sassa R, Taki T, et al. Relation of pancreatic duct hyperplasia to carcinoma. Cancer 1979;43:1418–28.
229. Lack EE, Cassady JR, Levey R, Vawter GF. Tumors of the exocrine pancreas in children and adolescents. A clinical and pathologic study of eight cases. Am J Surg Pathol 1983;7:319–27.
230. Lafler CJ, Hinerman DL. A morphologic study of pancreatic carcinoma with reference to multiple thrombi. Cancer 1961;14:944–52.
231. Leach WB. Carcinoma of the pancreas. A clinical and pathologic analysis of thirty-nine autopsied cases. Am J Pathology 1950;26:333–47.
232. Lee CS, Georgiou T, Rode J. Proliferating cell nuclear antigen (PCNA) in pancreatic adenocarcinoma. Path Res Pract 1993;189:527–9.
233. Lemoine NR, Jain S, Hughes CM, et al. Ki-ras oncogene activation in preinvasive pancreatic cancer. Gastroenterology 1992;102:230–6.
234. Levin DL, Connelly RR, Devesa SS. Demographic characteristics of cancer of the pancreas: mortality, incidence, and survival. Cancer 1981;47:1456–68.
235. Lewin K. Carcinoid tumors and the mixed (composite) glandular-endocrine cell carcinomas. Am J Surg Pathol 1987;11(Suppl):71–86.
236. Lin JT, Wang TH, Chen DS, et al. Pancreatic carcinoma associated with chronic calcifying pancreatitis in Taiwan: a case report and review of the literature. Pancreas 1988;3:111–4.
237. Lin RS, Kessler II. A multifactorial model for pancreatic cancer in man. JAMA 1981;245:147–52.
238. Lipponen PK, Eskelinen MJ, Collan Y, Marin S, Alhava E. Volume-corrected mitotic index in human pancreatic cancer. Relation to histologic grade, clinical stage, and prognosis. Scand J Gastroenterol 1990;25:548–54.
239. Longnecker DS. Carcinogenesis in the pancreas. Arch Pathol Lab Med 1983;107:4–8.
240. Lowenfels AB, Maisonneuve P, Cavallini G, et al. Pancreatitis and the risk of pancreatic cancer. The International Pancreatitis Study Group. N Engl J Med 1993;328:1433–7.
241. Lynch HT, Fusaro L, Lynch JF. Familial pancreatic cancer: a family study. Pancreas 1992;7:511–5.
242. Mack TM, Yu MC, Hanisch R, Henderson B. Pancreas cancer and smoking, beverage consumption, and past medical history. JNCI 1986;76:49–60.
243. MacMahon B, Yen S, Trichopoulos D, Warren K, Nardi G. Coffee and cancer of the pancreas. N Engl J Med 1981;304:630–3.
244. Manabe T, Miyashita T, Ohshio G, et al. Small carcinoma of the pancreas. Clinical and pathologic evaluation of 17 patients. Cancer 1988;62:135–41.
245. Mancuso TF, El-Attar AA. Cohort study of workers exposed to betanaphthylamine and benzidine. J Occup Med 1967;9:277–85.
246. Mannell A, van Heerden JA, Weiland LH, Ilstrup DM. Factors influencing survival after resection for ductal adenocarcinoma of the pancreas. Ann Surg 1986;203:403–7.
247. Matsuno S, Kato S, Kobari M, Sato T. Clinicopathological study of hematogenous metastasis of pancreatic cancer. Jpn J Surg 1986;16:406–11.
248. Mikal S, Campbell AJ. Carcinoma of the pancreas. Diagnostic and operative criteria based on one hundred consecutive autopsies. Surgery 1950;28:963–9.
249. Miller JR, Baggenstoss AH, Comfort MW. Carcinoma of the pancreas. Effect of histological type and grade of malignancy on its behavior. Cancer 1951;4:233–41.
250. Mills PK, Beeson WL, Abbey DE, Fraser GE, Phillips Rl. Dietary habits and past medical history as related to fatal pancreas cancer risk among adventists. Cancer 1988;61:2578–85.
251. Min KW, Gyorkey F, Sato C. Mucin-producing adenocarcinomas and nonbacterial thrombotic endocarditis: pathogenic role of tumor mucin. Cancer 1980;45:2374–82.
252. Mitchell ML, Bittner CA, Wills JS, Parker FP. Fine needle aspiration cytology of the pancreas. A retrospective study of 73 cases. Acta Cytologica 1988;32:447–51.
253. Monno S, Nagata A, Homma T, et al. Exocrine pancreatic cancer with humoral hypercalcemia. Am J Gastroenterol 1984;79:128–32.
254. Moossa AR, Levin B. The diagnosis of early pancreatic cancer. The University of Chicago experience. Cancer 1981;47:1688–97.

255. Morinaga S, Tsumuraya M, Nakajima T, Shimosato Y, Okazaki N. Ciliated-cell adenocarcinoma of the pancreas. Acta Pathol Jpn 1986;36:1905–10.
256. Morohoshi T, Held G, Klöppel G. Exocrine pancreatic tumours and their histological classification. A study based on 167 autopsy and 97 surgical cases. Histopathology 1983;7:645–61.
257. Morohoshi T, Kanda M, Horie A, et al. Immunocytochemical markers of uncommon pancreatic tumors. Acinar cell carcinoma, pancreatoblastoma and solid-cystic (papillary-cystic) tumor. Cancer 1987;59:739–47.
258. Motojima K, Tsunoda T, Kanematsu T, Nagata Y, Urano T, Shiku H. Distinguishing pancreatic carcinoma from other periampullary carcinomas by analysis of mutations in the Kirsten-ras oncogene. Ann Surg 1991;214:657–62.
259. Motojima K, Urano T, Nagata Y, Shiku H, Tsunoda T, Kanematsu T. Mutations in the Kirsten-ras oncogene are common but lack correlation with prognosis and tumor stage in human pancreatic carcinoma. Am J Gastroenterol 1991;86:1784–8.
260. Nagai H, Kuroda A, Morioka Y. Lymphatic and local spread of T1 and T2 pancreatic cancer. A study of autopsy material. Ann Surg 1986;204:65–71.
261. Nakaizumi A, Tatsuta M, Uehara H, et al. Cytologic examination of pure pancreatic juice in the diagnosis of pancreatic carcinoma. The endoscopic intraductal catheter aspiration cytologic technique. Cancer 1992;70:2610–14.
262. Nakao A, Ichihara T, Nonami T, et al. Clinicohistopathologic and immunohistochemical studies of intrapancreatic development of carcinoma of the head of the pancreas. Ann Surg 1989;209:181–7.
263. Niederau C, Grendell JH. Diagnosis of pancreatic carcinoma. Imaging techniques and tumor markers. Pancreas 1992;7:66–86.
264. Nonomura A, Kono N, Mizukami Y, Nakanuma Y, Matsubara F. Duct-acinar-islet cell tumor of the pancreas. Ultrastruct Pathol 1992;12:317–29.
265. Offerhaus GJ, Giardiello FM, Moore GW, Tersmette AC. Partial gastrectomy: a risk for carcinoma of the pancreas? Hum Pathol 1987;18:285–8.
266. Ohta T, Nagakawa T, Tsukioka Y, et al. Expression of argyrophilic nucleolar organizer regions in ductal adenocarcinoma of the pancreas and its relationship to prognosis. Int J Pancreatol 1993;13:193–200.
267. Ohtsuki Y, Yoshino T, Takahashi K, Sonobe H, Kohno K, Akagi T. Electron microscopic study of mucoepidermoid carcinoma in the pancreas. Acta Pathol Jpn 1987;37:1175–82.
268. Ornitz DM, Hammer RE, Messing A, Palmiter RD, Brinster RL. Pancreatic neoplasia induced by SV40 T-antigen expression in acinar cells of transgenic mice. Science 1987;238:188–93.
269. Osborn M, van Lessen G, Weber K, Klöppel G, Altmannsberger M. Differential diagnosis of gastrointestinal carcinomas by using monoclonal antibodies specific for individual keratin polypeptides. Lab Invest 1986;55:497–504.
270. Oster MW, Gray R, Panasci L, Perry MC. Chemotherapy for advanced pancreatic cancer. A comparison of 5-fluorouracil adriamycin and mitomycin (FAM) and 5-fluorouracil streptozotocin and mitomycin (FSM). Cancer 1986;57:29–33.
271. Pellegata NS, Sessa F, Renault B, et al. K-ras and p53 gene mutations in pancreatic cancer: Ductal and nonductal tumors progress through different genetic lesions. Cancer Res 1994;54:1556–60.
272. Permert J, Larsson J, Westermark GT, et al. Islet amyloid polypeptide in patients with pancreatic cancer and diabetes. N Engl J Med 1994;330:313–8.
273. Permert J, Mogaki M, Andrén-Sandberg A, Kazakoff K, Pour PM. Pancreatic mixed ductal-islet tumors. Is this an entity? Int J Pancreatol 1992;11:23–9.
274. Pettengill OS, Faris RA, Bell RH, Kuhlmann ET, Longnecker DS. Derivation of ductlike cell lines from a transplantable acinar cell carcinoma of the rat pancreas. Am J Pathol 1993;143:292–303.
275. Pipeleers D, Couturier E, Gepts W, Reynders J, Somers G. Five cases of somatostatinoma: clinical heterogeneity and diagnostic usefulness of basal and tolbutamide-induced hypersomatostatinemia. J Clin Endocrinol Metab 1983;56:1236–42.
276. Pour PM, Runge RG, Birt D, et al. Current knowledge of pancreatic carcinogenesis in the hamster and its relevance to the human disease. Cancer 1981;47:1573–87.
277. Reid JD, Yuh SL, Petrelli M, Jaffe R. Ductuloinsular tumors of the pancreas: a light, electron microscopic and immunohistochemical study. Cancer 1982;49:908–15.
278. Rosai J. Carcinoma of pancreas simulating giant cell tumor of bone. Electron-microscopic evidence of its acinar cell origin. Cancer 1968;22:333–44.
279. Satoh K, Sasano H, Shimosegawa T, et al. An immunohistochemical study of the c-erbB-2 oncogene product in intraductal mucin-hypersecreting neoplasms and in ductal cell carcinomas of the pancreas. Cancer 1993;72:51–6.
280. Scarpa A, Capelli P, Mukai K, et al. Pancreatic adenocarcinomas frequently show p53 gene mutations. Am J Pathol 1993;142:1534–43.
281. Scarpa A, Capelli P, Zamboni G, et al. Neoplasia of the ampulla of Vater. Ki-ras and p53 mutations. Am J Pathol 1993;142:1163–72.
282. Schaeffer BK, Glasner S, Kuhlmann E, Myles JL, Longnecker DS. Mutated c-K-ras in small pancreatic adenocarcinomas. Pancreas 1994;9:161–5.
283. Schron DS, Mendelsohn G. Pancreatic carcinoma with duct, endocrine, and acinar differentiation. Cancer 1984;54:1766–70.
284. Schüssler MH, Skoudy A, Ramaekers F, Real FX. Intermediate filaments as differentiation markers of normal pancreas and pancreas cancer. Am J Pathol 1992;140:559–68.
285. Sessa F, Bonato M, Frigerio B, et al. Ductal cancers of the pancreas frequently express markers of gastrointestinal epithelial cells. Gastroenterology 1990;98:1655–65.
286. Seymour AB, Hruban RH, Redston M, et al. Allelotype of pancreatic adenocarcinoma. Cancer Res 1994;54: 2761–4.
287. Smit VT, Boot AJ, Smits AM, Fleuren GJ, Cornelisse CJ, Bos JL. K-ras codon 12 mutations occur very frequently in pancreatic adenocarcinomas. Nucleic Acid Res 1988;16:7773–82.
288. Sommers SC, Meissner WA. Unusual carcinomas of the pancreas. Arch Pathol 1954;58:101–11.
289. Suda K, Hashimoto K. Argyrophil cells in the exocrine pancreas. Acta Pathol Jpn 1979;29:413–9.
290. Tabata T, Fujimori T, Maeda S, Yamamoto M, Saitoh Y. The role of ras mutation in pancreatic cancer, precancerous lesions, and chronic pancreatitis. Int J Pancreatol 1993;14:237–44.
291. Tada M, Omata M, Kawai S, et al. Detection of ras gene mutations in pancreatic juice and peripheral blood of patients with pancreatic adenocarcinoma. Cancer Res 1993;53:2472–4.

292. Takeda S, Nakao A, Ichihara T, et al. Serum concentration and immunohistochemical localization of SPAN-1 antigen in pancreatic cancer. A comparison with CA19-9 antigen. Hepatogastroenterology 1991;38:143–8.
293. Tanimura A, Yamamoto H, Shibata H, Sano E. Carcinoma in heterotopic gastric pancreas. Acta Pathol Jpn 1979;29:251–7.
294. Temellini F, Bavosi M, Lamarra M, Quagliarini P, Giuliani F. Pancreatic metastasis 25 years after nephrectomy for renal cancer. Tumori 1989;75:503–4.
295. Tempero M, Takasaki H, Uchida E, et al. Co-expression of CA 19-9, DU-PAN-2, CA 125, and TAG-72 in pancreatic adenocarcinoma. Am J Surg Pathol 1989;13(Suppl 1):89–95.
296. Tomita T, Bhatia P, Gourly W. Mucin producing islet cell adenoma. Hum Pathol 1981;12:850–3.
297. Tracey KJ, O'Brien MJ, Williams LF, et al. Signet ring carcinoma of the pancreas, a rare variant with very high CEA values. Immunohistologic comparison with adenocarcinoma. Dig Dis Sci 1984;29:573–6.
298. Trede M, Schwall G, Saeger HD. Survival after pancreatoduodenectomy. 118 consecutive resections without an operative mortality. Ann Surg 1990;211:447–58.
299. Tryka AF, Brooks JR. Histopathology in the evaluation of total pancreatectomy for ductal carcinoma. Ann Surg 1979;190:373–81.
300. Tschang TP, Garza-Garza R, Kissane JM. Pleomorphic carcinoma of the pancreas. An analysis of 15 cases. Cancer 1977;39:2114–26.
301. Tsuchiya R, Noda T, Harada N, et al. Collective review of small carcinomas of the pancreas. Ann Surg 1986;203:77–81.
302. Tsukimoto I, Watanabe K, Lin JB, Nakajima T. Pancreatic carcinoma in children in Japan. Cancer 1973;31:1203–7.
303. Tsunoda T, Ura K, Eto T, Matsumoto T, Tsuchiya R. UICC and Japanese stage classifications for carcinoma of the pancreas. Int J Pancreatol 1991;8:205–14.
304. Tsutsumi Y, Nagura H, Watanabe K. Immunohistochemical observations of carcinoembryonic antigen (CEA) and CEA-related substances in normal and neoplastic pancreas. Pitfalls and caveats in CEA immunohistochemistry. Am J Clin Pathol 1984;82:535–42.
305. Ulich T, Cheng L, Lewin KJ. Acinar-endocrine cell tumor of the pancreas. Report of a pancreatic tumor containing both zymogen and neuroendocrine granules. Cancer 1982;50:2099–105.
306. Urbanski SJ, Medline A. Giant cell carcinoma of pancreas with clear cell pattern in metastases. Hum Pathol 1982;13:1047–9.
307. van Heerden JA, ReMine WH, Weiland LH, McIlrath DC, Ilstrup DM. Total pancreatectomy for ductal adenocarcinoma of the pancreas. Mayo Clinic experience. Am J Surg 1981;142:308–11.
308. van Heerden JA. Pancreatic resection for carcinoma of the pancreas: Whipple versus total pancreatectomy—an institutional perspective. World J Surg 1984;8:880–8.
309. Warshaw AL, Fernandez-Del Castillo C. Pancreatic carcinoma. N Engl J Med 1992;326:455–65.
310. Weger AR, Falkmer UG, Schwab G, et al. Nuclear DNA distribution pattern of the parenchymal cells in adenocarcinomas of the pancreas and in chronic pancreatitis. A study of archival specimens using both image and flow cytometry. Gastroenterology 1990;99:237–42.
311. Wynder EL. An epidemiological evaluation of the causes of cancer of the pancreas. Cancer Res 1975;35:2228–33.,D%0
312. Yamanaka Y, Friess H, Kobrin MS, et al. Overexpression of HER2/neu oncogene in human pancreatic carcinoma. Hum Pathol 1993;24:1127–34.
313. Yanagisawa A, Ohtake K, Ohashi K, et al. Frequent c-Ki-ras oncogene activation in mucous cell hyperplasias of pancreas suffering from chronic inflammation. Cancer Res 1993;53:953–6.
314. Young RH, Hart WR. Metastases from carcinomas of the pancreas simulating primary mucinous tumors of the ovary. A report of seven cases. Am J Surg Pathol 1989;13:748–56.


**Osteoclast-like Giant Cell Tumor**


315. Berendt RC, Shnitka TK, Wiens E, Manickavel V, Jewell LD. The osteoclast-type giant cell tumor of the pancreas. Arch Pathol Lab Med 1987;111:43–8.
316. Cubilla AL, Fitzgerald PJ. Tumors of the exocrine pancreas. Atlas of Tumor Pathology. 2nd series, Fascicle 19. Washington, D.C.: Armed Forces Institute of Pathology, 1984;220:162.
317. Dworak O, Wittekind C. Osteoclastic giant cell tumor of the pancreas. An immunohistological study and review of the literature. Path Res Pract 1993;189:228–31.
318. Fischer HP, Altmannsberger M, Kracht J. Osteoclast-type giant cell tumour of the pancreas. Virchows Arch [A] 1988;412:247–53.
319. Goldberg RD, Michelassi F, Montag AG. Osteoclast-like giant cell tumor of the pancreas: immunophenotypic similarity to giant cell tumor of bone. Hum Pathol 1991;22:618–22.
320. Mentes A, Yüce G. Osteoclast-type giant cell tumor of the pancreas associated with mucinous cystadenoma. Eur J Surg Oncol 1993;19:84–6.
321. Newbould MJ, Benbow EW, Sene A, Young M, Taylor TV. Adenocarcinoma of the pancreas with osteoclast-like giant cells: a case report with immunocytochemistry. Pancreas 1992;7:611–5.
322. Nojima T, Nakamura F, Ishikura M, Inoue K, Nagashima K, Kato H. Pleomorphic carcinoma of the pancreas with osteoclast-like giant cells. Int J Pancreatol 1993;14:275–81.
323. Posen JA. Giant cell tumor of the pancreas of the osteoclastic type associated with a mucous secreting cystadenocarcinoma. Hum Pathol 1981;12:944–7.
324. Rosai J. Carcinoma of pancreas simulating giant cell tumor of bone. Electron-microscopic evidence of its acinar cell origin. Cancer 1968;22:333–44.
325. Suster S, Phillips M, Robinson MJ. Malignant fibrous histiocytoma (giant cell type) of the pancreas. A distinctive variant of osteoclast-type giant cell tumor of the pancreas. Cancer 1989;64:2303–8.
326. Trepeta RW, Mathur B, Lagin S, LiVolsi VA. Giant cell tumor (osteoclastoma) of the pancreas: a tumor of epithelial origin. Cancer 1981;48:2022–8

## Acinar Cell Carcinoma


327. Alcantara EN Jr. Functioning acinar cell carcinoma of the pancreas. Can Med Assoc J 1962;87:970–3.
328. Auger C. Acinous cell carcinoma of the pancreas with extensive fat necrosis. Arch Pathol 1947;43:400–5.
329. Belsky H, Cornell NW. Disseminated focal fat necrosis following radical pancreatoduodenectomy for acinous carcinoma of head of pancreas. Ann Surg 1955;141:556–62.
330. Berner O. Subkutane fettgewebenekrose. Virchows Arch [A] 1908;193:510–22
331. Burns WA, Matthews MJ, Hamosh M, Vander Weide G, Blum R, Johnson FB. Lipase-secreting acinar cell carcinoma of the pancreas with polyarthropathy. A light and electron microscopic, histochemical, and biochemical study. Cancer 1974;33:1002–9.
332. Cantrell BB, Cubilla AL, Erlandson RA, Fortner J, Fitzgerald PJ. Acinar cell cystadenocarcinoma of human pancreas. Cancer 1981;47:410–6.
333. Chen J, Baithun SI. Morphological study of 391 cases of exocrine pancreatic tumors with special reference to the classification of exocrine pancreatic carcinoma. J Pathol 1985;146:17–29.
334. Comfort MW, Butt HR, Baggenstoss AH, Osterberg AE, Priestley JT. Acinar cell carcinoma of pancreas: report of case in which function of carcinomatous cells was suspected. Ann Int Med 1943;19:808–16.
335. Cubilla AL, Fitzgerald PJ. Tumors of the exocrine pancreas. Atlas of Tumor Pathology. 2nd Series, Fascicle 19. Washington D.C.: Armed Forces Institute of Pathology, 1984:208–19.
336. di Sant Agnese PA. Acinar cell carcinoma of the pancreas. Ulrastruct Pathol 1991;15:573–7.
337. Feliu J, de la Gandara I, Garrido P, Gonzalez Baron M. Somatostatin analogues and pancreatic acinar cell carcinoma: an alternative in symptomatic treatment? Am J Gastroenterol 1990;85:1539–40.
338. Garcia H, Pelfrene A, Love LA. Pancreatic acinar adenomas [Letter]. Arch Pathol 1975;99:621.
339. Good AE, Schnitzer B, Kawanishi H, Demetropoulos KC, Rapp R. Acinar pancreatic tumor with metastatic fat necrosis: report of a case and revieg of rheumatic manifestations. Am J Dig Dis 197&;21:978–87.
340. Grosfeld JL, Clatworthy HW Jr, Hamoudi AB. Pancreatic malignancy in children. Arch Surg 1970;101:370–5.
341. Hassan MO, Gogate PA. Malignant mixed exocrine-endocrine tumor of the pancreas with unusual intracytoplasmic inclusions. Ultrastruct Pathol 1993; 17:483–93.
342. Hegler C, Wohlwill F. Fettgewebenekrosen in subcutis und knochenmark durch metastasen eines carcinoms des pankreasschwanzes. Virchows Arch [A] 1930;274:784–802.
343. Hewan-Lowe KO. Acinar cell carcinoma of the pancreas: metastases from an occult primary tumor. Arch Pathol Lab Med 1983;107:552–4.
344. Hoorens A, Gebhard F, Kraft K, Lemoine NR, Klöppel G. Pancreatoblastoma in an adult: its separation from acinar cell carcinoma. Virchows Arch [A] 1994;424:485–90.
345. Hoorens A, Lemoine NR, McLellan E, et al. Pancreatic acinar cell carcinoma. An analysis of cell lineage markers, p53 expression and Ki-ras mutations. Am J Pathol 1993;143:685–98.
346. Horie A, Morohoshi T, Klöppel G. Ultrastructural comparison of pancreatoblastoma, solid cystic tumor and acinar cell carcinoma. J Clin Electron Microscopy 1987;20:353–62.
347. Horie Y, Gomyoda M, Kishimoto Y, et al. Plasma carcinoembryonic antigen and acinar cell carcinoma of the pancreas. Cancer 1984;53:1137–42.
348. Hruban RH, Molina JM, Reddy MN, Boitnott JK. A neoplasm with pancreatic and hepatocellular differentiation presenting with subcutaneous fat necrosis. Am J Clin Pathol 1987;88:639–45.
349. Ishihara A, Sanda T, Takanari H, Yatani R, Liu PI. Elastase-1-secreting acinar cell carcinoma of the pancreas. A cytologic electron microscopic and histochemical study. Acta Cytol 1989;33:157–63.
350. Jackson SA, Savidge RS, Stein L, Varley H. Carcinoma of the pancreas associated with fat-necrosis. Lancet 1952;263:962–7.
351. Kakudo K, Sakurai M, Miyaji T, Ikeda Y, Sattani M, Manabe H. Pancreatic carcinoma in infancy. An electron microscopic study. Acta Pathol Jpn 1976;26:719–26.
352. Kawamoto S, Hiraoka T, Kanemitsu K, Kimura M, Miyauchi Y, Takeya M. Alpha-fetoprotein-producing pancreatic cancer—a case report and review of 28 cases. Hepatogastroenterology 1992;39:282–6.
353. Kimura N, Yonekura H, Okamoto H, Nagura H. Expression of human regenerating gene mRNA and its product in normal and neoplastic human pancreas. Cancer 1992;70:1857–63.
354. Kishi K, Nakamura K, Yoshimori M, et al. Morphology and pathological significance of focal acinar cell dysplasia of the human pancreas. Pancreas 1992;7:177–82.
355. Klimstra DS, Heffess CS, Oertel JE, Rosai J. Acinar cell carcinoma of the pancreas. A clinicopathologic study of 28 cases. Am J Surg Pathol 1992;16:815–37.
356. Klimstra DS, Rosai J, Heffess CS. Mixed acinar-endocrine carcinomas of the pancreas. Am J Surg Pathol 1994;18:765–78.
357. Klimstra DS, Wenig D, Heffess CS. Pancreatoblastoma: a clinicopathologic study [Abstract]. Mod Pathol 1994;7:133A
358. Klöppel G. Pancreatic, non-endocrine tumors. In: Klöppel G, Heitz PU, eds. Pancreatic pathology. New York: Churchill Livingstone, 1984:79–113.
359. Kodama T, Mori W. Atypical acinar cell nodules of the human pancreas. Acta Pathol Jpn 1983;33:701–14.
360. Lack EE, Levey R, Cassady JR, Vawter GF. Tumors of the exocrine pancreas in children and adolescents. A clinical and pathologic study of 8 cases. Am J Surg Pathol 1983;7:319–27.
361. Lim JH, Chung KB, Cho OK, Cho KS. Acinar cell carcinoma of the pancreas. Ultrasonography and computed tomography findings. Clin Imaging 1990;14:301–4.
362. Longnecker DS. Lesions induced in rodent pancreas by azaserine and other pancreatic carcinogens. Environ Health Perspect 1984;56:245–52.
363. Longnecker DS, Shinozuka H, Dekker A. Focal acinar cell dysplasia in human pancreas. Cancer 1980;45:534–40.
364. MacMahon HE, Brown PA, Shen EM. Acinar cell carcinoma of the pancreas with subcutaneous fat necrosis. Gastroenterology 1965;49:555–9.

365. Mah PT, Loo DC, Tock EP. Pancreatic acinar cell carcinoma in childhood. Am J Dis Child 1974;128:101–4.
366. Miller JR, Baggenstoss AH, Comfort MW. Carcinoma of the pancreas. Effect of histological type and grade of malignancy on its behavior. Cancer 1951;4:233–41.
367. Min KW, Cain GD, Györkey P, Kyörkey F. Myeloma-like lesions of the kidney. Occurrence in a case of acinic cell adenocarcinoma of the pancreas. Arch Intern Med 1976;136:1299–302.
368. Morohoshi T, Held G, Klöppel G. Exocrine pancreatic tumours and their histological classification. A study based on 167 autopsy and 97 surgical cases. Histopathology 1983;7:645–61.
369. Morohoshi T, Kanda M, Horie A, et al. Immunocytochemical markers of uncommon pancreatic tumors: acinar cell carcinoma, pancreatoblastoma, and solid cystic (papillary-cystic) tumor. Cancer 1987;59:739–47.
370. Moynan RW, Neerhort RC, Johnson TS. Pancreatic carcinoma in childhood. Case report and review. J Pediatr 1964;65:711–20.
371. Nojima T, Kojima T, Kato H, Sato T, Koito K, Nagashima K. Alpha-fetoprotein-producing acinar cell carcinoma of the pancreas. Hum Pathol 1992;23:828–30.
372. Oertel JE. The pancreas. Nonneoplastic alterations. Am J Surg Pathol 1989;13(Suppl 1):50–65.
373. Ono J, Sakamoto H, Sakoda K, et al. Acinar cell carcinoma of the pancreas with elevated serum alphafetoprotein. Int Surg 1984;69:361–4.
374. Osborne BM, Culbert SJ, Cangir A, MacKay B. Acinar cell carcinoma of the pancreas in a 9-year-old child: case report with electron microscopic observations. South Med J 1977;70:370–2.
375. Osborne RR. Functioning acinous cell carcinoma of the pancreas accompanied with widespread focal fat necrosis. Arch Intern Med 1950;85:933–43.
376. Pour PM, Sayed S, Sayed G. Hyperplastic, preneoplastic and neoplastic lesions found in 83 human pancreases. Am J Clin Pathol 1982;77:137–52.
377. Quaife CJ, Pinkert CA, Ornitz DM, Palmiter RD, Brinster RL. Pancreatic neoplasia induced by ras expression in acinar cells of transgenic mice. Cell 1987;48:1023–34.
378. Radin DR, Colletti PM, Forrester DM, Tang WW. Pancreatic acinar cell carcinoma with subcutaneous and intraosseous fat necrosis. Radiology 1986;158:67–8.
379. Reducka K, Gardiner GW, Sweet J, Vandenbroucke A, Bear R. Myeloma-like cast nephropathy associated with acinar cell carcinoma of the pancreas. Am J Nephrol 1988;8:421–4.
380. Robertson JC, Eeles GH. Syndrome associated with pancreatic acinar cell carcinoma. Br Med J 1970;2:708–9.
381. Rosewicz S, Vogt D, Harth N, et al. An amphicrine pancreatic cell line: AR42J cells combine exocrine and neuroendocrine properties. Eur J Cell Biol 1992;%9:80–91.
382. Sandgren EP, Quaife CJ, Paulovich AG, Palmiter RD, Brinster RL. Pancreatic tumor pathogenesis reflects the causative genetic lesion. Proc Natl Acad Sci USA 1991;88:93–7.
383. Scarpelli DG, Rao MS, Reddy JK. Studies of pancreatic carcinogenesis in different animal models. Environ Health Perspect 1984;56:219–27.
384. Schmid M. Über das Syndrom des sekretorisch aktiven, metastasierenden, exokrinen Pankreasadenoms. Z Klin Med 1957;154:439–55.
385. Schreiber D, Probst HJ. Sekretorisch aktives karzinom des exokrinen Pankreas. Fallbericht und literaturübersicht. Zbl allg Pathol u Pathol Anat 1977;121:114–21.
386. Schron DS, Mendelsohn G. Pancreatic carcinoma with duct, endocrine, and acinar differentiation. A histological, immunocytochemical, and ultrastructural study. Cancer 1984;54:1766–70.
387. Shinozuka H, Lee RE, Dunn JL, Longnecker DS. Multiple atypical acinar cell nodules of the pancreas. Hum Pathol 1980;11:389–91.
388. Stamm BH. Incidence and diagnostic significance of minor pathologic changes in the adult pancreas at autopsy. Hum Pathol 1984;15:677–83.
389. Stamm BH, Burger H, Hollinger A. Acinar cell cystadenocarcinoma of the pancreas. Cancer 1987;60:2542–7.
390. Tanaka T, Mori H, Williams GM. Atypical and neoplastic acinar cell lesions of the pancreas in an autopsy study of Japanese patients. Cancer 1988;61:2278–85.
391. Titone M. Über ungewöhnlich ausgebreitete fettgewebs- und gewebsnekrosen bei pankreaskrebs. Virchows Arch [A] 1936;277:416–24.
392. Tucker JA, Shelburne JD, Benning TL, Yacoub L, Federman M. Filamentous inclusions in acinar cell carcinoma of the pancreas. Ultrastruct Pathol 1994;18:279–86.
393. Ulich T, Cheng L, Lewin KJ. Acinar-endocrine cell tumor of the pancreas. Report of a pancreatic tumor containing both zymogen and neuroendocrine granules. Cancer 1982;50:2099–105.
394. van Klaveren RJ, de Mulder PH, Boerbooms AM, et al. Pancreatic carcinoma with polyarthritis, fat necrosis, and high serum lipase and trypsin activity. Gut 1990;31:953–5.
395. Webb JN. Acinar cell neoplasms of the exocrine pancreas. J Clin Pathol 1977;30:103–12.
396. Wilander E, Sundstrom C, Meurling S, Grotte G. A highly differentiated exocrine pancreatic tumor in a young boy. Acta Pediatr Scand 1976;65:769–72.
397. Wuketich ST, Pavlik F. Syndrom des metastasierenden lipasebildenden pankreasadenoms. Zugleich ein beitrag zur differentialdiagnose der Pfeifer-Weber-Christianschen krankheit. Arch Klin Exp Derm. 1963;216:412–26.

**Pancreatoblastoma**

398. Becker WF. Pancreatoduodenectomy for carcinoma of the pancreas in an infant: report of a case. Ann Surg 1957;145:864–72.
399. Benjamin E, Wright DH. Adenocarcinoma of the pancreas of childhood: a report of two cases. Histopathology 1980;4:87–104.
400. Buchino JJ, Castello FM, Nagaraj HS. Pancreatoblastoma: a histochemical and ultrastructural analysis. Cancer 1984;53:963–9.
401. Cooper JE, Lake BD. Use of enzyme histochemistry in the diagnosis of pancreatoblastoma. Histopathology 1989;15:407–14.

402. Cubilla AL, Fitzgerald PJ. Tumor of exocrine pancreas. Atlas of Tumor Pathology, 2nd Series, Fascicle 19. Washington, D.C.: Armed Forces Institute of Pathology, 1984.
403. Drut R, Jones MC. Congenital pancreatoblastoma in Beckwith-Wiedemann syndrome: an emerging association. Pediatr Pathol 1988;8:331–9.
404. Fonkalsrud EW, Wilkerson JA, Longmire WP. Pancreatoduodenectomy for islet-cell tumor of the pancreas in infancy and childhood. Case report with five-year survival. JAMA 1966;197:586–8.
405. Frable WJ, Still WJ, Kay S. Carcinoma of the pancreas, infantile type: a light and electron microscopic study. Cancer 1971;27:667–73.
406. Griffin BR, Wisbeck WM, Schaller RT, Benjamin DR. Radiotherapy for locally recurrent infantile pancreatic carcinoma (pancreatoblastoma). Cancer 1987;60:1734–6.
407. Grosfeld JL, Clatworthy HW, Hamoudi AB Jr. Pancreatic malignancy in children. Arch Surg 1970;101:370–5.
408. Hoorens A, Gebhard F, Kraft K, Lemoine N, Klöppel G. Pancreatoblastoma in an adult: its separation from acinar cell carcinoma. Virchows Arch 1994;424:485–90.
409. Hoorens A, Lemoine NR, McLellan E, et al. Pancreatic acinar cell carcinoma. An analysis of cell lineage markers, p53 expression and Ki-ras mutations. Am J Pathol 1993;143:685–98.
410. Horie A. Clinicopathological features of pancreatoblastoma. Tan to Sui 1988;9:1511–19.
411. Horie A. Pancreatoblastoma. Histopathologic criteria based upon a review of six cases. In: Humphrey GB, Grindey GB, Dehner LP, Acton LP, Pysher TJ, eds. Pancreatic tumors in children. The Hague: Martinus Nijhoff, 1982:159–66.
412. Horie A, Haratake J, Jimi A, Matsumoto M, Ishii N, Tsutsumi Y. Pancreatoblastoma in Japan, with differential diagnosis from papillary cystic tumor (ductuloacinar adenoma) of the pancreas. Acta Pathol Jpn 1987;37:47–63.
413. Horie A, Morohoshi T, Klöppel G. Ultrastructural comparison of pancreatoblastoma, solid-cystic tumor and acinar cell carcinoma. J Clinic Electron Microscopy 1987;20:353–62.
414. Horie A, Yano Y, Kotoo Y, Miwa A. Morphogenesis of pancreatoblastoma, infantile carcinoma of the pancreas: report of two cases. Cancer 1977;39:245–54.
415. Ichijima K, Akaishi K, Toyoda N, et al. Carcinoma of the pancreas with endocrine component in childhood. A case report. Am J Clin Pathol 1985;83:95–100.
416. Imamura M, Yokoyama S, Nishino C, Kikuchi T. A case of AFP-producing pancreatoblastoma. Pediatr Oncol 1984;20:212–3.
417. Iseki M, Suzuki T, Koizumi Y, et al. Alpha-fetoprotein-producing pancreatoblastoma: a case report. Cancer 1986;57:1833–5.
418. Kakudo K, Sakurai M, Miyaji T, Ikeda Y, Satani M, Manabe H. Pancreatic carcinoma in infancy. An electron microscopic study. Acta Pathol Jpn 1976;26:719.
419. Klimstra DS, Heffess CS, Oertel JE, Rosai J. Acinar cell carcinoma of the pancreas. A clinicopathologic study of 28 cases. Am J Surg Pathol 1992;16:815–37.
420. Klimstra DS, Wenig BM, Adair CF, Heffess CS. Pancreatoblastoma. A clinicopathologic study and review of the literature. Am J Surg Pathol 1995;19:371–89.
421. Koh TH, Cooper JE, Newman CL, Walker TM, Kiely EM, Hoffmann EB. Pancreatoblastoma in a neonate with Wiedemann-Beckwith syndrome. Eur J Pediatr 1986;145:435–8.
422. Lack EE, Levey R, Cassady JR, Vawter G. Tumors of the exocrine pancreas in children and adolescents: a clinical and pathologic study of eight cases. Am J Surg Pathol 1983;7:319–27.
423. Mah PT, Loo DC, Tock EP. Pancreatic acinar cell carcinoma in childhood. Am J Dis Child 1974;128:101–4.
424. Morohoshi T, Kanda M, Horie A. Immunocytochemical markers of uncommon pancreatic tumors. Acinar cell carcinoma, pancreatoblastoma and solid cystic (papillary-cystic) tumor. Cancer 1987;59:739–47.
425. Morohoshi T, Sagawa F, Mitsuya T. Pancreatoblastoma with marked elevation of serum alpha-fetoprotein. An autopsy case report with immunocytochemical study. Virchows Arch [A] 1990;416:265–70.
426. Morohoshi T, Shimizu K, Kanda M. Pancreatic tumors: their pathology and morphogenesis. Jpn J Cancer Dig Organs 1991;1:556–62.
427. Moynan RW, Neerhout RC, Johnson TS. Pancreatic carcinoma in childhood, case report and review. J Pediatr 1964;65:711–20.
428. Ohaki Y, Misugi K, Fukuda J, Okudaira M, Hirose M. Immunohistochemical study of pancreatoblastoma. Acta Pathol Jpn 1987;37:1581–90.
429. Ohaki Y, Misugi K, Sasaki Y, Okudaira M. Pancreatic carcinoma in childhood: report of an autopsy case and a review of the literature. Acta Pathol Jpn 1985;35:1543–54.
430. Ono J, Sakamoto H, Sakoda K. Acinar cell carcinoma of the pancreas with elevated serum alpha-fetoprotein. Int Surg 1984;69:361–4.
431. Osborne BM, Culbert SJ, Cangir A, MacKay B. Acinar cell carcinoma of the pancreas in a 9-year-old child: case report with electron microscopic observations. Southern Med J 1977;70:370–2.
432. Palosaari D, Clayton F, Seaman J. Pancreatoblastoma in an adult. Arch Pathol Lab Med 1986;110:650–2.
433. Potts SR, Brown S, O'Hara MD. Pancreatoblastoma in a neonate associated with Beckwith-Wiedemann syndrome. Z Kinderchir 1986;41:56–7.
434. Robey G, Daneman A, Martin DJ. Pancreatic carcinoma in a neonate. Pediatr Radiol 1983;13:284–6.
435. Sakaida N, Jho T, Hara F, et al. Two cases of pancreatoblastoma with various differentiation. Tr Soc Pathol Jpn 1992;81:150.
436. Sasaki M, Ueda M, Ito H. A case of pancreatoblastoma. Transactiones Sosietatis Pathol Japonicae 1987;76:220.
437. Shimizu K, Akiyama H. A case of infantile carcinoma of the pancreas. Pediatr Oncol 1984;20:206–8.
438. Silverman JF, Holbrook CT, Pories WJ, Kodroff MB, Joshi VV. Fine needle aspiration cytology of pancreatoblastoma with immunocytochemical and ultrastructural studies. Acta Cytol 1990;34:632–40.
439. Tsukimoto I, Watanabe K, Lin JB, Nakajima T. Pancreatic carcinoma in children in Japan. Cancer 1973;31:1203–7.
440. Wilander E, Sundstrom C, Meurling S, Grotte G. A highly differentiated exocrine pancreatic tumor in a young boy. Acta Pediatr Scand 1976;65:769–72.

**Solid-Pseudopapillary Tumor**


441. Benjamin E, Wright DH. Adenocarcinoma of the pancreas of childhood: a report of two cases. Histopathology 1980;4:87–104.
442. Bombi JA, Milla A, Badal JM, Piulachs J, Estape J, Cardesa A. Papillary-cystic neoplasm of the pancreas. Report of two cases and review of the literature. Cancer 1984;54:780–4.
443. Boor PJ, Swanson MR. Papillary-cystic neoplasm of the pancreas. Am J Surg Pathol 1979;3:69–75.
444. Cappellari JO, Geisinger KR, Albertson DA, Wolfman NT, Kute TE. Malignant papillary cystic tumor of the pancreas. Cancer 1990;66:193–8.
445. Carbone A, Ranelletti FO, Rinelli A, et al. Type II estrogen receptors in the papillary cystic tumor of the pancreas. Am J Clin Pathol 1989;92:572–6.
446. Choi BI, Kim KW, Han MC, Kim YI, Kim CW. Solid and papillary epithelial neoplasms of the pancreas: CT findings. Radiology 1988;166:413–6.
447. Chott A, Klöppel G, Buxbaum P, Heitz PU. Neuron specific enolase demonstration in the diagnosis of a solid-cystic (papillary cystic) tumour of the pancreas. Virchows Arch [A] 1987;410:397–402.
448. Cubilla AL, Fitzgerald PJ. Tumors of the exocrine pancreas. Atlas of Tumor Pathology, 2nd Series, Fascicle 19. Washington, D.C.: Armed Forces Institute of Pathology, 1984:201–7.
449. Duff P, Greene VP. Pregnancy complicated by solid-papillary epithelial tumor of the pancreas, pulmonary embolism, and pulmonary embolectomy. Am J Obstet Gynecol 1985;152:80–1.
450. Foote A, Simpson JS, Stewart RJ, Wakefield JJ, Buchanan A, Gupta RK. Diagnosis of the rare solid and papillary epithelial neoplasm of the pancreas by fine needle aspiration cytology. Acta Cytol 1986;30:519–22.
451. Frantz VK. Tumors of the pancreas. In: Atlas of Tumor Pathology, Fascicles 27 and 28. Washington, D.C.: Armed Forces Institute of Pathology, 1959:32–3.
452. Friedman AC, Lichtenstein JE, Fishman EK, Oertel JE, Dachman AH, Siegelman SS. Solid and papillary epithelial neoplasm of the pancreas. Radiology 1985;154:333–7.
453. Hamoudi AB, Misugi K, Grosfeld JL, Reiner CB. Papillary epithelial neoplasm of pancreas in a child. Report of a case with electron microscopy. Cancer 1970;26:1126–34.
454. Ishikawa O, Ishiguro S, Ohhigashi H, et al. Solid and papillary neoplasm arising from an ectopic pancreas in the mesocolon. Am J Gastroenterol 1990;85:597–601.
455. Jorgensen LJ, Hansen AB, Burcharth F, Philipsen E, Horn T. Solid and papillary neoplasm of the pancreas. Ultrastruct Pathol 1992;16:659–66.
456. Kamisawa T, Fukayama M, Koike M, Tabata I, Okamoto A. So-called papillary and cystic neoplasm of the 'ancreas. An immunohistochemical and ultrastructural study. Acta Pathol Jpn 1987;37:785–94.
457. Kim YI, Kim ST, Lee GK, Choi BI. Papillary cystic tumor of the liver. A case report with ultrastructural observation. Cancer 1990;65:2740–6.
458. Klöppel G. Pancreatic non-endocrine tumours. In: Klöppel G, Heitz PH, eds. Pancreatic pathology. Edinburgh: Churchill Livingstone, 1984:79–113.
459. Klöppel G, Maurer R, Hofmann E et al. Solid-cystic (papillary-cystic) tumours within and outside the pancreas in men: report of two patients. Virchows Arch [A] 1991;418:179–83.
460. Klöppel G, Morohoshi T, John HD, et al. Solid and cystic acinar cell tumour of the pancreas. A tumour in young women with favourable prognosis. Virchows Arch [A] 1981;392:171–83.
461. Kuo TT, Su IJ, Chien CH. Solid and papillary neoplasm of the pancreas. Report of three cases from Taiwan. Cancer 1984;54:1469–74.
462. Lack EE, Levey R, Cassady JR, Vawter GF. Tumors of the exocrine pancreas in children and adolescents. A clinical and pathologic study of eight cases. Am J Surg Pathol 1983;7:319–27.
463. Ladanyi M, Mulay S, Arseneau J, Bettez P. Estrogen and progesterone receptor determination in the papillary cystic neoplasm of the pancreas. With immunohistochemical and ultrastructural observations. Cancer 1987;60:1604–11.
464. Learmonth GM, Price SK, Visser AE, Emms M. Papillary and cystic neoplasm of the pancreas—an acinar cell tumour? Histopathology 1985;9:63–79.
465. Lieber MR, Lack EE, Roberts JR Jr, et al. Solid and papillary epithelial neoplasm of the pancreas. An ultrastructural and immunocytochemical study of six cases. Am J Surg Pathol 1987;11:85–93.
466. Matsunou H, Konishi F. Papillary-cystic neoplasm of the pancreas: a clinicopathologic study concerning the tumor aging and malignancy of nine cases. Cancer 1990;65:283–91.
467. Matsunou H, Konishi F, Yamamichi N, Takayanagi N, Mukai M. Solid, infiltrating variety of papillary cystic neoplasm of the pancreas. Cancer 1990;65:2747–57.
468. Miettinen M, Partanen S, Fräki O, Kivilaakso E. Papillary cystic tumor of the pancreas. An analysis of cellular differentiation by electron microscopy and immunohistochemistry. Am J Surg Pathol 1987;11:855–65.
469. Morohoshi T, Held G, Klöppel G. Exocrine pancreatic tumors and their histological classification. A study based on 167 autopsy and 97 surgical cases. Histopathology 1983;7:645–61.
470. Morohoshi T, Kanda M, Horie A, et al. Immunocytochemical markers of uncommon pancreatic tumors. Acinar cell carcinoma, pancreatoblastoma, and solid cystic (papillary cystic) tumor. Cancer 1987;59:739–47.
471. Morrison DM, Jewell LD, McCaughey WT, Danyluk J, Shnitka TK, Manickavel V. Papillary cystic tumor of the pancreas. Arch Pathol Lab Med 1984;108:723–7.
472. Murao T, Toda K, Tomiyama Y. Papillary and solid neoplasm of pancreas in a child. Report of a case in which acinar differentiation was demonstrated by immunohistochemistry and electron microscopy. Acta Pathol Jpn 1983;33:565–75.
473. Nishihara K, Nagoshi M, Tsuneyoshi M, Yamaguchi K, Hayashi I. Papillary cystic tumors of the pancreas. Assessment of their malignant potential. Cancer 1993;71:82–92.
474. Oertel JE, Mendelsohn G, Compagno J. Solid and papillary epithelial neoplasms of the pancreas. In: Humphrey GB, Grindey GB, Dehner LP, Acton RT, Pysher TJ, eds. Pancreatic tumors in children. Den Haag: Martinus Nijhoff, 1982:167–71.

475. Orlando CA, Bowman RL, Loose JH. Multicentric papillary-cystic neoplasm of the pancreas. Arch Pathol Lab Med 1991;115:958–60.
476. Persson M, Bisgaard C, Nielsen BB, Christiansen T, Kroustrup JP. Solid and papillary epithelial neoplasm of the pancreas presenting as a traumatic cyst. Case report. Acta Chir Scand 1986;152:223–6.
477. Rustin RB, Broughan TA, Hermann RE, Grundfest-Broniatowski SF, Petras RE, Hart WR. Papillary cystic epithelial neoplasms of the pancreas. A clinical study of four cases. Arch Surg 1986;121:1073–6.
478. Sanchez JA, Newman KD, Eichelberger MR, Nauta RJ. The papillary-cystic neoplasm of the pancreas. An increasingly recognized clinicopathologic entity. Arch Surg 1990;125:1502–5.
479. Sanfey H, Mendelsohn G, Cameron JL. Solid and papillary neoplasm of the pancreas. A potentially curable surgical lesion. Ann Surg 1983;197:272–5.
480. Schlosnagle DC, Campbell WG Jr. The papillary and solid neoplasm of the pancreas: a report of two cases with electron microscopy, one containing neurosecretory granules. Cancer 1981;47:2603–10.
481. Sclafani LM, Reuter VE, Coit DG, Brennan MF. The malignant nature of papillary and cystic neoplasm of the pancreas. Cancer 1991;68:153–8.
482. Stömmer P, Kraus J, Stolte M, Giedl J. Solid and cystic pancreatic tumors. Clinical, histochemical, and electron microscopic features in ten cases. Cancer 1991;67:1635–41.
483. Taxy JB. Adenocarcinoma of the pancreas in childhood. Report of a case and a review of the English language literature. Cancer 1976;37:1508–18.
484. Tsunoda T, Eto T, Tsurifune T, et al. Solid and cystic tumor of the pancreas in an adult male. Acta Pathol Jpn 1991;41:763–70.
485. von Herbay A, Sieg B, Otto HF. Solid-cystic tumour of the pancreas. Virchows Arch [A] 1990;416:535–8.
486. Wilson MB, Adams DB, Garen PD, Gansler TS. Aspiration cytologic, ultrastructural, and DNA cytometric findings of solid and papillary tumor of the pancreas. Cancer 1992;69:2235–43.
487. Wrba F, Chott A, Ludvik B, et al. Solid and cystic tumour of the pancreas: a hormonal-dependent neoplasm? Histopathology 1988;12:338–40.
488. Wrba F, Chott A, Schratter M, Ludvik B, Krisch K, Holzner JH. Feinnadelpunktionszytologie eines solid-zystischen Tumors des Pankreas. Pathologe 1988;9:340–4.
489. Yagihashi S, Sato I, Kaimori M, Matsumoto J, Nagai K. Papillary and cystic tumor of the pancreas. Two cases indistinguishable from islet cell tumor. Cancer 1988;61:1241–7.
490. Yamaguchi K, Hirakata R, Kitamura K. Papillary cystic neoplasm of the pancreas: radiological and pathological characteristics in 11 cases. Br J Surg 1990;77:1000–3.
491. Yamaguchi K, Miyagahara T, Tsuneyoshi M, et al. Papillary cystic tumor of the pancreas: an immunohistochemical and ultrastructural study of 14 patients. Jpn J Clin Oncol 1989;19:102–11.
492. Zamboni G, Bonetti F, Scarpa A, et al. Expression of progesterone receptor in solid cystic tumor of the pancreas: a clinicopathological, immunohistochemical and ultrastructural study of ten cases. Virchows Arch [A] 1993;423:425–31.
493. Zinner MJ, Shurbaji MS, Cameron JL. Solid and papillary epithelial neoplasms of the pancreas. Surgery 1990;108:475–80.

**Miscellaneous Carcinomas**

494. Bondeson L, Bondeson AG, Grimelius L, Kjellström UL. Oncocytic tumor of the pancreas. Report of a case with aspiration cytology. Acta Cytologica 1990;34:425–8.
495. Chen J, Baithun SI. Morphological study of 391 cases of exocrine pancreatic tumours with special reference to the classification of exocrine pancreatic carcinoma. J Pathol 1985;146:17–29.
496. Childs CC, Korsten MA, Choi HS, Schwarz R, Fisse RD. Pancreatic choriocarcinoma presenting as inflammatory pseudocyst. Gastroenterology 1985;89:426–31.
497. Friedman HD. Nonmucinous, glycogen-poor cystadenocarcinoma of the pancreas. Arch Pathol Lab Med 1990;114:888–91.
498. Huntrakoon M. Oncocytic carcinoma of the pancreas. Cancer 1983;51:332–36.
499. Nozawa Y, Abe M, Sakuma H, et al. A case of pancreatic oncocytic tumor. Acta Pathol Jpn 1990;40:367–70.
500. Sironi M, Radice F, Taccagni GL, Braga M, Zerbi M. Fine needle aspiration of a pancreatic oxyphilic carcinoma with pulmonary and subcutaneous metastases. Cytopathology 1991;2:303–9.
501. Zerbi A, De Nardi P, Braga M, Radice F, Sironi M, Di Carlo V. An oncocytic carcinoma of the pancreas with pulmonary and subcutaneous metastases. Pancreas 1993;8:116–19.

**Mature Teratoma**

502. Assawamatianont S, King AD. Dermoid cysts of the pancreas. Am J Surg 1977;43:503–4.
503. Iacono C, Zamboni G, DiMarcello R, et al. Dermoid cyst of the head of the pancreas area. Int J Pancreatol 1993;14:269–73.
504. Mester M, Trajber H, Compton CC, de Camargo HS, Cardoso de Almeida PC, Hoover HC Jr. Cystic teratomas of the pancreas. Arch Surg 1990;125:1215–8.

# 5
# TUMORS OF THE ENDOCRINE PANCREAS

Pancreatic endocrine tumors are benign or malignant epithelial tumors that show evidence of endocrine cell differentiation. According to conventional histologic appearance, pancreatic endocrine tumors are either well- to moderately differentiated (which are here called differentiated) or poorly differentiated (undifferentiated) tumors.

## DIFFERENTIATED ENDOCRINE TUMORS

**Definition.** These are benign or malignant low-grade tumors with prominent morphologic features of endocrine differentiation.

**General Features.** Pancreatic endocrine tumors of clinical relevance are relatively uncommon. In surgical series the annual incidence is 1 per 2 million population (37): in a study from Northern Ireland, the prevalence was 1 to 5 per million population per year for all pancreatic endocrine tumors (7) and in a study from the United States, it was less than 1 per 100,000 population for endocrine carcinomas (42). In Northern Ireland, the mortality rate for pancreatic cancer is 7 per 100,000 population per year (21). From our data, clinically relevant nonlethal forms of pancreatic neoplasia correspond to 10 to 20 percent of all tumors, of which 1 to 6 percent are endocrine tumors. Data from Brussels and Varese show that endocrine neoplasms represent 1 to 2 percent of all pancreatic tumors (unpublished findings, 1996).

The majority of clinically relevant pancreatic endocrine tumors are functional (32,36). Nonfunctioning tumors are found in 15 to 35 percent of surgical cases, and are usually associated with signs of an expanding mass (36,67). Incidental, clinically silent endocrine tumors have been reported in 0.4 to 1.6 percent of random autopsies in which only a few pancreatic sections were examined and in 10 percent of autopsies in which the whole organ was systematically investigated (25,34). They represent about 5 percent of pancreatic endocrine tumors in surgical series (67). In patients with type 1 multiple endocrine neoplasia (MEN 1), the pancreas is involved in 82 to 100 percent of cases (18,40).

Pancreatic endocrine tumors may occur at any age, although they are rare in children. Of 125 tumors studied by Heitz et al. (29), the age range was 12 to 78 (mean, 58) years. No significant sex difference has been observed.

No specific causes have been identified for human pancreatic endocrine tumors, apart from those arising in patients with type 1 MEN syndrome (see Multiple Endocrine Neoplasia, Type 1). A family history of diabetes has been reported in 20 to 30 percent of patients with insulinoma (46). It is not known, however, whether this indicates a common genetic trait favoring both dysfunction and growth of islet B cells. The involvement of BK virus infection in the pathogenesis of human insulinoma has been also suggested (14), while that of the "rat insulinoma gene" (*rig* gene, now identified with the "regenerating" [*rig*] gene and the pancreatic stone protein gene expressed by acinar cells) seems unlikely (33,48) Recently, von Hippel-Lindau disease gene has been implicated, together with other tumor-suppressor genes located on the short arm of chromosome 3, in the initiation or progression of some nonfunctioning endocrine tumors (44,54). On the contrary, no evidence has been obtained for a role of K-*ras* or p53 genes, two genes frequently mutated in pancreatic ductal cancers, in pancreatic endocrine tumorigenesis, apart from p53 gene mutation and p53 protein nuclear overaccumulation in small cell endocrine carcinomas (49).

The origin of pancreatic endocrine tumors from hypothetical multipotent ductular stem cells has been suggested by: 1) the observation of endocrine cell neogenesis (nesidioblastosis) in the ductules of pancreatic tissue surrounding endocrine tumors; 2) the well-known origin of islets from ductular outgrowths during fetal life as well as in infants with neonatal hyperinsulinemic hypoglycemia, with resultant ductuloinsular complexes; and 3) the frequent finding in pancreatic endocrine tumors of multiple types of endocrine cells including, on occasion, scattered ductular cells (3,27,34,46). However, ploidy studies have shown that, in contrast to pancreatic endocrine tumors, nesidioblastosis is an essentially euploid, nondysplastic growth process. Thus, tumor-associated nesidioblastosis may well be a secondary (rather than preneoplastic) change due to the trophic action of hormones and trophic factors released by the tumor itself (23, 50). In addition, as discussed below (see Tumors in Animals), both in vitro and in vivo experiments show the high plasticity of the mechanisms controlling endocrine cell differentiation in tumors, with frequent direct switching of insulin-producing tumor cells to pancreatic polypeptide (PP) cells, glucagon-producing cells, or even to cells producing nonislet "ectopic" hormones. Moreover, histologic patterns suggestive of an islet origin of tumors arising in MEN 1 syndrome have been observed (fig. 5-1) (67).

That at least part of pancreatic endocrine (islet cell) tumors are histogenetically related to intralobular, serous-type ductules is suggested by the common embryogenetic origin of islets, intralobular serous ductules, and centroacinar and acinar cells from primitive peripheral ducts (38); the concomitant growth in focal nesidioblastosis of islets and serous-type intralobular ductules to form ductuloinsular complexes inside residual acinar tissue (16,22); the intimate admixture of endocrine growth, serous ductules, and centroacinar cells in an occasional insulinoma (11); and the frequent occurrence of islet cells among tumors like acinar cell carcinoma and pancreatoblastoma. The ductular stem cell origin of pancreatic endocrine tumors remains an attractive, though unproven, hypothesis, whereas their origin from the transformation of mature islet cells has been proven in experimental transgenic tumors and seems likely in human MEN 1 syndrome.

An endocrine component has also been observed in some mucin-producing ductal carcinomas or cystadenocarcinomas. Both islet and nonislet, gut-related endocrine cells, such as gastrin- and serotonin-producing cells, are found in these cases, which may occasionally be associated with a Zollinger-Ellison syndrome due to gastrin hypersecretion (41). The histogenesis of such tumors is likely related to mucin-producing extralobular ducts and their gut-type metaplastic potential (64).

**Clinical Features.** See section, Clinicopathologic Profiles.

**Diagnosis.** In most cases the endocrine nature of a pancreatic tumor is suggested by its distinctive cellular and structural patterns. Relatively monomorphic, medium-sized cells arranged in trabeculae, microlobules, perivascular rosettes, tubules, and acini or solid sheets are observed in histologic preparations. A smear obtained by fine-needle aspiration shows rather small regular cells with pale and vacuolated cytoplasm (see Fine-Needle Aspiration in chapter 9). However, some nonendocrine tumors, including solid-pseudopapillary tumors or acinar cell carcinomas, may have structural patterns similar to those of endocrine tumors. Thus, confirmation of the endocrine nature of the tumor should be obtained with endocrine granule stains including argyrophil methods, lead hematoxylin, and aldehyde fuchsin (25,47,66), or with immunohistochemical tests for secretory proteins including chromogranins A, B, and C (65,72). The chromogranin proteins probably provide binding sites for the silver, lead, and basic dyes used in granule stains, as well as for biogenic amines (e.g., serotonin in enterochromaffin [EC] cell granules) (58). Granule membrane proteins such as synaptophysin (8,12), and cytosolic proteins including PGP9.5 protein (60) or neuron-specific enolase (10), are also useful markers for pancreatic endocrine tumors (see Table 3-1). Although neuron-specific enolase may be present in nonendocrine tumors (e.g., solid-pseudopapillary tumors) (43), cytosolic markers are useful for the recognition of agranular and poorly granular endocrine cells, especially from poorly differentiated carcinomas. Pancreatic endocrine tumors may also express cytokeratins 8 and 18 and neurofilaments (30,51). The detection of somatostatin receptors in tumor sections by autoradiography may help in tumor localization by scanning and in predicting the suppressive effects of somatostatin analogues on hormone release from the tumor (56).

In addition to conventional histologic criteria and general endocrine markers, functional characterization of tumor cells by hormone immunohistochemistry is also needed for a precise classification of pancreatic endocrine tumors. As the distribution of immunoreactive cells is often uneven and tumors frequently produce more than one, and sometimes several, hormones (3,27,45), immunohistochemical tumor diagnosis must rely on dominant populations of hormone-characterized cells in extensively sampled specimens. Hormone mRNA detection by in situ hybridization can be used to identify hormone expression

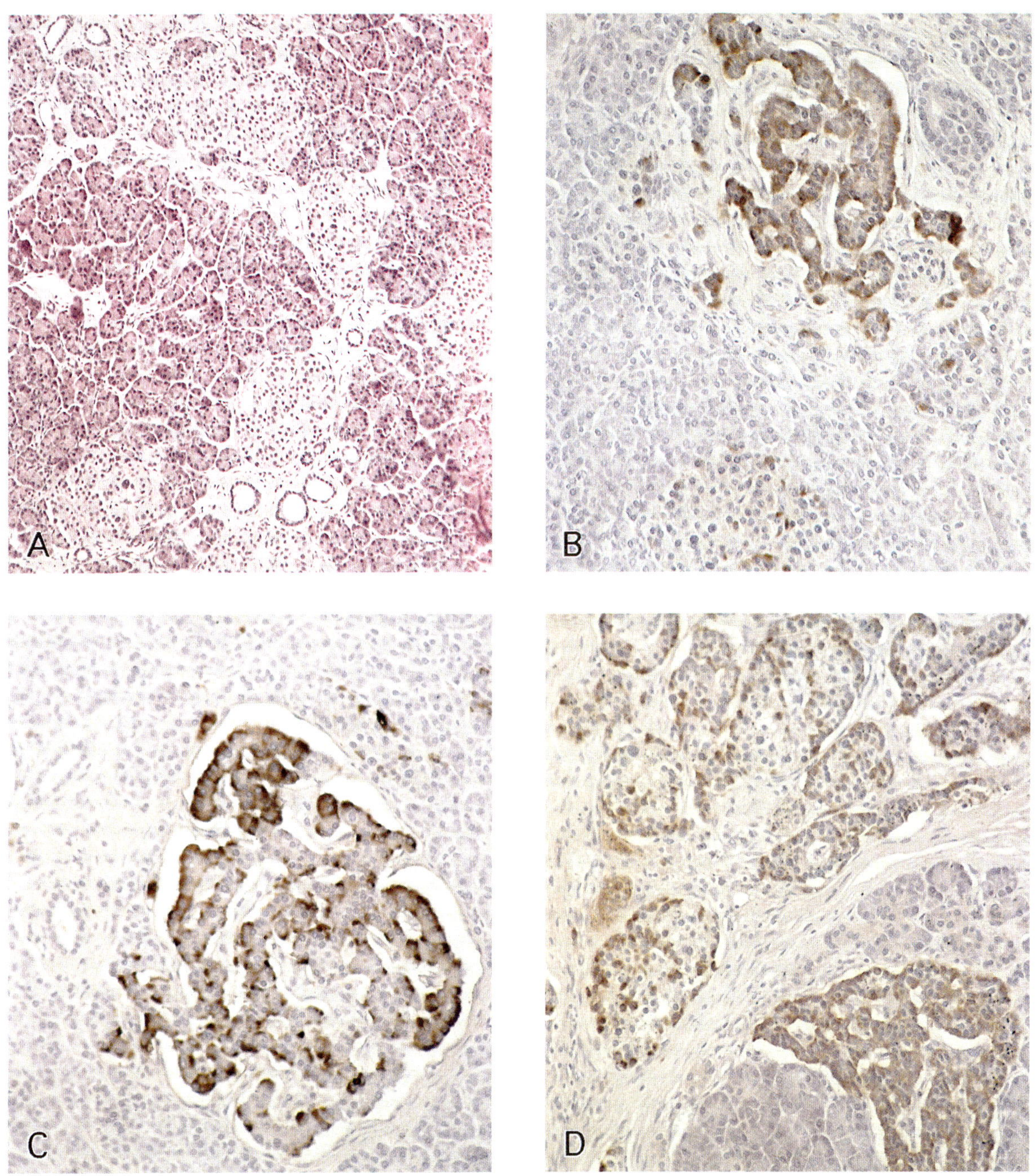


Figure 5-1

ENDOCRINE TUMORS: HISTOGENESIS

A: Admixture of newly formed islet-like structures and ductules in a focus of nesidioblastosis of pancreatic tissue adjacent to a sporadic gastrinoma. (Fig. 11 from Solcia E, Capella C, Buffa R, Frigerio B, Fiocca R. Pathology of the Zollinger-Ellison syndrome. Progr Surg Pathol 1980;1:119–33.)

B: Dysplastic lesion mostly composed of glucagon cells arranged in gyriform trabeculae separated by sclerotic strands of connective tissue. Note close contact, in the right middle part, with a small glucagon-negative endocrine microlobule, a remnant of the original islet. This is a MEN1 case. (Immunoperoxidase technique)

C: Minute microadenoma mainly composed of glucagon cells forming gyriform trabeculae.

D: Islet crowding in an area of exocrine tissue atrophy due to chronic pancreatitis (upper left). Note the glucagon cell microadenoma with a trabecular-gyriform structure in a surviving pancreatic lobule (bottom right). MEN1 case. (Immunoperoxidase technique)

at the cellular level in the occasional tumor in which hormone immunohistochemistry fails (52). This approach allows correlation between clinical signs of hormone hyperfunction or increased hormone levels in blood and their precise source in primary pancreatic tumors, tumor recurrences, metastases, or extrapancreatic tumors. It has been noted that all pancreatic endocrine tumors, with or without a hyperfunctional syndrome, that are composed of cells normally found in the pancreatic islets and produce islet hormones like insulin, glucagon, somatostatin, and PP have much lower malignancy rates (10 to 20 percent) than those producing "gut" hormones such as gastrin, vasoactive intestinal peptide (VIP), and neurotensin (60 to 80 percent) (27,45,46,65), or "ectopic" hormones such as adrenocorticotrophic hormone (ACTH), vasopressin, or parathyroid hormone (90 to 100 percent) (13). These data suggest that the tumor cells producing inappropriate hormones are more severely transformed and more aggressive.

From the systematic comparison of functionally characterized tumors with associated clinical syndromes, it appears that the various hormones or cell types have different potentials for producing clinically relevant symptoms. For instance, most patients with insulin-producing tumors, even when their tumors are smaller than 1 cm, develop the insulinoma syndrome, while only a small proportion of patients with glucagon-producing tumors, usually of large size (62), develop the glucagonoma syndrome. In the latter case it is likely that a larger tumor mass or a longer history is required for development of the hyperfunctional syndrome, thus selecting tumors of greater growth potential and lesser differentiation. This may explain the much higher malignancy rate (70 to 80 percent) of glucagon-producing tumors associated with the glucagonoma syndrome. Most of the glucagon-producing tumors lacking the syndrome are small benign adenomas discovered by chance at autopsy (25) or in surgical specimens (62,67).

Tumors composed of multiple cell types have a tendency to develop a single, well-defined, hyperfunctional syndrome, which often dominates the clinicopathologic pattern and is usually more predictive of the natural history of the tumor than are purely morphologic findings. Demonstration in tumor tissue of some cells producing the hormone causing the syndrome remains a necessary prerequisite for classifying the tumor according to the associated hyperfunctional syndrome. Indeed, multiple tumors with different hormonal expression, which are not infrequent (30 percent of gastrinomas and 13 percent of insulinomas), may lead to diagnostic mistakes, inappropriate surgery, and failure to cure the syndrome.

**Criteria for Malignancy.** Unequivocal evidence of malignancy is either gross invasion of adjacent organs; metastases to regional lymph nodes, liver, and other distant sites; or blood vessel invasion.

The size of the primary tumor is greater in metastatic versus nonmetastatic tumors (6,15, 19). Kenny and coworkers (33) recently confirmed that localized tumors (mean maximum diameter, 1.7 cm) are significantly smaller in size than metastatic tumors (mean, 6.4 cm), and comparable findings have been obtained from our research. In general, well-differentiated endocrine tumors less than 2 cm in size show a benign behavior while those above 3 cm are mainly (with many exceptions) malignant (9,37a). Tumors exceeding 6 cm in size should be considered malignant as 93 percent of a large series of proven carcinomas were of this size (15). However, in all series size overlap among benign and malignant tumors has been observed, and tumors as large as 15 cm have shown benign behavior (29). Size alone is an insufficient criterion for predicting malignancy of differentiated endocrine tumors, and should be coupled with other parameters (e.g., an associated clinical syndrome or an invasive pattern).

At present, the only histologic marker of malignancy is blood vessel invasion. Features suggestive of potential malignant behavior are high mitotic index, tumor necrosis, and definite invasion of tumor capsule, adjacent normal pancreas, lymphatics, or perineural spaces. Invasion of blood vessels, particularly veins located in the tumor capsule (fig. 5-2), and perineural spaces has been observed in 90 percent of our malignant cases associated with distant metastases (37a). Blood vessel invasion should be accepted as true only when the vessel wall is identified through factor VIII or CD31 antigen immunostaining, when tumor thrombi are attached to the vessel wall, or when an actual point of invasion into the vessel wall is recognized.

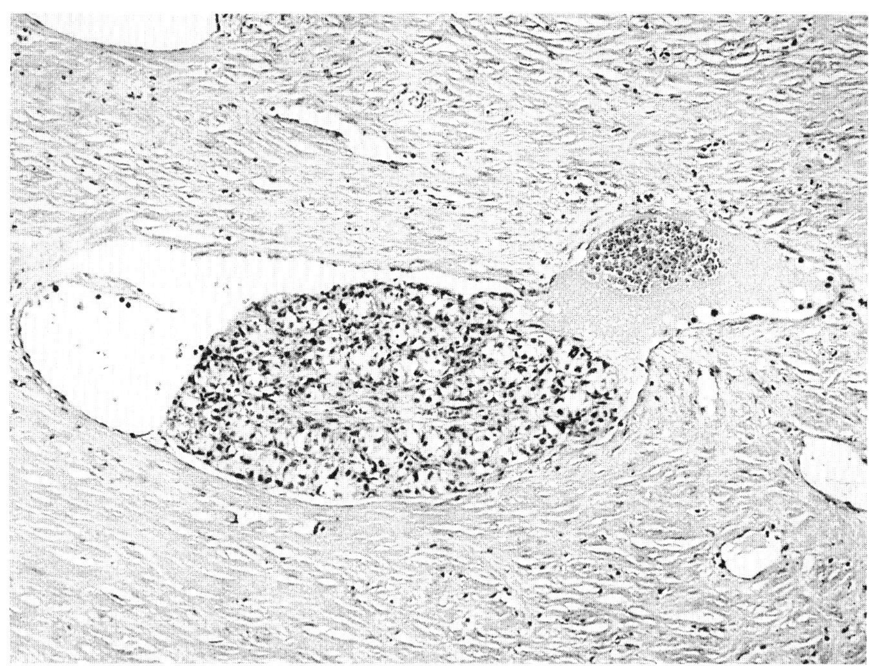

Figure 5-2
ENDOCRINE CARCINOMA: INVASION OF A BLOOD VESSEL IN TUMOR CAPSULE

This micrograph shows blood vessel invasion by a well-differentiated nonfunctioning endocrine carcinoma.

Tumor necrosis is a finding restricted to malignant cases; however, it occurs only rarely in differentiated endocrine tumors. It was found in only 2 out of a series of 31 differentiated endocrine tumors with malignancy proven by metastasis or gross local invasion (to be compared with 4 out of 5 small cell carcinomas and 0 of 25 benign or borderline tumors) investigated by two of the authors. A mitotic index above 2 or 4 per 10 high-power fields rules out an adenoma or a tumor of uncertain malignant potential, respectively, in our experience, with more than 80 percent accuracy; a mitotic index below these figures is of no predictive value. In fact, from our series, 13 out of 31 differentiated carcinomas, 6 of 9 tumors with uncertain malignancy, and 12 of 16 adenomas showed 0 or 1 mitosis per 10 high-power fields (37a).

There is general agreement among various authors (9,19,24,36,45,46,67) that histologic features alone, as seen in routinely stained sections, correlate poorly with the malignant potential of pancreatic endocrine tumors. Exceptions are: 1) the poor prognosis of a small group of tumors with a high grade of cellular anaplasia, focal or widespread necrosis, and high mitotic index (poorly differentiated endocrine or small cell carcinomas); 2) the higher metastatic rate of tumors with solid to diffuse, poorly defined histology (Soga's type D); and 3) the benign nature of tumors with gyriform, anastomosing ribbons consisting of one to two layers of small polygonal cells (type IIa structure of Nieuwenhuijzen Kruseman et al. [47]). Nuclear pleomorphism seems a particularly unreliable criterion.

Several attempts have been recently made to overcome the difficulties in assessing prognosis based on conventional histology alone. Suggested predictors of malignancy are: more than 1.5 nuclei per $mm^2$ coupled with a nuclear/cytoplasmic ratio of 30 percent or more (33); aneuploidy with a DNA index (relative DNA content of the aneuploid stemline as compared with diploid cells) of more than 1.5, especially when associated with multiploidy (1,36); Ha-*ras* oncogene overexpression (31); lack of the progesterone receptor immunoreactivity normally found in some islet cells (70); presence of human chorionic gonadotropin (HCG) or its alpha subunit (28); more than 5 mitoses per 10 high-power fields (33); more than 5 percent AgNOR (silver stained nucleolar organizer region)-rich cells (6 AgNORs per nucleus) (61); a PCNA (proliferating cell nuclear antigen) above 5 percent (50); and a Ki-67 index above 5 percent (37a).

The practical usefulness of these findings is limited by several drawbacks: many metastatic tumors had 0 to 2 mitoses per 10 high-power fields in their primary sites (37a); Ha-*ras* was also overexpressed in nonmetastatic tumors, although somewhat less than in metastatic ones (31); 36 percent of malignant tumors expressed the progesterone receptor and 28 percent of benign tumors failed to express it (70); 36 percent of malignant tumors showed less than 5 percent AgNOR-rich cells (61); and 30 to 40 percent of malignant tumors (especially insulinomas) had no HCG or its subunits (29) which, on the other hand, were found in up to 18 percent of benign tumors (4,61).

In addition, the efficacy of high DNA index aneuploidy in differentiating benign and malignant tumors by flow cytometry has not been evaluated in a sufficiently large series of cases. Most apparently benign insulinomas were also aneuploid, with a DNA index of less than 1.5 (1). Moreover, in several studies the predictive value of the associated clinical syndrome (rather than tumor cell immunostaining or serum hormone assays) has not been sufficiently considered. For instance, only apparently benign insulinomas were adequately represented among functioning tumors in the PCNA study (50), and all benign functioning tumors were insulinomas, while all gastrinomas were malignant in the morphometric study (33) (see above). As detailed below (see Clinicopathologic Profiles) clinical syndromes are per se predictive of tumor behavior, with metastatic rates ranging from around 10 percent for clinically silent incidental tumors and insulinomas to 60 to 90 percent for glucagonomas, somatostatinomas, VIPomas, gastrinomas, tumors associated with "ectopic" syndromes, and symptomatic nonfunctioning tumors (13,20,46,62,67,68,69).

Proliferative rate indexes, among which Ki-67 proved more reliable than PCNA in separating adenomas (0 to 2 percent Ki-67 versus 0 to 8.5 percent for PCNA-positive cells) from low-grade carcinomas (1 to 10 percent for both antigens) among our series of 61 nonfunctioning tumors (37a), remain to be tested for their capacity to discriminate between benign and malignant tumors within separate groups of functioning insulinomas, gastrinomas, glucagonomas, VIPomas, etc; i.e., independent of the clinical syndrome. The proportion of AgNOR-rich cells is a good predictor of prognosis in insulinoma (all 5 malignant cases and 10 of 11 benign cases were correcdly identified); this is less reliable for gastrinoma (10 of 15 malignant and 5 of 5 benign cases correctly identified) and other, mostly nonfunctioning cases (11 of 18 malignant and 6 of 6 benign cases identified) (61).

In our experience, a simple multiparametric approach, including size, angio/neuroinvasion, proliferative rate, type of hormone secretion, and presence or absence of hyperfunctional syndrome, is effective for the identification of tumors at higher risk of recurrence or metastasis (see Microscopic Findings and Table 5-1).

**Gross Findings.** Endocrine tumors arise with about the same frequency in all parts of the pancreas. However, different tumor subtypes may show a predilection for the body and tail (glucagonomas, VIPomas, insulinomas) or the head (locally symptomatic nonfunctioning tumors, gastrinomas, somatostatinomas). Tumors similar to those arising in the pancreas may also occur more or less frequently outside the pancreas, as for instance gastrin cell tumors in the duodenum, stomach, and upper jejunum; insulin-producing tumors in the duodenum and ileum; glucagon-enteroglucagon–producing tumors in the rectum, colon, and appendix; and somatostatin-producing tumors in the duodenum (see Clinicopathologic Profiles).

Careful, gentle palpation and systematic serial blocking in transverse sections 0.3 to 0.5 cm thick are required to identify small endocrine tumors within the pancreatic parenchyma. The tumor is usually slightly firmer than the adjacent parenchyma and is pinkish gray to pinkish white. Hemorrhagic foci (which may result from the tumor or from surgical trauma or excessive manipulation) impart a purple (fig. 5-3) to bluish black color, whereas a whitish color and firmer consistency are found in tumors with abundant fibrous or hyaline stroma, amyloid deposits, or calcification. Tumor necrosis and hemorrhage, seen in two thirds of malignant tumors (fig. 5-4), appear as softer foci of yellow to tan (15). Some tumors have a cystic appearance and have to be distinguished from exocrine tumors such as solid-pseudopapillary and serous cystic tumors (fig. 5-5).

The tumor nodules are multiple in 7.5 to 13 percent of insulinomas, 30 percent of gastrinomas, and nearly all MEN 1 cases (27,36,67,69). They have regular, well-demarcated borders suggesting an expansile type of growth. A fibrous pseudocapsule, often incomplete, usually surrounds the tumor. Patterns of direct local, intrapancreatic,

Table 5-1

**CLINICOPATHOLOGIC CORRELATIONS IN PANCREATIC ENDOCRINE TUMORS**

| Histologic Type | Cell Types* | Clinical Signs* |
|---|---|---|
| DIFFERENTIATED | | |
| Adenoma** (Mitoses: <2/10 HPF; Ki-67: <2%)† | | |
| Microadenoma (Size: < 0.5 cm) | Glucagon, PP, insulin, and somatostatin cells | Asymptomatic |
| Macroadenoma (Size: 0.5 to 2 cm) | Insulin, glucagon, PP, and/or somatostatin cells | Insulinoma syndrome; others: mostly asymptomatic |
| Borderline tumor‡ (Size: > 2 cm; mitoses: 0 to 3/10 HPF; Ki-67: 1 to 5%) | Gastrin, insulin, glucagon, PP, VIP, somatostatin, serotonin, GRF, and/or other cells | Gastrinoma, insulinoma, glucagonoma, VIPoma, somatostatinoma, carcinoid or acromegalic syndrome; nonfunctioning tumors: asymptomatic or locally symptomatic |
| Low-grade carcinoma (Size: > 3 cm; mitoses: 1 to 10/10 HPF; K-67: 1 to 10%) | Gastrin, insulin, glucagon, VIP, somatostatin, PP, serotonin, GRF, ACTH, neurotensin, parathirin, and/or calcitonin cells | Gastrinoma, insulinoma, glucagonoma, VIPoma, somatostatinoma, and Cushing, carcinoid, acromegalic, or hypercalcemic syndromes; nonfunctioning tumors: signs of slow growing tumor |
| UNDIFFERENTIATED | | |
| Small cell carcinoma (Mitoses: >10/10 HPF; Ki-67: >10%) | Endocrine cells with various, usually scarce, hormone immunoreactivities | Signs of rapidily progressing tumor without hormonal symptons; rarely: Cushing, carcinoid, hypercalcemic, or multiple syndromes |

*Common cell types and associated clinical signs (in order of frequency).
**Microadenomas, macroadenoma(s), and/or low-grade carcinoma may coexist in the pancreas of MEN 1 patients.
†Criteria in parentheses are helpful although not strictly diagnostic.
‡Tumors with uncertain malignant potential.

or extrapancreatic (duodenum, retroperitoneal soft tissues, and blood vessels) tumor invasion are rarely observed macroscopically.

Metastases are usually found in the liver (mainly with diffuse multifocal involvement of both lobes) and abdominal lymph nodes (predominantly affecting peripancreatic, hepatic, para-aortic-paracaval, and mesenteric nodes, and sometimes involving mediastinal, neck, or axillary nodes). Bone, peritoneum, lung, kidney, and thyroid are involved only occasionally. Interestingly, tumor types arising preferentially in the tail and body (glucagonomas, VIPomas, insulinomas) show a striking predilection for hematogenous spread, whereas pancreatic gastrinomas (and even more their duodenal counterpart) prefer the lymphatic route. As liver metastasis implies a worse prognosis than regional lymph node metastasis (17,20,68) these differences are prognostically relevant.

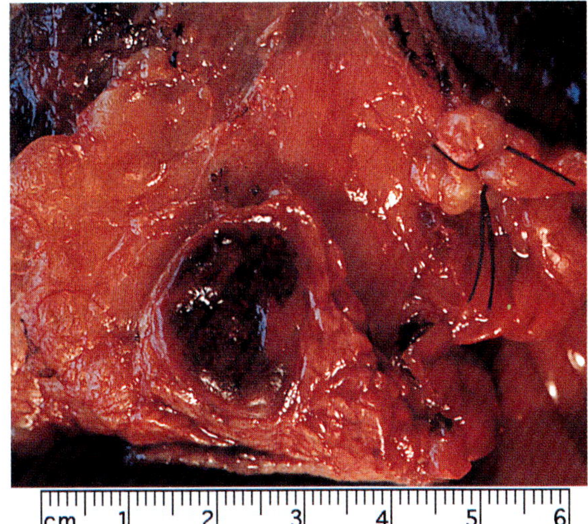


Figure 5-3
ENDOCRINE ADENOMA
Small (2 cm in diameter) intrapancreatic tumor with expansile margins showing a relatively homogeneous, deep red, hemorrhagic appearance.

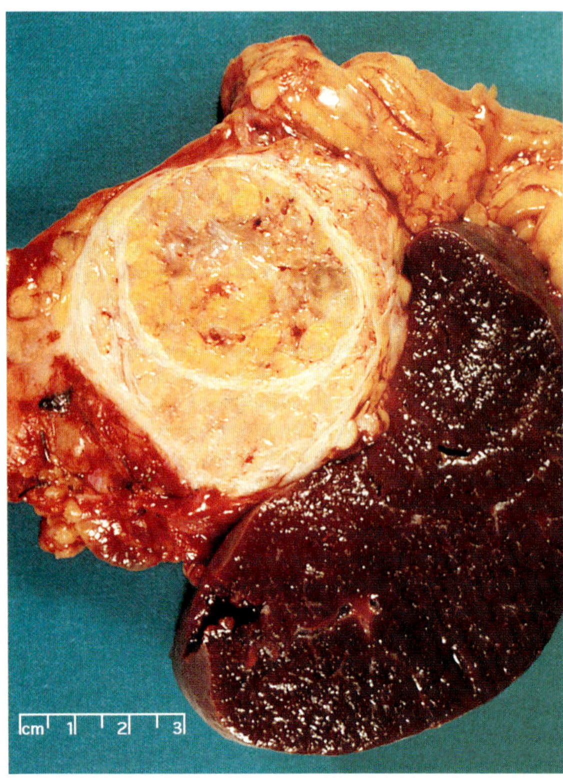


Figure 5-4
ENDOCRINE CARCINOMA
This rather large (6 cm) tumor invades the splenic capsule and contains minute foci of hemorrhage.

**Microscopic Findings.** Differentiated pancreatic endocrine tumors are composed of epithelial cells of small to medium size and mild to moderate atypia, forming trabeculae, ribbons, solid nests with or without vascular pseudorosettes, tubules and acini, or more diffuse sheets. Three main structural patterns have been recognized (19,24,27,45,47).

The trabecular pattern (figs. 5-6, 5-7) is characterized by cell cords, with or without a gyriform arrangement. Gyriform festoons composed of cellular monolayers or bilayers separated by highly vascular stroma are typical of small glucagon cell tumors (fig. 5-8). Parallel thin trabeculae formed by the palisading of cells are frequently observed in PP-cell tumors. Less prominent, larger, gyriform trabeculae or lobular nests separated by strands of vascular stroma, sometimes with amyloid deposits, may be found in insulin-producing tumors. The glandular pattern (fig. 5-9) is formed by tubules and acini with true lumina, often containing secretory material. This pattern is more frequently observed in gastrinomas and VIPomas. Admixed are poorly formed trabeculae or solid nests often containing vascular pseudorosettes. The medullary (or solid) pattern (fig. 5-10) shows nodular to diffuse cellular growth with scant intervening stroma partly separating large sheets of cells.

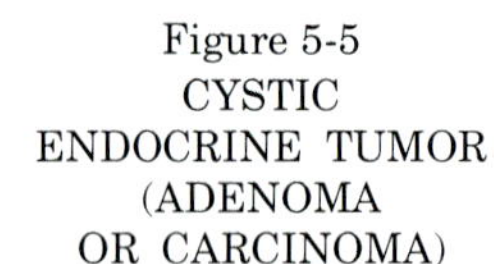

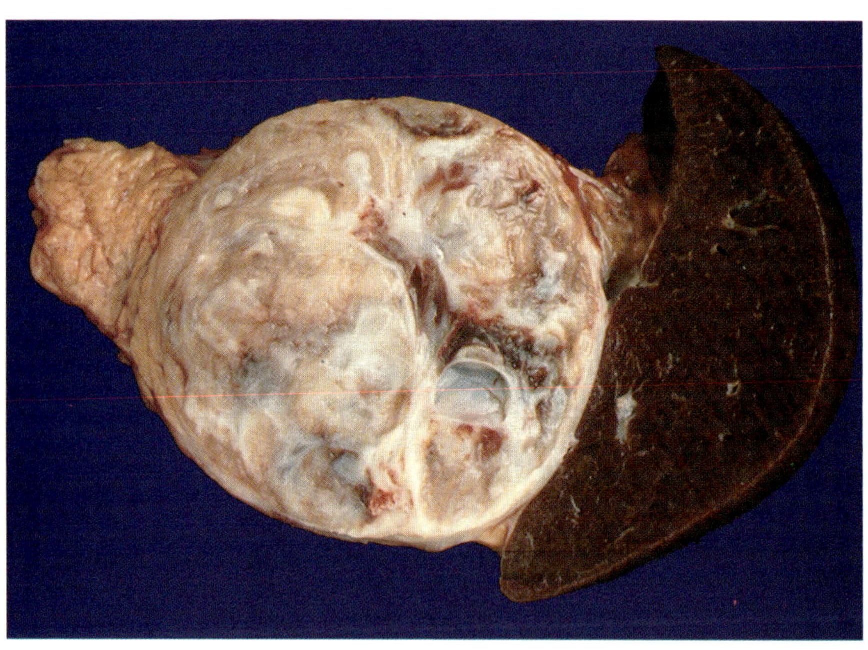

Figure 5-5
CYSTIC
ENDOCRINE TUMOR
(ADENOMA
OR CARCINOMA)
Cut surface of a large (8 cm), expansile endocrine tumor with cystic pattern.

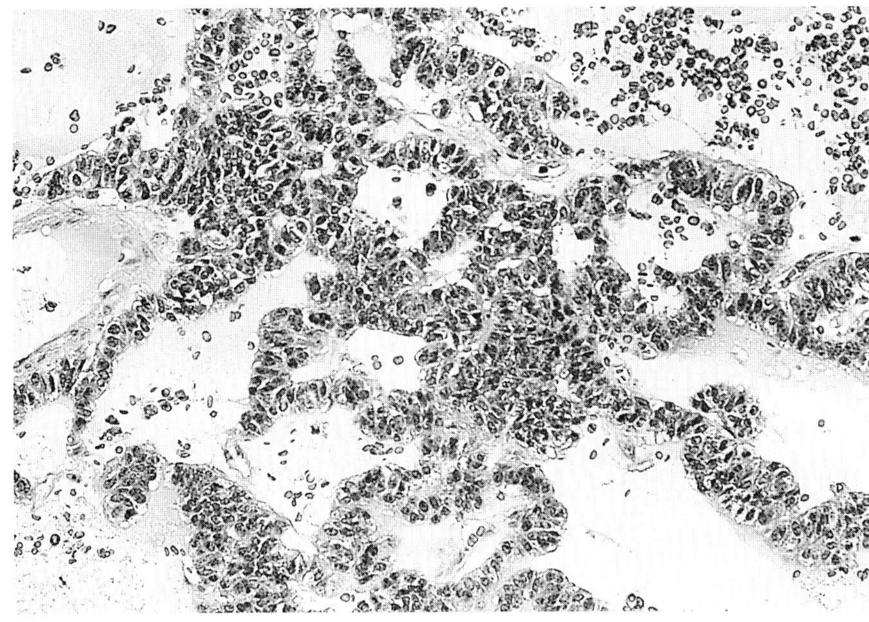

Figure 5-6
ENDOCRINE TUMOR WITH TRABECULAR PATTERN
Nonfunctioning PP-cell tumor showing ribbons and festoons of tumor cells present throughout the neoplasm, separated by loose fibrovascular stroma.

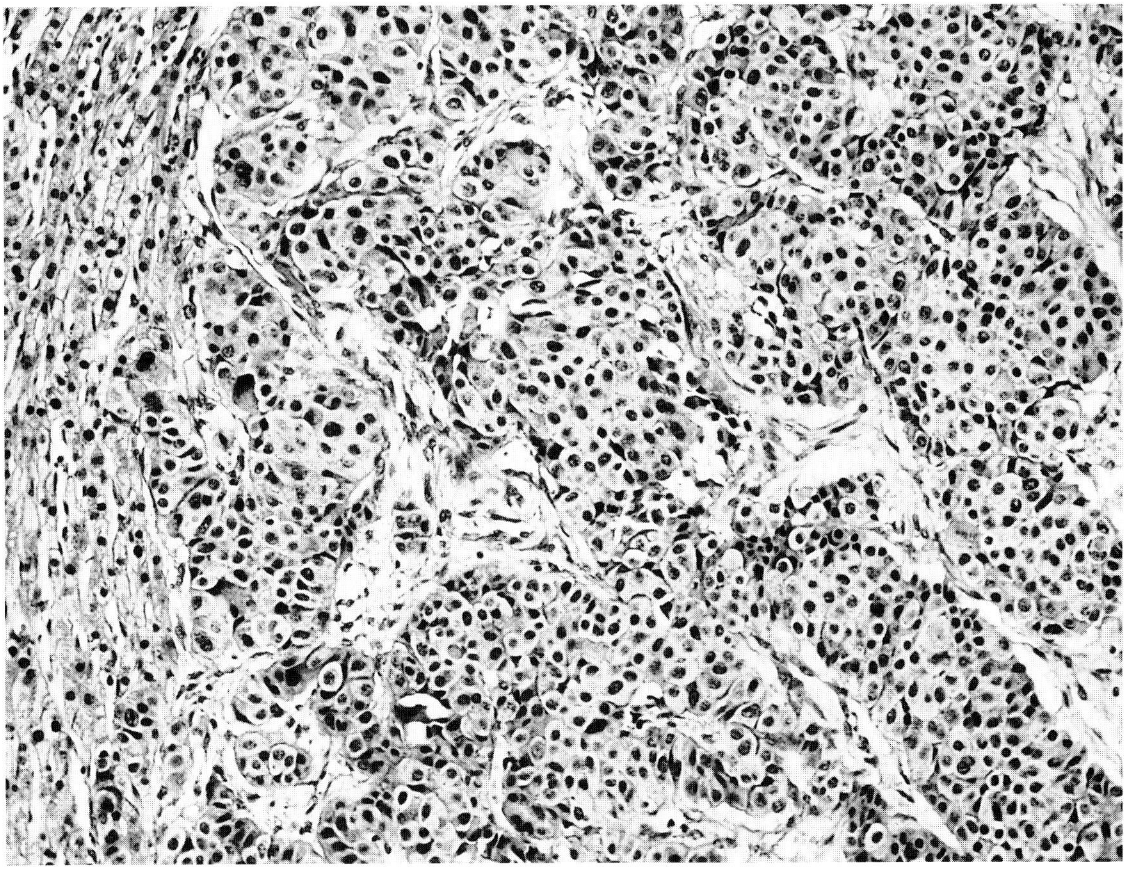

Figure 5-7
ENDOCRINE CARCINOMA WITH TRABECULAR AND LOBULAR PATTERN
Large trabeculae and lobules in a well-differentiated malignant insulinoma metastatic to the liver.

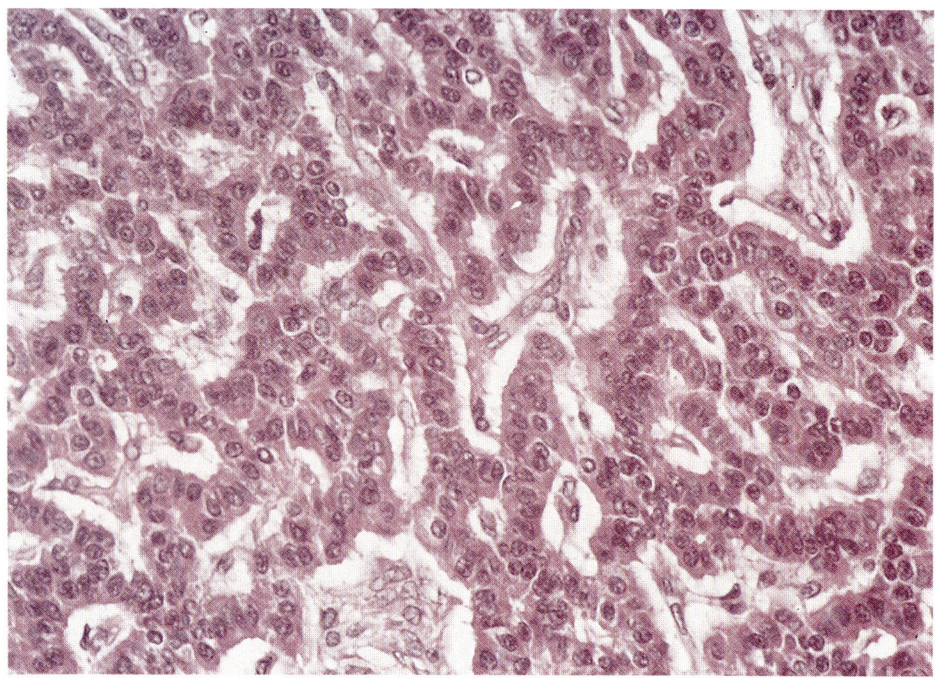

Figure 5-8
ENDOCRINE ADENOMA WITH GYRIFORM ARRANGEMENT
Gyriform festoons separated by highly vascular stroma in a clinically nonfunctioning adenoma which was immunohistochemically glucagon-positive.

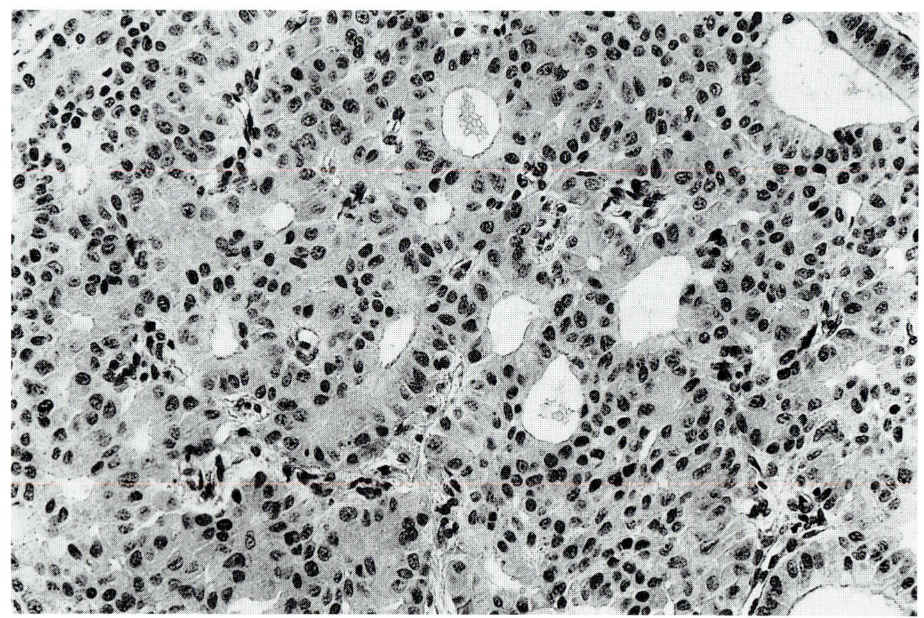

Figure 5-9
ENDOCRINE CARCINOMA WITH GLANDULAR PATTERN
Small regular glands are present throughout a malignant VIPoma.

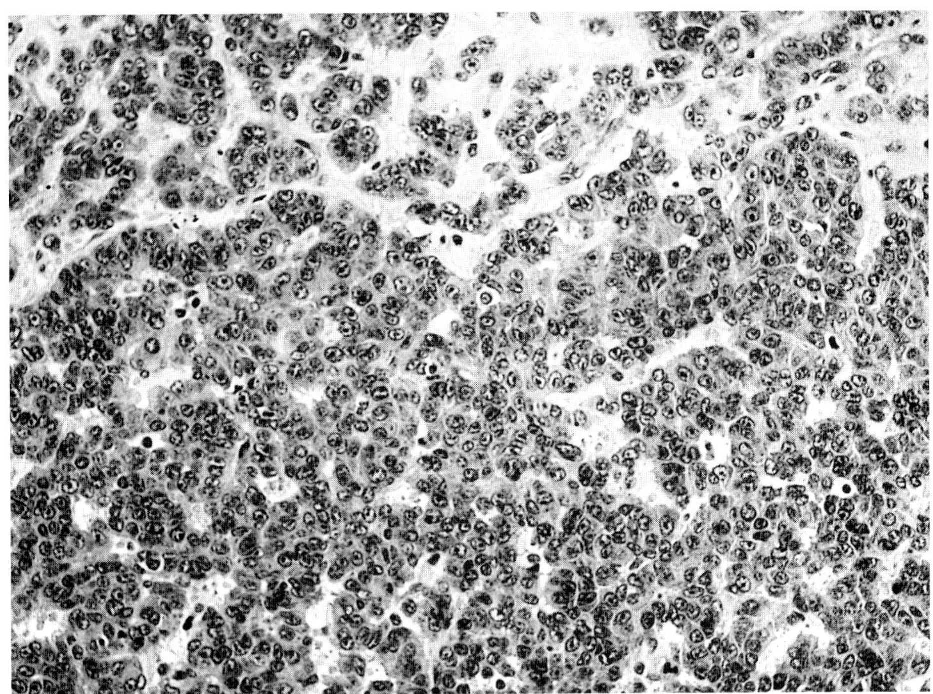

Figure 5-10
ENDOCRINE CARCINOMA WITH MEDULLARY PATTERN
Sheets and ill-defined nests of cells in a nonfunctioning endocrine carcinoma. Note nuclear crowding.

The trabecular pattern is more frequently found in benign tumors, while malignant tumors more often have the other two patterns. In general, the relationship between histologic structure and tumor cell type has been found to be rather poor (27,45,46,67): admixtures of patterns are frequently observed in the same tumor and are often independent of the cell types forming them or the associated clinical syndromes. However, the presence of abundant amyloid deposits in direct contact with tumor cells seems to be fairly distinctive of insulin-producing tumors (fig. 5-11) while foci of calcified amyloid or even psammoma bodies, which are diagnostic for somatostatin cell tumors in the duodenum, have been reported in pancreatic insulinomas. Although the histologic patterns have little value in individual cases, they sometimes predict cell type or hormones to be detected by subsequent immunohistochemistry.

Intense, diffuse reactivity for endocrine granule markers like Grimelius silver (fig. 5-12); chromogranins A, B (fig. 5-13), or C; and synaptophysin is regularly found in well-differentiated tumors. Electron microscopy may confirm the relative abundance of secretory granules and the differentiated pattern of cellular organelles. Secretory granules with a distinctive substructure are frequently found in neoplastic glucagon or insulin cells. Somatostatin, PP, or gastrin cells of pancreatic tumors are less often detected at the ultrastructural level; hormone immunohistochemistry is a better method of detection. Nonendocrine tumor cell components, such as agranular ductular-centroacinar cells, can be recognized with electron microscopy.

Most differentiated endocrine tumors are well circumscribed and show an expansile type of growth. They may be single or multiple and range in size from 0.5 mm to up to 20 cm, with obviously different clinical behavior. Based on size, proliferative rate, invasive pattern, and metastases (see above section) the tumor can be classified as an adenoma, a tumor of uncertain malignant potential, or a low-grade carcinoma (Table 5-1). A few moderately differentiated carcinomas have a poor prognosis; however, their precise clinicopathologic profiles require further investigation.

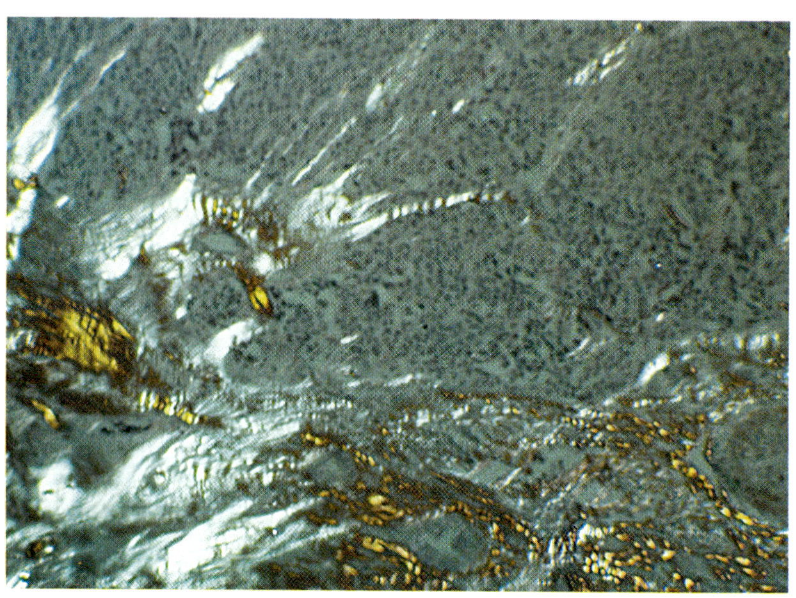

Figure 5-11
AMYLOID IN AN INSULINOMA
This tumor was stained with Congo red and photographed in polarized light. The amyloid deposits exhibit green birefringence.

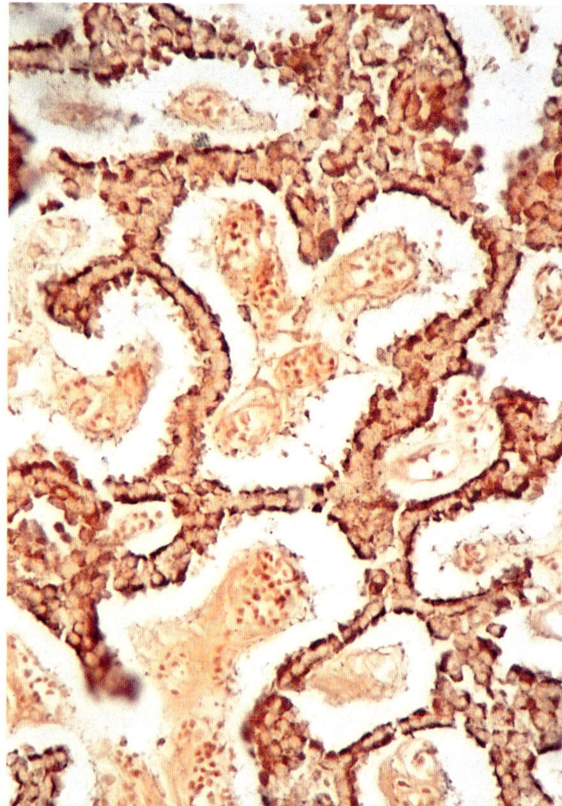

Figure 5-12
ENDOCRINE ADENOMA STAINED WITH GRIMELIUS SILVER
Most of the tumor cells in this gyriform, nonfunctioning A-cell adenoma contain argyrophilic granules.

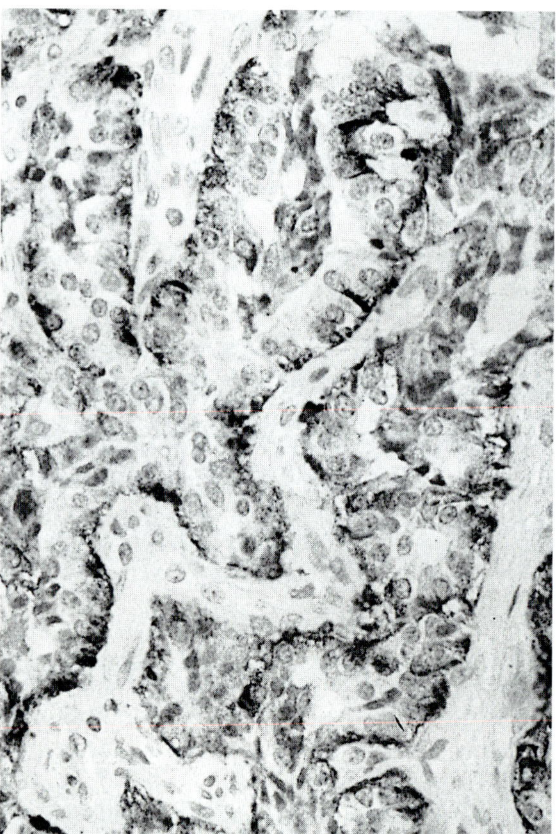

Figure 5-13
ENDOCRINE TUMOR IMMUNOSTAINED FOR SECRETORY PROTEINS
Intense chromogranin B staining in a serotonin-producing tumor.

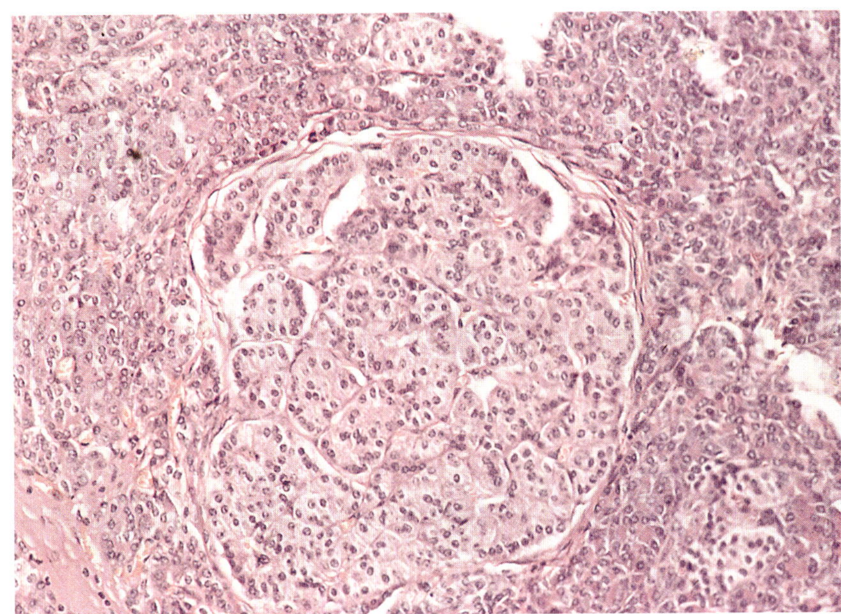

Figure 5-14
MICROADENOMA
Well-demarcated, partly encapsulated growth of uniform cells forming regular microlobules. Compare with islet in the lower right corner.

*Adenomas.* These are well-differentiated endocrine tumors with an abundance of cytoplasmic granules and intense reactivity to endocrine markers. Most tumors with benign morphology and behavior are less than 3 cm in size and have very low proliferative rates: 0 to 2 mitoses per 10 high-power fields and Ki-67-positive tumors cells of 2 percent or less. Cellular atypia is absent or minimal. There are no metastases, and no gross, vascular, or neural invasion. Tumors less than 2 cm in size can confidently be diagnosed as adenomas (37a). *Microadenomas* (fig. 5-14), ranging in size from 0.5 mm to 0.5 cm, can be separated from the remaining adenomas (macroadenomas). Microadenomas often form prominent lobules and ribbons, with or without cellular palisades, which are separated by more or less abundant fibrotic stroma. They occur either sporadically, as occasional findings in autopsy or surgical specimens, or in association with MEN 1 syndrome, where they often coexist with islet dysplasia, with or without signs of nesidioblastosis. Enlarged or irregularly shaped dysplastic islets in which there is a prominent switch from a microlobular to a trabecular structure and an abnormal increase in A, B, and PP cells should be distinguished from the minute monomorphous, essentially monohormonal growths of neoplastic nature forming microadenomas. As a rule, microadenomas are clinically silent despite their often high hormone content, especially of glucagon and PP. Coexisting macrotumors usually account for any associated hyperfunctional syndrome. *Macroadenomas* are well-circumscribed, completely or partly encapsulated tumors measuring more than 0.5 cm. They lack signs of vascular or perineural space invasion, although misleading patterns suggestive of invasion through an incomplete pseudocapsule are observed. The abundant secretory granules of macroadenomas have a relatively high content of endocrine markers and islet hormones (figs. 5-12, 5-13). Ectopic or gut-related hormones are only rarely expressed. Macroadenomas may be functioning, when secreting insulin, or nonfunctioning. Functioning tumors other than insulinomas are better classified as "of uncertain malignant potential."

In the old literature (19) a diagnosis of "questionably malignant tumor" was based on: 1) capsule invasion or incomplete capsule; 2) cellular variation and bizarre pattern; 3) blood vessel invasion; and 4) high mitotic rate. Long-term follow-up of these tumors after surgery has been mostly uneventful (53). Of the above criteria, capsular (pseudo)invasion and cellular pleomorphism are no longer considered suspicious for malignancy; when found alone, they do not distinguish an otherwise benign-looking tumor from an adenoma.

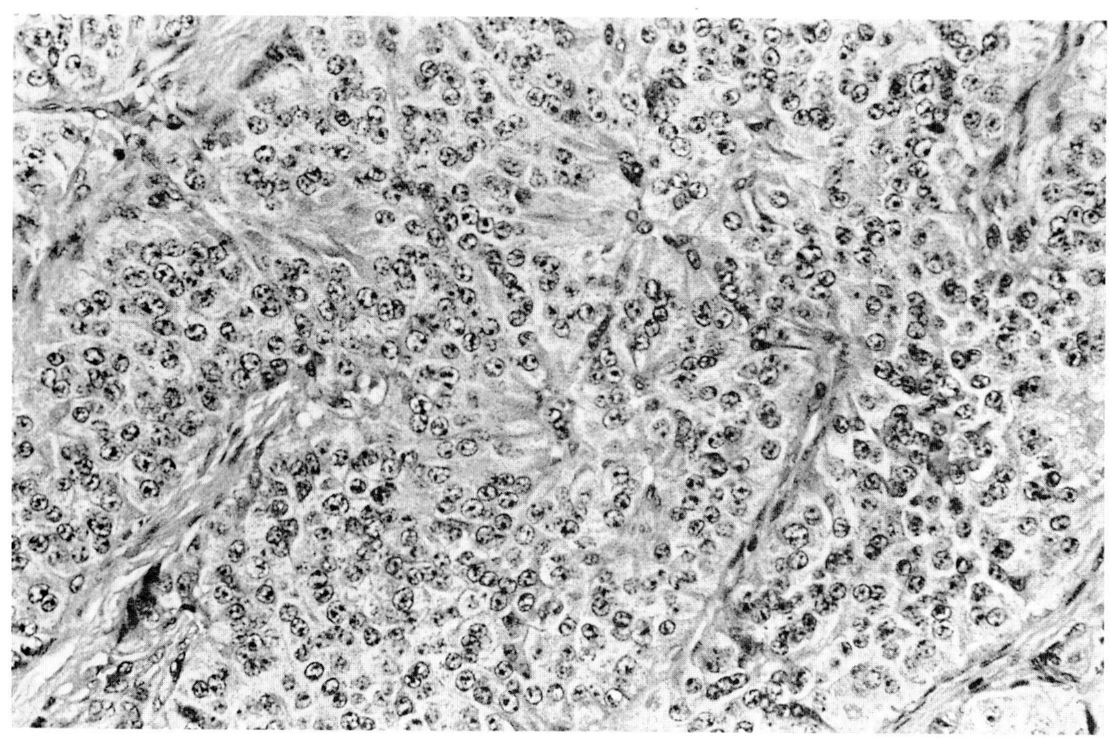

Figure 5-15
TUMOR OF UNCERTAIN MALIGNANT POTENTIAL
In this nonfunctioning somatostatin cell tumor cells show moderate nuclear crowding with evident nucleoli. The tumor is 3 cm in size and nonangioinvasive. Tumor recurred locally 14 years later with gross invasion and somatostatinoma syndrome.

*Tumors of Uncertain Malignant Potential.* These tumors have a well-differentiated histologic pattern. They are greater than 2 cm (mean, 5 to 6 cm) in size and may show mild cellular atypia, with nucleolar enlargement, an increased nuclear/cytoplasmic ratio (more than 30 percent), and nuclear crowding (more than 1500 nuclei/mm$^2$). There may be a slightly increased proliferative rate and histologic findings suggesting capsular, peritumor tissue, or venular invasion (fig. 5-15). The tumors may be associated with various kinds of hormone expression, with or without an associated syndrome of endocrine hyperfunction or signs of an expanding mass. All functioning tumors, other than insulinomas, that lack signs of malignancy fit in this group.

*Low-Grade Carcinomas.* These are large (most greater than 3 cm; mean, 6 cm), partly encapsulated tumors which grossly invade parapancreatic tissues, large vessels, or adjacent organs (see fig. 5-4). Low-grade carcinomas may resemble adenomas in their expansile type of growth and differentiated histologic structure (fig. 5-16), although diffuse cellular sheets and large, poorly defined trabeculae and pseudoglandular structures are formed more frequently. Common features of low-grade carcinomas are mild to moderate cellular atypia, evident nucleoli, an increased nuclear/cytoplasmic ratio, nuclear crowding, mitotic figures (1 to 10 per 10 high-power fields; mean, 3), and expression of proliferative markers (1 to 10 percent Ki-67; mean, 5 percent) (fig. 5-17). In most cases these features alone do not allow separation of tumors with uncertain malignant potential. However, we have found histologic signs of venular, lymphatic (fig. 5-18), or perineural invasion of capsular and parenchymal tissues surrounding the primary tumor in up to 90 percent of metastatic or grossly invasive tumors and in less than 30 percent of nonmetastatic noninvasive ones (37a).

Like tumors of uncertain malignant potential, low-grade carcinomas have various patterns of hormone expression, with or without endocrine

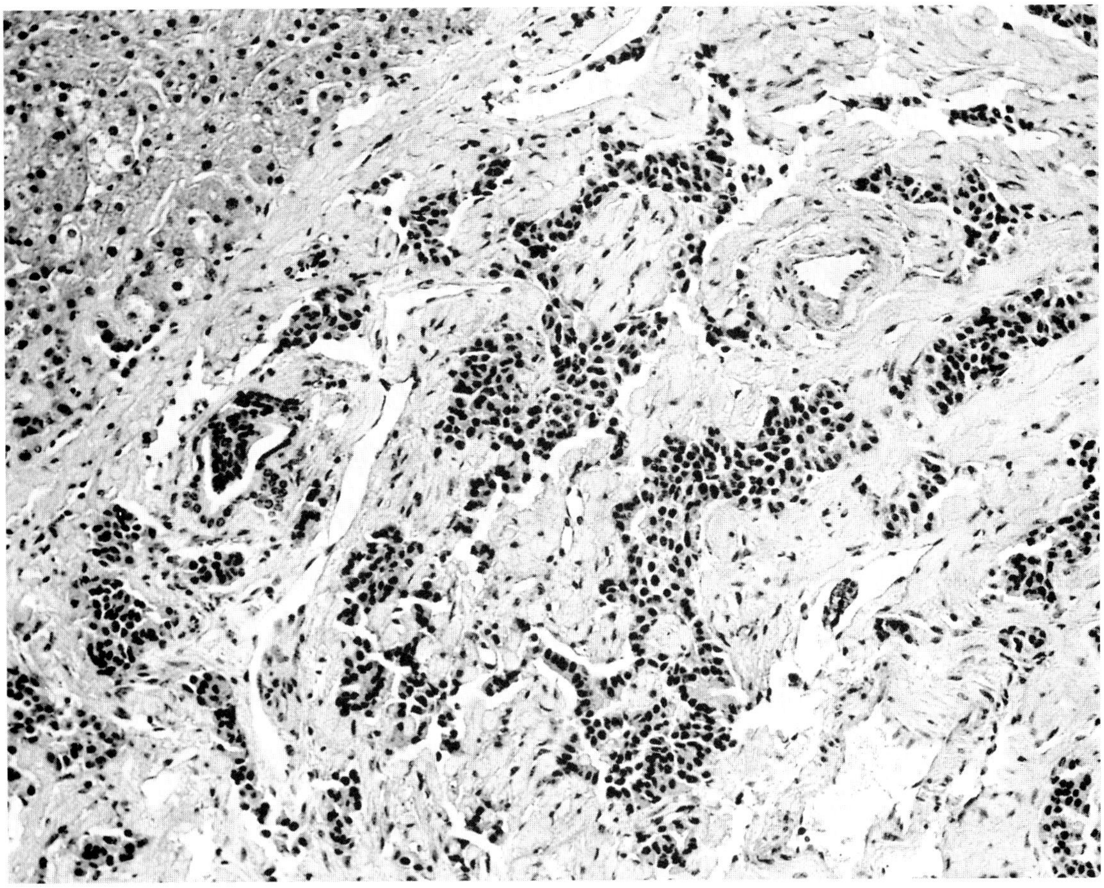

Figure 5-16
WELL-DIFFERENTIATED ENDOCRINE CARCINOMA WITH METASTASES
Malignant glucagonoma with a trabecular, partly gyriform pattern, metastatic to the liver.

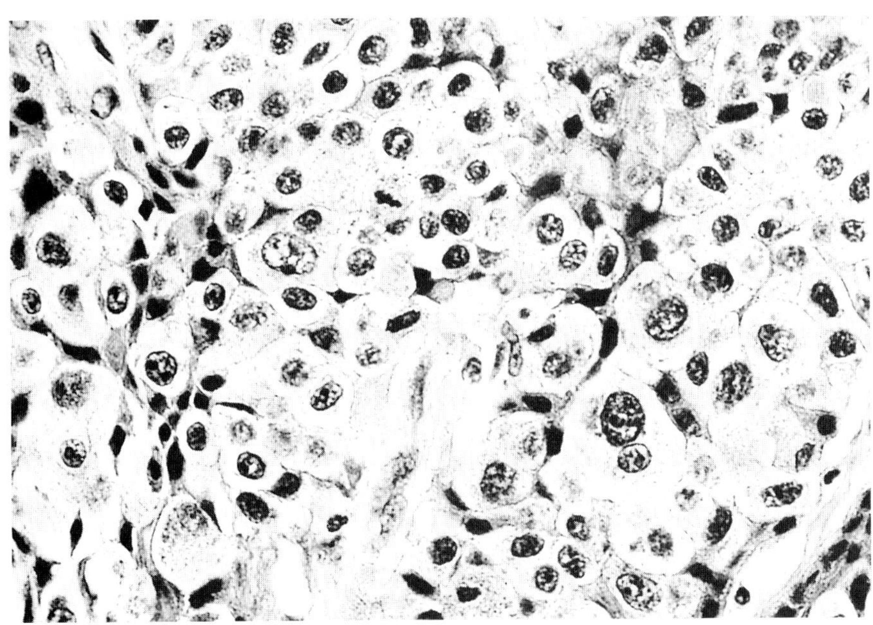

Figure 5-17
WELL-DIFFERENTIATED ENDOCRINE CARCINOMA WITH CELLULAR ATYPIA
Malignant insulinoma metastatic to the liver showing several cells with enlarged, hyperchromatic nuclei and conspicuous nucleoli.

Figure 5-18
ENDOCRINE CARCINOMA WITH LYMPHATIC INVASION
Neoplastic thrombi in a lymphatic vessel of peritumoral pancreatic tissue.

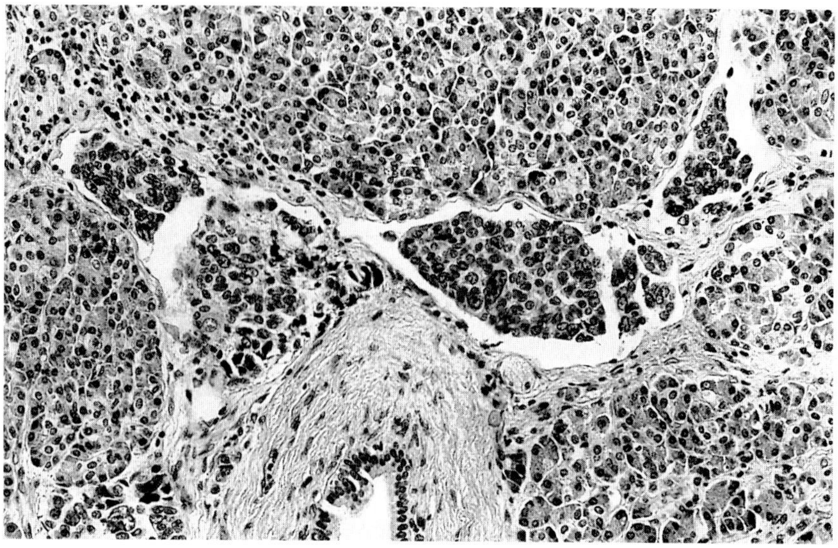

hyperfunction or an expanding mass. Malignant insulinomas, glucagonomas, and VIPomas arise more frequently in the body/tail, while malignant gastrinomas and nonfunctioning tumors are concentrated in the head of the gland. Aggressive surgical treatment of primary tumors, recurrences, and metastases in regional lymph nodes or liver is curative in about 30 percent of cases and prolongs survival up to a mean of 5 years for patients with malignant insulinoma (17). Comparable findings may be obtained with malignant gastrinoma, glucagonoma, VIPoma, and nonfunctioning tumors. In general, overall survival is several years.

A few moderately differentiated endocrine carcinomas have been also observed. They are characterized by relatively high mitotic (10 or more mitoses per 10 high-power fields) and proliferative marker (more than 10 percent Ki-67-positive cells) rates; a high nuclear/cytoplasmic ratio with moderate nuclear atypia (relatively large, pleomorphic, often vesicular nuclei with prominent nucleoli); a histologic pattern prevalently of solid to diffuse sheets; evident angio/neuroinvasion; and obvious malignancy proven by metastasis or gross local invasion. Tumor necrosis and the severe cellular atypia characteristic of poorly differentiated, highly malignant tumors are not present. Many of the pancreatic tumors that cause Cushing's, hypercalcemic, and carcinoid syndromes and most multisyndromic tumors, known to be associated with a shorter survival period than other more common functioning tumors, may also fit in the moderately differentiated carcinoma category. More evidence is needed to clearly define these tumors as a distinct morphologic entity with a poorer prognosis.

**Histochemical and Ultrastructural Findings.** The general histochemical features of pancreatic endocrine tumors are discussed in the sections Diagnosis and Microscopic Findings in this chapter. Specific histochemical features of the various functional subtypes of these tumors are reported in the next section, Clinicopathologic Profiles.

Ultrastructurally, the endocrine cells of pancreatic tumors are essentially characterized by their small secretory granules, mostly ranging from 100 to 400 nm in size. They have a dense core, with (as in insulin granules) or without a crystalline or other kind of regular substructure, enveloped by a thin membrane with or without intervening space. Subtle differences in the substructure of the secretory granules allow identification of tumor cell type and pertinent hormone secretion (see next section). However, in most cases this is more easily achieved by immunohistochemical tests.

**Differential Diagnosis.** Included in the differential diagnosis of pancreatic endocrine tumors are small cell carcinoma, islet aggregation and neogenesis in chronic pancreatitis, solid-pseudopapillary tumor, acinar cell carcinoma, and pancreatoblastoma. In the latter three essentially nonendocrine tumors minor populations of endocrine cells occur frequently, as single scattered cells or minute aggregates. Truly mixed tumors with roughly equal endocrine and exocrine components are rare (see Mixed Ductal-Endocrine and Acinar-Endocrine Tumors). Findings pointing to a poorly differentiated small or intermediate cell endocrine carcinoma, while ruling out a well-differentiated endocrine tumor, are cellular anaplasia with a high nuclear/cytoplasmic ratio; focal or extensive cell necrosis; poor or only focal reactivity with hormone and secretory granule markers; more than 10 mitoses per 10 high-power fields; more than 10 percent of cells expressing Ki-67 or PCNA antigen; prominent local invasion involving pancreatic and parapancreatic tissues, blood or lymphatic vessels, and perineural spaces; and clinical evidence of rapidly progressive disease with terminal widespread, abdominal and extra-abdominal metastases.

At least partial retention of islet individuality and inner structure, including persistence of the four main cell types, and close topographic association with atrophic acinar tissue clearly separate most cases of massive islet crowding and neogenesis in chronic pancreatitis from true, morphologically distinct endocrine tumors. Care must be taken not to misinterpret small endocrine nests and cords entrapped in desmoplastic tissue, sometimes in a perineural position, as evidence of invasion (2).

Endocrine tumors may mimic a solid-pseudopapillary tumor when there is a solid-medullary histologic structure formed by small to medium size monomorphous cells. However, the widespread degenerative changes usually found in solid-pseudopapillary tumors are generally lacking in endocrine tumors. Reactivity for endocrine granule stains (Grimelius silver) or markers (chromogranins, synaptophysin) and for hormone immunohistochemistry supports a diagnosis of endocrine tumor, while an intense, multifocal positivity for alpha-1-antitrypsin favors a solid-pseudopapillary tumor. However, the interpretation of some immunohistochemical tests requires cautiousness since immunoreactivity for alpha-1-antitrypsin has also been reported in endocrine tumors while reactivity for neuron-specific enolase may also occur in solid-pseudopapillary tumors (43). Electron microscopy can distinguish the small, regular secretory granules with distinctive inner structure typical of endocrine cells from the few, large, often irregularly shaped granules of solid-pseudopapillary tumors. Moreover, mitochondria-rich oncocytoid cells are more frequently found in solid-pseudopapillary than in endocrine tumors.

Distinguishing endocrine tumors from acinar cell carcinomas is important because of the generally worse prognosis of the latter. An acinar cell carcinoma showing solid to trabecular histology in the absence of acinar structures may be easily misinterpreted as an endocrine tumor. The presence of an even restricted area of acinar differentiation or larger tumor cells with large nuclei, prominent nucleoli, and abundant cytoplasm with PAS-positive granules favors a diagnosis of acinar cell carcinoma. Positive immunostaining for pancreatic enzymes like trypsin or lipase and lack of staining for general endocrine markers like chromogranins or synaptophysin are the main distinctive immunohistochemical features of acinar cell carcinoma (35); diagnostic ultrastructural criteria are tumor cells with large (500 to 700 mm) zymogen granules, arrangement of cells in poorly formed acinar configurations around minute submicroscopic microlumina, and absence of typical, small endocrine granules.

Endocrine tumors with a solid structure should also be distinguished from pancreatoblastoma, although endocrine tumors are rare during the first decade of life, a period when most pancreatoblastomas occur. The presence of squamoid nests, an acinar structure, or alpha-fetoprotein supports a diagnosis of pancreatoblastoma (43), while widespread reactivity for general endocrine or specific hormonal markers is diagnostic of an endocrine tumor.

**Tumors in Animals.** Islet cell tumors have been induced in rats by irradiation (5), injection of certain plant derived pyrolizidine alkaloids (63), and with application of a streptozotocin-nicotinamide combination (5,71). Streptozotocin-induced tumors resemble spontaneous human endocrine pancreatic tumors. They contain, in addition to insulin-producing cells, other endocrine cell types such as glucagon, somatostatin, and PP cells. An additional analogy with human tumors is the usually reduced hormone content of the neoplastic cells compared to normal islet cells, reflecting reduced storage capacity. However, unlike human pancreatic endocrine tumors, these experimentally induced neoplasms do not express gastrin.

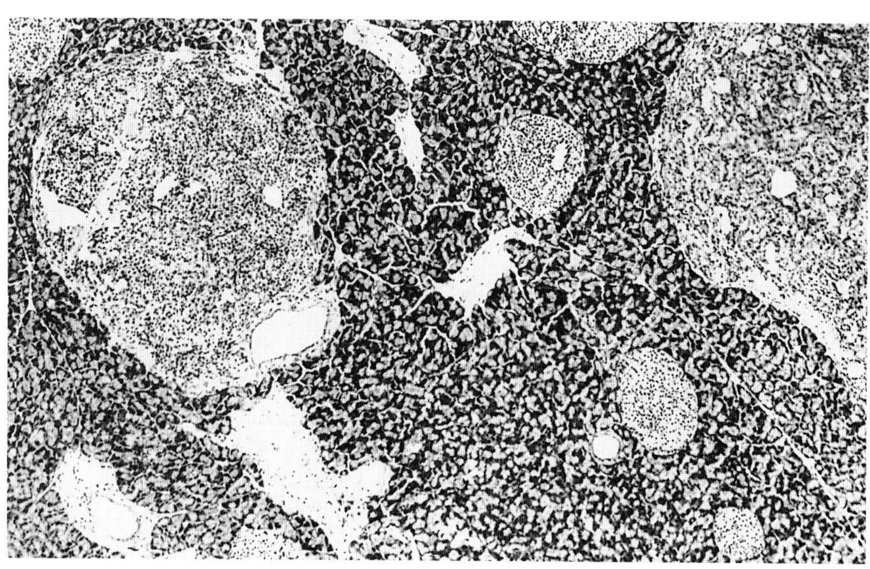

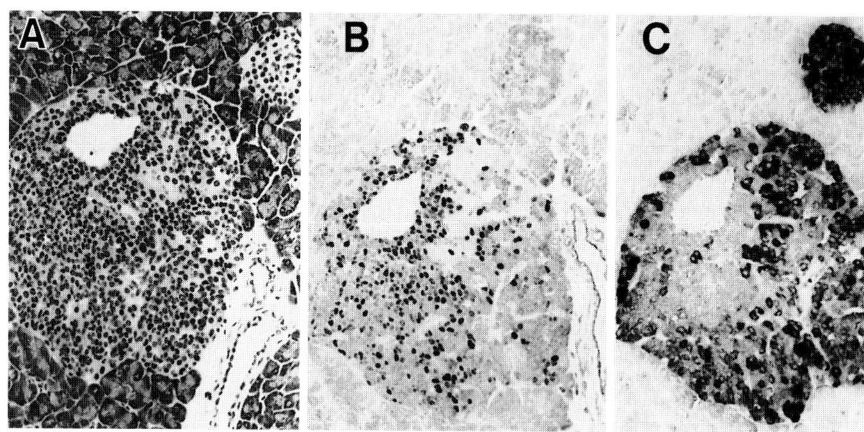


Figure 5-19
ENDOCRINE ADENOMATOSIS IN A TRANSGENIC MOUSE

Top: This 100-day-old mouse has an insulin/SV40 transgene. General view of pancreatic tissue shows endocrine tumors as well as larger dysplastic islets and smaller normal islets. The multiple tumors were identified as insulinomas because of the insulin immunoreactivity of the tumor cells and associated hyperinsulinemic hypoglycemia.

Bottom: A 50-day-old mouse with an insulin/SV40 transgene. A dysplastic islet (A–C) is adjacent to a small normal islet (A–C, top right) and an interlobular duct (A-C, bottom right). The dysplastic islet shows focal cell crowding with hyperchromatic nuclei (A) expressing the nuclear transforming protein large T antigen encoded by the SV40 genome (B: immunoperoxidase). Note the lack of T antigen expression in the normal islet as well as in the duct. Many transformed islet cells have lowered insulin immunoreactivity (C: immunoperoxidase). (Figs. 1A and 7A, B, C from Rindi G, Bishop AE, Murphy D, Solcia E, Hogan B, Polak JM. A morphological analysis of endocrine tumour genesis in pancreas and anterior pituitary of AVP/ SV40 transgenic mice. Virchows Arch [A] 1988;412:255–66.)

Pancreatic endocrine neoplasms have recently been induced in mice rendered transgenic for the hybrid insulin/simian virus (SV)4O or glucagon/ SV4O oncogene (26,57,59). The site of expression of the SV4O genome encoding the potent oncoprotein large T antigen is specifically directed to islet B cells by the insulin gene promoter and to islet A cells by the glucagon gene promoter. The result is selective transformation and growth of islet B or A cells, and all subsequent steps can be followed, from minute foci of intrainsular hyperplastic-dysplastic changes, to multiple B- or A-cell microadenomas (fig. 5-19), to macroadenomas with additional islet cell subpopulations, to metastatic tumors with islet as well as nonislet (inappropriate or "ectopic") tumor cell populations (57,59). Progressive transition from a strictly monotypic growth exclusively composed of transformed A or B cells to tumors with multiple endocrine phenotypes has been observed. These experiments prove the in vivo origin, through an early monotypic growth, of multitypic ("multicellular") endocrine tumors from transformation of intrainsular mature cells, in keeping with previous in vitro experiments showing multidirectional differentiation of monoclonal tumors derived from single cell growths (39). In addition, no evidence of intraductal cell transformation has been obtained (fig. 5-19), thus not supporting the hypothesis that pancreatic endocrine tumors result from transformation and growth of multipotent ductular stem cells.

Table 5-2

**INTRAPANCREATIC LOCALIZATION OF FUNCTIONALLY CHARACTERIZED ENDOCRINE TUMORS**

| Tumor Type (Reference) | Head No.(%) | Body and Tail No.(%) | Total* |
|---|---|---|---|
| Insulinoma (79,85,88) | 525 (35) | 994 (65) | 1519 |
| Gastrinoma (124,142, and personal cases) | 40 (71) | 16 (29) | 56 |
| Glucagonoma (95) | 16 (25) | 49 (75) | 65 |
| VIPoma (152 and literature to 1991) | 15 (23) | 51 (77) | 66 |
| Somatostatinoma (110) | 13 (59) | 9 (41) | 22 |
| Nonfunctioning (207,209,210, 213,217,220) | 53 (65) | 29 (35) | 82 |

* Excluding cases involving both sites or with localization not given.

Table 5-3

**FREQUENCY OF LIVER AND LYMPH NODE METASTASES OF FUNCTIONALLY CHARACTERIZED ENDOCRINE TUMORS**

| Tumor Type (Reference) | No. of Cases | Metastases Lymph Nodes No.(%) | Metastases Liver No.(%) |
|---|---|---|---|
| Insulinoma (177) | 62 | 20 (32) | 49 (79) |
| Gastrinoma (122,125,142) | 137 | 100 (73) | 89 (65) |
| Glucagonoma (95) | 66 | 19 (29) | 52 (79) |
| VIPoma (152 and literature to 1991) | 36 | 11 (31) | 31 (86) |
| Somatostatinoma (110) | 23 | 8 (35) | 16 (69) |
| Nonfunctioning (206,208,210) | 48 | 29 (60) | 36 (75) |

## CLINICOPATHOLOGIC PROFILES OF WELL-DIFFERENTIATED ENDOCRINE TUMORS

As a rule, pancreatic endocrine tumors causing a given hyperfunctional syndrome represent a fairly homogeneous tumor group, with distinctive patterns of intrapancreatic and extrapancreatic distribution (Tables 5-2, 5-3) and a well-defined clinicopathologic profile requiring specific medical and surgical therapies. To establish the nature and predict the behavior of tumor growth, it is necessary to establish a correlation between clinical syndrome and hormonal products of tumor cells whenever possible. Tumors proven to sustain an endocrine syndrome (functioning syndromic tumors) are labeled according to the hormonal syndrome, such as insulinoma, glucagonoma, somatostatinoma, gastrinoma, or VIPoma. Cytologically and hormonally characterized tumors not associated with a hyperfunctional syndrome (nonfunctioning nonsyndromic tumors) are named after their tumor cell type(s): A or glucagon cell tumor, PP cell tumor, D or somatostatin cell tumor, B or insulin cell tumor, G or gastrin cell tumor, etc. The behavior of tumors causing increased blood levels of hormonal products in the absence of a definite clinical syndrome of endocrine hyperfunction (functioning nonsyndromic tumors) is insufficiently known. In general, they seem to resemble more nonfunctioning than syndromic tumors, especially when increased hormonal levels only appear in blood after appropriate stimulation tests.

### Insulinoma

**Definition.** An insulinoma is a predominantly benign endocrine tumor of the pancreas showing evidence of B-cell differentiation and producing severe fasting hyperinsulinemic hypoglycemia. Synonyms and related terms are: *islet cell tumor associated with persistent hyperinsulinemic hypoglycemia, insulin-producing pancreatic endocrine tumor,* and *functioning B-cell tumor.*

**Incidence.** Insulinomas are the most common type of functioning pancreatic endocrine tumor (75,81). At our department (ES, CC), 144 insulinomas, 85 gastrinomas, 43 VIPomas, 29 glucagonomas, and only 3 somatostatinomas were collected during a 30-year period (80,87). Nevertheless, even the insulinomas are relatively rare tumors, and hypoglycemia is often due to other causes. The tumors occur at all ages;

most patients, however, are between 30 and 60 years of age. Children below 15 years are rarely affected. Newborn hypoglycemia is usually due to nesidioblastosis, a proliferative-malformative process diffusely or focally affecting the endocrine pancreas. Insulinomas are slightly more frequent in women (58 percent of all cases) (79,88).

**Clinical Features.** The well-known symptoms associated with hypoglycemia and inappropriate plasma insulin levels occur after periods of fasting. Headache, weakness, dizziness, dysarthria, incoherence, convulsion, and coma are due to the deleterious effect of hypoglycemia on brain function. The simulation of almost any neurologic or psychiatric syndrome is possible and is often responsible for a diagnostic delay. Most features of the insulinoma syndrome can be directly attributed to the uncontrolled release of insulin and proinsulin by the tumor cells (76,84).

Hypoglycemia (less than 40 mg/dL) due to inappropriate levels of circulating insulin is crucial for the clinical diagnosis of insulinoma. Prolonged fasting is the most useful provocative test: over 90 percent of patients with proven insulinoma become hypoglycemic after a 15-hour fast, and many of the remaining patients respond to longer periods of fasting. Fasting concentrations of immunoreactive proinsulin are also elevated in the majority of patients with insulinoma, a finding reflecting the elevated levels of proinsulin in comparison to insulin detected in extracts of human insulinomas (76).

**Gross Findings.** Insulinomas occur in any part of the pancreas, with a fairly uniform distribution (85). Their higher incidence in the body-tail reflects the preponderance of pancreatic tissue there (Table 5-2). Extrapancreatic insulinomas (less than 1 percent of the cases) have been reported in the wall of the duodenum, adjacent to the pancreas, in the hilus of the spleen, in the gastrosplenic ligament, and in the gastric wall, jejunum, ileum, lung, or cervix (81). The tumor is single in the majority of cases, but multiple tumors may coexist (10 percent), a finding which must prompt an investigation for MEN 1.

Insulinomas are usually small: about 50 percent are less than 1.5 cm and they rarely exceed 3 cm, with the exception of malignant cases. The behavior of an insulinoma measuring between 2 and 3 cm is often difficult to predict. There is no relationship between size and severity of clinical symptoms. Clinically significant tumors usually weigh more than 2 g, but single tumors as small as 0.5 g have been detected in patients with the insulinoma syndrome. The tumors are well circumscribed, at least partially encapsulated, and vary from firm to soft and from gray-white to mottled red or deep red. Tumors with a red appearance and soft consistency may be misinterpreted as accessory spleens. Since insulinomas vary considerably in gross appearance and since many symptomatic tumors are small, preoperative localization with imaging procedures and selective arteriography, dynamic computerized tomography, or intraoperative ultrasonography are useful in guiding the surgeon (85).

**Histologic and Histochemical Findings.** The architectural pattern of insulinomas may be trabecular-gyriform, lobular, solid, diffuse, or mixed and does not permit their confident separation from other functional types of pancreatic endocrine neoplasms (fig. 5-20). A peculiar histologic finding more often observed in insulinomas than in the other types is the presence of amyloid in the fibrovascular stroma and in close proximity to the tumor cells (see fig. 5-11). Such deposits, which are congophilic and show green birefringence in polarized light, are usually seen as hyaline areas within the stroma or, less often, as crystalline structures. A major component of amyloid has been extracted and sequenced by Westermark et al. (89). The insulinoma (or islet) amyloid polypeptide (IAPP) was composed of 37 amino acids and shared a 40 percent sequence homology with calcitonin-gene related peptide (CGRP). The finding of amyloid in contact with insulinoma cells suggests secretion of IAPP by tumor cells.

A well-defined capsule is commonly found in larger tumors, while most microadenomas are not encapsulated. The fibrous capsule is often incomplete, a finding not to be interpreted as a sign of invasive growth. Tumor nuclei are generally round or ovoid, with a fairly distinctive, finely stippled chromatin pattern and an inconspicuous nucleolus. Large (polyploid) nuclei are sometimes found in insulinomas; however, their presence, as well as DNA ploidy analysis, is unlikely to provide useful prognostic information for most patients with insulinomas (73,78). In contrast, however, the presence of more than 5 percent AgNOR-rich cells (6 AgNORs per nucleolus) seems to be predictive of malignancy

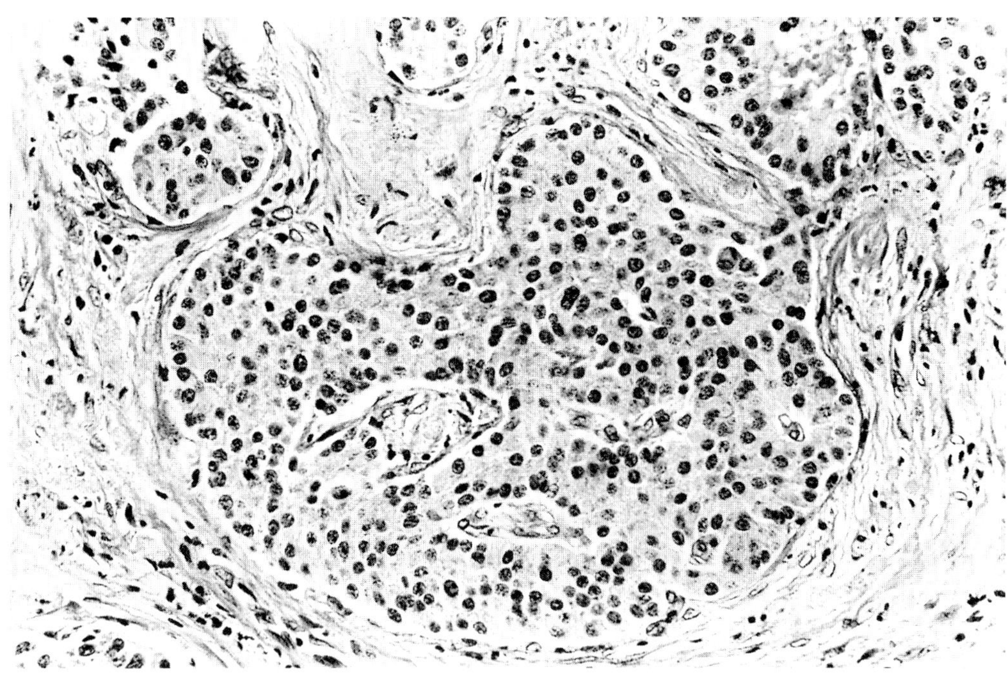

Figure 5-20
BENIGN INSULINOMA
Tumor trabeculae and microlobuli separated by abundant hyalinized stroma.

(86). Insulinomas with no signs of invasion; moderate cellular atypia (nucleolar enlargement, increased nuclear/cytoplasmic ratio, nuclear crowding); mitoses between 2 and 5 per 10 high-power fields; and Ki-67- or PCNA-positive cells between 2 and 5 percent should be considered of uncertain biologic behavior, especially when they are larger than 2 cm. Tumors above 3 cm in size with 5 or more mitoses per 10 high-power fields and more than 5 percent Ki-67- or PCNA-positive cells are more likely to be malignant and should be carefully investigated for angio/neuro-invasion, gross local invasion, or metastases.

Some selective B-cell stains, such as aldehyde fuchsin and aldehyde thioneine, may give positive results in up to 15 percent of insulinomas. Such staining reactions are frequently weaker than in normal B cells, possibly due to the lower insulin content of the tumor cells. The Grimelius silver reaction demonstrates a variable number of positive cells in about 40 percent of insulinomas, although normal B cells are unreactive to this technique.

With immunoperoxidase stains, insulin and proinsulin can be found in almost all tumors (81), including those in which selective stains for beta-granules are negative (fig. 5-21). The number, staining intensity, and distribution of immunoreactive cells varies remarkably, not only from tumor to tumor, but also from block to block in the same tumor. About half of the insulinomas are multihormonal, and cells positive for glucagon, somatostatin, PP, gastrin, ACTH, and calcitonin have been described (82,83). In most cases, hormones other than insulin are localized in cells that do not contain insulin.

**Ultrastructural Findings.** By electron microscopy, well-granulated cells with typical crystalline-type beta-granules; cells with solid, round to slightly pleomorphic granules; and poorly granulated cells have been described (fig. 5-22). In addition, cells with typical A and PP granules may be identified. Based on the presence and amount of typical and atypical B cells, two working classifications for insulinomas have been proposed (74,76). According to Creutzfeldt's classification, type 1 (typical beta-granules only) and type 2 (with typical as well as nontypical granules) insulinomas are immunocytochemically well granulated and have the highest insulin content, but only a moderate elevation of the

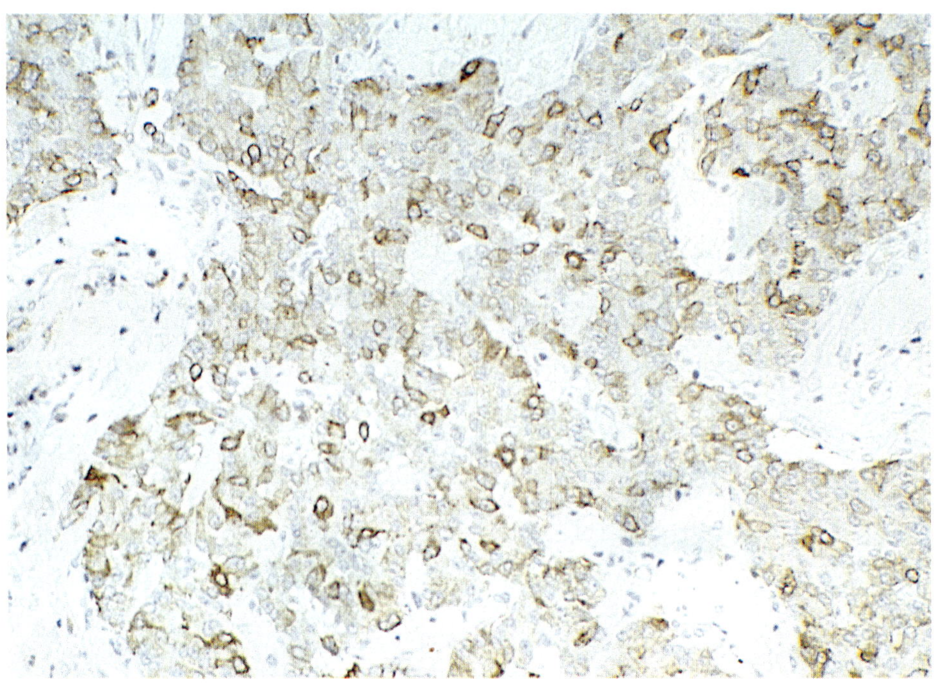

Figure 5-21
INSULINOMA
Most tumor cells are stained for insulin with the immunoperoxidase technique.

proinsulin/insulin ratio. These insulinoma types correspond to group A tumors of Berger's classification, which are further characterized histologically by the trabecular arrangement of their tumor cells and functionally by their good response to diazoxide and somatostatin treatment. In contrast, Creutzfeldt's type 3 (with nontypical granules only) and type 4 (with virtually agranular cells) insulinomas, which correspond to Berger's group B tumors, show the lowest insulin concentrations, the highest proinsulin/ insulin ratio, a solid-medullary pattern, patchy immunoreactivity for insulin, and usually no response to diazoxide or somatostatin treatment.

**Prognosis, Natural History, and Treatment.** Unlike other types of clinically relevant pancreatic endocrine tumors, about 90 to 95 percent of insulinomas are benign at the time of diagnosis (79,88). Since there are no histologic criteria or histochemical markers that permit conclusive separation of benign and malignant tumors, an unquestionable diagnosis of malignant insulinoma can be made only in the presence of metastasis or gross local invasion. At the time of first diagnosis, patients with malignant insulinomas usually have a single tumor which is larger in diameter (mean diameter of 6.2 cm according to Danforth et al. [77], versus 1.5 for benign tumors) than those found in patients with adenomas, although there is no difference in age and sex, or tumors' topographic distribution. Metastases from these tumors are most commonly found in the liver (79 percent of cases) or regional lymph nodes (parapancreatic, hepatic or celiac, periaortic, paracaval: 32 percent cases); dissemination to other distant sites is unusual (Table 5-3) (77).

The treatment of choice for insulin-producing tumors is surgical excision, which is curative for most of the patients without metastases (85). For patients in whom curative resection is not possible because of distant metastases or poor general health conditions, options available are: antihormonal therapy (diazoxide, somatostatin and its derivatives), cytotoxic therapy (streptozotocin in combination with 5-fluorouracil), hepatic arterial embolization, and radiotherapy (84). Malignant insulinomas often grow slowly: the median survival period of patients with metastasis undergoing palliative resection is 4 years (77).

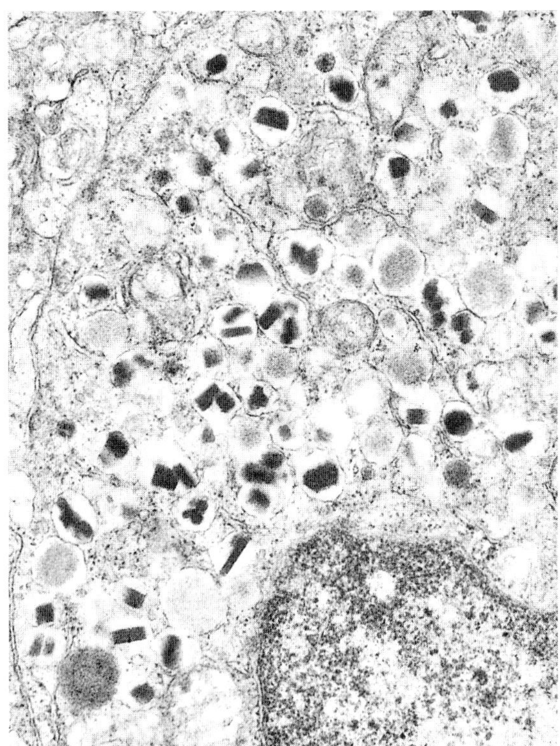

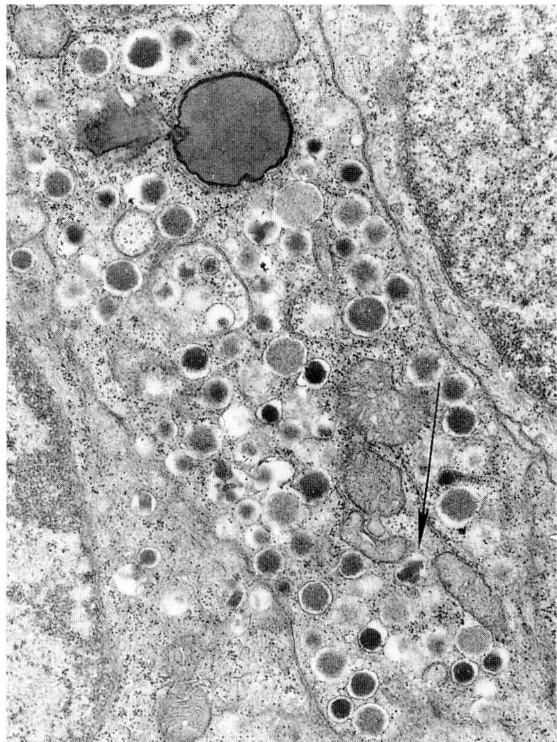

Figure 5-22
ULTRASTRUCTURAL APPEARANCE OF INSULINOMAS

Left: This tumor contains a sufficient number of crystalline granules for diagnostic identification (X28,000).

Right: Insulinoma with a prevalence of round haloed granules of low density. Note, in addition, occasional crystalloid granules (arrow) (X28,000).

## Glucagonoma

**Definition.** This is a predominantly malignant pancreatic endocrine tumor with A-cell differentiation and glucagon production, which causes a clinical syndrome of skin rash, stomatitis, diabetes, weight loss, and anemia. The tumor is also called *pancreatic A-cell tumor associated with the glucagonoma syndrome.* Nonfunctioning endocrine tumors with A-cell differentiation are dealt with in the chapter on nonfunctioning tumors.

**Incidence.** Guillausseau et al. in 1982 (95) reviewed 92 cases of glucagonoma reported in the literature (by now the number is considerably higher [about 200 cases]). Glucagonomas represent about 5 percent of all clinically relevant pancreatic endocrine tumors and 8 percent of functioning tumors. They occur most often in patients between 40 and 70 years of age (mean, 55 years), and are slightly more common in women (55 percent of the cases). Glucagonomas are occasionally part of the MEN 1 syndrome (94). One family has been reported in which five persons had hyperglucagonemia (90).

**Clinical Features.** The glucagonoma syndrome includes a skin rash (necrolytic migratory erythema), stomatitis, angular cheilitis, glossitis, mild diabetes mellitus, normochromic normocytic anemia, weight loss, depression, and a tendency to develop deep vein thrombosis (98). Not all of these features are found in every patient.

The dermatitis is certainly the most striking sign of the glucagonoma syndrome and is often the key to the diagnosis. The main features of the rash are macules or barely palpable light brown papules giving an eczematous psoriasiform appearance, which develop into bullae with superficial epidermal spongiosis and intraepidermal clefts. The blisters progress to central crusting and healing, followed by hyperpigmentation 7 to 14 days after the beginning of the rash. The skin lesions occur symmetrically on the buttocks, groin, perineum, thighs, and distal extremities. Bacterial or fungal overgrowth is a common complication (fig. 5-23). The rash is intermittent and moves from one area to the next, while healing at the initial site. On initial evaluation, the eruption is often mistaken for an eczematous dermatitis or for a bullous dermatitis such as pemphigus foliaceous or pemphigoid. The pathogenesis of the skin lesions is unknown, although low blood levels of amino acids may play some role in it. The diabetes is usually mild, and diabetic complications such as ketoacidosis have been only rarely reported. Anemia and weight loss may be attributed to the catabolic action of glucagon.

The diagnosis of glucagonoma is readily confirmed by finding elevated plasma glucagon concentrations in association with hyperglycemia. Gel filtration analysis of plasma from patients with glucagonoma frequently reveals unusual molecular forms of the hormone. Greater immunoreactivity is often localized in the high molecular weight position, due to a defect in prohormone processing (99). Hypoaminoacidemia is a frequent and perhaps universal feature in patients with the glucagonoma syndrome. This is probably due to the increased hepatic gluconeogenesis and ureogenesis induced by high glucagon levels.

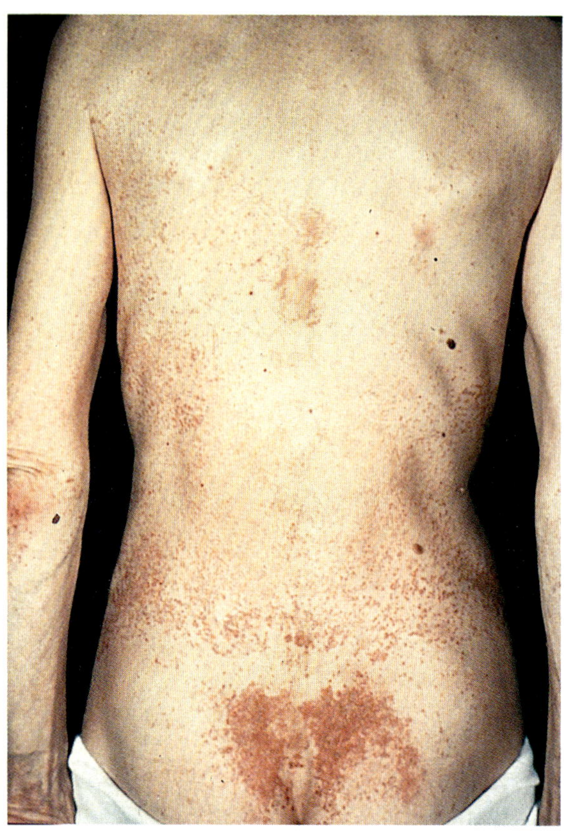

Figure 5-23
SKIN LESION IN GLUCAGONOMA
Necrolytic migratory erythema in a patient with pancreatic glucagonoma. The lesion disappeared after tumor resection.

**Gross Findings.** Most glucagonomas are localized to the distal portion of the pancreas (Table 5-2). Of 79 cases in which tumor site was indicated, 30 (38 percent) were confined to the tail, 19 (24 percent) were in the body or body-tail region, 3 (4 percent) in the head and body-tail, and 16 (20 percent) were confined to the head. In 11 cases (14 percent), diffuse involvement of the pancreas by a single mass was described (95). At least two extrapancreatic glucagon-producing tumors associated with the typical glucagonoma syndrome have been described: one was in the proximal duodenum (100) and the other in the upper lobe of the left lung (97).

Glucagonomas are generally single pancreatic tumors of considerable size: the mean length of the major axis equaled 7.6 cm (range, 0.2 to 35 cm) in 29 discretely localized neoplasms (101). Among these cases, malignant glucagonomas showed a mean diameter of 9.3 cm, while nonmetastatic and nonlocally invasive forms displayed a mean diameter of 6.1 cm. More than half are invasive, either locally or through metastatic spread; the most common metastatic site is the liver (79 percent of metastatic cases), followed by regional lymph nodes (29 percent).

**Histologic and Histochemical Findings.** Glucagonomas display architectural features which do not differ substantially from those of other endocrine pancreatic tumors. They usually show an irregular association of trabecular (see fig. 5-16) and diffuse patterns of growth, with the latter often predominant. Tumor cells are polygonal and have faintly granular, often abundant cytoplasm (fig. 5-24). The malignant potential of glucagonomas is difficult to establish by examining the primary tumor. Focal invasion of vascular and neural structures by tumor cells is not uncommon, mitoses are noted infrequently, and prominent nuclear atypia is rare. The presence of metastases or gross local invasion is the most reliable criterion of malignancy.

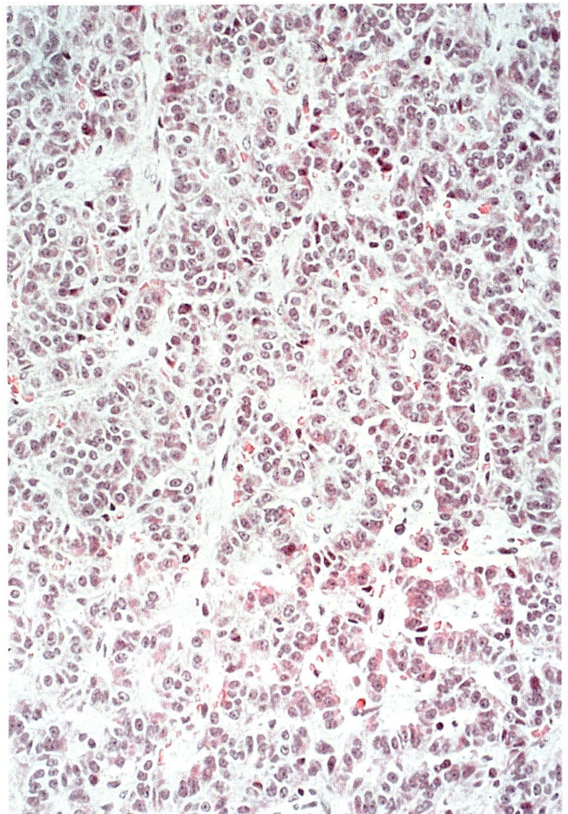

Figure 5-24
GLUCAGONOMA
This tumor shows a characteristic partly monolayered gyriform pattern. Malignancy cannot be determined from the morphologic appearance of the tumor.

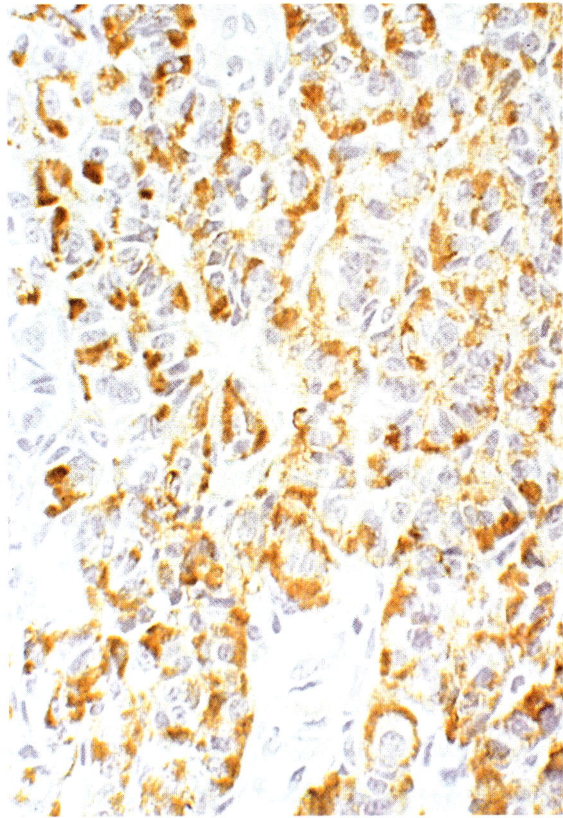

Figure 5-25
GLUCAGONOMA
Most tumor cells are stained for glucagon with the immunoperoxidase technique.

In contrast to insulinomas, amyloid deposits are rarely reported in glucagonomas. The tumor cells are nonargentaffin and show argyrophilia with the Bodian and Grimelius techniques.

Immunohistochemical localization of glucagon within the tumor cells is the only reliable morphologic means to establish the diagnosis in these tumors (fig. 5-25). In addition to glucagon, these tumors show immunoreactivity for one or more peptides derived from proglucagon, including glicentin and the glucagon-like peptides (GLP)-1 and -2 (96,99). Comparison of serial sections immunostained for glucagon, glicentin, GLP-1, and GLP-2 showed co-localization of two or more of the peptides in a proportion of tumor cells; separate localization of the peptides was observed only infrequently (96). The intensity of immunoreactivity and the number of reactive tumor cells are variable, depending on the granularity of the tumor and on the molecular forms produced by a given tumor. In general, GLP-2 appears to be the more reliable marker for active glucagonoma, while glucagon is restricted to a smaller percentage of cells, with the reaction product mainly localized at the capillary pole of the cells (101). Apart from proglucagon-related peptides, glucagonomas may also contain PP cells and, in declining order, somatostatin and insulin cells. In addition, a case of mixed glucagon- and VIP-producing tumor associated with a combined glucagonoma and VIPoma syndrome has been reported (92).

**Ultrastructural Findings.** Conventional electron microscopy reveals relatively few well-granulated cells. At least three types of secretory granules have been identified in glucagonomas (91,93): 1) typical A-cell granules, 180 to 300 nm in diameter, with a characteristic dense inner

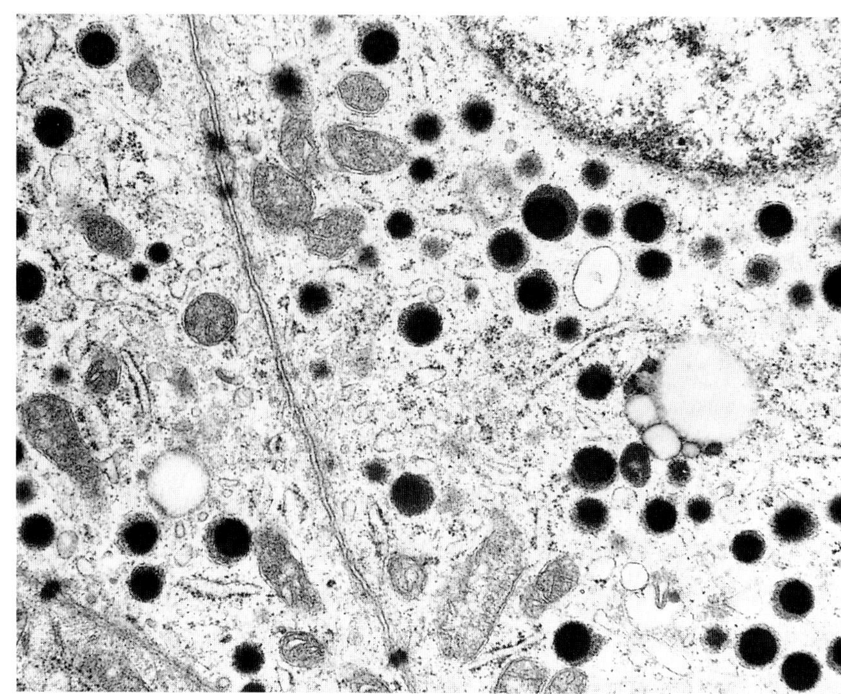

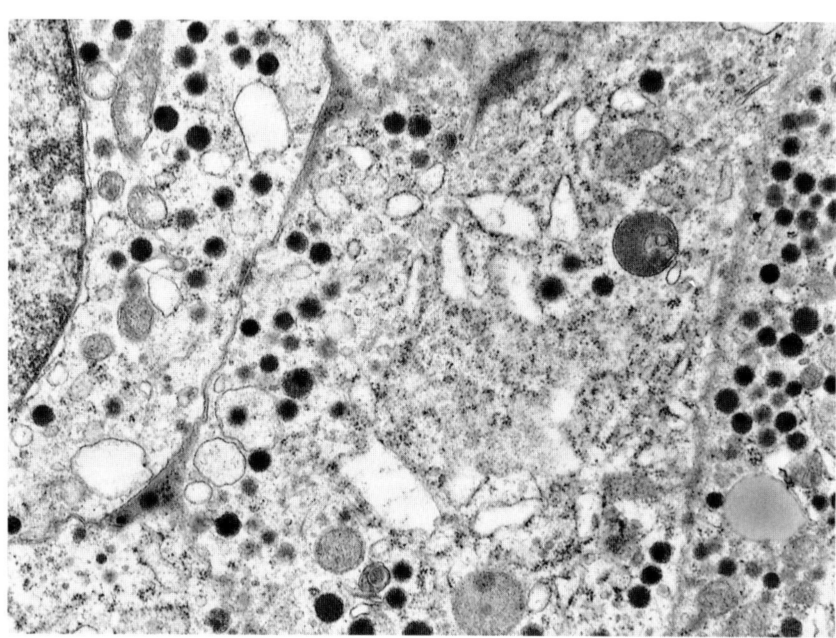

Figure 5-26
ULTRASTRUCTURAL APPEARANCE OF GLUCAGONOMA

Top: Glucagonoma showing diagnostic secretory granules with a central dense core encircled by a less dense matrix (X28,000).

Bottom: Glucagonoma with nondiagnostic, round, homogeneous dense granules (X28,000).

core surrounded by a mantle of lower density (fig. 5-26, top); 2) "atypical" or "unspecific" small to medium-sized (130 to 250 nm) round granules with a uniform core of various density (fig. 5-26, bottom), sometimes separated from the limiting membrane by a narrow space; and 3) medium-sized (180 to 260 nm) granules resembling alpha-granules in the fetal human islets, characterized by an inner core of lower density and a surrounding denser mantle. Type 2 and 3 granules are prevalent in the majority of glucagonomas, while typical, diagnostic, mature alpha-granules, which are prominent in nonfunctioning A-cell adenomas, are seldom observed in glucagonomas.

**Prognosis, Natural History, and Treatment.** Approximately 80 percent of glucagonomas causing the syndrome are malignant; 70 percent are metastatic at the time of diagnosis, with preference for hematogenous spread to the liver (95,101). As in the case of malignant insulinomas, glucagon-producing carcinomas tend to grow slowly, and patients have survived for up to a decade with malignant disease.

Development of a second, or even a third, hyperfunctional syndrome has been observed by Wynick et al. (102) in 11 of 42 patients with glucagonomas (26 percent) followed for a mean of 19 months. In 8 of the 11 cases a gastrinoma syndrome was found. During the same period, only 3 out of 86 (3.5 percent) insulinoma patients developed a second or third syndrome.

Surgical removal of a glucagonoma and as much metastatic tissue as possible results in dramatic clinical improvement, including regression of the rash. In nonresectable tumors a favorable response to streptozotocin (sometimes combined with fluorouracil) has been reported (99). Long-acting somatostatin analogues are also used to reduce glucagon secretion.

### Somatostatinoma

**Definition.** This pancreatic endocrine tumor is composed of somatostatin D cells and is associated with a complex of symptoms (somatostatinoma syndrome) likely caused by the hypersomatostatinemia induced by the tumor.

**Incidence.** As yet only a small number of somatostatinomas have been described. They represent less than 1 percent of active endocrine tumors of the pancreas. All tumors so far reported have been in adults between 30 and 84 years of age (mean, 53.9 years) (110); the majority occur between the fourth and sixth decade, with a slight prevalence in females (108,110). No case of pancreatic somatostatinoma associated with MEN 1 cyndrome has been reported so far. A combined pancreatic and duodenal somatostadinoma and a duodenal case have been observed in patients with celiac disease (106,112).

**Clinical Features.** Clinical findings associated with pancreatic somatostatinoma include diabetes mellitus, cholelithiasis, diarrhea with or without steatorrhea, hypochlorhydria, weight loss, and anemia. These features can be ascribed to the inhibitory actions of somatostatin on endocrine cells that produce insulin, secretin, cholecystokinin, and gastrin, as well as on gastric parietal cells, pancreatic acinar cells, intestinal absorbing cells, and gallbladder muscle cells.

The diagnosis, suspected on clinical grounds, has to be proven by radioimmunoassay of plasma to detect hypersomatostatinemia (10 to 100 times the normal level). As in the case of insulinomas, glucagonomas, and other polypeptide-secreting pancreatic tumors, the recognition, by gel-filtration chromatography, of forms of somatostatin immunoreactivity with high molecular weight may aid in the diagnosis of hypersomatostatinemia of neoplastic origin. Additional diagnostic features in patients with somatostatinoma are depressed serum concentrations of both immunoreactive insulin and glucagon.

**Gross Findings.** Pancreatic somatostatinomas are more commonly located in the region of the head (56.5 percent), although they may arise anywhere within the pancreas: 8.7 percent in the body, 30.4 percent in the tail, and 4.4 percent in the entire pancreas (110). They are usually large, the mean length of the major axis being 6.7 cm (range, 3.5 to 11 cm) in our 8 neoplasms. The tumors are single, well circumscribed but not encapsulated, and generally soft in consistency.

**Histologic and Histochemical Findings.** These tumors show the usual histologic features common to all pancreatic endocrine tumors, with cells forming solid sheets (fig. 5-27), anastomosing trabeculae, and acinar structures. Signs of histologic malignancy, including cellular polymorphism, increased mitotic activity, and extensive necrosis, are generally lacking.

Staining with somatostatin antibodies is positive in significant populations of tumor cells (fig. 5-28). In agreement with the multihormonality of other types of pancreatic endocrine tumors, some somatostatinomas contain calcitonin, adrenocorticotropin, and gastrin. Calcitonin and somatostatin immunoreactive material coexist in the secretory granules of a few tumor cells (111).

**Ultrastructural Findings.** Ultrastructural examination of tumor cells shows large numbers of secretory granules of two populations: 1) large (250 to 450 nm) granules with homogeneous, variably electron-dense cores closely bound by limiting membranes, resembling the mature granules of normal D cells (fig. 5-29) and 2)

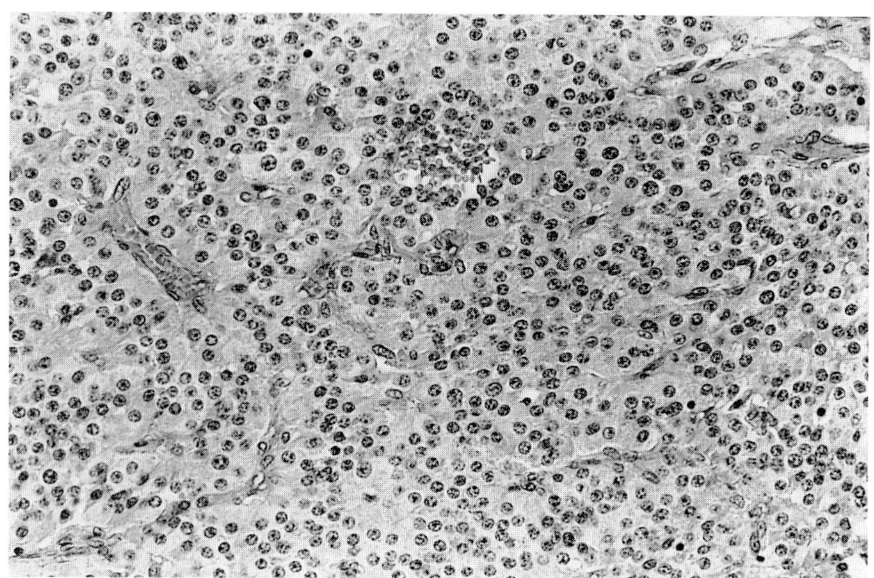

Figure 5-27
PANCREATIC
SOMATOSTATINOMA

This locally invasive tumor shows a medullary pattern and no significant cellular atypia. (Figures 5-27 and 5-28 are from the same case.)

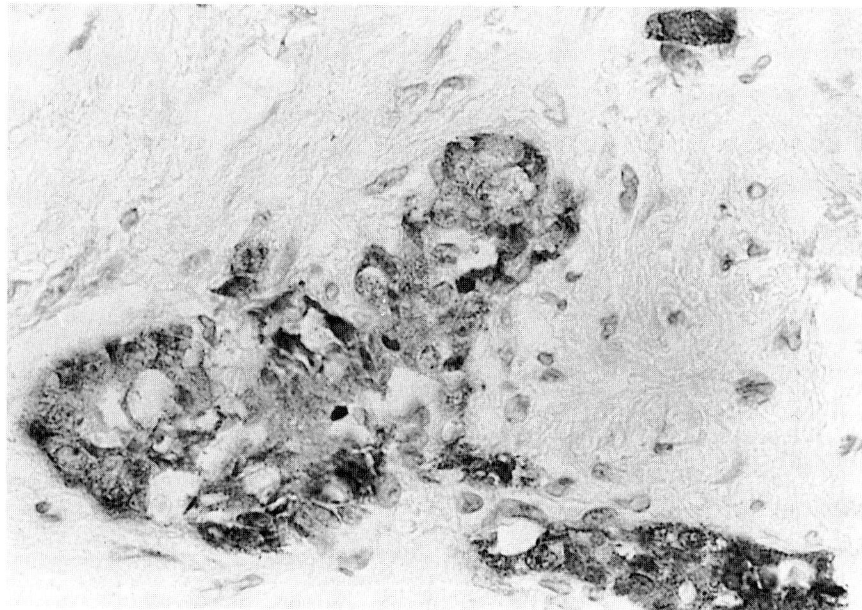

Figure 5-28
PANCREATIC
SOMATOSTATINOMA

Immunostaining for somatostatin in an invasive tumor cell cluster.

smaller (150 to 300) granules with dense cores surrounded by a thin peripheral halo. The heterogeneity in granule morphology has been related either to differences in the maturity of the granules or to costorage of secretory products different from somatostatin, as for example calcitonin (108,111).

**Prognosis, Natural History, and Treatment.** Seventy-four percent of 23 pancreatic somatostatinomas reviewed by Konomi et al. (110) were malignant tumors that were locally invasive or had metastasized to the liver (69.5 percent of cases) and regional lymph nodes (34.8 percent) by the time they were diagnosed. Extensive distant metastases to bones, skin, ovaries, adrenals, and thyroid have also been described in some cases (103,114). Patients with large lesions of the head of the pancreas may require pancreatoduodenectomy. Other patients have been treated with distal pancreatectomy or tumor excision. Chemotherapy with streptozotocin and 5-fluorouracil is used in cases of widespread or residual disease.

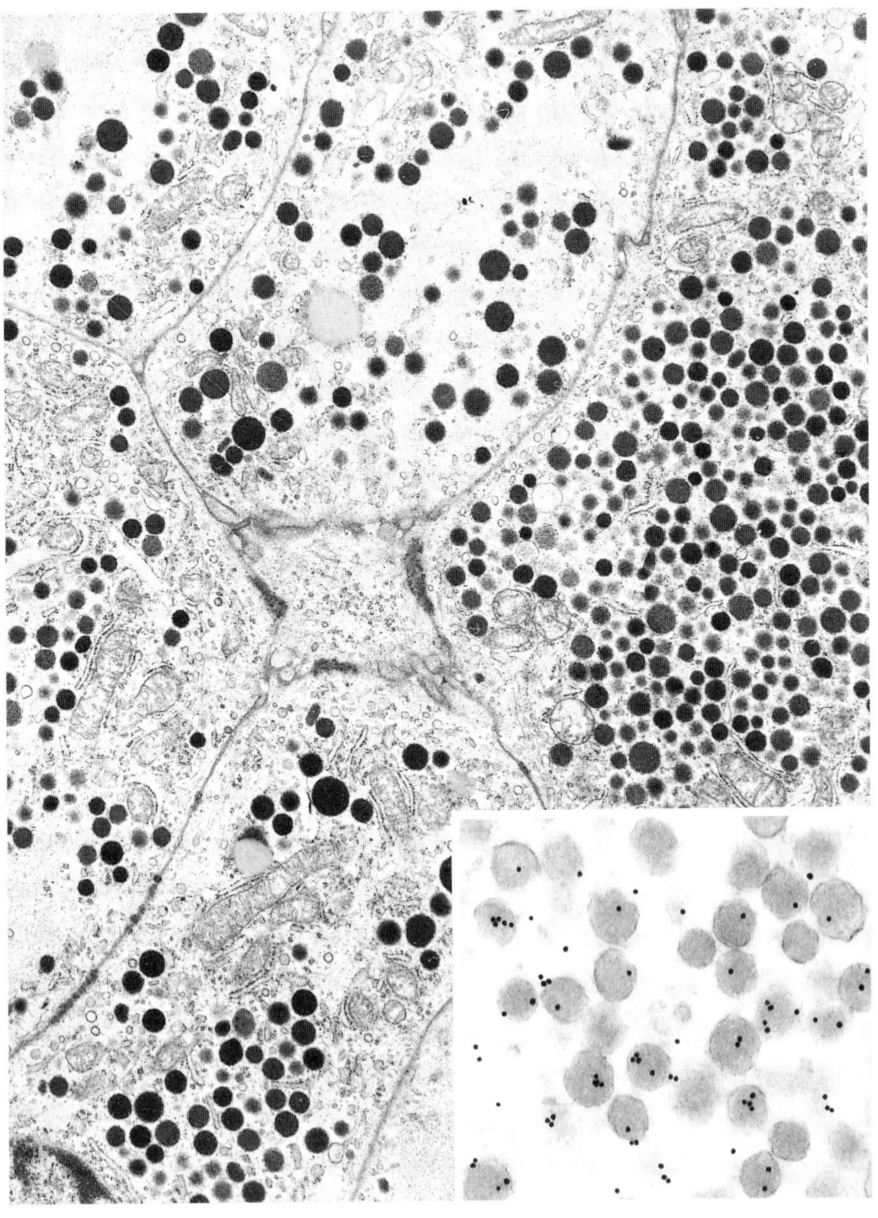

Figure 5-29
ULTRASTRUCTURAL APPEARANCE OF SOMATOSTATINOMA

D-cell granules in cells of somatostatinoma (X28,000). Inset: The immunogold reactivity with somatostatin antibodies is seen (X45,000).

The prognosis of patients with pancreatic somatostatinomas depends on the site, extension, and resectability of the tumor. Of 13 patients with sufficient follow-up information, only 3 were considered cured, with persistent complete remission 2.5 and 14 years after surgery (108). Most of the remaining patients died within 2 years of the diagnosis or were under treatment with chemotherapy.

**Somatostatin Cell Tumors of the Duodenum.** According to recently reported series (104, 106,108), somatostatin cell tumors of the upper small intestine appear to be more frequent than pancreatic somatostatinomas. Most of them occur between the fourth and sixth decades of life, with a slight prevalence in males. They show a relatively strong association with von Recklinghausen disease (neurofibromatosis type 1) (105, 107,109). This association seems to be rare in pancreatic somatostatinomas, since only one case has thus far been reported (108). With rare exceptions, duodenal somatostatin cell tumors do not express the full-blown features of the somatostatinoma syndrome. Patients present with symptoms and signs that depend on the anatomic location of the tumor: epigastric pain, nausea, vomiting, weight loss, gastrointestinal bleeding, or obstructive jaundice and pancreatitis.

Most tumors arise in the ampullary or periampullary area (106,113,115). Grossly, they may present ac intramucosal or submucosal elevated lesions, or may grow intraluminally as a fungating mass. They usually range from 1 to 4 cm in size and often invade the duodenal wall deeply.

Most duodenal somatostatin cell tumors show a mixed histologic pattern, with characteristic prevalence of the acinar (glandular) component. The acinar areas are composed of tubular glands often containing eosinophilic homogeneous secretions. These areas have to be differentiated from, and not misdiagnosed as, low-grade adenocarcinoma. Psammoma bodies are frequently found, either within the glandular lumina or in connective tissue septa. Immunohistochemical tests and electron microscopy show a uniform population of well-differentiated somatostatin D cells with very few, if any, cells of other enteropancreatic endocrine types. Despite the fact that duodenal somatostatin cell tumors are frequently malignant, with metastases to regional lymph nodes in more than 50 percent of cases at the time of first diagnosis, patients have a better prognosis than with the pancreatic tumors that cause the somatostatinoma syndrome.

## Gastrinoma

**Definition.** Gastrinoma is a predominantly malignant endocrine tumor of the pancreas or extrapancreatic sites (duodenum, upper jejunum, stomach) which causes unregulated hypergastrinemia and the Zollinger-Ellison syndrome (ZES).

This chapter primarily deals with pancreatic tumors. However, epidemiologic and clinical data cover both pancreatic and extrapancreatic tumors; in addition, the morphology of extrapancreatic tumors is also concisely described.

**Incidence.** Buchanan et al. (118) calculated an incidence of approximately 0.5 gastrinomas per year per 1 million population, based on their series of pancreatic and extrapancreatic tumors associated with ZES analyzed during a 10-year period in Northern Ireland. Incidences of 1.5 patients and 2 to 4 patients per million population per year were calculated in Denmark (130) and in Switzerland (143), respectively. This incidence may be underestimated since efficient treatment of peptic ulcers with H2-receptor blockers and proton-pump inhibitors may obscure the diagnosis of some gastrinomas that cause milder peptic ulcer disease. Gastrinomas account for about 20 percent of all pancreatic endocrine tumors and 30 percent of functioning tumors, and are second in frequency only to insulinomas. The male to female ratio is 3 to 2; the age range is from 7 to 83 years (mean, 38 years). Evidence of MEN 1 was found in 21 percent of 522 patients with ZES syndrome from six clinical institutions with special interest in the field (131).

**Clinical Features.** Massive gastric acid hypersecretion and peptic ulceration are the predominant features. The ulcers may be multiple, unusual in site, and rapidly recurrent. Often heartburn due to gastroesophageal reflux and severe esophagitis is noted. Diarrhea occurs frequently and may even precede the manifestation of ulcers; diarrhea depends on acid overload to the intestine, since aspiration of the gastric secretion or total gastrectomy stops it in most patients. The acid load may act through pH-dependent inactivation of pancreatic digestive enzymes or by directly irritating the intestinal mucosa. Sometimes the disease is discovered by sudden hematemesis or perforation of an unsuspected ulcer.

**Laboratory Tests.** Gastric secretion studies in gastrinoma patients generally show a basal acid output above 5 mmol per hour, a basal to maximal acid output ratio greater than 0.6, and an overnight 12-hour acid secretion level of more than 10 mmol. A gastric hypersecretory state associated with basal serum gastrin levels above 200 pmol/L is highly indicative of ZES. Conditions such as pernicious anemia and renal failure may also elevate plasma gastrin levels; however, these conditions are usually associated with low gastric acidity. Since about half the patients with gastrinoma have nondiagnostic fasting serum gastrin values, provocative tests, like the secretin injection test, have been developed to give additional information in suspected cases (131,147).

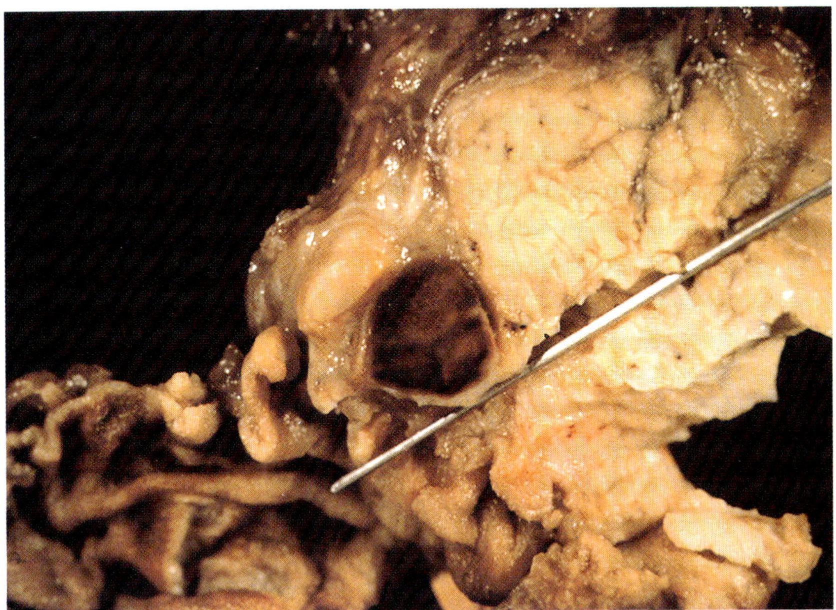

Figure 5-30
GASTRINOMA
IN A LYMPH NODE

Biggest (2.5 cm) of five pancreato-duodenal lymph nodes with endocrine tumor tissue (immunoreactive for gastrin at histologic level) found in a Whipple resection specimen from a 57-year-old man with ZES. No tumor was found in the pancreas or in the duodenum, despite careful search. The patient had undergone Billroth II gastric resection 12 years before.

**Gross Findings.** The pancreas is the organ most frequently involved by gastrinoma. Of 800 patients with ZES in the Zollinger-Ellison Tumor Registry up to 1973, 53 percent had tumors localized to the pancreas and 13 percent to the duodenum or upper jejunum (126). In 7 percent of the cases only metastatic tissue was found whereas in as much as 27 percent no tumor was detected. Among 262 cases collected from five studies from 1974 to 1983, 40 percent showed tumor in the pancreas, 15 percent in the duodenum, and 11 percent in metastatic or other sites. In 34 percent of patients, no gastrin-producing tumor was detected despite careful preoperative and intraoperative search (131). Occult duodenal microgastrinomas, which may be as small as 1 to 2 mm and very difficult to detect, may account for a substantial proportion of these undetected gastrinomas as well as for apparently "primary" lymph node tumors (123,138,140). Sites of extraenteropancreatic gastrinomas in which surgical removal cured the ZES, with normalization of serum gastrin levels, include paraduodenal, peripancreatic, paracholedochal, perigastric, and mesenteric lymph nodes (fig. 5-30) (116). Many of these patients had had a previous gastrectomy involving the proximal duodenal bulb, a frequent site of minute, occult gastrinomas that may have been overlooked (119); the subsequent lymph node metastasis was then erroneously interpreted as "primary" gastrinoma (145). In fact, recent clinical and pathologic investigations (119,138,145,146) suggest that the relative proportion of duodenal versus pancreatic gastrinomas is higher than previously reported. Ten of 26 (38 percent) sporadic gastrinomas proved to be of duodenal origin and 16 of pancreatic origin, while of 18 MEN 1 gastrinomas, 9 (50 percent) were detected in the duodenum, 1 (6 percent) in the pancreas, 2 (11 percent) in metastatic sites only, and 6 (33 percent) remained unlocalized (124).

*Pancreatic Tumors.* Pancreatic gastrinomas are well-circumscribed but nonencapsulated tumors that push the surrounding parenchyma. Their consistency varies from soft to firm depending on the amount of fibrous stroma. As many as 50 percent of ZES-associated tumors from the old Zollinger-Ellison Tumor Registry were multiple (125). However, 30 percent of the tumors were in patients with MEN 1, in which case growth is usually multiple and, in the pancreas, mostly nongastrin producing. Present evidence suggests that most ZES-associated pancreatic sporadic tumors proven to produce gastrin are single and larger than 2 cm (146).

Inside the pancreas, gastrinomas have been reported to be uniformly distributed (125) or concentrated mostly in the head (142): half of the sporadic tumors from various pathology series

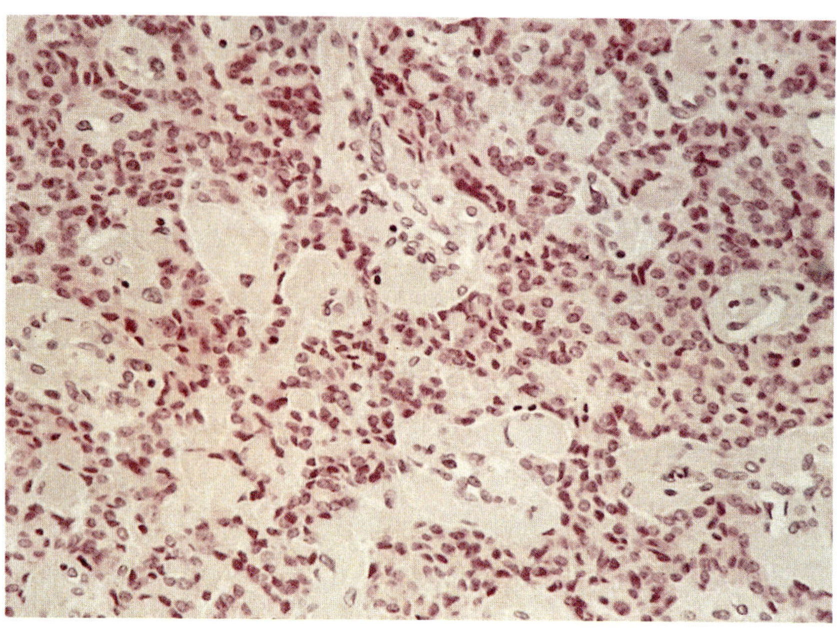

Figure 5-31
PANCREATIC GASTRINOMA
Pancreatic malignant gastrinoma showing a trabecular pattern. Note the presence of hyaline and fibrous tissue between epithelial cell cords.

were concentrated in the head (Table 5-3). Available data suggest that appropriate resection of the proximal pancreas, duodenum, and periduodenal-peripancreatic soft tissues and lymph nodes (the "gastrinoma triangle"), removes most gastrinomas (Table 5-2) (124,141,142,146). By contrast, distal "blind" pancreatectomy, a procedure used in the past by surgeons for ZES, is usually unsuccessful.

*Gastrointestinal Tumors.* Gastrinomas from the duodenum and jejunum account for 30 percent of the 42 overt ZES-associated tumors from our files, although representing only 40 percent of the 30 gastrin cell tumors that arose in the intestine. In fact, unlike their pancreatic counterparts which are practically all functional, the majority of duodenojejunal gastrin cell tumors are nonfunctioning (40 percent) or associated with signs of mild hyperfunction (20 percent) that may not be the result of gastrin hypersecretion by the tumor (119). ZES-associated tumors (gastrinomas) differ from their nonfunctioning counterparts (gastrin cell tumors) by arising earlier in life (median 40 years as opposed to 60 to 70 years) and showing a higher incidence of deeply infiltrative growth involving the muscularis propria (60 percent compared to no or only occasional cases), metastases (25 to 50 compared to 0 percent), and distal (nonbulbar) localization (119).

Duodenal gastrinomas may appear as circumscribed, relatively soft, mucosal-submucosal nodules, sometimes involving the muscular layer. In about three fourths of cases they are less than 1 cm in diameter. Microgastrinomas less than 0.5 cm in size may not be palpable through the intestinal wall. Often, they are detected only after duodenotomy and careful inspection and palpation of the everted mucosa, with the help of intestinal wall transillumination.

*Tumors Outside the Pancreas and Gastrointestinal Tract.* Proven, though rare, sites of primary gastrinomas include the gastric wall, with special reference to the antropyloric mucosa, gallbladder, biliary tree, liver, and possibly kidney (131). In addition, mucinous cystadenomas or cystadenocarcinomas of the pancreas and ovary may show pyloric type differentiation with gastrin cells (139,144). In the absence of the acid-mediated inhibition normally operating in the stomach, such gastrin cells may hyperfunction and occasionally cause severe hypergastrinemia and ZES (121,133).

**Microscopic, Histochemical, and Ultrastructural Findings.** Pancreatic gastrinomas, extrapancreatic tumors, and changes in nontumor tissues are described separately.

*Pancreatic Gastrinomas.* The histologic appearance of pancreatic gastrinomas includes all the patterns classically associated with pancreatic endocrine tumors. The most common arrangement of cells is the formation of trabeculae

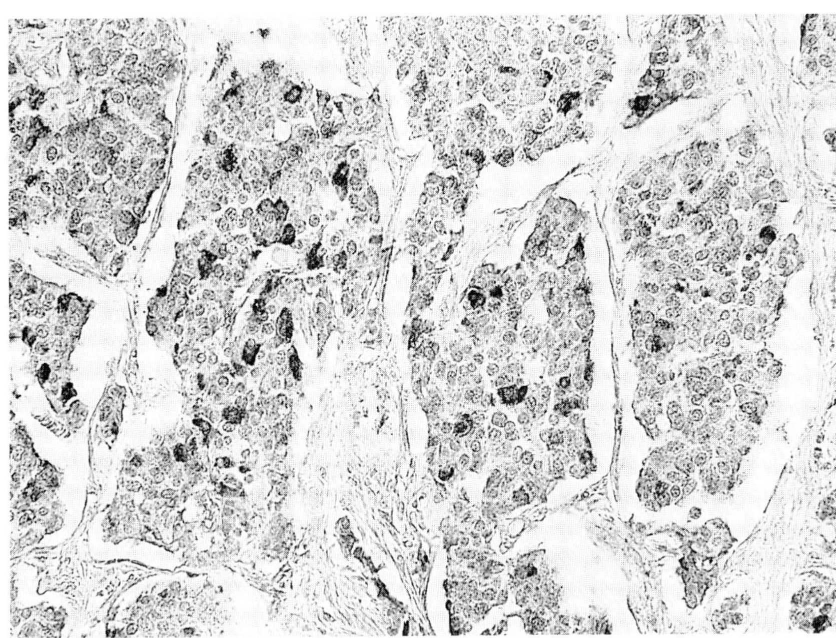

Figure 5-32
PANCREATIC GASTRINOMA
This tumor shows a lobular-trabecular pattern and scattered gastrin immunoreactive cells.

(fig. 5-31): this was found in about two thirds of tumors in our series (124,140). Trabecular tumors showed a marked tendency to contain areas with solid sheets or nests of cells. Tubuloacinar structures were seldom observed. The tumor cells generally had round or ovoid nuclei that were notably uniform and showed minimal atypia. Mitotic figures were rarely found. In most cases, it was impossible to predict, on purely histologic grounds, the frequently malignant behavior of pancreatic gastrinomas. Invasion of large blood vessels or gross infiltration into peripancreatic tissues, two reliable criteria of malignancy, were rarely observed. Invasion of the peritumoral lymphatics and small blood vessels, considered to be a suggestive sign of malignancy, was found more frequently.

Gastrinoma cells stain for general endocrine markers like Grimelius silver and chromogranin A or B. Gastrin immunohistochemistry (fig. 5-32) is essential for diagnosis. In the case of negative findings in a ZES-associated tumor, a panel of antibodies of differing specificities, directed against different parts of the gastrin molecule (C-terminus and non-C-terminus gastrin-17, N-terminus gastrin-34, extended C-terminus, etc.) should be used before excluding a diagnosis of gastrinoma. In many pancreatic tumors, a large population of cells remains gastrin unreactive, possibly due to defective hormone synthesis, processing, or storage. Gastrin mRNA detection by in situ hybridization is important in suspected gastrinomas that fail to react with gastrin antibodies. In addition to gastrin cells, a number of other cell types have been identified in pancreatic gastrinomas, including PP, glucagon, insulin, somatostatin, ACTH, and serotonin cells (122,128,135,140).

Ultrastructurally, gastrinomas are composed of variable proportions of granular and agranular cells. The granules are often heterogeneous in size and shape; a reliable diagnosis can therefore seldom be made on the basis of electron microscopic findings. Based on the morphologic characteristics of secretory granules, Creutzfeldt et al. (122) subdivided gastrinomas into four groups: type 1 in which granular cells contain "typical" G-cell granules (fig. 5-33, left); type 2 in which some cells resemble typical G cells and other cells contain small (150 to 200 nm), round "atypical" granules (fig. 5-33, right); type 3 in which cells contain only "atypical" granules; and type 4 which includes additional nongastrin cell types.

*Extrapancreatic Tumors.* Broad gyriform trabeculae and vascular pseudorosettes are the dominant histologic pattern of most duodenojejunal gastrin cell tumors, with or without an associated gastrinoma syndrome (fig. 5-34). In duodenal, jejunal, and gastric gastrinomas, more or less abundant somatostatin cells are frequently found, admixed with gastrin cells. In addition, a

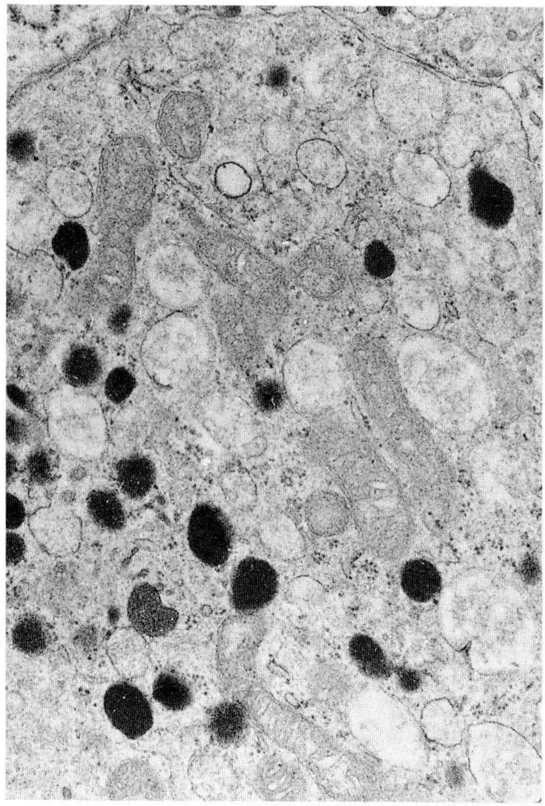

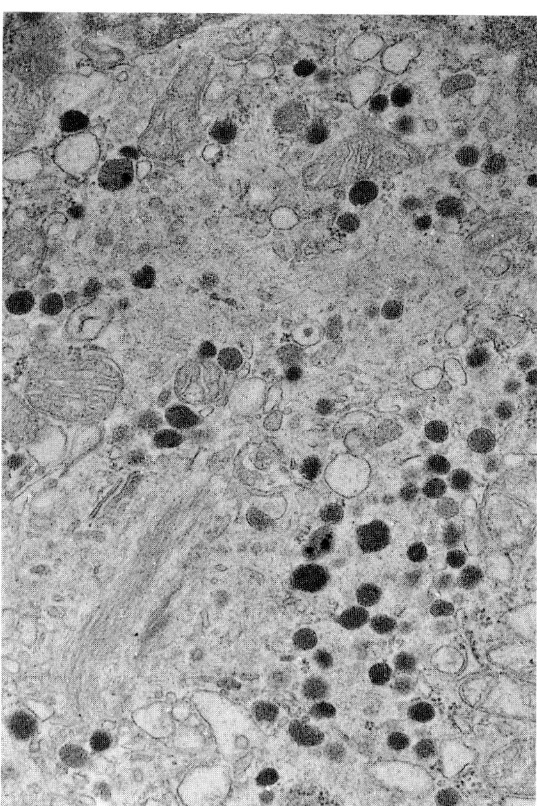

Figure 5-33
PANCREATIC GASTRINOMA

Left: As seen in this electron micrograph, tumor cells contain typical vesicular G-cell granules as well as nondiagnostic dense granules (X28,000).

Right: The cells of this tumor contain small, nondiagnostic secretory granules (X28,000).

few serotonin, insulin, and cholecystokinin cells have been observed (119). Duodenal gastrinomas do not differ ultrastructurally from pancreatic gastrinomas, except in greater granularity and differentiation of the tumor cells.

*Nontumor Tissues.* Varying degrees of chronic pancreatitis (probably secondary to duct obstruction by large gastrinomas) and centroacinar-ductular cell hyperplasia may be observed in nontumor pancreatic tissue. Islet hyperplasia and neogenesis of endocrine tissue from duct epithelium (nesidioblastosis) have been reported in the nontumor pancreas of patients with ZES (122,125). Islet hyperplasia is not a proven cause of ZES since gastrin cells have not been identified in the normal human pancreas, and hyperproduction of gastrin by hyperplastic islets has never been convincingly demonstrated (122,143). Some of the earlier reports of "islet hyperplasia" can now be reinterpreted as microadenomatosis, mostly composed of glucagon and PP cells and characteristic of MEN 1. Recent quantitative morphometric studies do not confirm significant islet hyperplasia in patients with sporadic gastrinoma (143). On the contrary, primary gastrin cell hyperplasia of the antropyloric mucosa may represent a potential source of hypergastrinemia coupled with peptic ulcer disease (132,140).

In the gastric mucosa of oxyntic type, a hypertrophic gastropathy is usually observed; this may be so prominent that macroscopically a giant rugae pattern is seen. The parietal cell mass may become three to six times larger than normal (136). Argyrophil endocrine cells of the oxyntic glands also show prominent hyperplasia. Most hyperplastic endocrine cells are enterochromaffin-like (ECL) cells, which are gastrin dependent and secrete histamine.

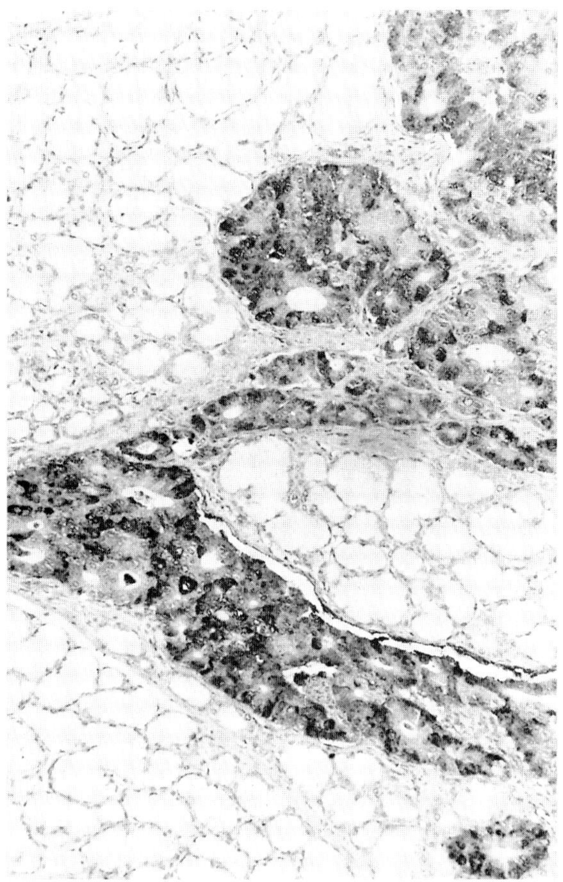

Figure 5-34
DUODENAL GASTRINOMA
Diffuse gastrin immunoreactivity of tumor cells in a gastrinoma infiltrating the Brunner glands.

Brunner gland hyperplasia and hypertrophy is frequently detected in the duodenum. Atrophy and distortion of the villi, with hyperemia and inflammation of the stroma, may contribute to the malabsorption and diarrhea observed in some patients with gastrinoma. The villus epithelium of the proximal duodenum is progressively replaced by gastric epithelium of surface type (gastric metaplasia), which can be easily recognized because it is periodic acid–Schiff positive.

**Prognosis, Natural History, and Treatment.** Both pancreatic and duodenal gastrinomas are slow-growing tumors, and long survival is not exceptional even in the presence of metastases. Since proton-pump inhibitors and histamine H2-receptor antagonists suppress acid hypersecretion and prevent the severe, often fatal, ulcer complications of ZES, progressive tumor growth is the most frequent cause of death in these patients. The prognosis of a gastrinoma is based upon the slow growth of the tumor and the late onset of metastases. Patients must be followed for decades after surgery. The malignancy rate of duodenal gastrinomas (25 to 57 percent [119,143]) is lower than that of pancreatic gastrinomas (68 to 84 percent [125,142]). This may be due in part to the earlier detection of duodenal tumors, although duodenal gastrinomas can metastasize while still very small; 5 of 11 duodenal gastrinomas smaller than 1 cm in diameter were already associated with lymph node metastasis (137). In several cases the primary duodenal or jejunal tumor was detected years after the resection of a paraduodenal lymph node metastasis (119,123). These cases demonstrate that the assumption of gastrinoma arising in a lymph node is misleading. The main metastatic sites of gastrinomas are the regional lymph nodes and liver (Table 5-3). The frequency of liver metastases increases with size and pancreatic location of the primary tumor and decreases with the presence of MEN 1 at the initial presentation. Metastases to the lymph nodes do not depend on these factors (146). In rare cases, metastases have been reported to occur in the lung, pleura, skin, bone, and spleen (143).

Revised published series (Table 5-4) show that patients with duodenal gastrinomas develop regional lymph node metastases in 32 percent (62 of 191) of cases, a figure only slightly lower than the 40 percent (120 of 301) for those with pancreatic gastrinomas. However, only 3 percent of duodenal tumors metastasize to liver as compared to 30 percent of pancreatic tumors. Considering

Table 5-4

**FREQUENCY OF LIVER AND LYMPH NODE METASTASES OF DUODENAL AND PANCREATIC GASTRINOMAS**

| Organ (Ref. no.) | No. of Cases | Metastases: Lymph nodes No. (%) | Metastases: Liver No. (%) |
|---|---|---|---|
| Pancreas (122, (125,142,146) | 301 | 120 (40) | 91 (30) |
| Duodenum (117, 119,122,129,137, | 191 | 62 (32) | 6 (3) |

that metastases from duodenal gastrinomas restricted to regional lymph nodes do not affect survival once surgically removed (123,146), and that for pancreatic gastrinomas the presence of liver metastases is the main predictor of worse prognosis (126,146), it is clear why patients with duodenal gastrinoma have a better survival rate than those with pancreatic tumors (123,137,145). Most of our patients are alive 2 to 16 years after surgery or died from unrelated disease (119).

Only 4 percent of patients with pancreatic gastrinomas followed for a mean of 19 months by Wynick et al. (148) developed a second syndrome of endocrine hyperfunction. Simultaneously, 8 percent of patients with functioning pancreatic tumors other than gastrinomas (including 22 percent with glucagonomas and 3 percent with insulinomas) developed ZES as a second syndrome. A combination of ZES and Cushing's syndrome caused by the same pancreatic tumor has been found in 5 percent of ZES patients (134) and 14 percent of those with Cushing's disease (120). Nearly all the tumors were large, metastatic, resistant to medical therapy, and associated with a rapidly worsening clinical course.

Streptozotocin, 5-fluorouracil, adriamycin, and alpha interferon are beneficial for less than half of the patients with metastatic gastrinoma. In general, patients with gastrinoma survive long term. The 10-year survival rate is better in patients with MEN 1 (93 percent) than in patients with sporadic gastrinoma (74 percent) (146). The mean survival period for patients with gastrinoma and liver metastasis is about 7 years (127).

## VIPoma

**Definition.** This is an endocrine tumor predominantly occurring in the pancreas which produces the Verner-Morrison or WDHA (watery diarrhea, hypokalemia, achlorhydria) syndrome through secretion of vasoactive intestinal peptide (VIP), peptide histidine methionine (PHM), and other hormone-like substances. Synonyms include *diarrheogenic tumor of the pancreas* and *islet cell tumor of the pancreas with watery diarrhea.*

**Incidence.** Pancreatic VIPomas are rare neoplasms. They comprise about 8 percent of all pancreatic endocrine tumors (159). The incidence in several large series of cases is slightly higher in females than in males (63 females, 52 males) (152,165,166). Patients range in age from 19 to 79 years (mean, 48 years). A family history is usually absent; however, an association of pancreatic VIPomas with MEN 1 has been reported in at least 15 cases (157,167,168).

**Clinical Features.** Secretory diarrhea (0.5 to 6.0 L per 24 hours), hypokalemia, hypochlorhydria, alkalosis, flushing, hypercalcemia, abnormal glucose tolerance test, tetany, and a dilated gallbladder are the distinctive clinical features. Diarrhea is always the most prominent symptom at presentation. The volume of stool is usually 700 ml or more daily and may reach several liters per day with severe loss of potassium and bicarbonate, resulting in metabolic acidosis and dehydration (157). The stool resembles dilute tea and there is usually no steatorrhea. The clinical picture is dominated by dehydration and hypotension. Most patients are hypochlorhydric rather than achlorhydric (165). Hypercalcemia with normal levels of serum parathormone and hyperglycemia are found in about 50 percent of patients (175). Although flushing of the face and chest is reported in some patients, the excretion of serotonin and its metabolites is only occasionally increased. Gallbladder distention and dilute bile have been reported in several patients. Tetany is rare and might be explained by hypomagnesemia with normal or elevated levels of serum calcium (161).

For some patients with fatal WDHA syndrome, apparently benign pancreatic VIPomas were first diagnosed at autopsy, emphasizing the importance of early diagnosis.

**Hormonal Mediators of the WDHA Syndrome.** High concentrations of VIP have been detected in tumors associated with WDHA syndrome. The biologic actions of VIP include stimulation of intestinal secretion, inhibition of gastric acid secretion, dilation of the gallbladder, and promotion of glycogenolysis with consequent hyperglycemia and dilation of peripheral blood vessels leading to hypotension and flushing. Since all these actions closely parallel the clinical features of the WDHA syndrome, it seems likely that VIP is the main mediator of the syndrome. Recently, the tumors have been shown to cosecrete a peptide (P) with an amino terminal histidine (H) and a carboxyl terminal methionine (M). PHM shares a common precursor (prepro-VIP) with VIP as well as some pharmacologic effects

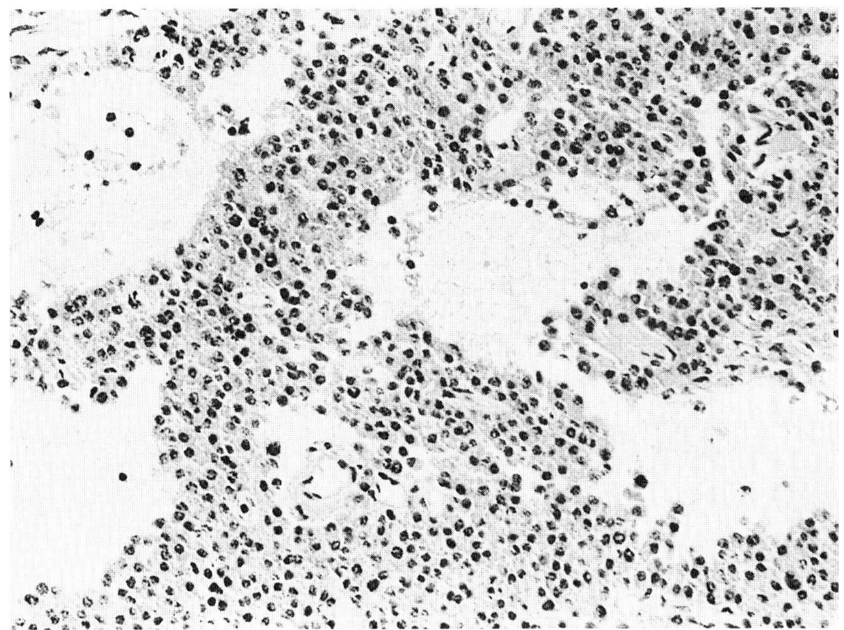

Figure 5-35
PANCREATIC VIPOMA
Solid arrangement of uniform epithelial cells with faintly stained cytoplasm, interrupted by cystic spaces filled with weakly eosinophilic serum-like material.

(177). About 75 percent of VIPomas also produce pancreatic polypeptide (PP) and increased serum fasting PP levels; however, there is no evidence supporting a role for PP in the pathogenesis of the WDHA syndrome. Two other diarrheogenic peptides, neurotensin and calcitonin, have been detected in a few cases (149). High plasma levels of diarrheogenic prostaglandins have been also reported in some patients with the WDHA syndrome (158).

A VIP assay should be performed in all patients with severe secretory diarrhea. VIP plasma levels in patients with VIPomas are usually above 60 pmol/L. Diagnosis may be facilitated by evaluation of PHM levels in plasma, which are high due to the high circulating concentrations and greater resistance to proteolysis of this peptide (150).

**Gross Findings.** Early reports of pancreatic pathology associated with the WDHA syndrome described a well-defined tumor within the pancreas in 85 percent of patients, while no evident gross lesion could be detected in the remaining cases (165). In more recent series, all patients with VIP hypersecretion and the WDHA syndrome had a tumor (152,159). Careful review of 66 cases from the literature up to 1991 (149,152, 168,175) in which the exact tumor site was known indicates that the tumor is usually solitary, with sharply defined margins. The tumors are most often located in the tail (47 percent), followed by the head (23 percent), body (19 percent), and body and tail together (11 percent). Pancreatic VIPomas range in size from 1.5 to 20 cm, with a median diameter of 4.5 cm, which is much larger than insulinomas (1.5 to 2 cm) and about the same size as gastrinomas and glucagonomas. Tumor size is an important but not absolute criterion for distinguishing benign from malignant VIPomas since tumors less than 2 cm do metastasize, while tumors measuring up to 7 cm in diameter are apparently benign. Other gross features, such as type of border, color, and consistency, are indistinguishable from those of other functional pancreatic endocrine tumors.

**Microscopic Findings.** The pancreatic tumors show histologic features of three main structural patterns of epithelial endocrine growth: solid, broad trabecular, and tubuloacinar, in order of decreasing frequency (figs. 5-35, 5-36). The solid pattern is sometimes interrupted by irregular cystic spaces filled with weakly eosinophilic material. The tubuloacinar pattern is generally seen admixed with trabecular or solid patterns. Individual tumor cells have faintly granular eosinophilic or clear, relatively abundant cytoplasm. They are polygonal in shape or, when within tubules and trabeculae, cylindric and cuboidal. The nuclei are hyperchromatic and polymorphic in the majority of cases; the polymorphism is slight in

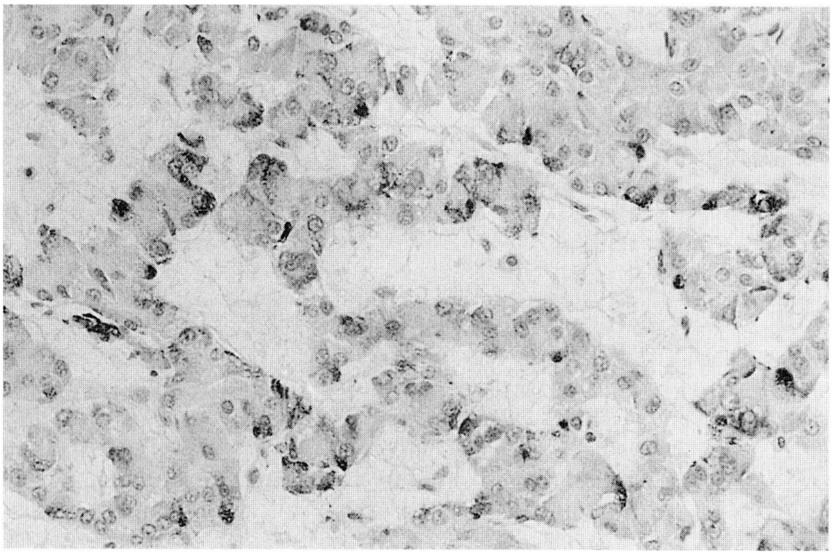

Figure 5-36
PANCREATIC VIPOMA
Trabeculae of epithelial cells with fairly abundant cytoplasm separated by loose stroma. Scattered tumor cells show VIP immunostaining.

about one third of cases and fairly prominent in the remainder. In addition, frequent, often atypical mitoses are observed in one eighth of the cases. Vascular and perineural invasion at the periphery of the tumor are present in about half the cases, most of which have lymph node or liver metastases. Although the amount of stroma varies from case to case, it is often abundant and richly vascularized. About 70 percent of cases have some Grimelius-reactive argyrophil cells. These are more numerous and stain intensely in tissue specimens fixed with Bouin's fluid.

Although islet cell hyperplasia has been reported as a cause of WDHA syndrome (174), this is unlikely since in the non-neoplastic pancreas, VIP is present in autonomic nerves but not in islet cells. In fact, no convincing case of WDHA syndrome due to islet hyperplasia has been reported in the recent literature. Microscopic lesions of the exocrine pancreas, especially focal centroacinar and ductular hyperplasia, have been also detected. The precise meaning of these changes is unclear. They might be secondary to VIP-induced overstimulation of ductular-centroacinar cells, whose secretory activity is known to be enhanced by VIP.

**Immunohistochemical Findings.** In 28 pancreatic tumors studied by the authors (172), immunohistochemical tests showed reactivity for the following markers of epithelial endocrine cells: neuron-specific enolase (95 percent of cases), cytokeratin A (61 percent), synaptophysin (93 percent), chromogranin A (45 percent), and alpha-1-antitrypsin (33 percent). No consistent staining of tumor cells was obtained with antibodies against serotonin, microtubule-associated protein (MAP2), and S-100 protein. Present were the neuroendocrine peptides VIP (87 percent of the cases), PHM (57 percent), growth hormone-releasing hormone (GRH; 50 percent), PP (53 percent), alpha chain of human chorionic gonadotropin (alpha- hCG; 48 percent), insulin (17 percent), neurotensin (18 percent), glucagon (10 percent), somatostatin (15 percent), and met-enkephalin (8 percent) (figs. 5-37, 5-38). In the majority of tumors associated with WDHA syndrome, only a few tumor cells reacted with VIP antibodies, in keeping with the sparsely granular ultrastructural pattern of most tumor cells (152,172). Both findings suggest a defective hormonal storage mechanism, which may imply a rapid release of synthesized hormone which reaches high levels in blood even when at a low level in tumor cells.

Immunohistochemical staining for VIP and PP has been reported in a mucinous adenocarcinoma (170), and for PP alone in a mucinous islet cell (amphicrine) carcinoma (169). Both were pancreatic and associated with WDHA syndrome.

Pancreatic tumor production of VIP and PHM (normally present only in neuroectodermal cells [162]) may be attributed to the increased plasticity in differentiation shown by tumor cell lines. In fact, epithelial endocrine cells undergoing

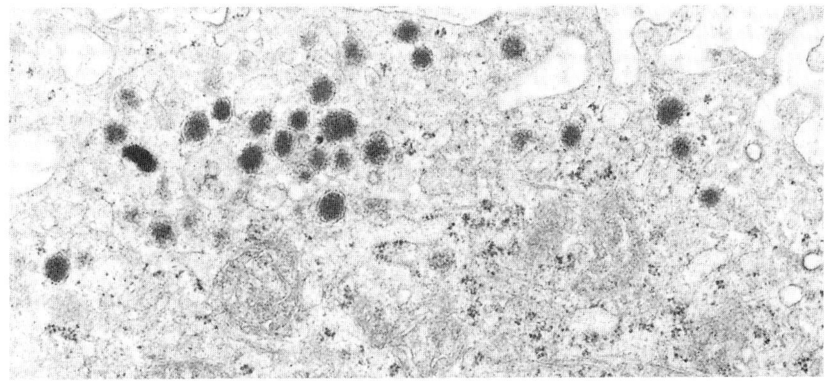

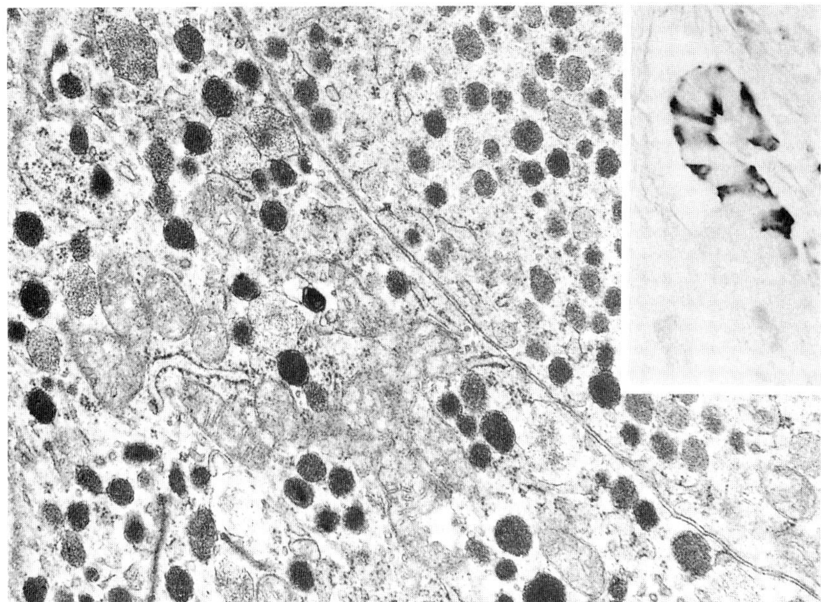

Figure 5-37
PANCREATIC VIPOMA

Top: Small secretory granules in a pancreatic tumor with scattered VIP-immunoreactive cells and associated WDHA syndrome (X28,000).

Bottom: Electron microscopy of a pancreatic VIPoma. Abundant secretory granules of variable size, shape, and density in a pancreatic tumor with WDHA syndrome. Abundant PP- and a few VIP-immunoreactive cells (inset) were detected by light microscopic immunohistochemistry of the same tumor (X28,000).

neoplastic transformation have been found to increase their spectrum of differentiation to include some "neurogenic" markers, for instance the neurofilament 68K protein, which is absent in the corresponding normal cells. The frequent presence of PP-producing cells in pancreatic VIPomas and the occasional finding of both PP and VIP immunoreactivity in the same tumor cells suggest that a cell line somewhat akin to that of dorsal pancreas PP cells might be involved in the histogenesis of these tumors (172).

**Ultrastructural Findings.** Ultrastructural studies have confirmed the epithelial nature of the tumors. Most tumors are primarily composed of sparsely granulated or agranular cells, with a fairly developed endoplasmic reticulum and Golgi complex. Secretory granules (fig. 5-37) are usually round and small (120 to 190 nm). Two types of secretory granules are seen: 1) smaller (120 to 160 nm), thin-haloed granules containing a moderately dense core, and which react with VIP antibodies in electron immunocytochemical tests, and 2) slightly larger (140 to 190), more solid granules which react with anti-PP antibodies and resemble those of PP cells in pancreatic tissue of dorsal pouch origin (152,155).

In a minority of tumors, well-granulated endocrine cells with abundant rough endoplasmic reticulum that often forms parallel cisternae filled with secretory material have been found (fig. 5-37). Their granules vary in shape (round to ovoid, angular, pear-shaped, or comma-shaped), and size (from 150 to 200 nm mean diameter), thus resembling those of F-type PP cells that form the PP-rich

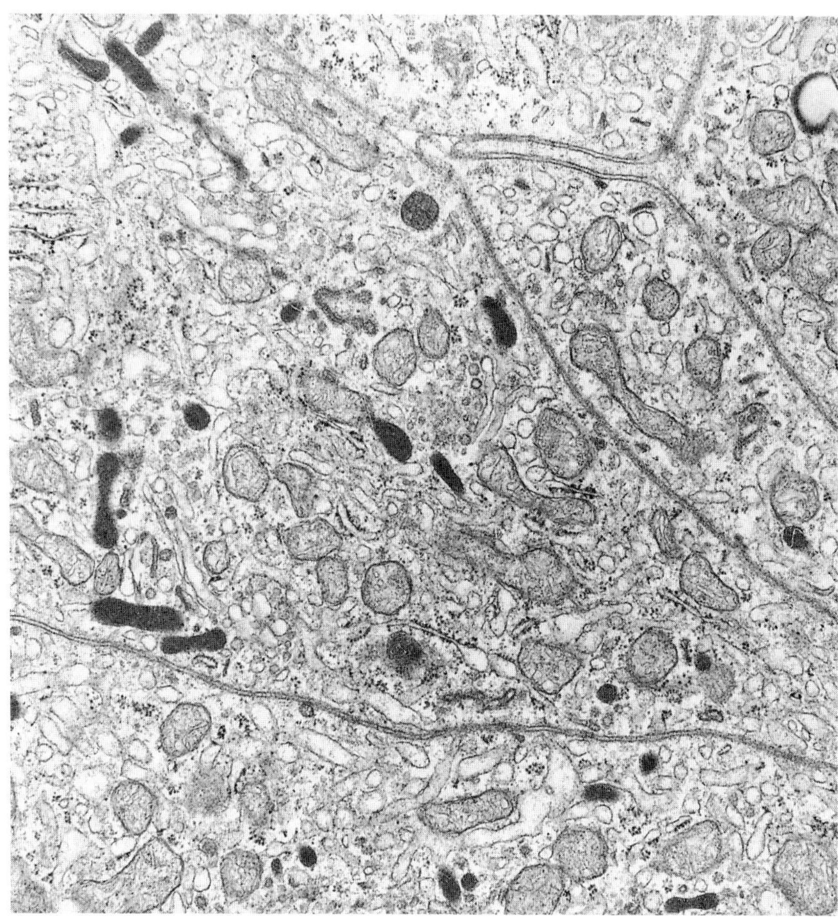

Figure 5-38
PANCREATIC VIPOMA
Cells with a few, round, small granules; well-developed reticulum and Golgi complex; and scattered elongated dense bodies (X28,000).

irregular islets of the posterior head (155). The PP-cell nature of the latter tumors, which usually have a prominent trabecular structure, has been confirmed immunohistochemically.

Elongated, electron-dense bodies of peculiar shape, resembling that of endosomal tubulovesicles, have also been observed in a number of pancreatic VIPomas (fig. 5-38) (152,153). They are more prominent in tumors having few endocrine granules and extensively developed small clear tubulovesicles in a clear cytoplasm. Immunohistochemically, these tumors are characterized by their reactivity for alpha-1-antitrypsin and poor reactivity for neuroendocrine markers.

Tumor areas with a tubuloacinar structure consist of agranular or poorly granular cells with clear cytoplasm, abundant smooth tubulovesicles, and elongated, thin microvilli. In most cases these microvilli lack the long cytoplasmic rootlets seen in cells of large pancreatic ducts, but closely resemble the microvilli of intralobular ductules. The tubuloacinar areas show no or only minimal immunoreactivity for endocrine markers but stain strongly with epithelial membrane antigen (EMA) antibodies.

**Prognosis, Natural History, and Treatment.** From a review of our cases and those collected by Morrison (165), it appears that 54 percent of 107 pancreatic tumors associated with the WDHA syndrome were malignant at presentation. Most metastases were in the liver (86 percent of metastatic cases) and regional lymph nodes (31 percent) (Table 5-2). The exact behavior of some of the remaining tumors remained uncertain, due to equivocal histologic findings or lack of follow-up. Cases with proven or potential malignancy represent a consistent majority of such tumors. Both the malignancy rate and mean tumor size (4.5 cm) of pancreatic VIPomas resemble those of gastrin-producing tumors, while sharply differing from those of insulinomas, most of which are benign and small (1 to 3 cm).

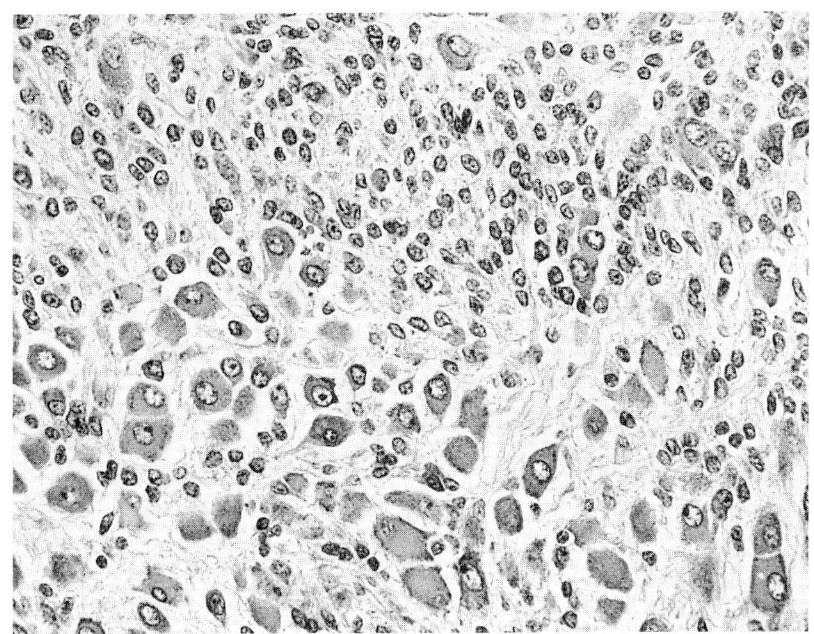

Figure 5-39
RETROPERITONEAL GANGLIONEUROBLASTOMA
Well-differentiated ganglion cells and nerve fibers in a retroperitoneal diarrheogenic ganglioneuroblastoma.

Fluids and electrolytes, particularly potassium, should be replaced before surgical treatment. The possible cardiovascular and renal complications of hypokalemia must be considered and controlled. Surgical resection of a localized tumor usually suppresses or alleviates diarrhea, with concomitant correction of hypokalemia and reduction of plasma VIP/PHM levels. When complete surgical excision is not feasible, tumor debulking and ischemic shrinkage of liver metastases by arterial embolization are useful palliatives. Streptozotocin and, more recently, interferon have proved effective in obtaining good remissions (150).

**Extrapancreatic Tumors Associated with the WDHA Syndrome.** Both epithelial and, especially, neurogenic tumors have been reported in association with the diarrheogenic syndrome.

*Epithelial Tumors.* At least three cases of extrapancreatic VIP-producing epithelial tumors associated with the classic WDHA syndrome have been reported so far: a malignant jejunal endocrine tumor that metastasized to the liver in a 47-year-old woman (152); a mixed-cell (squamous/small cell) carcinoma of the esophagus in a 50-year-old woman (176) which was large and metastasized to supraclavicular lymph nodes, bones, and skin; and a large intracapsular endocrine tumor of the lower pole of the left kidney in a 64-year-old woman (156).

*Neurogenic Tumors.* The occurrence of diarrhea in association with neurogenic tumors of the ganglioneuroma-ganglioneuroblastoma type is well documented in the pediatric literature. The incidence of this association varies from 9 to 25 percent of reported tumors (160,171). Besides diarrhea, patients with neural tumors usually have hypertension and elevated urinary excretion of norepinephrine and its metabolites. About 60 percent of neurogenic tumors are benign (ganglioneuromas) and the rest malignant (neuroblastomas and ganglioneuroblastomas). About one third of the tumors are located in the mediastinum and two thirds in the abdomen, usually arising near an adrenal gland or the aortic bifurcation.

Adults with neurogenic tumors and profuse diarrhea have also been reported (151,154). The production of VIP and PHM by neurogenic tumors is in keeping with the fact that these peptides are normal products of nerve tissue where they may act as neuromodulators or neurotransmitters (162). Diarrheogenic ganglioneuroblastomas have neuroblastic foci, ganglion cells, axons, nerve fibers, and Schwann-like cells (fig. 5-39). Several cases of pheochromocytoma associated with the WDHA syndrome have been reported (163,164), including a case of mixed retroperitoneal ganglioneuroma-pheochromocytoma (173).

Immunohistochemically, VIP, PHM, neuropeptide Y, enkephalins, somatostatin, NSE, microtubule-associated protein (MAP2), and synaptophysin are more or less widely represented in nerve cell bodies and fibers as well as in pheochromocytes. S-100 protein is detected in Schwann and sustentacular cells. Unlike pancreatic VIPomas, neurogenic tumors show no reactivity with PP or cytokeratin A antibodies.

Most of the VIP-producing ganglioneuroblastomas so far reported in the literature were well-encapsulated neoplasms that do not recur following complete surgical excision.

### Enterochromaffin Cell Tumor Causing the Carcinoid Syndrome

**Definition.** Enterochromaffin (EC) cell tumor is a predominantly malignant endocrine tumor that has enterochromaffin cell differentiation and produces the carcinoid syndrome. The tumor is extremely rare: only 17 cases were traced in the literature.

**Clinicopathologic Features.** Diarrhea, cutaneous flushing, hypotension, bronchospasm, right heart endocardial fibrosis, and mesenteric and retroperitoneal fibrosis are all components of the carcinoid syndrome caused by excessive secretion of a variety of tumor factors. These factors include serotonin, kallikreins (which in turn release bradykinin), substance P and other tachykinins, and prostaglandins.

Among serotonin-producing pancreatic endocrine tumors causing the carcinoid syndrome, well-differentiated argentaffin or EC cell tumors (carcinoids) are characterized by abundant argentaffin-positive, serotonin-storing, pleomorphic granules; minimal cellular atypia; and a solid alveolar to trabecular structure with peripheral palisading of cells (fig. 5-40) (179,180). Other tumors are less differentiated, with relatively few secretory granules of low serotonin content, more obvious cellular atypia, mitoses, and a solid to diffuse structure with or without focal necrosis (178,180,183); these tumors have the morphologic pattern of the intermediate cell variant of small cell endocrine carcinoma. Although 5 of 10 well-differentiated EC cell tumors reported were metastatic, they were less aggressive than intermediate cell carcinomas, the majority of which were highly invasive. Fifteen of 17 pancreatic endocrine tumors associated with the carcinoid syndrome were metastatic, mostly to the liver and regional lymph nodes (182). A few small, well-differentiated argentaffin EC cell tumors not associated with the carcinoid syndrome (nonfunctioning EC cell tumors) were not metastatic (181,184).

### Tumors Producing Acromegaly, Cushing's Syndrome, or Hypercalcemia

These are predominantly malignant endocrine tumors of the pancreas which produce growth hormone–releasing factor/growth hormone (GRF/GH), ACTH, parathyroid hormone (PTH), or parathirin and cause, respectively, acromegaly, Cushing's syndrome, or hyperparathyroidism-like hypercalcemia. They are discussed together, apart from other pancreatic tumors, as they have a higher malignancy potential and higher propensity for multiple hormone expression, with or without multiple endocrine syndromes.

Several pancreatic tumors that produce growth hormone–releasing factors (GRF, somatoliberin) and cause acromegaly through pituitary GH hypersecretion from hyperplastic pituitary GH cells have been reported (186,196,197). Histologically, these tumors have a trabecular, whorl-like meningotheliomatous or even paraganglioid "zellballen" structure. They are large tumors, with proven liver or lymph node metastases in 3 of the 7 cases in which pertinent information was given (186,196,197). They arose in relatively young patients (median, 34 years), and were associated with MEN 1 syndrome in two cases. The tumors are characterized histochemically by their GRF immunoreactivity. Ultrastructural investigation reveals small (100 to 180 nm), round, secretory granules. A single case of GH-producing pancreatic endocrine carcinoma with acromegaly and liver metastasis has been reported (190).

Pancreatic tumors that produce ACTH and biosynthetically related melanocyte stimulating hormone (MSH) or opioid peptides as well as Cushing's syndrome or hypokalemic alkalosis are well documented in the literature. They correspond to about 10 percent of ectopic Cushing's syndrome cases, 64 percent of which are found in women (187,191,192). The tumors are firm, nodular masses, 2 to 12 cm in diameter, distributed randomly in the pancreas. Most (88 percent of 42 cases) are metastatic to regional lymph nodes and

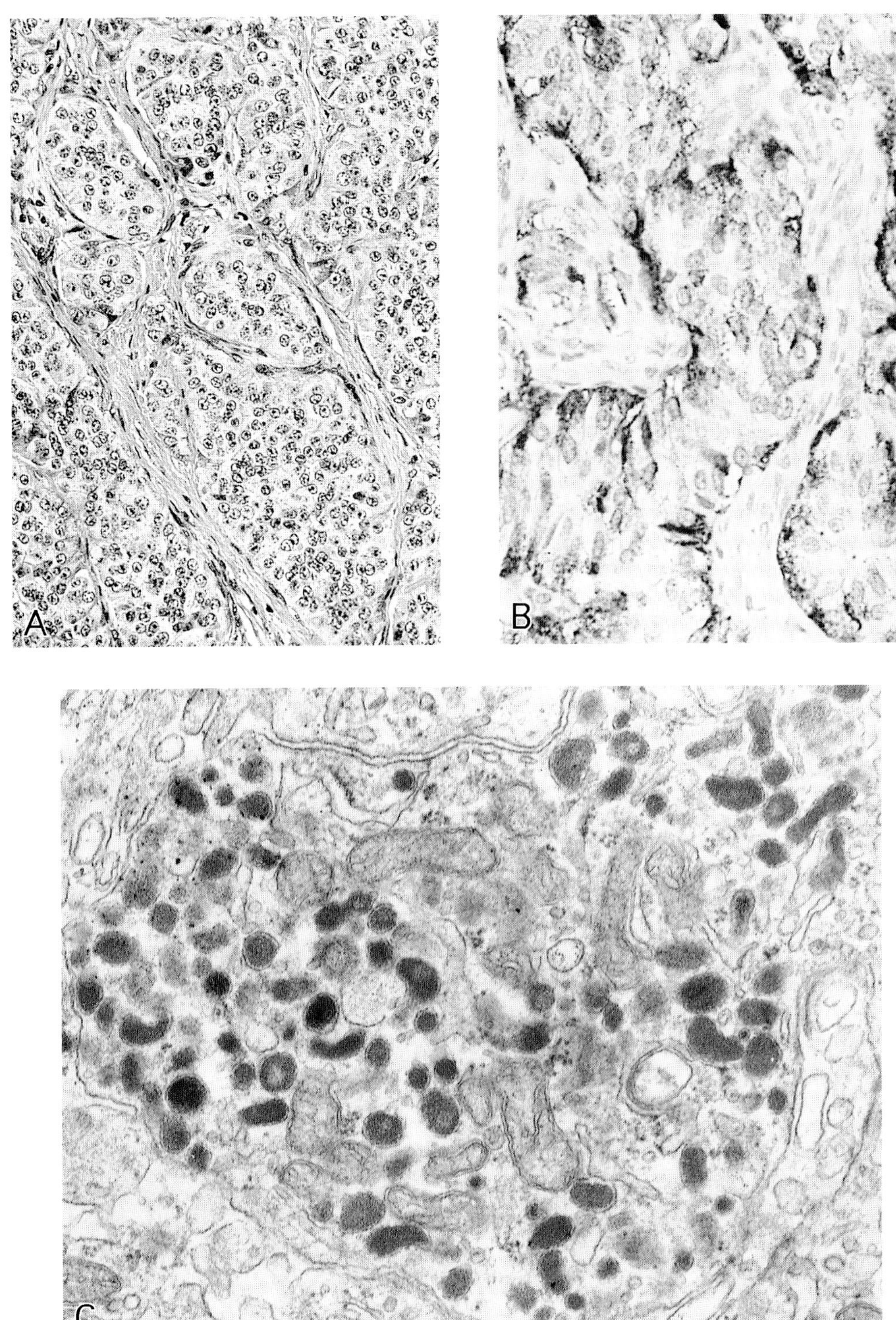


Figure 5-40
PANCREATIC ENTEROCHROMAFFIN CELL TUMOR

A: The tumor is composed of polygonal cells arranged in solid nests.

B: The cells are immunoreactive for serotonin.

C: Electron microscopy shows tumor cells containing irregularly shaped dense granules, characteristic of enterochromaffin (EC) cells (X28,000).

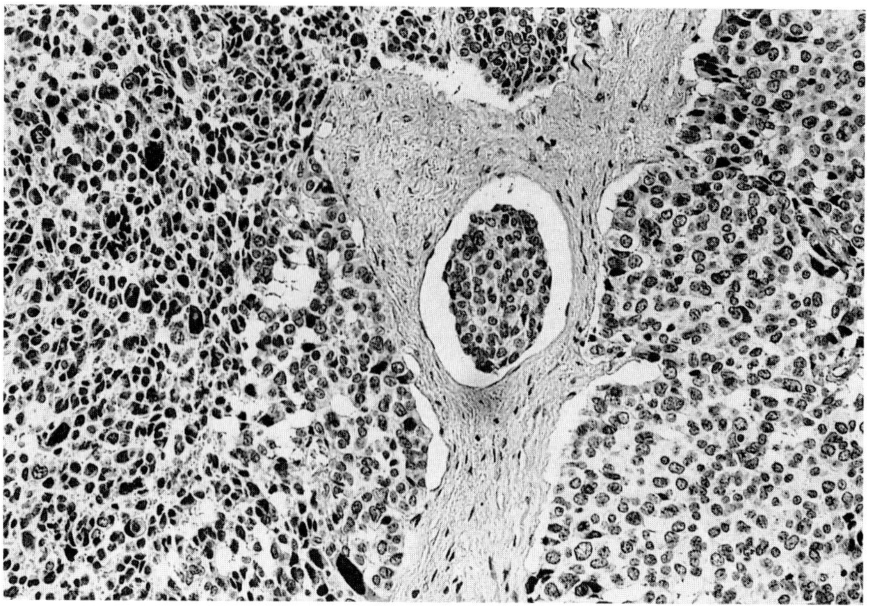

Figure 5-41
ACTH-PRODUCING TUMOR WITH CUSHING'S SYNDROME
Moderately differentiated tumor with consistent cellular atypia, solid growth pattern, and lymphatic invasion.

liver, and often involve the kidney, thyroid, peritoneum, and bone (187). Massive direct invasion of peripancreatic tissues is frequent in larger tumors, whereas smaller tumors are well circumscribed. Histologically, most tumors have small to medium-sized, moderately atypical cells arranged in broad trabeculae, acini, or as solid growth separated by fairly abundant fibrous stroma (fig. 5-41). Many of these histologically well- to moderately differentiated pancreatic endocrine carcinomas associated with Cushing's syndrome are aggressive tumors, with a 2-year survival rate of 40 percent. In addition, rare, poorly differentiated tumors with histologic patterns mimicking those of small cell carcinomas (poorly differentiated endocrine carcinomas) have been reported (188). They are more likely to be associated with short survival and hypokalemic alkalosis, rather than with full-blown Cushing's syndrome.

In several cases the same tumor produces an associated Cushing's syndrome and ZES in which both ACTH and gastrin immunoreactive cells are found. The prognosis in this case is usually worse (187,193). This association occurs in 5 percent of ZES cases and 14 percent of Cushing cases due to pancreatic tumor. ACTH immunoreactive cells have been detected in several tumors lacking an association with Cushing's syndrome, including 14 gastrinomas (189).

A few pancreatic endocrine carcinomas causing a hypercalcemic and hyperparathyroid type syndrome have been described. In 3 of 10 cases reported, there was evidence of production of PTH by the tumor cells (185). In other cases, the lack of evidence of PTH secretion by the pancreatic tumor indicated involvement of a hypercalcemic peptide with PTH-like activity (parathirin) (195). Hypercalcemia-inducing pancreatic endocrine tumors should be distinguished from adenocarcinomas of the exocrine pancreas that result in paraneoplastic hypercalcemia (194).

### Tumors with Multiple Syndromes

A usually malignant pancreatic endocrine tumor that causes, synchronously or metachronously, two or more hormonal syndromes is referred to as a tumor with multiple syndromes.

The presence in the same tumor of two or more endocrine cell types, producing distinct hormones, is a common finding in pancreatic endocrine tumors. Often (but not invariably) minority subpopulations of cells are involved, which in most cases do not cause any endocrine symptom, either with or without an associated increase of pertinent hormone levels in blood (201). However, a combination in the same patient, at the same or different times, of two or more syndromes of endocrine hyperfunction is rare (199–201,203, 204). Sometimes, transition from one syndrome to another occurs during chemotherapy, apparently due to the selective response of the different cell types. Only 7 percent of a large series of patients with pancreatic tumors followed for a mean of 19 months by Wynick et al. (205) developed a second syndrome, usually a glucagonoma syndrome at presentation and ZES as the second syndrome. An association of ZES and Cushing's syndrome caused by the same pancreatic tumor has been found in 5 percent of ZES patients (202) and 14 percent of Cushing's cases (198).

Nearly all bisyndromic or multisyndromic tumors are large, metastatic, resistant to medical therapy, and associated with a rapidly progressing clinical course. Median survival of patients after diagnosis of the second syndrome is 5 to 7 months.

### Nonfunctioning Tumors (Including PP-Cell Tumors)

**Definition.** Nonfunctioning tumors are pancreatic tumors with endocrine differentiation in the absence of a clinical syndrome of hormone hyperfunction. They include nearly all PP-cell tumors and a majority of A- and D-cell tumors. Many of these tumors lack evidence of (or investigation for) increased hormonal levels in blood, which is why they are labeled "nonfunctioning" tumors, even when hormones are found in the tumor cells. Tumors producing increased hormone levels in blood without evidence of a hyperfunctional syndrome, which in principle should be called "functioning nonsyndromic tumors," are also currently reported as nonfunctioning tumors. Among nonfunctioning tumors, those presenting with symptoms of an expanding mass in the upper abdomen should be separated from clinically silent tumors.

**Incidence.** Clinically silent endocrine tumors have been detected in 0.3 to 1.6 percent of unselected autopsies in which only a few sections of the pancreas were examined, and in up to 10 percent of autopsies in which the whole pancreas was systematically investigated both grossly and microscopically. Most tumors were in elderly patients (mean age, 70 years), small (less than 1 cm, often a few millimeters), mainly composed of well-granulated islet A and PP cells, and benign (clinically silent A- and PP-cell microadenomas) (211,214). The majority of patients with nonfunctioning tumors from surgical series have malignant tumors and present with symptoms of an expanding mass or metastatic growth (nonfunctioning low-grade carcinomas, locally symptomatic). A few incidentally found, smaller and often benign tumors have also been reported (209). Of 39 patients with nonfunctioning tumors (30 percent of 132 surgical cases), 25 (64 percent) had local symptoms, 6 (15 percent) had incidentally found tumors, and 8 (21 percent) had MEN 1 syndrome (221).

The proportion of nonfunctioning tumors has varied over the years: it was 41 percent in the large series of pancreatic endocrine tumors reviewed by Howard et al. in 1950 (212); 15 percent of the 168 cases collected by Kent and coworkers in 1981 (213); 25 percent of the 84 cases studied by Broughan and coworkers in 1986 (207); and 36 percent of the 365 cases investigated by Klöppel and Heitz in 1988 (215). Different diagnostic procedures (with special reference to the extent of hormone measurements) and referral patterns of the various institutions involved may account for these different figures. Taken together, the above surgical series of nonfunctioning tumors suggests an overall incidence of about 30 to 35 percent (65 percent with symptoms of a growing mass) in the present decade, a figure second only to that of insulinomas (about 40 percent) and higher than that of all remaining tumor types. Among endocrine carcinoma series, nonfunctioning tumors account for 21 to 83 percent of all cases (206,218). Nonfunctioning tumors of surgical series are equally distributed among sexes.

**Clinicopathologic Features.** In surgical series, clinically symptomatic, nonfunctioning endocrine tumors arise more frequently in the head of the pancreas (Table 5-3). This may be due in part to the more prominent local symptoms produced by tumors in the head of the gland rather than in the body or tail. The most frequent presenting signs and symptoms are pain, jaundice, a palpable abdominal mass, ascites, steatorrhea, and intestinal bleeding. The size of the primary tumor was more than 5 cm (with a maximum of 20 cm) in 72 percent of cases from the Mayo Clinic series (213).

Sixty to 100 percent of cases have their malignancy proven by the presence of metastases or local invasion (207,209,213,215,217,220). These figures increase further if incidentally found tumors are excluded. Of the 25 nonfunctioning tumors investigated by Kent and coworkers (213), 18 (72 percent) had histologically proven

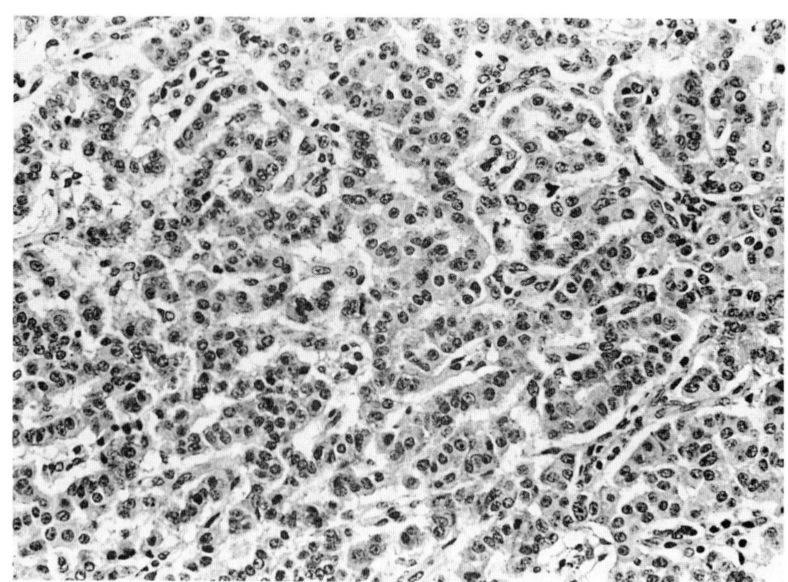

Figure 5-42
PANCREATIC NONFUNCTIONING ENDOCRINE ADENOMA

This tumor showing a gyriform pattern was an incidental finding during abdominal surgery. The tumor was glucagon immunoreactive. (Figures 5-42 and 5-43 are from the same case.)

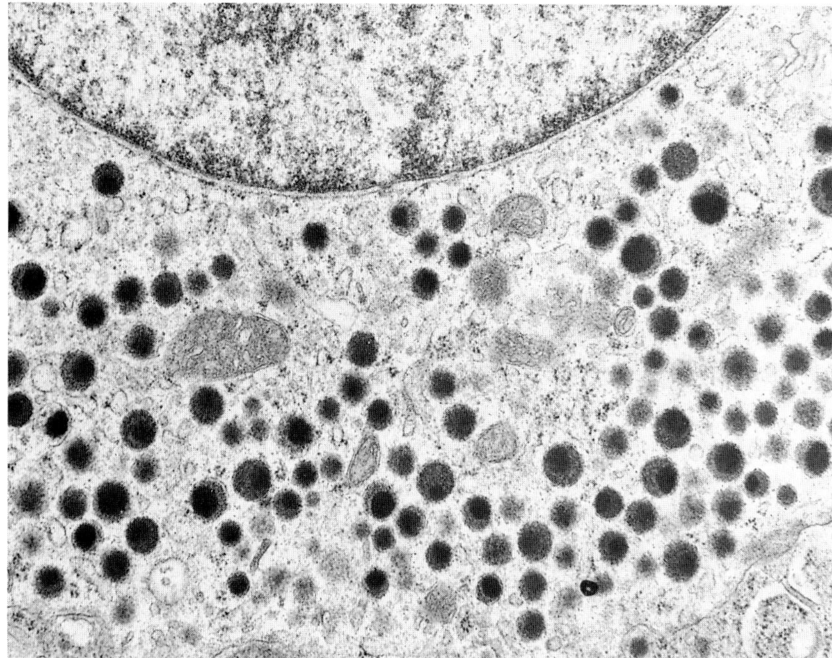

Figure 5-43
PANCREATIC NONFUNCTIONING ENDOCRINE ADENOMA

In this electron micrograph tumor cells contain characteristic alpha granules with a central dense core and a peripheral, less dense mantle (X28,000).

metastases; 5 (20 percent) showed perineural or vascular invasion in the absence of metastases (a pattern highly suggestive of malignancy, although not universally accepted as proof of it); and only 2 (8 percent), which had been found incidentally, were diagnosed as benign tumors.

**Histologic, Histochemical, and Ultrastructural Findings.** No differences in histologic pattern have been found in nonfunctioning as compared to functioning tumors. Well-granulated tumors may have some distinctive structural features, such as the thin gyriform ribbons of A-cell tumors or the parallel, palisading trabeculae of PP-cell tumors (figs. 5-42–5-45). Poorly granular tumors usually have a moderately defined, solid to broadly trabecular pattern formed by monomorphic, small to medium-sized, mildly atypical cells (fig. 4-46).

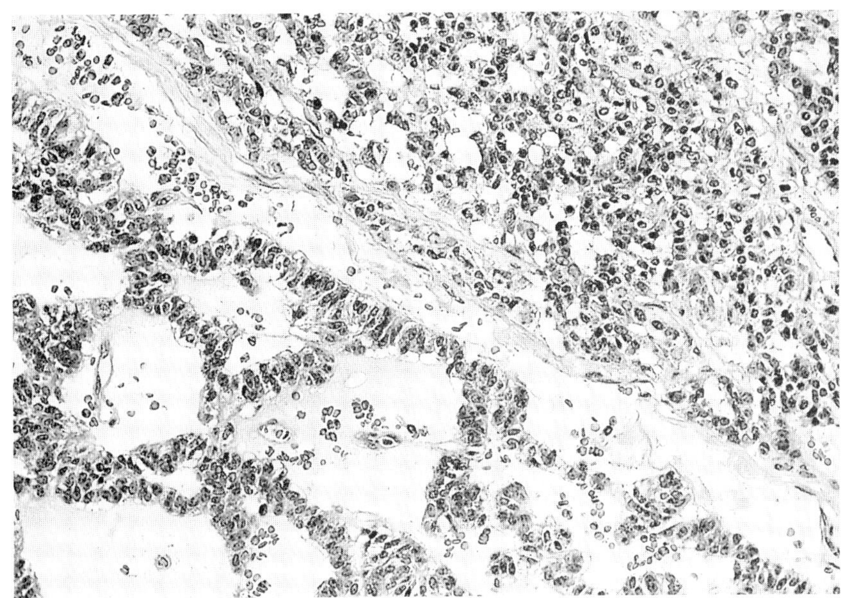

Figure 5-44
PANCREATIC NONFUNCTIONING ENDOCRINE TUMOR

This tumor has a partly trabecular structure with palisading of cells, and partly a solid pattern. The tumor was large (5.5 cm in diameter), endocrinologically nonfunctioning, and was associated with clinical symptoms due to local compression. (Figures 5-44 and 5-45 are from the same case.)

In a series of 61 nonfunctioning tumors investigated by two of the authors (215a), PP immunoreactivity was detected in 35 percent of cases, with a mean of 33 percent of all tumor cells; glucagon was found in 30 percent of cases and 30 percent of cells; somatostatin in 15 percent of cases and 20 percent of cells; serotonin in 20 percent of cases and 36 percent of cells; calcitonin in 20 percent of cases and 10 percent of cells; neurotensin in 8 percent of cases and 8 percent of cells; and insulin in 15 percent of cases and 2 percent of cells. No gastrin or VIP immunoreactivity was detected. It seems clear that tumors producing PP, glucagon, somatostatin, calcitonin, or serotonin are more likely to remain nonsyndromic than are those producing clinically powerful hormones such as insulin, gastrin, or VIP. Hormonally unreactive cells have been found frequently (215,219,221); they accounted for most tumor cells in 15 of our 61 cases, including most of the larger, poorly granular and malignant cases.

In many hormone-poor cases, the reactivity for granule markers like Grimelius silver, lead hematoxylin, chromogranins A and B, synaptophysin, or PGP9.5 exceeds hormone immunoreactivities. This suggests defective hormone biosynthesis by tumor cells, even when they retain, to some extent, the ability to produce and store secretory granules, as shown by parallel electron microscopy investigations. Electron microscopy can help diagnose well-granulated tumors, but is usually of no help in diagnosing poorly granulated tumors apart from confirming their endocrine nature (fig. 5-43).

The same general criteria used for endocrine tumors can distinguish benign from malignant nonfunctioning tumors (see Criteria for Malignancy, chapter 4). In particular, size below 2 cm, well-defined histologic structure and cytologic differentiation (high granularity), absence of mitoses or angioinvasion, and less than 2 percent Ki-67 nuclear antigen expression were distinctive markers of adenomas in our series of nonfunctioning tumors. Malignant potential was indicated by size above 4 cm; angioinvasion and invasion of perineural spaces; mitoses above 3 per 10 high-power fields; and 7 percent or more Ki-67 antigen expression. However, tumor behavior remained uncertain in 15 percent of our cases, which showed features in between those of benign and malignant cases (215a).

**Prognosis and Treatment.** Small (less than 3 cm) nonfunctioning tumors with well-granulated, hormone-rich cells have a favorable prognosis. On the contrary, larger tumors having a prevalence of poorly granulated, hormone-poor cells are usually of low-grade malignancy. These

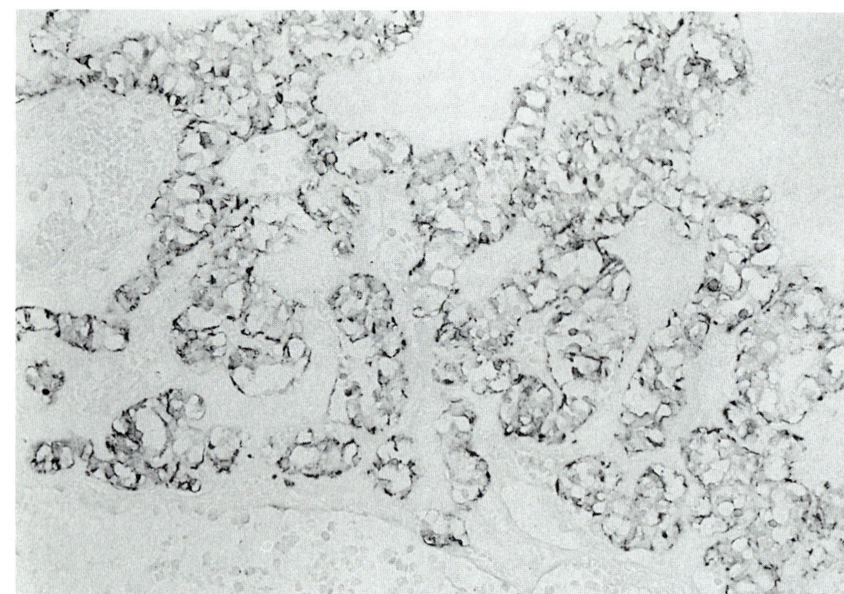

Figure 5-45
PANCREATIC NONFUNCTIONING ENDOCRINE TUMOR

There is intense immunostaining for pancreatic polypeptide (PP).

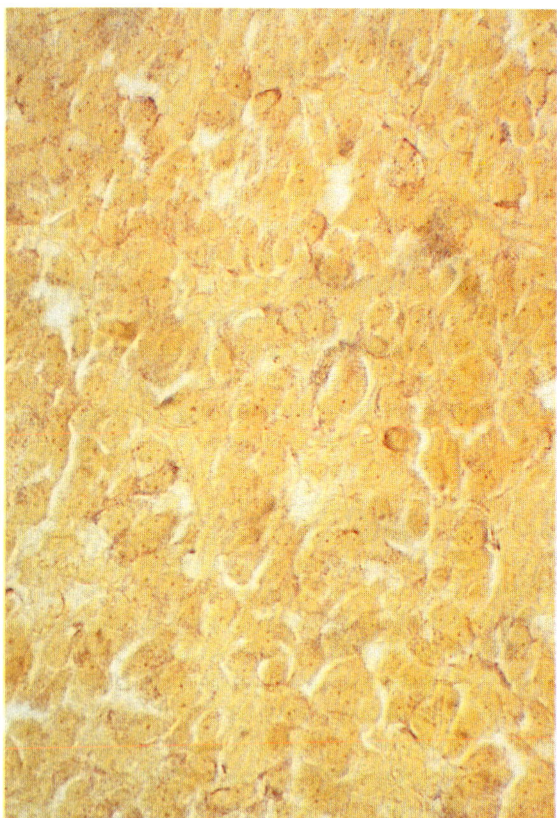

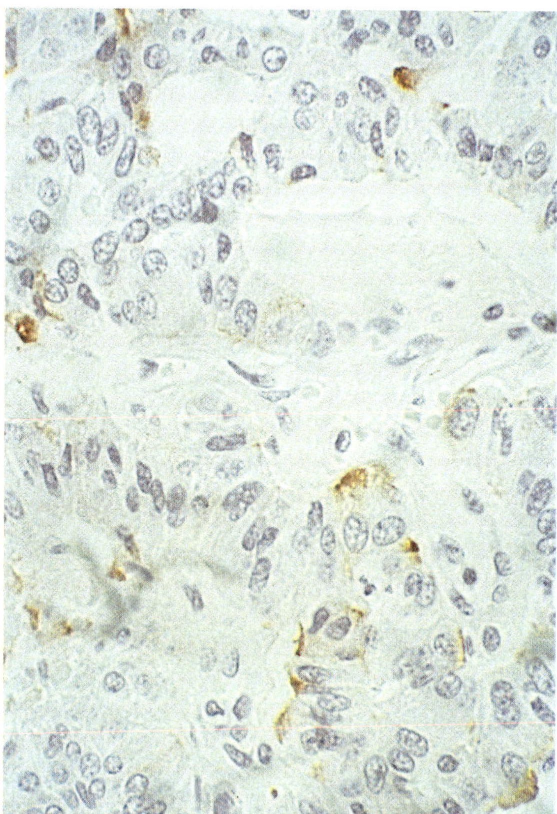

Figure 5-46
NONFUNCTIONING ENDOCRINE CARCINOMA

Left: Scattered Grimelius-positive tumor cells in a nonfunctioning malignant neoplasm metastatic to regional lymph nodes.

Right: The field shown is stained for chromogranin A with the immunoperoxidase technique. Few cells show granular cytoplasmic staining.

are slow-growing tumors which, whenever possible, should be treated by appropriate resection. Approximately 60 percent respond to streptozotocin and fluorouracil therapy (206,218). The mean survival time of patients with nonfunctioning pancreatic endocrine carcinoma ranges from 23 months to 4.3 years, longer than that of malignant functioning tumors from the same series (208,210). However, according to Venkatesh et al. (225), when matched for age, sex, and extent of disease, survival does not differ significantly between functioning and nonfunctioning carcinomas. The 10-year survival rate for all tumors (benign and malignant) is 55 percent for nonfunctioning lesions, 68 percent for gastrinomas, and 92 percent for insulinomas, due to the high incidence of benign growth among the latter tumors (207).

**PP-Cell Tumors.** Most tumors mainly composed of PP immunoreactive cells (fig. 5-45), with or without other subsets of hormone-producing cells, are nonfunctioning. Occasionally, PP-cell tumors with increased PP serum levels have been reported in association with a watery diarrhea, hypokalemia, and achlorhydria (WDHA) syndrome undistinguishable from that usually associated with VIP-producing tumors (216,222). However, no evidence supports a role for PP in the pathogenesis of the diarrheogenic syndrome and the possibility remains that concomitant VIP or prostaglandin E2 secretion by the same tumor is involved. Indeed, large PP-cell tumors producing extremely high PP serum levels have been reported in the absence of any sign of endocrine hyperfunction (223). No distinctive "PPoma syndrome" has been identified so far, and the diagnosis of "PP cell tumor" is preferred to the misleading term "PPoma" used by some authors.

Among PP-cell tumors, clinically silent, well-granulated, prominently trabecular, and small tumors are invariably benign. The few malignant PP-cell tumors observed are usually large (5 cm or larger), histologically more solid, and poorly granulated. In a review by Tomita et al. (224) the mean size of 5 tumors that metastasized was 8.1 cm (range, 4 to 15 cm); that of 3 tumors associated with watery diarrhea, 6.3 cm (range 5 to 9); and that of 7 nonmetastatic nondiarrheogenic tumors, 4.3 cm (0.8 to 15 cm). All tumors less than 2 cm in size were nonmetastatic.

## MULTIPLE ENDOCRINE NEOPLASIA TYPE 1

**Definition.** This disorder is characterized by the synchronous or metachronous development of endocrine lesions involving the parathyroid gland, pancreas, anterior pituitary gland, gastrointestinal tract, and, less commonly, the thymus, lung, thyroid gland, and adrenal gland.

**General Features.** The syndrome may be inherited as an autosomal dominant trait or may occur sporadically as a result of new mutation. The multiple endocrine neoplasia (MEN) 1 gene, probably an antioncogene, has been mapped to the long arm of chromosome 11, at the 11q13 locus (235). Germ-line heterozygous loss of genetic material at this site has been documented in various cells of patients who inherit the MEN 1 trait. Subsequently, acquired somatic mutation of the remaining wild type allele that selectively affects the endocrine cells, leads to their unrestricted proliferation, ultimately resulting in endocrine neoplasia. Increased serum levels of fibroblast growth factor (FGF)–like material have been documented in MEN 1 patients. This factor may promote endocrine growth, especially in the parathyroid gland (228).

Type 1 MEN, or Wermer's syndrome, must be distinguished from another dominantly inherited familial endocrine neoplasia syndrome, type 2 MEN, which involves thyroid calcitonin C cells and the adrenal medulla. The appearance of parathyroid hyperplasia or adenoma, in addition to thyroid medullary carcinoma and pheochromocytoma, rather than ocular, mucocutaneous, and gastrointestinal ganglioneuromas distinguishes type 2A MEN, or Sipple's syndrome, from type 2B (or 3) MEN. An inherited germ-line mutation involving chromosome 10 may be the initial event in MEN 2.

**Incidence.** The prevalence of type 1 MEN in the general population is unknown. Features suggestive of the syndrome have been found in 0.25 percent of unselected autopsies (238). The average age at clinical presentation is the third to fourth decade. In individuals with an established diagnosis of MEN 1, 90 to 97 percent have hyperparathyroidism, 30 to 80 percent have evidence of pancreatic endocrine tumors, and 15 to 50 percent have pituitary abnormalities. There is a remarkable variability in clinical manifestations in different kindreds and, less prominently, among individuals of the same kindred (228,230).

**Clinicopathologic Features.** Only tumors arising in the pancreas and gastroduodenal tract are discussed here.

*Pancreas.* The rate of involvement of the various endocrine tissues in the MEN 1 syndrome varies considerably depending upon whether autopsy findings, clinical presentation, or hormone measurements are considered. This is especially true in the pancreas, where up to 100 percent of individuals have evidence of pancreatic involvement, as reported in the autopsy study of Majewski and Wilson (239). Thirty to 80 percent of patients present with evidence of pancreatic tumors. This discrepancy reflects the nonfunctioning nature of many pancreatic neoplasms associated with the syndrome (246).

In fact, small (less than 0.5 cm), clinically silent endocrine tumors are usually numerous in the pancreas of patients having type 1 MEN syndrome, with or without coexistent functioning tumors in the pancreas or elsewhere. Similar to solitary microadenomas found at autopsy, nonfunctioning microadenomas in MEN 1 patients (fig. 5-47) are composed mainly of non-B islet cells, particularly glucagon, and PP cells. In addition to microadenomas, larger, discrete adenomas, composed mainly of PP cells and sometimes of glucagon or insulin cells, have been found. Although increased blood levels of glucagon and PP are frequently detected in such patients, as a rule, related clinical syndromes have seldom or never been observed (233,234,240). Most clinically nonfunctioning pancreatic tumors in patients with MEN 1 syndrome have benign histologic patterns and behavior.

Among the hyperfunctional syndromes of pancreatic origin observed in MEN 1 patients, ZES predominates, followed by insulinoma, VIPoma, glucagonoma, and growth hormone-releasing factor (GRF)–induced acromegaly. Hyperinsulinism has been found in about one fourth of patients. In many cases it was cured by excision of a discrete insulin-producing tumor. However, in MEN cases, a recurrence rate of 42 percent versus 3 percent in patients with sporadic benign insulinoma has been reported (247), a difference probably reflecting the multifocality (rather than higher malignancy) of insulin-producing tumors in the MEN syndrome.

Gastrin hypersecretion has been documented in more than 50 percent of patients with type 1 MEN. In most cases gastrin cells are absent from the microadenomas, even when concomitant hypergastrinemia and ZES were found. Separate, larger pancreatic gastrinomas, usually located in the head, or small duodenal gastrinomas may account for the ZES in these patients. Distal resection of the pancreas in a patient with combined ZES/MEN 1 syndromes is more likely to remove benign, clinically nonfunctioning A- or PP-cell adenomas than potentially malignant gastrin-producing tumors causing the ZES. Direct evidence of gastrin production by body-tail tumors should be a prerequisite for such surgery. Interestingly, there seems to be a lower potential for metastatic spread and a better survival rate for patients with gastrinoma associated with the MEN 1 syndrome compared to those with sporadic gastrinoma (248).

*Duodenum.* Little information is available on the prevalence of extrapancreatic gastrinomas in MEN patients. A high prevalence rate of duodenal gastrinomas in MEN-associated ZES is suggested by the findings of Pipeleers-Marichal et al. (231, 241). Generally, duodenal gastrin cell tumors are small nodules arising in the deep crypts or Brunner glands and growing in the submucosa (fig. 5-48). Some of them may infiltrate the muscularis propria and give rise to local lymph node metastases; however, as a whole, they seem to be less malignant than corresponding pancreatic tumors. Those coupled with the MEN 1 syndrome are characterized by tumor multifocality as well as hyperplasia (or even dysplasia) of gastrin cells in the intervening nontumor mucosa. Their frequently small size (0.5 cm or less) may prevent effective radiologic, endoscopic, and even surgical detection. Systematic histologic and histochemical investigation of all surgical and biopsy specimens is mandatory in such cases (229,231). Apart from a single, minute PP-cell tumor, no endocrine tumor other than gastrinoma has been reported so far in the duodenum of MEN 1 patients, despite the large endocrine cell population normally present at this site (229).

*Stomach.* Diffuse and micronodular hyperplasia of pyloric gastrin cells has been reported in occasional patients with ZES/MEN 1 syndromes (244). No gastrinoma has been found in the stomach of these patients, although a multifocal antroduodenal tumor was reported in an 11-year-old

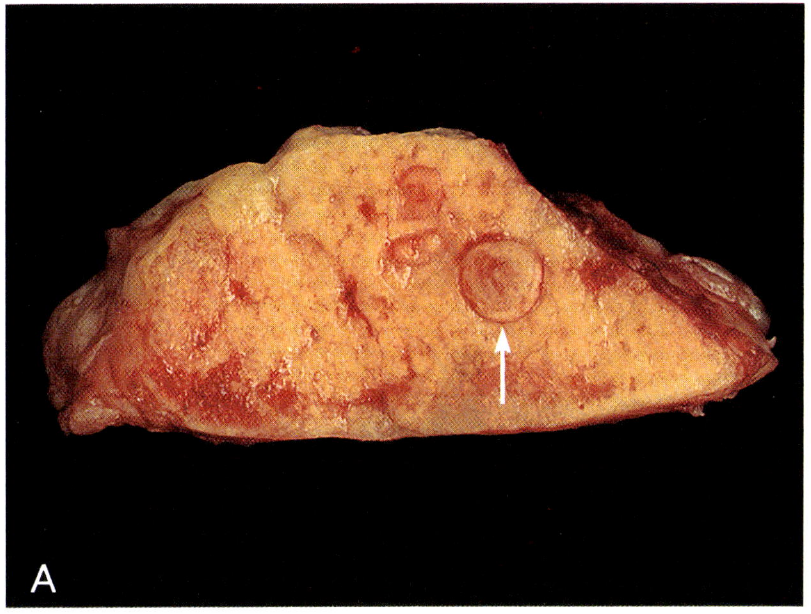


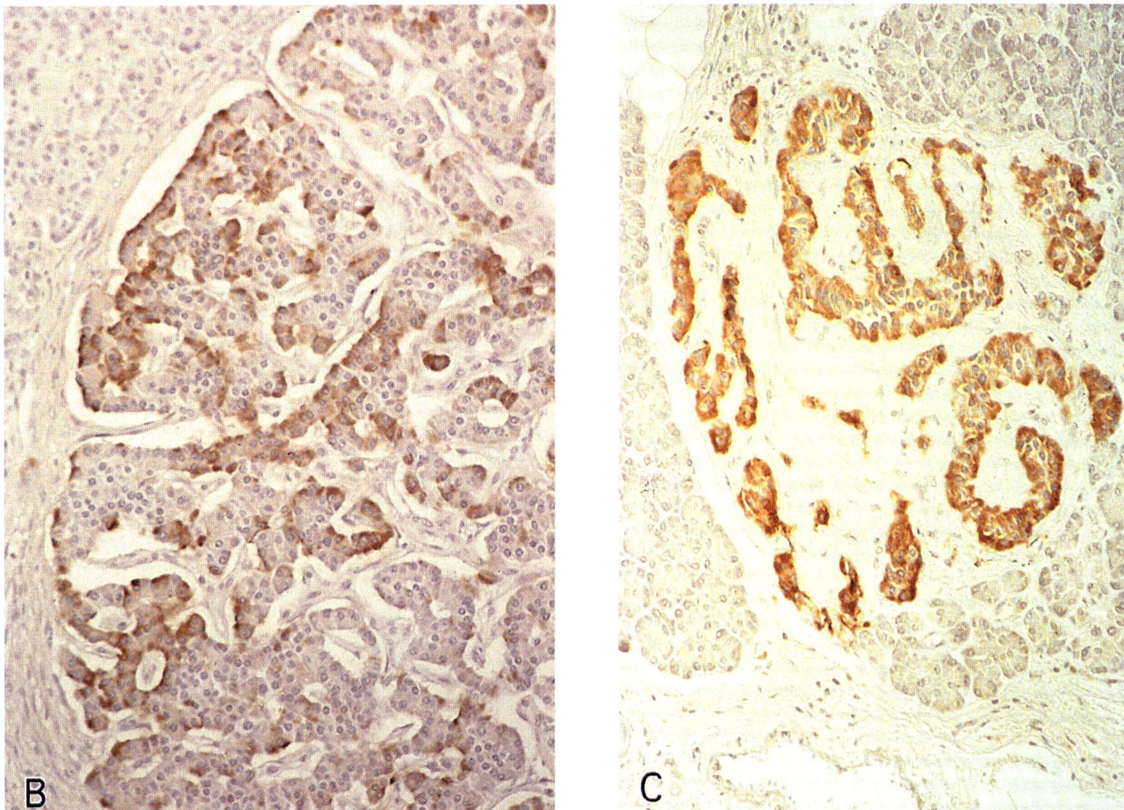


Figure 5-47

PANCREATIC MICROADENOMAS IN PATIENTS WITH MEN 1

A: Nonfunctioning microadenoma of the pancreas (arrow) in a 39-year-old patient with the Zollinger-Ellison syndrome.

B: Nonfunctioning glucagon-producing microadenoma. (Immunoperoxidase technique)

C: Nonfunctioning insulin-producing microadenoma. (Immunoperoxidase technique, insulin-antibodies) (Fig. 1 from Solcia E, Capella C, Fiocca R, Rindi G, Rosai J. Gastric argyrophil carcinoidosis in patients with Zollinger-Ellison syndrome due to type 1 multiple endocrine neoplasia. A newly recognized association. Am J Surg Pathol 1990;14:503–13.)

boy with nonfamilial ZES (226). Patients with gastrin cell hyperplasia and hyperfunction have a positive familial background (232,237). Normal or slightly reduced numbers of gastrin cells have been observed in the antropyloric mucosa of patients with sporadic type ZES.

Diffuse and linear hyperplasia of argyrophil endocrine cells, mainly of enterochromaffin-like (ECL) type, are found regularly in the hypertrophic oxyntic glands of patients with ZES with longstanding severe hypergastrinemia (227,236, 243,244). *Argyrophil ECL cell carcinoids* have been described in a few of these patients, mostly among those with MEN 1 syndrome (236,245). Of 28 patients with argyrophilic carcinoids (mean age 45 years; no sex preference) presently known from personal investigation or review of the literature, 24 had proven MEN 1 with at least hyperparathyroidism in addition to ZES, 2 had unassessed MEN status, and only 2 had apparently sporadic ZES (242). As MEN/ZES accounts for one fourth to one fifth of all ZES cases, it seems clear that the argyrophil carcinoids are closely linked to MEN/ZES, and occur in 10 to 20 percent of such cases (236,242). Indeed, both severe, longstanding hypergastrinemia and the genetic trait inherent to MEN 1 syndrome are required for the genesis of such tumors (245).

Nearly all argyrophil carcinoids in MEN/ZES are multiple and associated with innumerable, minute intramucosal growths (microcarcinoidosis): 25 percent are intramucosal, 70 percent mucosal-submucosal, and one case infiltrated the muscularis propria. Only 3 cases (12 percent) were metastatic, all to local lymph nodes; no patient developed the carcinoid syndrome; and no patient died because of the carcinoid tumor. Tumor nodules range from 0.5 mm to 4 cm (median, 5 to 6 mm). They appear as sessile polypoid lesions covered with normal, hyperplastic, or eroded mucosa and may be difficult to detect macroscopically due to the often coexisting enlarged gastric folds (figs. 5-49, 5-50) (236,245). Microscopically, a regular growth of small to medium-sized, uniform cells arranged in minute solid microlobules or microtubules, or thin trabeculae separated by scarce, fairly vascular stroma is found in most cases (figs. 5-51, 5-52). Only occasional mitoses (0 to 0.1 per high-power field) are observed, and cellular atypia is mild. Intense argyrophilia with Grimelius or Sevier-Munger silver stains and chromogranin A immunoreactivity in the absence of (or with only a few) gastrin, somatostatin, and serotonin immunoreactive cells are distinctive features of these gastric body-fundus argyrophil carcinoids, whose ECL cell nature can only be ascertained by electron microscopy (fig. 5-53) or histamine immunohistochemistry.

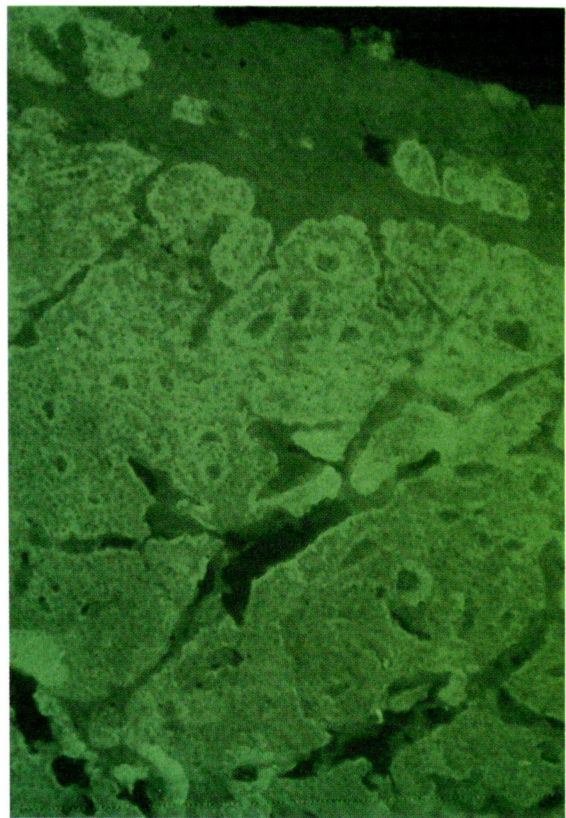

Figure 5-48
GUT TUMORS IN MEN 1–ASSOCIATED ZES
Duodenal gastrinoma arising in the deep crypts of the mucosa and invading the submucosa deeply. (Immunofluorescence technique)

## POORLY DIFFERENTIATED (SMALL CELL) CARCINOMA

**Definition.** Small cell carcinoma is a poorly differentiated pancreatic tumor composed of small to intermediate-sized cells with endocrine features.

Until recently, small cell carcinomas were classified as exocrine tumors (250,256,258). Recent investigations, however, have disclosed variable degrees of reactivity for hormones or endocrine markers in these tumors, and some patients have

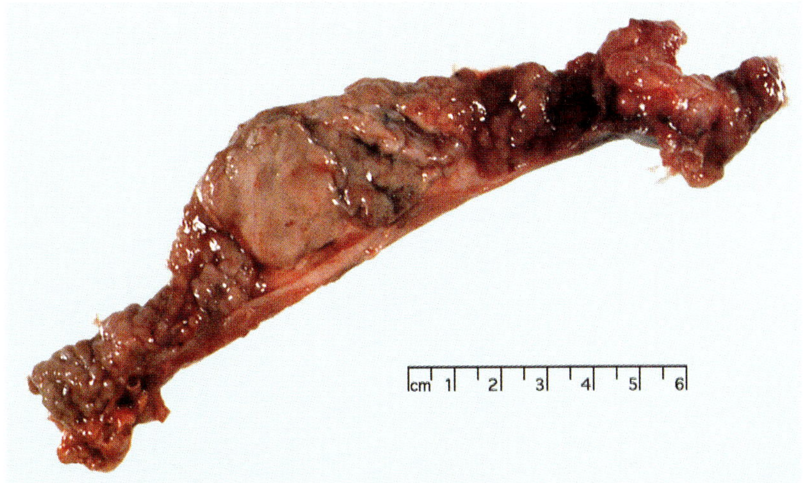


Figure 5-49
GUT TUMORS IN
MEN 1–ASSOCIATED ZES

Cut section of this hypertrophic gastropathy specimen reveals intramucosal tumor nodules. (Courtesy of Dr Juan Rosai, Memorial Sloan-Kettering Cancer Center, New York.)

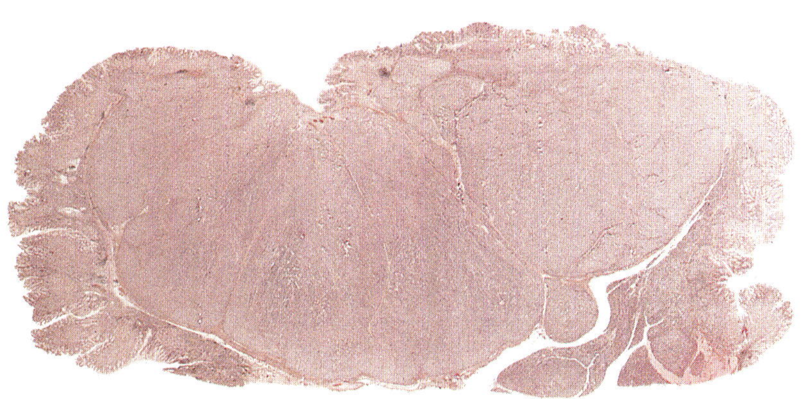

Figure 5-50
GUT TUMORS IN
MEN 1–ASSOCIATED ZES

Low magnification histology of one of the tumor nodules from the same case shown in figure 5-49. The tumor nodule is surrounded by hypertrophic (left and right) and eroded (top) mucosa. (Courtesy of Dr Juan Rosai, Memorial Sloan-Kettering Cancer Center, New York.)

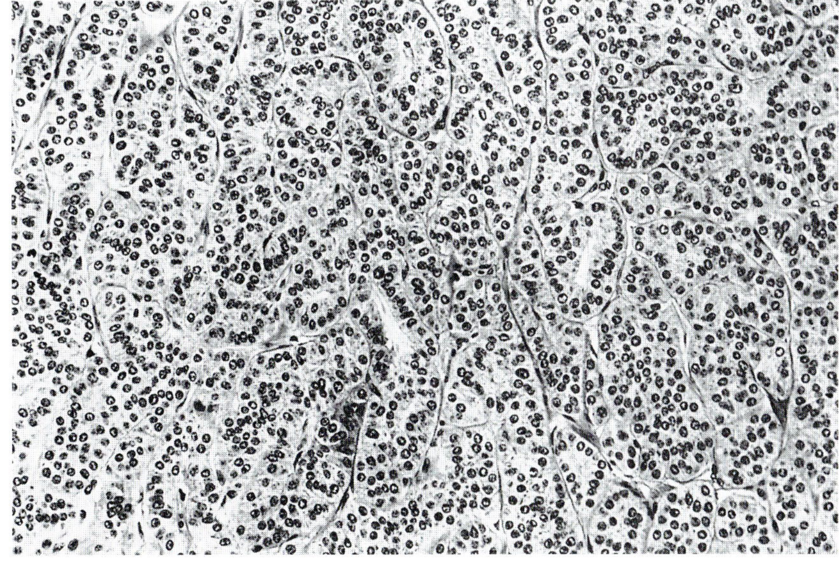

Figure 5-51
GASTRIC CARCINOID IN
MEN 1–ASSOCIATED ZES

Mosaic-like pattern of solid cords and microlobules separated by very thin stromal septa.

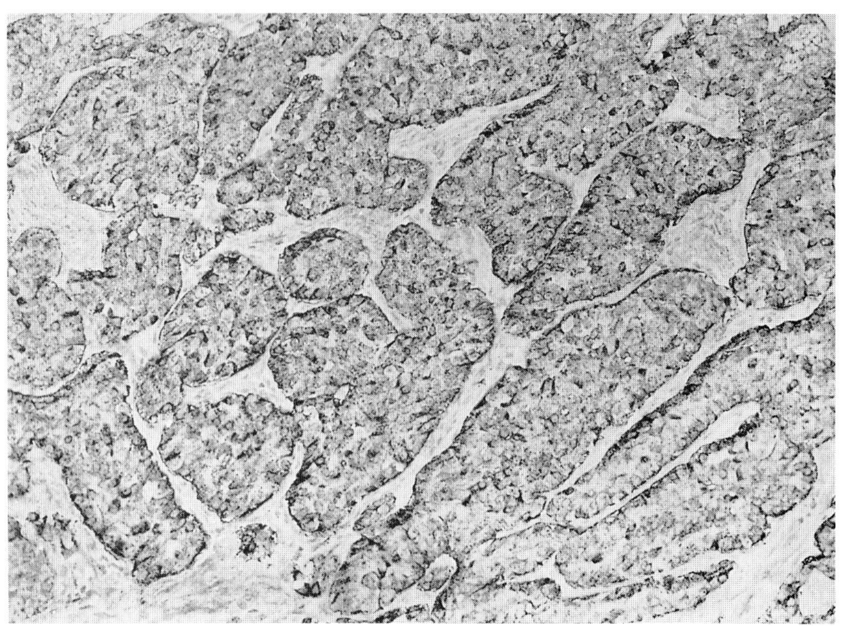

Figure 5-52
ARGYROPHILIA OF GASTRIC CARCINOID IN MEN 1–ASSOCIATED ZES

Note the intense and diffuse staining of tumor cells with Grimelius silver. (Fig. 7 from Solcia E, Bordi C, Creutzeldt W, et al. Histopathological classification of nonantral gastric endocrine growths in man. Digestion 1988;41:185–200.)

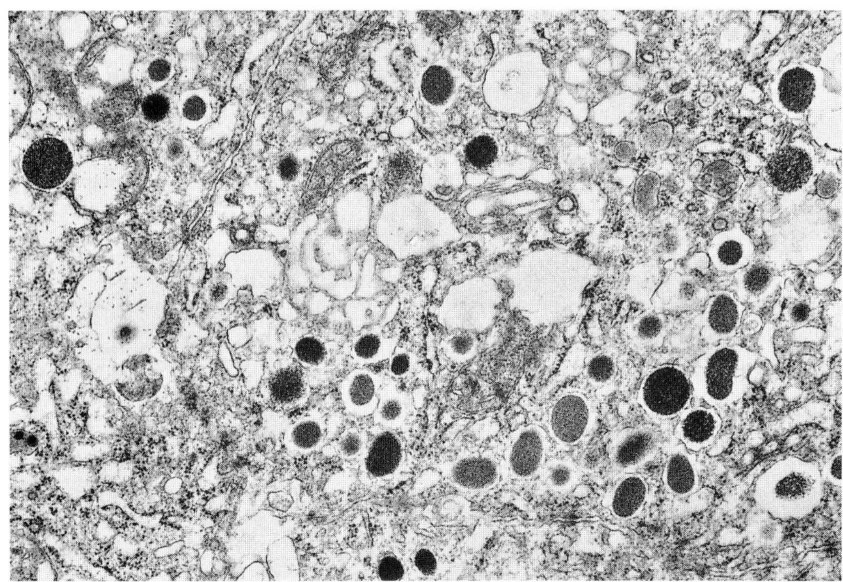

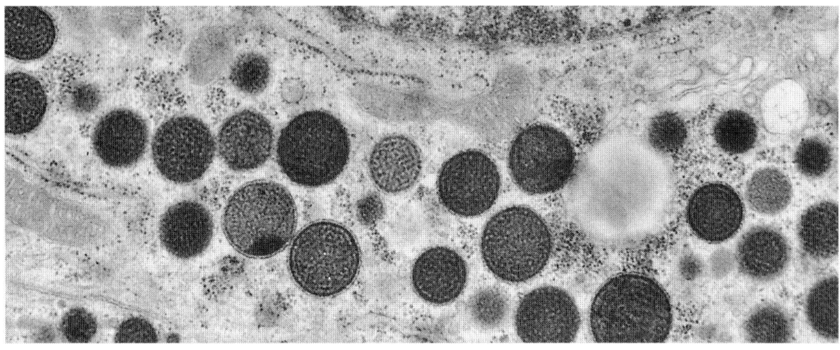

Figure 5-53
ELECTRON MICROSCOPY OF ARGYROPHIL GASTRIC CARCINOID

ECL-type vesicular granules (top) and solid granules (bottom) with cerebroid punctate structure (atypical ECL cell granules?) in gastric carcinoids.

increased serum levels of such substances and ultrastructural features indicating scattered or abortive endocrine differentiation. Additionally, small cell carcinomas lack reactivity for markers of exocrine tumors (249,253,254,259). Therefore, it seems more appropriate to consider this tumor as a poorly differentiated endocrine carcinoma. Its morphology and natural history closely resemble those of pulmonary and extrapulmonary small to intermediate cell carcinomas showing evidence of poor endocrine differentiation, so-called neuroendocrine carcinomas.

**Incidence.** Poorly differentiated, small to intermediate cell endocrine carcinomas make up about 1 percent of all pancreatic malignant tumors (257) and about 2 to 3 percent of all pancreatic endocrine tumors from surgical series (260).

**Clinical Features.** Small cell carcinoma occurs predominantly in men aged between 40 and 75 years (257,258). The patient usually presents with symptoms of advanced malignant disease, including weight loss, jaundice, and metastases. Paraneoplastic hormonal syndromes, which are relatively common in pulmonary small cell carcinoma, are rare in pancreatic tumors. To date, only one ACTH-producing tumor and a tumor associated with hypercalcemia have been reported (249,253). However, occasional tumors associated with carcinoid syndrome and short survival, which were reported as pancreatic carcinoid tumors (251,252), showed histologic features suggestive of small to intermediate cell carcinoma.

The tumors can be detected easily with ultrasonography and CT coupled with fine-needle biopsy. Among tumor markers that can be detected in serum, excessive levels of neuron-specific enolase (NSE) have been observed (257).

**Gross Findings.** The tumors are usually large by the time they are diagnosed (mean diameter, 4.2 cm), and are poorly demarcated. On cut surface, they are grey-white and show areas of necrosis and hemorrhage. Most tumors are located in the head of the pancreas and invade adjacent organs. Metastases are widespread and may involve intra- and extra-abdominal sites (258), a pattern contrasting with the essentially intra-abdominal (liver plus regional lymph nodes) metastases of differentiated endocrine carcinomas.

**Histologic, Histochemical, and Ultrastructural Findings.** The histologic appearance of the tumor (figs. 5-54, 5-55) is indistinguishable from that of small cell carcinoma of the lung. There are sheets and nests of small to medium-sized cells with markedly hyperchromatic round to oval nuclei, inconspicuous nucleoli, and poorly defined cytoplasmic borders. Occasional areas with glandular differentiation may be present (249). In addition, there may be trabecular arrangements within a delicate fibrous stroma. Mitoses are numerous (more than 10 per 10 high-power fields), 10 percent or more of the cells express Ki-67 or PCNA proliferative markers, and there are degenerative changes with widespread or multifocal areas of necrosis. The center of solid nests is a preferred site of focal necrosis. At the ultrastructural level, tumor cells contain small amounts of granular endoplasmic reticulum, fairly abundant scattered ribosomes, bundles of intermediate filaments and, as the most diagnostic feature, membrane-bound electron-dense granules measuring 100 to 200 nm in diameter. Small cell carcinomas are negative for mucin stains. Their diffuse, fairly intense reactivity for cytosolic neuroendocrine markers such as NSE (fig. 5-55B), synaptophysin, or PGP9.5 contrasts with their moderate to scarce, often focal and scanty reactivity with granule markers such as chromogranins or Grimelius silver, and their usually poor (fig. 5-55C) or absent immunostaining for hormonal products, among which calcitonin and ACTH have been occasionally detected (257,259). Extensive nuclear accumulation of p53 oncoprotein is a frequent finding in pancreatic as well as nonpancreatic small cell carcinomas. Globular perinuclear immunostaining for keratin may also be found.

Based on the relative abundance of cytoplasm, cytoplasmic organelles, secretory granules, and granule marker immunoreactivity, and on the frequent presence of hormone immunoreactivity, an intermediate cell variant may be separated from truly small cell carcinoma. Occasional tumors associated with an endocrine syndrome due to overproduction of ACTH, parathirin, vasopressin, or serotonin fit in the intermediate cell subgroup.

**Differential Diagnosis.** The diagnosis of small cell carcinoma of the pancreas is made after the possibility of metastasis of the same type of tumor originating from other sites, especially from the lung, is excluded (254). As the small cell carcinoma of bronchogenic and extrapulmonary origin share the same histologic features, diagnosis of a primary small cell carcinoma of the

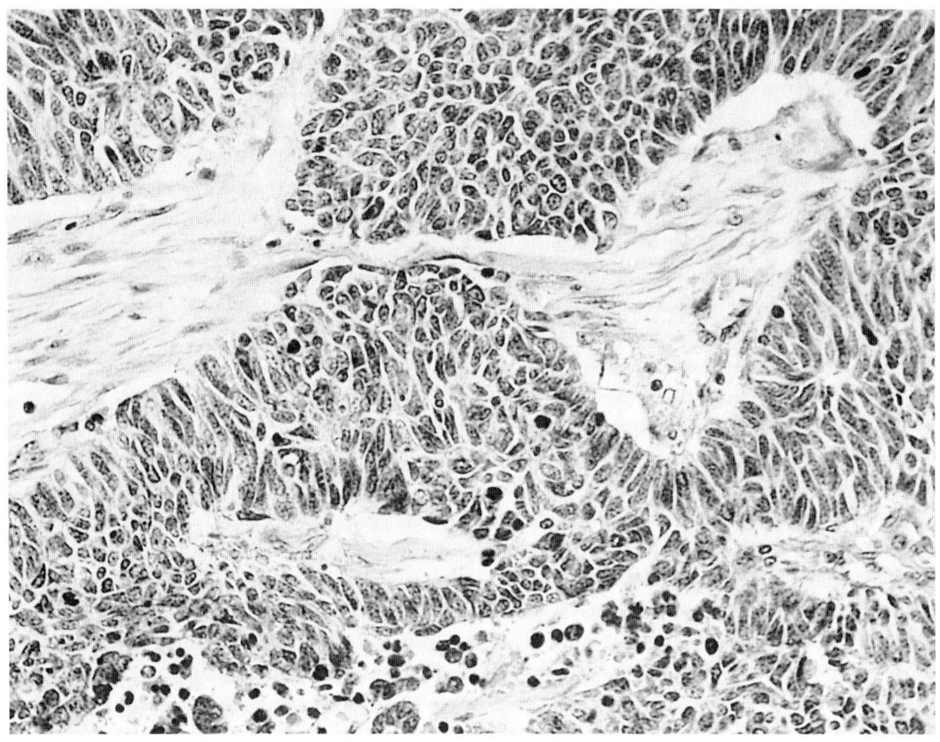

Figure 5-54
POORLY DIFFERENTIATED ENDOCRINE CARCINOMA
Intermediate cell endocrine carcinoma showing a large number of poorly differentiated fusiform cells and focal necrosis.

pancreas relies entirely on the exclusion of a primary tumor outside the pancreas. This is, in most cases, only possible by a meticulous postmortem examination.

The intermediate cell variant of small cell carcinoma may show a trabecular arrangement of cells with fairly abundant cytoplasm, thus mimicking the histology of some low-grade, well-differentiated pancreatic endocrine tumors. In this case, the presence of prominent nuclear atypia, focal cellular degeneration, and necrosis (especially in the center of solid nests); a mitotic rate of more than 10 per 10 high-power fields; more than 10 percent Ki-67 or PCNA positive cells; and extensive nuclear p53 accumulation are diagnostic for intermediate cell carcinoma, whereas abundance of secretory granules and related markers (chromogranins, silver stains) or hormones point to low-grade tumors. However, paucity of secretory granules and poor reactivity for granule markers and hormones are of no value per se in assessing the grade of malignant nonfunctioning tumors.

Small cell carcinoma of the pancreas may be confused histologically with non-Hodgkin's lymphoma. The latter neoplasm, however, is distinguished by a positive immunoreaction to common leukocyte antigen and negative staining for keratin, a marker constellation that is reversed in small cell carcinoma.

**Prognosis and Survival.** All small cell carcinomas described so far presented with metastases to the liver, lymph nodes, and other organs or invasion to adjacent tissues. As tumor resection was impossible in these instances, the patients were treated by chemotherapy, which resulted in partial and even complete tumor remission (with up to 50 months' survival), particularly when etoposide and cisplatin were used (255,257). When patients with small cell carcinomas of the pancreas received supportive treatment only, prognosis was poor, with a survival between 1 and 2 months. Patients with tumors fitting in the intermediate cell group and associated with hyperfunctional syndromes had slightly longer survival periods of 6 months to 1 year (251,252).

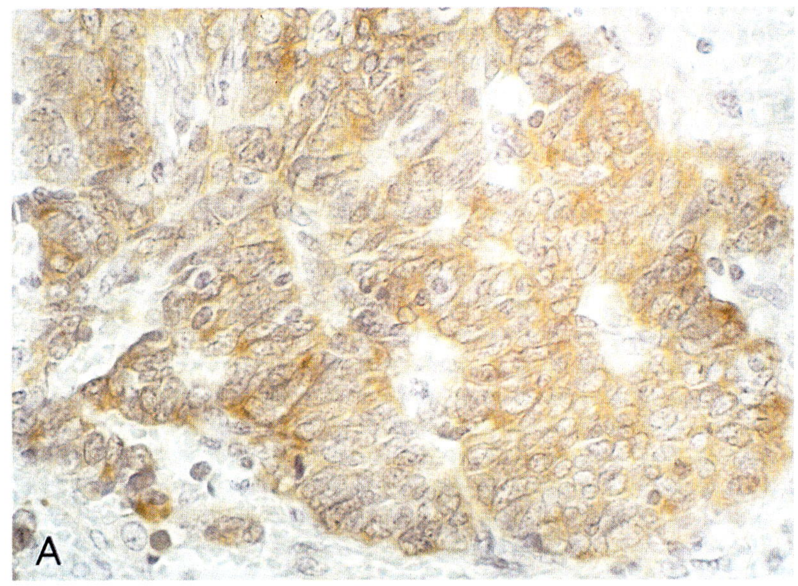


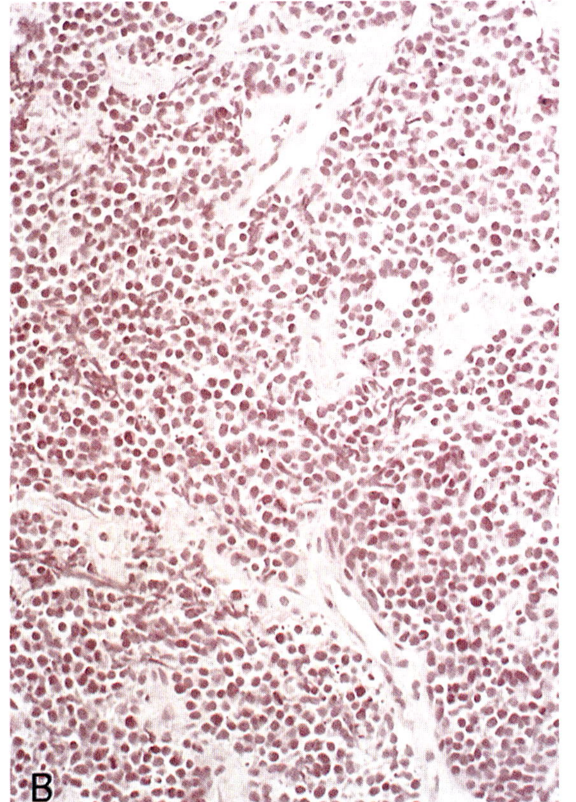


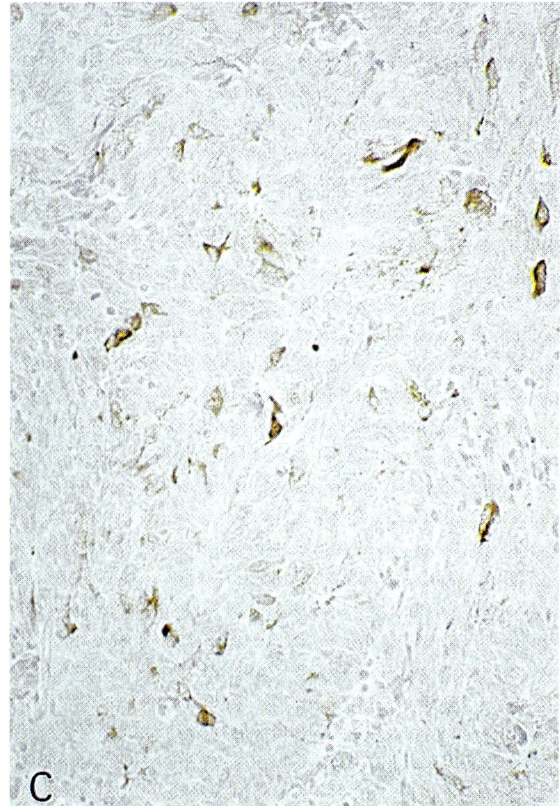


Figure 5-55
SMALL CELL CARCINOMA

A: Intense immunostaining for NSE in an intermediate cell endocrine carcinoma.
B: Solid-diffuse pattern in a small cell endocrine carcinoma.
C: Scattered somatostatin-immunoreactive cells in the same tumor shown in A.

## REFERENCES

### Differentiated Endocrine Tumors


1. Alanen KA, Joensun H, Klemi PJ, Marin D, Alavaikko M, Nevalainen TJ. DNA ploidy in pancreatic neuroendocrine tumors. Am J Clin Pathol 1990;93:784–8.
2. Bartow SA, Mukai K, Rosai J. Pseudoneoplastic proliferation of endocrine cells in pancreatic fibrosis. Cancer 1981;47:2627–33.
3. Bordi C, Bussolati G. Immunofluorescence, histochemical and ultrastructural studies for the detection of multiple endocrine polypeptide tumors of the pancreas. Virchows Arch [Cell Pathol] 1974;17:13–27.
4. Bordi C, Pilato FP, D'Adda T. Comparative study of seven neuroendocrine markers in pancreatic endocrine tumors. Virchows Arch [A] 1988;413:387–98.
5. Boschetti AE, Maloney WC. Observations on pancreatic islet cell and other radiation-induced tumors in the rat. Lab Invest 1966;15:565–75.
6. Broder LE, Carter SK. Pancreatic islet cell carcinoma. I. Clinical features of 52 patients. Am Intern Med 1973;79:101–7.
7. Buchanan KD, Johnson CF, O'Hare M, et al. Neuroendocrine tumors. A European view. Am J Med 1986;81(Suppl 6B):14–22.
8. Buffa R, Rindi G, Sessa F, et al. Synaptophysin immunoreactivity and small clear vesicles in neuroendocrine cells and related tumors. Mole Cell Probes 1987;1:367–81.
9. Capella C, Heitz PU, Höfler H, Solcia E, Klöppel G. Revised classification of neuroendocrine tumors of the lung, pancreas and gut. Virchows Arch [A] 1995;425:547–60.
10. Carlei F, Polak JM. Antibodies to neuron-specific enolase for the delineation of the entire diffuse neuroendocrine system in health and disease. Semin Diagn Pathol 1984;1:59.
11. Carney CN. Congenital insulinoma (nesidioblastoma): ultrastructural evidence for histogenesis from pancreatic ductal epithelium. Arch Pathol Lab Med 1976;100:352–6.
12. Chejfec G, Falkmer S, Grimelius L, et al. Synaptophysin. A new marker for pancreatic neuroendocrine tumors. Am J Surg Pathol 1987;11:241–7.
13. Clark ES, Carney JA. Pancreatic islet cell tumor associated with Cushing's syndrome. Am J Surg Pathol 1984;8:917–24.
14. Corallini A, Pagnani M, Viadana P, et al. Association of BK virus with human brain tumors and tumors of pancreatic islets. Int J Cancer 1987;39:60–7.
15. Cubilla AL, Hajdu SI. Islet cell carcinoma of the pancreas. Arch Pathol 1975;99:204–7.
16. Dahms BB, Lippe BM, Dakake C, Fonkalsurd EW, Mirra JM. The occurrence in a neonate of a pancreatic adenoma with nesidioblastosis in the tumor. Am J Clin Pathol 1976;65:462–6.
17. Danforth DN Jr, Gorden P, Brennan MF. Metastatic insulin-secreting carcinoma of the pancreas: clinical course and the role of surgery. Surgery 1984;96:1027–37.
18. Eberle F, Grun R. Multiple endocrine neoplasia, type I (MEN I). Erge Inn Med Kinderheil 1981;46:76–149.
19. Frantz VK. Tumors of the pancreas. Atlas of Tumor Pathology, 1st Series, Fascicle 27-28. Washington, D.C.: Armed Forces Institute of Pathology, 1959:79–149.
20. Friesen SR. Treatment of the Zollinger-Ellison syndrome: a 25 year assessment. Am J Surg 1982;143:331–8.
21. Gordis L, Gold EB. Epidemiology and etiology of pancreatic cancer. In: Go VL, Gardner JD, Brooks FP, Lebenthal E, DiMagno EP, Scheele EP, eds. The exocrine pancreas: biology, pathology and diseases. New York: Raven Press, 1986:621–36.
22. Goossens A, Heitz PU, Klöppel G. Pancreatic endocrine cells and their non-neoplastic proliferations. In: Dayal Y, ed. Endocrine pathology of the gut and pancreas. Boca Raton: CRC Press, 1991:69–104.
23. Goudswaard WB, Houthoff HJ, Koudstaal J, Zwierstra RP. Nesidioblastosis and endocrine hyperplasia of the pancreas: a secondary phenomenon. Hum Pathol 1986;17:46–54.
24. Greider MH, Rosai J, McGuigan JE. The human pancreatic islet cells and their tumors. II. Ulcerogenic and diarrheogenic tumors. Cancer 1974;33:1423–43.
25. Grimelius L, Hultquist GT, Stenkvist B. Cytological differentiation of asymptomatic pancreatic islet cell tumors in autopsy material. Virchows Arch [A] 1975;365;275–88.
26. Hanahan D. Heritable formation of pancreatic B-cell tumors in transgenic mice expressing recombinant insulin simian virus 40 oncogenes. Nature 1985;315:115–22.
27. Heitz PU. Pancreatic endocrine tumours. In: Klöppel G, Heitz PU, eds. Pancreatic pathology. Edinburgh: Churchill-Livingstone, 1984:206 32.
28. Heitz PU, Kasper M, Klöppel G, Polak JM, Vaitukaitis JL. Glycoprotein-hormone alpha-chain production by pancreatic endocrine tumors: a specific marker for malignancy. Immunocytochemical analysis of tumors of 155 patients. Cancer 1983;51:277–82.
29. Heitz PU, Kasper M, Polak JM, Klöppel G. Pancreatic endocrine tumors. Hum Pathol 1982;13:263–71.
30. Höfler H, Denk H, Lackinger E, Helleis G, Polak JM, Heitz PU. Immunocytochemical demonstration of intermediate filament cytoskeleton proteins in human endocrine tissues and (neuro-) endocrine tumours. Virchows Arch [A] 1986;409:609–26.
31. Höfler H, Ruhri C, Putz B, Wirnsberger G, Hauser H. Oncogene expression in endocrine pancreatic tumors. Virchow Arch [Cell Pathol] 1988;55:355–61.
32. Howard JN, Moss NH, Rhoads JE. Collective review: hyperinsulinism and islet cell tumors of the pancreas. Int Abstr Surg 1950;90:417–55.
33. Kenny BD, Sloan JM, Hamilton PW, Watt PC, Johnston CF, Buchanan KD. The role of morphometry in predicting prognosis in pancreatic islet cell tumors. Cancer 1989;64:460–5.

33a. Kimura N, Yonekura H, Okamoto H, Nagura H. Expression of human regenerating gene mRNA and its product in normal and neoplastic human pancreas. Cancer 1992;70:1857–63.

34. Kimura W, Kuroda A, Morioka Y. Clinical pathology of endocrine tumors of the pancreas. Analysis of autopsy cases. Dig Dis Sc 1991;36:933–42.
35. Klimstra DS, Heffess CS, Oertel JE, Rosai J. Acinar cell carcinoma of the pancreas. A clinicopathologic study of 28 cases. Am J Surg Pathol 1992;16:815–37.

36. Klöppel G, Heitz PU. Pancreatic endocrine tumors in man. In: Polak JM, ed. Diagnostic histopathology of neuroendocrine tumors. Edinburg: Churchill Livingstone, 1993:91–121.
37. Kümmerle F, Rückert K. Chirurgie des endokrinen Pancreas in der Bundesrepublik: Ergebnis einer Umfrage. Dtsch Med Wochenschr 1978;103:729–32.
37a. La Rosa S, Sessa F, Capella C, et al. Prognostic criteria in nonfunctioning pancreatic endocrine tumors. Virchows Arch, 1996;429:323–33.
38. Liu HM, Potter EL. Development of the human pancreas. Arch Pathol 1962;74:439–52.
39. Madsen OD, Larsson LI, Rehfeld JF, et al. Cloned cell lines from a transplantable islet cell tumor are heterogeneous and express cholecystokinin in addition to islet hormones. J Cell Biol 1986;103:2025–34.
40. Majewski JT, Wilson SD. The MEN-I syndrome: an all or none phenomenon. Surgery 1979;86:475–84.
41. Margolis RM, Jang N. Zollinger-Ellison syndrome associated with pancreatic cystadenocarcinoma [Letter]. N Engl J Med 1984;2:1380–1.
42. Moldow RE, Connelly RR. Epidemiology of pancreatic cancer in Connecticut. Gastroenterology 1968;55:677–86.
43. Morohoshi T, Kanda M, Horie A, et al. Immunocytochemical markers of uncommon pancreatic tumors. Acinar cell carcinoma, pancreatoblastoma and solid-cystic (papillary-cystic) tumor. Cancer 1987;59:739–47.
44. Mount SL, Weaver DL, Taatjes DJ, McKinnon WC, Herbert JC. Von Hippel-Lindau disease presenting as pancreatic neuroendocrine tumor. Virchows Arch 1995;426:523–28.
45. Mukai K, Grotting JC, Greider MH, Rosai J. Retrospective study of 77 pancreatic endocrine tumors using the immunoperoxidase method. Am J Surg Pathol 1982;6:387–99.
46. Nauck M, Creutzfeldt W. Insulin producing tumors and the insulinoma syndrome. In: Dayal Y, ed. Endocrine pathology of the gut and pancreas. Boca Raton: CRC Press, 1991:195–225.
47. Nieuwenhuijzen Kruseman AC, Knijnenburg G, Brutel De La Riviere G, Bosman FT. Morphology and immunohistochemically-defined endocrine function of pancreatic islet cells tumours. Histopathology 1978;2:389–99.
48. Okamoto H. Rig and reg: novel genes activated in insulinomas and in regenerating islets. In: Larkins RG, Zimmet PZ, Chisholm DJ, eds. Excerpta Medica Congress Series. Amsterdam: Elsevier, 1989:55-64.
49. Pellegata NS, Sessa F, Renault B, et al. K-ras and p53 gene mutation in pancreatic cancer: ductal and nonductal tumors progress through different genetic lesions. Cancer Res 1994;54:1556–60.
50. Pelosi G, Zamboni G, Doglioni C, et al. Immunodetection of proliferating cell nuclear antigen assesses the growth fraction and predicts malignancy in endocrine tumors of the pancreas. Am J Surg Pathol 1992;16:1215–25.
51. Perez MA, Saul HS, Trojanowski JQ. Neurofilament and chromogranin expression in normal and neoplastic neuroendocrine cells of the human gastrointestinal tract and pancreas. Cancer 1990;65:1219–27.
52. Perkins PL, McLeod MK, Fukuuchi A, Cho KJ, Thomson NW, Lloyd RV. Analysis of gastrinomas by immunohistochemistry and in situ hybridization histochemistry. Diagn Mol Pathol 1992;1:155–64.
53. Porter MR, Frantz VK. Tumors associated with hypoglycemia—pancreatic and extrapancreatic. Am J Med 1956;21:944–61.
54. Probst A, Lotz M, Heitz PU. Von Hippel-Lindau's disease, syringomyelia and multiple endocrine tumours: a complex neuroendocrinopathy. Virchows Arch [A] 1978;378:265–72.
55. Rakieten N, Gordon BS, Beaty A, Cooney DA, Davis RD, Schein PS. Pancreatic islet cell tumors produced by the combined action of streptozotocin and nicotinamide. Proc Soc Exp Biol 1971;137:260-73.
56. Reubi JC, Hacki WH, Lamberts SW. Hormone-producing gastrointestinal tumors contain a high density of somatostatin receptors. J Clin Endocrinol Metab 1987;65:1127–34.
57. Rindi G, Bishop AE, Murphy D, Solcia E, Hogan B, Polak JM. A morphological analysis of endocrine tumor genesis in pancreas and anterior pituitary of AVP/SV40 transgenic mice. Virchows Arch [A] 1988;412:255–66.
58. Rindi G, Buffa R, Sessa F, Tortora O, Solcia E. Chromogranin A, B and C immunoreactivities of mammalian endocrine cells. Distribution, distinction from costored hormones/prohormones and relationship with the argyrophil component of secretory granules. Histochemistry 1986;85:19–28.
59. Rindi G, Efrat S, Ghatei MA, Bloom SR, Solcia E, Polak JM. Glucagonomas of transgenic mice express a wide range of general neuroendocrine markers and bioactive peptides. Virchows Arch [A] 1991;419:115–29.
60. Rode J, Dhillon AP, Doran JF. PGP9.5, a new marker for human neuroendocrine tumours. Histopathology 1985;9:147–58.
61. Rüschoff J, Willemer S, Brunzel M, et al. Nucleolar organizer regions and glycoprotein-hormone alpha-chain reaction as markers of malignancy in endocrine tumors of the pancreas. Histopathology 1993;22:51–7.
62. Ruttmann E, Klöppel G, Bommer G, Kiehn M, Heitz PU. Pancreatic glucagonomas with and without syndrome. Immunocytochemical study of 5 tumour cases and review of the literature. Virchow Arch [A] 1980;388:51–67.
63. Schoental R, Fowler ME, Coady A. Islet cell tumors of the pancreas found in rats given pyrrolizidine alkaloids from Amsinekia intermedia Fisch and Mey and from Heliotropium supinum L. Cancer Res 1970;30:2127–31.
64. Sessa F, Bonato M, Frigerio B, et al. Ductal cancers of the pancreas frequently express markers of gastrointestinal epithelial cells. Gastroenterology, 1990;98:1655–65.
65. Solcia E, Capella C, Buffa R, Tenti P, Rindi G, Cornaggia M. Antigenic markers of neuroendocrine tumors: their diagnostic and prognostic value. In: Fenoglio CM, Weinstein RS, Kaufman N, eds. New concepts in neoplasia as applied to diagnostic pathology. Int Acad Pathol Monograph No 27. Baltimore: Williams & Wilkins, 1986: 242–61.
66. Solcia E, Capella C, Vassallo G. Lead-haematoxylin as a stain of endocrine cells. Significance of staining and comparison with other selective methods. Histochemie 1969;20:116–26.
67. Solcia E, Sessa F, Rindi G, Bonato M, Capella C. Pancreatic endocrine tumors: non-functioning tumors and tumors with uncommon function. In: Dayal Y, ed. Endocrine pathology of the gut and pancreas. Boca Raton: CRC Press, 1991:105–32.
68. Stabile BE, Passaro E Jr. Benign and malignant gastrinoma. Am J Surg 1985;149;144–50.

69. Stefanini P, Carboni M, Patrassi N, Basoli A. Beta-islet cell tumours of the pancreas: results of a statistical study on 1,067 cases collected. Surgery 1974;75:597–609.
70. Viale G, Doglioni C, Gambacorta M, Zamboni G, Coggi G, Bordi C. Progesterone receptor immunoreactivity in pancreatic endocrine tumors. An immunocytochemical study of 156 neuroendocrine tumors of pancreas, gastrointestinal and respiratory tracts, and skin. Cancer 1992;70:2268–77.
71. Volk BH, Wellmann KF, Brancato P. Fine structure of rat islet cell tumors induced by streptozotocin and nicotinamide. Diabetologia 1973;10:37–44.
72. Wilson BS, Lloyd RV. Detection of chromogranin in neuroendocrine cells with a monoclonal antibody. Am J Pathol 1984;115:458–68.

**Insulinoma**

73. Alanen KA, Joensum H, Klemi PJ, Marin D, Alavaikko M, Nevalainen TJ. DNA ploidy in pancreatic neuroendocrine tumors. Am J Clin Pathol 1990;93:784–8.
74. Berger M, Bordi C, Cupper HY, et al. Functional and morphologic characterization of human insulinomas. Diabetes 1983;32:921–31.
75. Broughan TA, Leslie JD, Soto JM, Hermann RE. Pancreatic islet cell tumors. Surgery 1986;99:671–8.
76. Creutzfeldt W, Arnold R, Creutzfeldt C, Deuticke U, Frerichs H, Track NS. Biochemical and morphological investigations of 30 human insulinomas. Correlation between the tumor content of insulin and proinsulin-like components and the histological and ultrastructural appearance. Diabetologia 1973;9:217–31.
77. Danforth DN Jr, Gorden P, Brennan MF. Metastatic insulin-secreting carcinoma of the pancreas: clinical course and the role of surgery. Surgery 1984;96:1027–37.
78. Graeme-Cook F, Bell DA, Flotte TJ, et al. Aneuploidy in pancreatic insulinomas does not predict malignancy. Cancer 1990;66:2365–8.
79. Howard JN, Moss NH, Rhoads JE. Collective review: hyperinsulinism and islet cell tumors of the pancreas. Int Abstr Surg 1950;90:417–55.
80. Klöppel G, Heitz PU. Pancreatic endocrine tumors. Path Res Pract 1988;183:155–68.
81. Klöppel G, Höfler H, Heitz PU. Pancreatic endocrine tumors in man. In: Polak JM, ed. Diagnostic histopathology of neuroendocrine tumors. Edinburgh: Churchill Livingstone, 1993:91–121.
82. Lin TH, Tseng HC, Zhu Y, Zhang SX, Chen J, Cui QC. Insulinoma. An immunocytochemical and morphologic analysis of 95 cases. Cancer 1985;56:1420–9.
83. Mukai K, Grotting JC, Greider MH, Rosai J. Retrospective study of 77 pancreatic endocrine tumors using the immunoperoxidase method. Am J Surg Pathol 1982;6:387–99.
84. Nauck M, Creutzfeldt W. Insulin-producing tumors and the insulinoma syndrome. In: Dayal Y, ed. Endocrine pathology of the gut and pancreas. Boca Raton: CRC Press, 1991:195–225.
85. Rothmund M, Angelini L, Breust M, et al. Surgery for benign insulinoma: an international review. World J Surg 1990;14:398–9.
86. Ruschoff J, Willemer S, Brunzel M, et al. Nucleolar organizer regions and glycoprotein-hormone alpha-chain reaction as markers of malignancy in endocrine tumors of the pancreas. Histopathology 1993;22:51–7.
87. Solcia E, Sessa F, Rindi G, Bonato M, Capella C. Pancreatic endocrine tumors: general concepts; nonfunctioning tumors and tumors with uncommon function. In: Dayal Y, ed. Endocrine pathology of the gut and pancreas. Boca Raton: CRC Press, 1991:105–32.
88. Stefanini P, Carboni M, Patrassi N, Basoli A. Beta-islet cell tumors of the pancreas: results of a study on 1,067 cases. Surgery 1974;75:597–609.
89. Westermark P, Wernstedt C, Wilander E, Sletten K. A novel peptide in the calcitonin gene related peptide family as an amyloid fibril protein in the endocrine pancreas. Biochem Biophys Res Commun 1986;140:827–31.

**Glucagonoma**

90. Boden G, Owen OE. Familial hyperglucagonemia—an autosomal dominant disorder. N Engl J Med 1977; 296:534–8.
91. Bordi C, Ravazzola M, Baetens D, Gorden P, Unger RH, Orci L. A study of glucagonomas by light and electron microscopy and immunofluorescence. Diabetes 1979; 28:925–36.
92. Cavallo-Perin P, De Paoli M, Guiso G, et al. A combined glucagonoma and VIPoma syndrome. First pathologic and clinical report. Cancer 1988;62:2576–9.
93. Creutzfeldt W. Endocrine tumors of the pancreas. In: Volk BW, Wellman KF, eds. The diabetic pancreas. New York: Plenum Publishing, 1977:551–90.
94. Croughs RJ, Hulsmans HA, Israel DE, Hackeng WH, Schopman W. Glucagonoma as a part of the polyglandular syndrome. Am J Med 1972;52:690–8.
95. Guillausseau PJ, Guillausseau C, Villet R. Les glucagonomes. Aspects cliniques, biologiques, anatomopathologiques et therapeutiques (revue generale de 130 cases). Gastroenterol Clin Biol 1982;6:1029–41.
96. Hamid QA, Bishop AE, Sikri KL, Varndell IM, Bloom SR, Polak JM. Immunocytochemical characterization of 10 pancreatic tumours, associated with the glucagonoma syndrome, using antibodies to separate regions of the pro-glucagon molecule and other neuroendocrine markers. Histopathology 1986;10:119–33.
97. Hunstein W, Trumper LH, Dummer R, Schwechheimer K. Glucagonoma syndrome and bronchial carcinoma. Ann Int Med 1988;109:920–1.
98. Mallinson CN, Bloom SR, Warin AP, Salmon PR, Cox B. A glucagonoma syndrome. Lancet 1974;2:1–5.
99. Polak JM, Bloom SR. Glucagon-producing tumors and the glucagonoma syndrome. In: Dayal Y, ed. Endocrine pathology of the gut and pancreas. Boca Raton: CRC Press, 1991:227–40.
100. Roggli VL, Judge DM, McGavran MD. Duodenal glucagonoma: a case report. Hum Pathol 1979;10:350-3.
101. Ruttmann E, Klöppel G, Klehn M, Heitz PU. Pancreatic glucagonoma with and without the syndrome. Immunocytochemical study of 5 tumour cases and review of the literature. Virchows Arch [A] 1980;388:51–67.
102. Wynick D, Williams SJ, Bloom SR. Symptomatic secondary hormone syndromes in patients with established malignant pancreatic endocrine tumors. N Engl J Med 1988;319:605–7.

**Somatostatinoma**

103. Axelrod L, Bush MA, Hirsch HJ, Loo SW. Malignant somatostatinoma: clinical features and metabolic studies. J Clin Endocrinol Metabol 1981;52:886–96.
104. Burke AP, Sobin LH, Shekitka KM, Federspiel BH, Helwig EB. Somatostatin-producing duodenal carcinoids in patients with von Recklinghausen's neurofibromatosis. A predilection for black patients. Cancer 1990;65:1591–5.
105. Cantor AM, Rigby CC, Beck PR, Mangion D. Neurofibromatosis, pheochromocytoma, and somatostatinoma. Br Med J 1982;285:1618–9.
106. Capella C, Riva C, Rindi G, et al. Histopathology, hormone products, and clinicopathological profile of endocrine tumors of the upper small intestine: a study of 44 cases. Endocr Pathol 1991;2:92-110.
107. Dayal Y, Doos WG, O'Brien MJ, Nunnemacher G, De Lellis RA, Wolfe HJ. Psammomatous somatostatinomas of the duodenum. Am J Surg Pathol 1983;7:653–65.
108. Dayal Y, Ganda Om P. Somatostatin producing tumors. In: Dayal Y, ed. Endocrine pathology of the gut and pancreas. Boca Raton: CRC Press, 1991:241–77.
109. Griffiths DF, Jasani B, Newman GR, Williams ED, Williams GT. Glandular duodenal carcinoid—a somatostatin rich tumour with neuroendocrine associations. J Clin Pathol 1984;37:163–9.
110. Konomi K, Chijiiwa K, Katsuta T, Yamaguchi K. Pancreatic somatostatinoma: a case report and review of the literature. I Surg Oncol 1990;43:259–65.
111. Krejis GJ, Orci L, Conlon JM, et al. Somatostatinoma syndrome. Biochemical, morphologic and clinical features. N Engl J Med 1979;301:285–92.
112. Levi S, Bjarnason I, Swinson CM, Polak JM, Murray W, Levi AJ. Malignant pancreatic somatostatinoma in a patient with dermatitis herpetiformis and coeliac disease. Digestion 1988;39:1–6.
113. Murayama H, Imai T, Kikuchi M, Kamio A. Duodenal carcinoid (APUDoma) with psammoma bodies: a light and electron microscopic study. Cancer 1979;43:1411–7.
114. Shirouzu K, Miyamoto Y, Shiramizu T, Morimatsu M. Somatostatinoma of the pancreas. Acta Pathol Jpn 1985;35:1285–92.
115. Stamm B, Hedinger CE, Saremaslani P. Duodenal and ampullary carcinoid tumors. A report of 12 cases with pathological characteristics, polypeptide content and relation to the MEN-1 syndrome and von Recklinghausen's disease (neurofibromatosis). Virchows Arch [A] 1986;408:475–89.

**Gastrinoma**

116. Bhagavan BS, Slavin RE, Goldberg J, Rao RN. Ectopic gastrinoma and Zollinger-Ellison syndrome. Hum Pathol 1986;17:584–92.
117. Bonfils S, Landor JH, Mignon M, Hervoir P. Results of surgical management in 92 consecutive patients with Zollinger-Ellison syndrome. Ann Surg 1981;194:692–7.
118. Buchanan KD, Johnson CF, O'Hare M, et al. Neuroendocrine tumors. A European view. Am J Med 1986;81(Suppl 6B):14–22.
119. Capella C, Riva C, Rindi G, et al. Histopathology, hormone products, and clinicopathological profile of endocrine tumors of the upper small intestine: a study of 44 cases. Endocr Pathol 1991;2:92–110.
120. Clark ES, Carney JA. Pancreatic islet cell tumor associated with Cushing's syndrome. Am J Surg Pathol 1984;8:917–24.
121. Cocco AE, Conway SJ. Zollinger-Ellison syndrome associated with ovarian mucinous cystadenocarcinoma. N Engl J Med 1975;293:485–6.
122. Creutzfeldt W, Arnold R, Creutzfeldt C, Track NS. Pathomorphologic, biochemical, and diagnostic aspects of gastrinomas (Zollinger-Ellison syndrome). Hum Pathol 1975;6:47–76.
123. Delcore R Jr, Cheung LY, Friesen SR. Outcome of lymph node involvement in patients with the Zollinger-Ellison syndrome. Ann Surg 1988;208:291–8.
124. Donow C, Pipeleers-Marichal M, Schröder S, Stamm B, Heitz PU, Klöppel G. Surgical pathology of gastrinoma. Site, size, multicentricity, association with multiple endocrine neoplasia type I, and malignancy. Cancer 1991;68:1329–34.
125. Ellison EH, Wilson SD. The Zollinger-Ellison syndrome: reappraisal and evaluation of 260 registered cases. Ann Surg 1964;160:512–28.
126. Fox PS, Hoffmann JW, Wilson SD, De Cosse JJ. Surgical management of the Zollinger-Ellison syndrome. Surg Clin North Am 1974;54:395–407.
127. Friesen SR. Treatment of the Zollinger-Ellison syndrome. A 25-year assessment. Am J Surg 1982;143:331–8.
128. Heitz PU, Kasper M, Polak JM, Klöppel G. Pancreatic endocrine tumors. Hum Pathol 1982;13:263–71.
129. Hofmann JD, Fox PS, Wilson SD. Duodenal wall tumors and the Zollinger-Ellison syndrome. Arch Surg 1973;107:334–9
130. Jacobsen O, Bardram L, Rehfeld JF. The requirement for gastrin measurements. Scand J Clin Lab Invest 1986;46:423–6.
131. Jensen RT, Doppman JL, Gardner JD. Gastrinoma. In: Go VL, Gardner JD, Brooks FP, Lebenthal E, DiMagno EP, Scheele GA, eds. The exocrine pancreas: biology, pathobiology, and disease. New York: Raven Press, 1986:727-44.
132. Lewin KJ, Yang K, Ulich T, Elashoff JD, Walsh J. Primary gastrin cell hyperplasia. Report of five cases and a review of the literature. Am J Surg Pathol 1984;8:821–32.
133. Margolis RM, Jang N. Zollinger-Ellison syndrome associated with pancreatic cystadenocarcinoma [Letter]. N Eng J Med 1984;311:1380–1.
134. Maton PN, Gardner JD, Jensen RT. Cushing's syndrome in patients with the Zollinger-Ellison syndrome. N Engl J Med 1986;315:1–5.
135. Mukai K, Grotting JC, Greider MH, Rosai J. Retrospective study of 77 pancreatic endocrine tumors using the immunoperoxidase method. Am J Surg Pathol 1982;6:387–99.

136. Neuburger P, Lewin M, Bonfils S. Parietal and chief cell populations in four cases of the Zollinger-Ellison syndrome. Gastroenterology 1972;63:937–42.
137. Oberhelman HA Jr. Excisional therapy for ulcerogenic tumors of the duodenum. Long-term results. Arch Surg 1972;104:447–53.
138. Pipeleers-Marichal M, Somers G, Willems G, et al. Gastrinomas in the duodenums of patients with multiple endocrine neoplasia type 1 and the Zollinger-Ellison syndrome. N Engl J Med 1990;322:723–7.
139. Sessa F, Bonato M, Frigerio B, et al. Ductal cancers of the pancreas frequently express markers of gastrointestinal epithelial cells. Gastroenterology 1990;98:1655–65.
140. Solcia E, Capella C, Buffa R, Frigerio B, Fiocca R. Pathology of the Zollinger-Ellison syndrome. Prog Surg Pathol 1980;1:119–33.
141. Solcia E, Sessa F, Rindi G, Bonato M, Capella C. Pancreatic endocrine tumors: general concepts; nonfunctioning tumors and tumors with uncommon function. In: Dayal Y, ed. Endocrine pathology of the gut and pancreas. Boca Raton: CRC Press, 1991:105–32.
142. Stabile BE, Morrow DJ, Passaro E Jr. The gastrinoma triangle: operative implications. Am J Surg 1984;147:25–31.
143. Stamm B, Hacki WH, Klöppel G, Heitz PU. Gastrin-producing tumors and the Zollinger-Ellison syndrome. In: Dayal Y, ed. Endocrine pathology of the gut and pancreas. Boca Raton: CRC Press, 1991:155–94.
144. Tenti P, Aguzzi A, Riva C, et al. Ovarian mucinous tumors frequently express markers of gastric, intestinal, and pancreatobiliary epithelial cells. Cancer 1992;69:2131–42.
145. Thompson NW, Vinik AI, Eckhauser FE. Microgastrinomas of the duodenum. A cause of failed operations for the Zollinger-Ellison syndrome. Ann Surg 1989;209:396–404.
146. Weber HC, Venzon DY, Lin JT, et al. Determinants of survival in patients with Zollinger-Ellison syndrome: a prospective long-term study. Gastroenterology 1995;108:1637–49.
147. Wolfe MM, Jensen RT. Zollinger-Ellison syndrome. Current concepts in diagnosis and management. N Engl J Med 1987;317:1200–9.
148. Wynick D, Williams SJ, Bloom SR. Symptomatic secondary hormone syndromes in patients with established malignant pancreatic endocrine tumors. N Engl J Med 1988;319:605–7.

**VIPoma**

149. Bloom SR, Lee YC, Lacroite JM, et al. Two patients with pancreatic apudomas secreting neurotensin and VIP. Gut 1983;24:448–52.
150. Bloom SR, Yangou Y, Polak JM. Vasoactive intestinal peptide secreting tumors. Pathophysiological and clinical correlation. Ann NY Acad Sci 1988;527:518–27.
151. Cameron DG, Warnez HA, Szabo AJ. Chronic diarrhea in an adult with hypokalemic nephropathy and osteomalacia due to functioning ganglioneuroblastoma. Am J Med Sci 1967;253:417–24.
152. Capella C, Polak JM, Buffa R, et al. Morphologic patterns and diagnostic criteria of VIP-producing endocrine tumors. A histologic, histochemical, ultrastructural and biochemical study of 32 cases. Cancer 1983;52:1860–74.
153. Creutzfeldt W. Endocrine tumors of the pancreas. In: Volk BW, Arquilla ER, eds. The diabetic pancreas, 2nd ed. New York: Plenum Press, 1985:543–86.
154. Fausa O, Fretheim B, Elgjo K, Semb LS, Gjone E. Intractable watery diarrhoea, hypokalaemia and achlorhydria associated with non-pancreatic retroperitoneal neurogenous tumor containing vasoactive intestinal peptide (VIP). Scand J Gastroenterol 1973;8:713–7.
155. Fiocca R, Sessa F, Tenti P, et al. Pancreatic polypeptide (PP) cells in the PP-rich lobe of the human pancreas are identified ultrastructurally and immunocytochemically as F cells. Histochemistry 1983; 77:511–23.
156. Hamilton I, Reis L, Bilimoria S, Long RG. A renal VIPoma. Brit Med J 1980;281:1323–4.
157. Hutcheon DF, Bayless TM, Cameron JL, Baylin SB. Hormone-mediated watery diarrhea in a family with multiple endocrine neoplasms. Ann Intern Med 1979; 90:932–4.
158. Jaffe BM, Kopen DF, De Schryver Kecskemeti K, Gingerich RL, Greider M. Indomethacin-responsive pancreatic cholera. N Engl J Med 1977;297:817–21.
159. Klöppel G, Heitz PU. Pancreatic endocrine tumors. Path Res Pract 1988;183:155–68.
160. Kogut MD, Kaplan SA. Systemic manifestations of neurogenic tumors. J Pediatr 1962;60:694–704.
161. Krejs GJ. VIPoma syndrome. Am J Med 1987;82(Suppl 5B):37–48.
162. Larsson LI, Polak JM, Buffa R, Sundler F, Solcia E. On the immunocytochemical localization of the vasoactive intestinal peptide. J Histochem Cytochem 1979;27:936–8.
163. Matta MK, Prorok JJ, Trimpi HD, Sheets JA, Stasik JJ, Khubchandani IT. WDHA syndrome caused by pheochromocytoma: report of a case. Dis Colon Rectum 1978;31:297–301.
164. Mendelsohn G. Vasoactive intestinal polypeptide (VIP) and the spectrum of tumors producing the watery diarrhea syndrome. Prog Surg Pathol 1982;4:199–216.
165. Morrison AB. Islet cell tumors and the diarrheogenic syndrome. In: Fitzgerald PJ, Morrison AB, eds. The pancreas. Baltimore: Williams & Wilkins, 1978:185–207.
166. Morrison AB, Rawson AJ, Fitts WT Jr. The syndrome of refractory watery diarrhea and hypokalemia in patients with a non-insulin-secreting islet cell tumor. A further case study and review of the literature. Am J Med 1962;32:119–27.
167. Mukai KM, Greider HH, Grotting JC, Rosai J. Retrospective study of 77 pancreatic endocrine tumors using the immunoperoxidase method. Am J Surg Pathol 1982;6:387–99.
168. Ooi A, Kameya T, Tsumaraia M, et al. Pancreatic endocrine tumors associated with WDHA syndrome. An immunohistochemical and electron microscopic study. Virchows Arch [A] 1985;405:311–23.
169. Ordonez NG, Balsaver AM, Mackay B. Mucinous islet cell (amphicrine) carcinoma of the pancreas associated with watery diarrhea and hypokalemia syndrome. Hum Pathol 1988;19:1458-61

170. Rood RP, De Lellis RA, Dayal Y, Donowitz M. Pancreatic cholera syndrome due to a vasoactive intestinal polypeptide-producing tumor: further insights into the pathophysiology. Gastroenterology 1988;94:813–8.
171. Rosenstein BJ, Engelman K. Diarrhea in a child with a catecholamine secreting ganglioneuroblastoma. J Pediatr 1963;63:217–26.
172. Solcia E, Capella C, Riva C, Rindi G, Polak JM. The morphology and neuroendocrine profile of pancreatic epithelial VIPomas and extrapancreatic, VIP-producing, neurogenic tumors. Ann NY Acad Sci 1988;527:508–17.
173. Trump DA, Livingston JN, Baylin SB. Watery diarrhea syndrome in an adult with ganglioneuroma-pheochromocytoma: identification of vasoactive intestinal peptide, calcitonin, and catecholamines and assessment of their biologic activity. Cancer 1977;40:1526–32.
174. Verner JV, Morrison AB. Endocrine pancreatic islet disease with diarrhea. Report of a case due to diffuse hyperplasia of non-beta islet tissue with a review of 54 additional cases. Arch Intern Med 1974;133:492–500.
175. Verner JV, Morrison AB. Non-beta islet tumors and the syndrome of watery diarrhea, hypokalemia, and hypochlorhydria. Clin Gastroenterol 1974;3:595–608.
176. Watson KJ, Shulkes A, Smallwood RA, et al. Watery diarrhea-hypokalemia-achlorhydria syndrome and carcinoma of the esophagus. Gastroenterology 1988;88:798–803.
177. Yiangou Y, Williams SJ, Bishop AE, Polak JM, Bloom SR. Peptide histidine-methionine immunoreactivity in plasma and tissue from patients with vasoactive intestinal peptide-secreting tumors and watery diarrhea syndrome. J Clin Endocrinol Metab 1987;64:131–9.

**Enterochromaffin Cell Tumor with Carcinoid Syndrome**

178. Dollinger MR, Ratner LH, Shamoian CA, Blackbourne BD. Carcinoid syndrome associated with pancreatic tumors. Arch Intern Med 1967;120:575–80.
179. Ordonez NG, Manning JT, Raymod AK. Argentaffin endocrine carcinoma (carcinoid) of the pancreas with concomitant breast metastasis: an immunohistochemical and electron microscopic study. Hum Pathol 1985;16:746–51.
180. Patchefsky AS, Solit R, Phillips LD, et al. Hydroxyindole-producing tumors of the pancreas. Carcinoid islet cell tumor and oat cell carcinoma. Ann Intern Med 1972;77:53–61.
181. Persaud V, Walrond ER. Carcinoid tumor and cystadenoma of the pancreas. Arch Pathol 1971;92:28–30.
182. Solcia E, Sessa F, Rindi G, Bonato M, Capella C. Pancreatic endocrine tumors: general concepts; nonfunctioning tumors and tumors with uncommon function. In: Dayal Y, ed. Endocrine pathology of the gut and pancreas. Boca Raton: CRC Press, 1991:105–31.
183. Van Der Sluys Veer J, Choufoer JC, Querido A, Van Der Heul RO, Hollander CF, Van Rijssel TG. Metastasizing islet-cell tumour of the pancreas associated with hypoglycaemia and carcinoid syndrome. Lancet 1964;1:1416–9.
184. Wilander E, El-Salhy M, Willen R, Grimelius L. Immunocytochemistry and electron microscopy of an argentaffin endocrine tumor of the pancreas. Virchows Arch [A] 1981;392:263–9.

**Tumors Producing Acromegaly, Cushing's Syndrome, or Hypercalcemia**

185. Arps H, Dietel M, Schulz A, Janzarik H, Kloppel G. Pancreatic endocrine carcinoma with ectopic PTH-production and paraneoplastic hypercalcaemia. Virchows Arch [A] 1986;408:497–503.
186. Caplan RH, Koob L, Abellera RM, Kovacs K, Randall RV. Cure of acromegaly by operative removal of an islet cell tumor of the pancreas. Am J Med 1978;64:874–82.
187. Clark ES, Carney JA. Pancreatic islet cell tumor associated with Cushings syndrome. Am J Surg Pathol 1984;8:917–24.
188. Corrin B, Gilby ED, Jones NF, Patrick J. Oat cell carcinoma of the pancreas with ectopic ACTH secretion. Cancer 1973;31:1523–7.
189. Creutzfeldt W. Endocrine tumors of the pancreas. In: Volk BW, Arquilla ER, eds, The diabetic pancreas, 2nd ed. New York: Plenum Press, 1985:543–86.
190. Ezzat S, Ezrin C, Yamashita S, Melmed S. Recurrent acromegaly resulting from ectopic growth hormone gene expression by a metastatic pancreatic tumor. Cancer 1993;71:66–70.
191. Heitz PU, Klöppel G, Polak JM, Staub JJ. Ectopic hormone production by endocrine tumors: localization of hormones at the cellular level by immunocytochemistry. Cancer 1981;48:2029–37.
192. Liddle GW, Givens JR, Nicholson WE, Island DP. The ectopic ACTH syndrome. Cancer Res 1965;25:1057–61.
193. Maton PN, Gardner JD, Jensen RT. Cushing's syndrome in patients with the Zollinger-Ellison syndrome. N Engl J Med 1986;315:1–5.
194. Monno S, Nagata A, Homma T, et al. Exocrine pancreatic cancer with humoral hypercalcemia. Am J Gastroenterol 1984;79:128–32.
195. Rasbach DA, Hammond JM. Pancreatic islet cell carcinoma with hypercalcemia. Primary hyperparathyroidism or humoral hypercalcemia of malignancy. Am J Med 1985;78:337–42.
196. Saeger W, Schulte HM, Klöppel G. Morphology of a GHRH producing pancreatic islet cell tumor causing acromegaly. Virchows Arch [A] 1986;409:547–54.
197. Sano T, Yamasaki R, Saito H, et al. Growth hormone-releasing hormone (GHRH)-secreting pancreatic tumor in a patient with multiple endocrine neoplasia type I. Am J Surg Pathol 1987;11:810–9.

**Tumors with Multiple Syndromes**

198. Clark ES, Carney JA. Pancreatic islet cell tumor associated with Cushing's syndrome. Am J Surg Pathol 1984;8:917–24.
199. Cryer PH, Hill GJ. Pancreatic islet cell carcinoma with hypercalcemia and hypergastrinemia. Response to streptozotocin. Cancer 1976;38:2217–21.

200. Hammar S, Sale G. Multiple hormone producing islet cell carcinomas of the pancreas. Hum Pathol 1975;6:349–62.
201. Heitz PU, Kasper M, Polak JM, Klöppel G. Pancreatic endocrine tumors. Hum Pathol 1982;13:263–71.
202. Maton PN, Gardner JD, Jensen RT. Cushing's syndrome in patients with the Zollinger-Ellison syndrome. N Engl J Med 1986;315:1–5.
203. Ohneda A, Otsuki M, Fujiya H, Yaginuma N, Kokubo T, Othani H. A malignant insulinoma transformed into a glucagonoma syndrome. Diabetes 1979;28:962–9.
204. O'Neal LW, Kipnis DM, Luse SA, Lacy PE, Jarrett L. Secretion of various endocrine substances by ACTH-secreting tumours—gastrin, melanotropin, norepinephrine, serotonin, parathormone, vasopressin, glucagon. Cancer 1968;21:1219–32.
205. Wynick D, Williams SJ, Bloom SR. Symptomatic secondary hormone syndromes in patients with established malignant pancreatic endocrine tumors. N Engl J Med 1988;319:605–7.

**Nonfunctioning Tumors**

206. Broder LE, Carter SK. Pancreatic islet cell carinoma II. Results of treatment with streptozotocin in 52 patients. Ann Intern Med 1973;79:108–18.
207. Broughan TA, Leslie JD, Soto JM, Hermann RE. Pancreatic islet cell tumors. Surgery 1986;99:671–8.
208. Cubilla AL, Hajdu SI. Islet cell carcinoma of the pancreas. Arch Pathol 1975;99:204–7.
209. Dial PF, Braasch JW, Rossi RL, Lee AK, Jin G. Management of nonfunctioning islet cell tumors of the pancreas. Surg Clin North Am 1985;65:291–9.
210. Eckhauser FE, Cheung PS, Vinik AI, Strodel WE, Lloyd RV, Thompson NW. Nonfunctioning malignant neuroendocrine tumors of the pancreas. Surgery 1986;100:978–88.
211. Grimelius L, Hultquist GT, Stenkvist B. Cytological differentiation of asymptomatic pancreatic islet cell tumors in autopsy material. Virchows Arch [A] 1975;365:275–88.
212. Howard JN, Moss NH, Rhoads JE. Collective review: hyperinsulinism and islet cell tumors of the pancreas. Int Abstr Surg 1950;90:417–55.
213. Kent RB, van Heerden JA, Weiland LH. Nonfunctioning islet cell tumors. Ann Surg 1981;193:185–90.
214. Kimura W, Kuroda A, Morioka Y. Clinical pathology of endocrine tumors of the pancreas. Analysis of autopsy cases. Dig Dis Sci 1991;36:933–42.
215. Klöppel G, Heitz PU. Pancreatic endocrine tumors. Pathol Res Pract 1988;183:155–68.
215a. La Rosa S, Sessa F, Capella C, et al. Prognostic criteria in nonfunctioning pancreatic endocrine tumors. Virchows Arch, 1996;429:323–33.
216. Lundqvist G, Krause U, Larsson LI, et al. A pancreatic polypeptide producing tumor associated with the WDHA syndrome. Scand J Gastroenterol 1978;13:715–8.
217. Marchal G, Seguin C. Les tumeures endocrines du pancreas. Lyon Chir 1980;76:217–26.
218. Moertel GC, Hanley JA, Johnson LA. Streptozotocin alone compared with streptozotocin plus fluorouracil in the treatment of advanced islet-cell carcinoma. N Engl J Med 1980;303:1189–94.
219. Mukai K, Grotting JC, Greider MH, Rosai J. Retrospective study of 77 pancreatic endocrine tumors using the immunoperoxidase method. Am J Surg Pathol 1982;6:387–99.
220. Prinz RA, Badrinath K, Cheifec G, Freeark K, Greenlee HB. Nonfunctioning islet cell carcinoma of the pancreas. Am Surg 1983;49:345–9.
221. Solcia E, Sessa F, Rindi G, Bonato M, Capella C. Pancreatic endocrine tumors: general concepts; nonfunctioning tumors and tumors with uncommon function. In: Dayal Y, ed. Endrocrine pathology of the gut and pancreas. Boca Raton: CRC Press, 1991:105–31.
222. Strodel WE, Vinik AI, Lloyd RV, et al. Pancreatic polypeptide-producing tumors. Silent lesions of the pancreas? Arch Surg 1984;119:508–14
223. Tomita T, Friesen SR, Kimmel JR, Doull V, Pollock NG. Pancreatic polypeptide-secreting islet-cell tumors. A study of three cases. Am J Pathol 1983;113:134–42.
224. Tomita T, Friesen SR, Pollock HG. PP-producing tumors (PPomas). In Dayal Y, ed. Endocrine pathology of the gut and pancreas. Boca Raton: CRC Press, 1991:279–304.
225. Venkatesh S, Ordonez NG, Ajani J, et al. Islet cell carcinoma of the pancreas. A study of 98 patients. Cancer 1990;65:354–7.

**Multiple Endocrine Neoplasia Type 1**

226. Bhagavan BS, Hofkin GA, Woel GM, Koss LG. Zollinger-Ellison syndrome. Ultrastructural and histochemical observations in a child with endocrine tumorlets of gastric antrum. Arch Pathol 1974;98:217–22.
227. Bordi C, Cocconi G, Togni R, Vezzadini P, Missale G. Gastric endocrine cell proliferation. Association with Zollinger-Ellison syndrome. Arch Pathol 1974;98:274–8.
228. Brandi ML, Marx SJ, Aurbach GK, Fitzpatrick LA. Familial multiple endocrine neoplasia type I: a new look at pathophysiology. Endocr Rev 1987;8:391–405.
229. Capella C, Riva C, Rindi G, et al. Histopathology, hormone products, and clinico-pathological profile of endocrine tumors of the upper small intestine: a study of 44 cases. Endocr Pathol 1991;2:92–110.
230. DeLellis RA, Dayal Y, Tischler AS, Lee AK, Wolfe HJ. Multiple endocrine neoplasia (MEN) syndromes: cellular origins and interrelationships. Int Rev Exp Pathol 1986;28:163–215.
231. Donow C, Pipeleers-Marichal M, Schröder S, Stamm B, Heitz PU, Klöppel G. Surgical pathology of gastrinoma. Site, size, multicentricity, association with multiple endocrine neoplasia type 1 and malignancy. Cancer 1991;68:1329–34.
232. Friesen SR, Schimke RN. Pearse AG. Genetic aspects of Zollinger-Ellison syndrome: prospective studies in two kindreds: antral gastrin cell hyperplasia. Ann Surg 1972;176:370–83.

233. Friesen SR, Tomita T, Kimmel JR. Pancreatic polypeptide update: its roles in detection of the trait for multiple endocrine adenopathy syndrome type I and pancreatic-polypeptide-secreting tumors. Surgery 1983;94:1028-37.

234. Klöppel G, Willemer S, Stamm B, Hacki WH, Heitz PU. Pancreatic lesions and hormonal profile of pancreatic tumors in multiple endocrine neoplasia type I. An immunocytochemical study of nine patients. Cancer 1986;57:1824–32.

235. Larsson C, Skogseid B, Oberg K, Nakamura Y, Nordenskjold M. Multiple endocrine neoplasia maps to chromosome 11 and is lost in insulinoma. Nature 1988;332:85–7.

236. Lehy T, Cadiot G, Mignon M, Ruszniewski P, Bonfils S. Influence of multiple endocrine neoplasia type 1 on gastric endocrine cells in patients with the Zollinger-Ellison syndrome. Gut 1992;33:1275–9.

237. Lewin KJ, Yang K, Ulich T, Elashoff JD, Walsh J. Primary gastrin cell hyperplasia. Report of five cases and a review of the literature. Am J Surg Pathol 1984; 8:821–32.

238. Lips CJ, Vasen HF, Lamers CB. Multiple endocrine neoplasia syndromes. CRC Crit Rev Oncol/Hematol 1984;2:117–84.

239. Majewski JT, Wilson SD. The MEA-I syndrome: an all or none phenomenon? Surgery 1979;86:475–84.

240. Pilato FP, D'Adda T, Banchini E, Bordi C. Nonrandom expression of polypeptide hormones in pancreatic endocrine tumors. An immunohistochemical study in a case of multiple islet cell neoplasia. Cancer 1988; 61:1815–20.

241. Pipeleers-Marichal M, Somers G, Willems G, et al. Gastrinomas in the duodenums of patients with multiple endocrine neoplasia type 1 and the Zollinger-Ellison syndrome. N Engl J Med 1990;322:723–7.

242. Rindi G, Luinetti O, Cornaggia M, Capella C, Solcia E. Three subtypes of gastric argyrophil carcinoid and the gastric neuroendocrine carcinoma: a clinicopathologic study. Gastroenterology 1993;104:994–1006.

243. Solcia E, Bordi C, Creutzeldt W, et al. Histopathological classification of nonantral gastric endocrine growths in man. Digestion 1988;41:185–200.

244. Solcia E, Capella C, Buffa R, Frigerio B, Fiocca R. Pathology of the Zollinger-Ellison syndrome. Prog Surg Pathol 1980;1:119–33.

245. Solcia E, Capella C, Fiocca R, Rindi G, Rosai J. Gastric argyrophil carcinoidosis in patients with Zollinger-Ellison syndrome due to type 1 multipe endocrine neoplasia. A newly recognized association. Am J Surg Pathol 1990;14:503–13.

246. Solcia E, Sessa F, Rindi G, Bonato M, Capella C. Pancreatic endocrine tumors: general concepts; nonfunctioning tumors and tumors with uncommon function. In: Dayal Y, ed. Endocrine pathology of the gut and pancreas. Boca Raton: CRC Press, 1991:105–31.

247. Van Heerden JA, Edis AJ, Service FJ. The surgical aspects of insulinomas. Ann Surg 1979;189:677–82.

248. Zollinger RM, Ellison EC, O'Dorisio TM, Sparks J. Thirty years' experience with gastrinomas. World J Surg 1984;8:427–35.

**Small Cell Carcinoma**

249. Corrin B, Gilby ED, Jones NF, Patrick J. Oat cell carcinoma of the pancreas with ectopic ACTH secretion. Cancer 1973;31:1523–7.

250. Cubilla AL, Fitzgerald PJ. Tumors of the exocrine pancreas. In: Atlas of Tumor Pathology, 2nd Series, Fascicle 19. Washington, D.C.: Armed Forces Institute of Pathology, 1984.

251. Dollinger MR, Ratner LH, Shamoian CA, Blackbourne BD. Carcinoid syndrome associated with pancreatic tumors. Arch Intern Med 1967;120:575–80.

252. Gordon DL, Lo MC, Schwartz MA. Carcinoid of the pancreas. Am J Med 1971;51:412–5.

253. Hobbs RD, Stewart AF, Ravin ND, Carter D. Hypercalcemia in small cell carcinoma of the pancreas. Cancer 1984;53:1552–4.

254. Ibrahim NB, Briggs JC, Corbishley CM. Extrapulmonary oat cell carcinoma. Cancer 1984;54:1645–61.

255. Morant R, Bruckner HW. Complete remission of refractory small cell carcinoma of the pancreas with cisplatin and etoposide. Cancer 1989;64:2007–9.

256. Morohoshi T, Held G, Klöppel G. Exocrine pancreatic tumours and their histological classification. A study based on 167 autopsy and 97 surgical cases. Histopathology 1983;7:645–61.

257. O'Connor TP, Wade TP, Sunwoo YC, et al. Small cell undifferentiated carcinoma of the pancreas. Report of a patient with tumor marker studies. Cancer 1992;70:1514–9.

258. Reyes CV, Wang T. Undifferentiated small cell carcinoma of the pancreas: a report of five cases. Cancer 1981;47:2500–2.

259. Sessa F, Bonato M, Frigerio B, et al. Ductal cancers of the pancreas frequently express markers of gastrointestinal epithelial cells. Gastroenterology 1990;98:1655–65.

260. Solcia E, Sessa F, Rindi G, Bonato M, Capella C. Pancreatic endocrine tumors: general concepts; nonfunctioning tumors and tumors with uncommon function. In: Dayal Y, ed. Endocrine pathology of the gut and pancreas. Boca Raton: CRC Press, 1991:105–31.

# 6
# NONEPITHELIAL AND SECONDARY TUMORS

## NONEPITHELIAL TUMORS

The primary nonepithelial tumors of the pancreas include benign and malignant soft tissue tumors as well as malignant lymphomas. All of these neoplasms are exceedingly rare in the pancreas (4,7,9,21) and do not differ in structure from those seen in other organs. Most reports are of single cases.

### Benign Soft Tissue Tumors

Benign soft tissue tumors of the pancreas that have been reported are benign fibrous histiocytoma (9), juvenile hemangioendothelioma (8, 35), benign schwannoma (10a), granular cell tumor (33), and lymphangioma (15,19). The lymphangioma reported by Pack et al. (27) most likely represents a serous microcystic adenoma.

### Malignant Soft Tissue Tumors

Some of the earlier reported malignant soft tissue tumors of the pancreas probably represent undifferentiated (sarcomatoid) carcinoma or secondary involvement of the pancreas by primarily retroperitoneal sarcomas (21). The tumors reported in the recent literature include leiomyosarcoma (11,22), malignant schwannoma (12, 24), fibrosarcoma (7,25), malignant fibrous histiocytoma (2,9,28), liposarcoma (14), rhabdomyosarcoma (20), malignant hemangiopericytoma (9), primitive neuroectodermal tumor (10), and clear cell “sugar” tumor of the pancreas (36a). Among these tumors leiomyosarcoma is the most frequent (11). Also, there is a variant of malignant fibrous histiocytoma with osteoclast-like giant cells (34) which probably belongs to the neoplastic lesions included under osteoclast-like giant cell tumors of the pancreas (see Osteoclast-Like Giant Cell Tumor).

Sarcomas with a pleomorphic or spindle cell pattern and malignant fibrous histiocytomas may be difficult to distinguish from undifferentiated (anaplastic) carcinomas. Usually sarcomas are positive for vimentin and negative for cytokeratins; however, an occasional undifferentiated carcinoma may be positive for vimentin, in addition to keratin, while a leiomyosarcoma may be positive for keratin in addition to actin and desmin. Large pancreatic soft tissue tumors are often cystic (22) and can therefore be difficult to differentiate from other cystic tumors of the pancreas. Features of sarcoma are central necrosis and lack of epithelial cells in the still intact tumor component.

Secondary involvement of the pancreas by retroperitoneal soft tissue tumors may resemble a primary pancreatic tumor (26). The pancreas was the main site in 3 of 19 cases of the recently described intra-abdominal desmoplastic small round cell tumor (18).

### Malignant Lymphoma

While secondary involvement of the pancreas by advanced Hodgkin’s disease, non-Hodgkin’s lymphoma, multiple myeloma, or extramedullary plasmacytoma is not uncommon (3,5,13,16, 17,21, 30), few lymphomas have been reported that arise primarily within the pancreas (6,23, 29,31,32,36). Most primary pancreatic lymphomas present with the symptoms of carcinoma of the pancreatic head. Grossly, the lymphomas produce large, soft, nodular masses, ranging from 4 to 14 cm in diameter, which most commonly occur in the head of the pancreas (31). The pancreatic duct system may be displaced but is usually not destroyed.

Non-Hodgkin lymphomas must be distinguished from undifferentiated carcinomas, including small cell carcinoma (1). The latter tumors are positive for keratins and endocrine markers, while lymphomas stain for common leukocyte antigen.

## SECONDARY TUMORS

Relatively few extrapancreatic neoplasms involve the pancreas by direct invasion: only 0.6 percent of 2,587 autopsies from the files of Memorial Hospital, New York, from 1973 to 1978 (37). Hematogenous metastases are more frequent: 10 percent in the Memorial Hospital series. The pancreas can also be involved by systemic

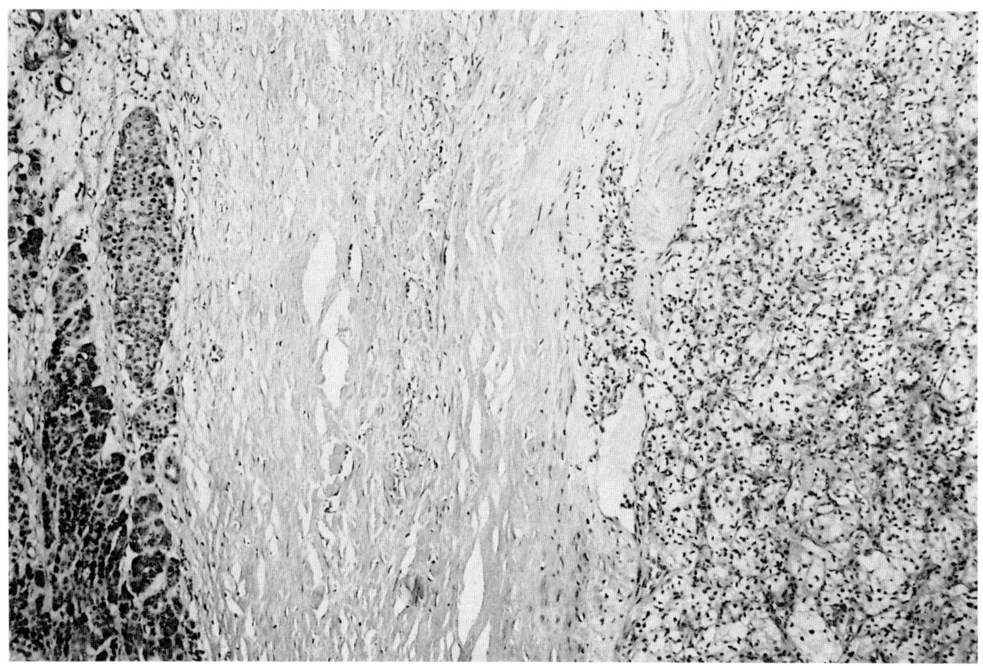

Figure 6-1
SECONDARY TUMOR
The illustration shows a metastasis (right) from a renal cell carcinoma which had been removed 5 years before. The tumor in the pancreas was originally diagnosed as an endocrine tumor.

malignant neoplasms such as malignant lymphomas and leukemias.

Primary cancers of adjacent organs that extend to the pancreas are mainly adenocarcinomas of the stomach, intestine, or biliary tract. Histologically, distinguishing a primary duct cell pancreatic adenocarcinoma from a gastric or intestinal adenocarcinoma may be difficult, since architectural features, cytologic details, and expression of tumor marker are similar (42). The finding of in situ areas can help establish the site of tumor origin. A peculiar feature of pancreatic invasion from a gastric cancer is lymphangiosis carcinomatosa which is seen in signet ring cell carcinoma.

The most frequent sites of origin of bloodborne metastases to the pancreas are breast, lung, skin (melanoma), and kidney (fig. 6-1). In patients with melanoma the development of pancreatic metastases, in association with diffuse gastrointestinal involvement, is common and has been reported in 53 percent of autopsies (38). However, involvement of the pancreas as a single metastatic organ is rare (less than 1 percent) in patients with melanoma of cutaneous origin (41).

Secondary tumors in the pancreas are rarely clinically evident (37,40). Acute pancreatitis has been particularly observed in metastatic small cell lung carcinoma (39,40).

In the Memorial Hospital series (37), malignant lymphomas (including 7 cases of Hodgkin's disease and 1 of multiple myeloma) involving the pancreas were found in 48 patients (1.9 percent). In 19 patients (0.7 percent) the pancreas was involved by different types of leukemia (including chronic myelogenous, acute lymphoblastic, chronic lymphocytic, acute myelomonocytic) infiltrating the glandular parenchyma.

## REFERENCES

### Nonepithelial Tumors


1. Ackerman NB, Aust JC, Bredenberg CE, Hanson VA Jr, Rogers LS. Problems in differentiating between pancreatic lymphoma and anaplastic carcinoma and their management. Ann Surg 1976;184:705–8.
2. Allen KB, Skandalakis LJ, Brown BC, Gray SW, Skandalakis JE. Malignant fibrous histiocytoma of the pancreas. Am Surg 1990;56:364–8.
3. Banks PM, Arseneau JC, Gralnick HR, Canellos GP, DeVita VT Jr, Berard CW. American Burkitt's lymphoma. A clinicopathologic study of 30 cases. II. Pathologic correlations. Am J Med 1975;58:322–9.
4. Baylor SM, Berg JW. Cross classification and survival characteristic of 5000 cases of cancer of the pancreas. J Surg Oncol 1973;5:355–8.
5. Bell HG, David R, Shamsuddin AM. Extrahepatic biliary obstruction and liver failure secondary to myeloma of the pancreas. Hum Pathol 1982;13:940–2.
6. Borgia G, Ciampi R, Nappa S, Iovinella V, Crowell J. Pancreatic plasmacytoma: an unusual cause of obstructive jaundice. Arch Pathol Lab Med 1984;108:773–4.
7. Brooke WS, Maxwell JG. Primary sarcoma of the pancreas. Eight year survival after pancreatoduodenectomy. Am J Surg 1966;112:657–61.
8. Chappell JS. Case reports. Benign hemangioendothelioma of the head of the pancreas treated by pancreaticoduodenectomy. J Pediatr Surg 1973;8:431–2.
9. Cubilla AL, Fitzgerald PJ. Tumors of the exocrine pancreas. Atlas of Tumor Pathology, 2nd Series, Fascicle 19. Washington, D.C.: Armed Forces Institute of Pathology. 1984:1–287.
10. Danner DB, Hruban RH, Pitt HA, Hayashi R, Griffin CA, Perlman EJ. Primitive neuroectodermal tumor arising in the pancreas. Mod Path 1994;7:200–4.

10a. David S, Barkin JS. Pancreatic schwannoma [Letter]. Pancreas 1993;8:274–6.

11. de Alva E, Torramadé J, Vazquez JJ. Leiomyosarcoma of the pancreas. Virchows Arch [A] 1993;422:419–22.
12. Eggermont A, Vuzeuski V, Huisman M, DeJang K, Jeekel J. Solitary malignant schwannoma of the pancreas: report of a case and ultrastructural examination. J Surg Oncol 1987;36:21–5.
13. Ehrlich AN, Stalder G, Geller W, Sherlock P. Gastrointestinal manifestations of malignant lymphoma. Gastroenterology 1968;54:1115–21.
14. Elliott TE, Albertazzi VJ, Danto LA. Pancreatic liposarcoma: case report with review of retroperitoneal liposarcoma. Cancer 1980;45:1720–3.
15. Epstein HS, Berman R. Mesenteric and pancreatic lymphangioma presenting as a right adnexal mass. Am J Obstet Gynecol 1975;121:117–8.
16. Fischer A, Suhrland MJ, Vogl SE. Myeloma of the head of the pancreas. A case report. Cancer 1991;67:681–3.
17. Frantz VK. Tumors of the pancreas. Atlas of Tumor Pathology, 1st Series, Fascicles 27 and 28. Washington, D.C.: Armed Forces Institute of Pathology, 1959.
18. Gerald WL, Miller HK, Battifora H, Miettinen M, Silva EG, Rosai J. Intra-abdominal desmoplastic small round-cell tumor. Report of 19 cases of a distinctive type of high-grade polyphenotypic malignancy affecting young individuals. Am J Surg Pathol 1991;15:499–513.
19. Gregory IL. Lymphangioma of pancreas. NY J Med 1976;76:289–91.
20. Grosfeld JL, Clatworthy HW Jr, Hamoudi AB. Pancreatic malignancy in children. Arch Surg 1970;101:370–5.
21. Gruber GB. Pathologie der bauchspeicheldrüse. In: Henke F, Lubarsch O, eds. Handbuch der speziellen pathologischen anatomie und histologie, Vol. 5, Teil 2. Berlin: Springer, 1929.
22. Ishikawa O, Matsui Y, Aoki Y, Iwanaga T, Terasawa T, Wada A. Leiomyosarcoma of the pancreas: report of a case and review of the literature. Am J Surg Pathol 1981;5:597–602.
23. Joly I, David A, Payan MJ, Sahel J, Sarles H. A case of primary non-Hodgkin lymphoma of the pancreas. Pancreas 1992;7:118–20.
24. Moller-Pederson VM, Hedes A, Graem N. A solitary malignant schwannoma mimicking a pancreatic pseudocyst. Acta Chir Scand 1982;148:697–8.
25. Neibling HA. Primary sarcoma of the pancreas. Am Surg 1968;34:690–3.
26. Nordback I, Mattila J, Tarkka M. Resectable leiomyosarcoma of inferior vena cava presenting as carcinoma of the pancreas. Case report. Acta Chir Scand 1990;156:577–80.
27. Pack GT, Trinidad SS, Lisa JR. Rare primary somatic tumors of the pancreas. Arch Surg 1958;77:1000–3.
28. Pascal RR, Sullivan L, Hauser L, Ferzli G. Primary malignant fibrous histiocytoma of the pancreas. Hum Pathol 1989;20:1215–7.
29. Richards WG, Katzmann FS, Coleman FC. Extramedullary plasmacytoma arising in the head of the pancreas. Report of a case. Cancer 1958;11:649–52.
30. Rosenbergh SA, Diamond HD, Jaslowitz B, Craver LF. Lymphosarcoma: a review of 1269 cases. Medicine 1961;40:31–84.
31. Satake K, Arimoto Y, Fujimoto Y, et al. Malignant T-cell lymphoma of the pancreas. Pancreas 1991;6:120–4.
32. Scheiman J, Elta G, Francis I. Biliary obstruction secondary to an extramedullary plasmacytoma of the pancreas: confusion with pancreatitis on computed tomography. Pancreas 1987;2:237–9.
33. Seidler A, Burstein S, Drweiga W, Goldberg M. Granular cell tumor of the pancreas. J Clin Gastroenterol 1986;8:207–9.
34. Suster S, Phillips M, Robinson MJ. Malignant fibrous histiocytoma (giant cell type) of the pancreas. A distinctive variant of osteoclast-type giant cell tumor of the pancreas. Cancer 1989;64:2303–8.
35. Tunell WP. Hemangioendothelioma of the pancreas obstructing the common bile duct and duodenum. J Pediatr Surg 1976;11:827–30.
36. Webb TH, Lillemoe KD, Pitt HA, Jones RJ, Cameron JL. Pancreatic lymphoma. Is surgery mandatory for diagnosis or treatment? Ann Surg 1989;209:25–30.

36a. Zamboni G, Pea M, Martignoni G. et al. Clear cell sugar tumor of the pancreas. A novel member of the family of lesions characterized by the presence of perivascular epithelioid cells. Am J Surg Pathol 1996;20:722–30.

**Secondary Tumors**

37. Cubilla A, Fitzgerald PJ. Tumors of the exocrine pancreas. Atlas of Tumor Pathology, 2nd Series, Fascicle 19. Washington, D.C.: Armed Forces Institute of Pathology, 1984.
38. Das Gupta TK, Brasfield RD. Metastatic melanoma of the gastrointestinal tract. Arch Surg 1964;88:969–73.
39. Lankisch PG, Löhr A, Kunze E. Matastasen-induzierte akute Pankreatitis beim Bronchialkarzinom. Dtsch Med Wschr 1987;112:1335–7.
40. Niccolini DG, Graham JH, Banks PA. Tumor-induced acute pancreatitis. Gastroenterology 1976;71:142–5.
41. Patel JK, Didolkar MS, Pickren JW, Moore RH. Metastatic pattern of malignant melanoma. A study of 216 autopsy cases. Am J Surg 1978;135:807–10.
42. Sessa F, Bonato M, Frigerio B, et al. Ductal cancers of the pancreas frequently express markers of gastrointestinal epithelial cells. Gastroenterology 1990;98:1655–65.

# 7
# TUMOR-LIKE LESIONS OF THE EXOCRINE PANCREAS

Although the pancreatic disorders classified as tumor-like lesions are heterogeneous, common to all is the possibility of misinterpretation as a neoplastic condition.

## CHRONIC PANCREATITIS

Chronic pancreatitis is the disease that most often results in a mistaken clinical, and sometimes also morphologic, diagnosis of pancreatic carcinoma.

**Definition.** Chronic pancreatitis is irreversible and irregular fibrotic destruction of the glandular parenchyma of the pancreas due to a variety of necrotizing and inflammatory processes. In Western countries most cases of chronic pancreatitis appear to be the result of severe and relapsing acute autodigestive pancreatitis caused by chronic alcoholism (24,25). Comparable pancreatic changes are seen in the hereditary (autosomal dominant) form of chronic pancreatitis (31). A similar type of chronic pancreatitis which occurs in tropical countries seems to be related to malnutrition. Rarely, chronic pancreatitis is associated with autoimmune sialadenitis or primary sclerosing cholangitis and appears to be of autoimmune origin (25). The diffuse atrophy and fibrosis of the pancreas that follows obstruction of the main duct in the head of the pancreas by tumor, scar, or stone is called obstructive chronic pancreatitis.

**Gross Findings.** In early chronic pancreatitis the gland is always unevenly affected. The affected part is usually enlarged and may be indurated to such an extent that it gives the impression of a "rock hard" mass (fig. 7-1). On sectioning, there is focal nodular or segmental sclerosis. The involved ducts may be distorted and occasionally may contain calculi (calcified protein plugs). In many cases, extrapancreatic pseudocysts are found in the vicinity of the sclerotic areas. These often thick-walled pseudocysts vary in size (range, 3 to 10 cm) and are filled with necrotic hemorrhagic debris.

In advanced chronic pancreatitis, the entire pancreas is hard, has an irregular contour, and appears to be shrunken. On sectioning, the main duct shows irregular dilatations and distortions and usually contains varying sized calculi (fig. 7-2) that may be impacted and therefore difficult to remove. The scarring in the head of the pancreas may lead to tubular stenosis of the intrapancreatic part of the bile duct (fig. 7-1).

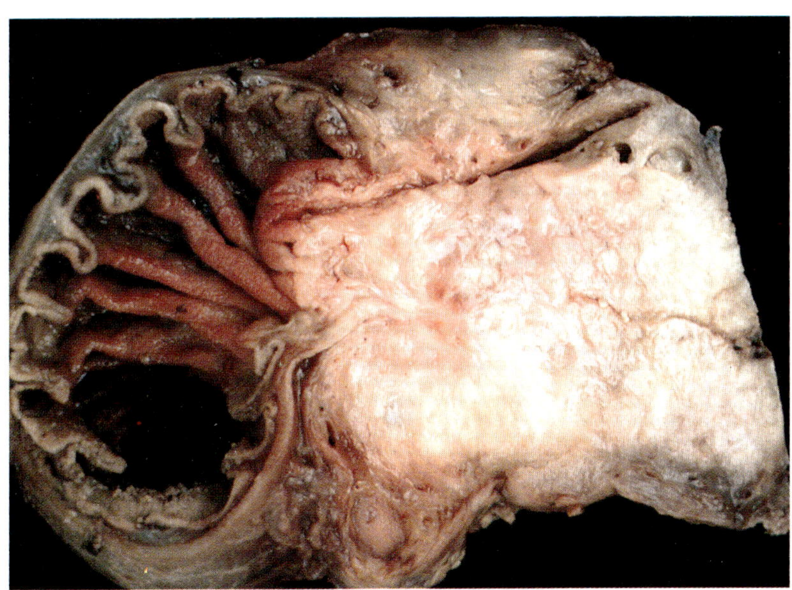

Figure 7-1
CHRONIC PANCREATITIS
Whipple resection specimen from a patient with chronic pancreatitis. The cut surface of the pancreas head shows diffuse sclerosis with small calculi in the main pancreatic duct. The sclerosis of the tissue gives the impression of a "rock hard" tumor mass. Note the tubular stenosis of the bile duct in the upper portion of the pancreatic head.

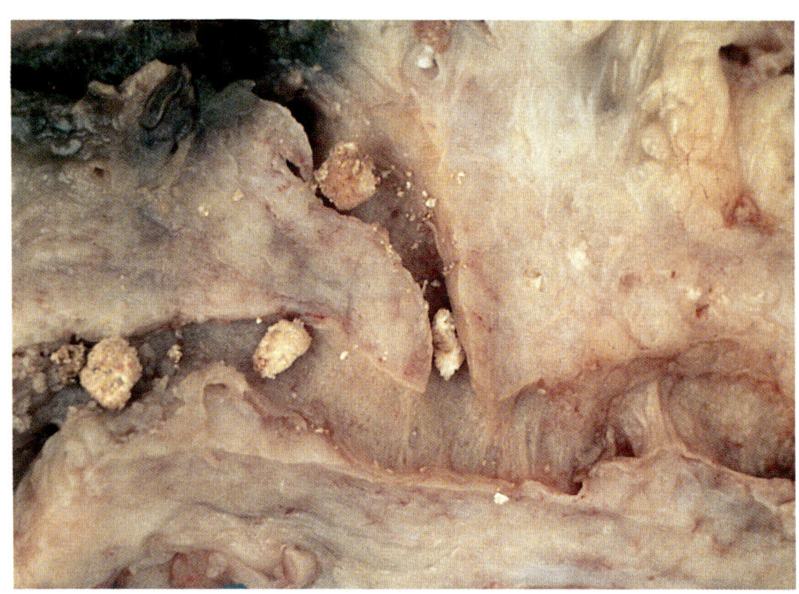

Figure 7-2
CHRONIC PANCREATITIS
The cut surface of a segment of the main pancreatic duct in the head-body region of the pancreas is seen. Note the irregular dilatation of the duct which contains varying sized calculi.

In obstructive chronic pancreatitis due to an occlusion of the main pancreatic duct in the head of the gland, there is a marked dilatation of the duct system upstream of the stenosis, combined with fibrotic atrophy of the parenchyma. As a rule, calculi are not found in this condition.

**Microscopic Findings.** In the early stages of the disease, fibrotic foci are found adjacent to relatively normal or completely normal pancreatic tissue. The affected parts show distinct interlobular (perilobular) fibrosis which tends to develop into the lobules (intralobular fibrosis) but, at this stage of the disease, only occasionally form a complete fibrotic nodule without any remaining acinar tissue (fig. 7-3). The interlobular ducts, which are embedded in fibrous tissue, are distorted and focally ectatic; they may contain eosinophilic proteinaceous material. Their epithelium is cuboidal and sometimes hyperplastic or metaplastic (see Duct Changes). Moderate numbers of lymphocytes, plasma cells, and macrophages are present, either in local collections or scattered diffusely throughout the fibrous tissue. Within the perilobular areas there may be patches of resolving fat necrosis surrounded by macrophages, granulocytes, and proliferating fibroblasts; this change is usually seen in the vicinity of extrapancreatic pseudocysts (see Pseudocysts).

In advanced chronic pancreatitis, large areas of the pancreas not only show perilobular but also intralobular fibrosis. In these areas the acinar cells are more or less replaced by fibrotic tissue and groups of dilated ductules (fig. 7-4) admixed with disorderly arranged and varying sized islets (fig. 7-5). The islets may become so prominent that they are mistaken for components of a solid (endocrine) tumor (fig. 7-5). The remaining interlobular ducts are distorted and ectatic, and their lumens are often filled with protein plugs or calculi (fig. 7-6). The duct epithelium lacks signs of severe cellular atypia (fig. 7-7), but may be atrophic or, around impacted calculi, completely replaced by fibrous inflammatory tissue. Occasionally, severe duct dilatation may evolve into a small retention cyst. The fibrous tissue contains thick-walled arteries, prominent nerve trunks, and a scant, predominantly periductal, lymphocytic infiltration.

Obstructive chronic pancreatitis is histologically difficult or even impossible (if only small pieces of pancreatic tissue are available as in an intraoperative biopsy) to distinguish from the primary chronic pancreatitis described above. However, in large specimens that contain the dilated main pancreatic duct it is obvious that the parenchyma is more evenly affected by fibrosis which, in addition, appears to be more pronounced in the central region of the gland around the main pancreatic duct than in the periphery.

**Differential Diagnosis.** In a resection specimen from the pancreas, chronic pancreatitis usually does not present a significant diagnostic problem. However, in a frozen section from a

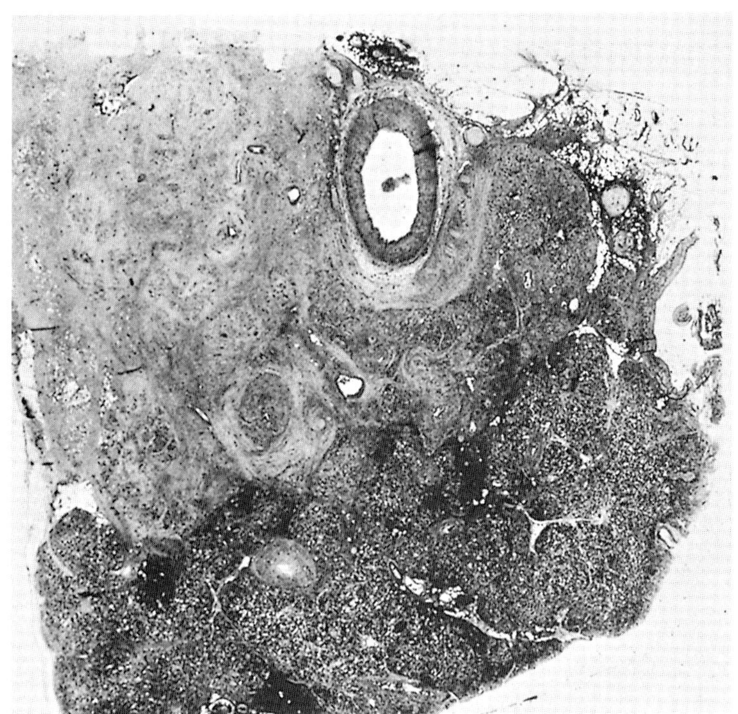

Figure 7-3
FOCAL FIBROSIS IN
CHRONIC PANCREATITIS

Focal fibrosis of the pancreatic parenchyma (upper left). The surgeon at operation and the pathologist at gross examination considered this nodule of scarring to be a carcinoma. No carcinoma was present. (Fig. 50 from Fascicle 19, Second Series.)

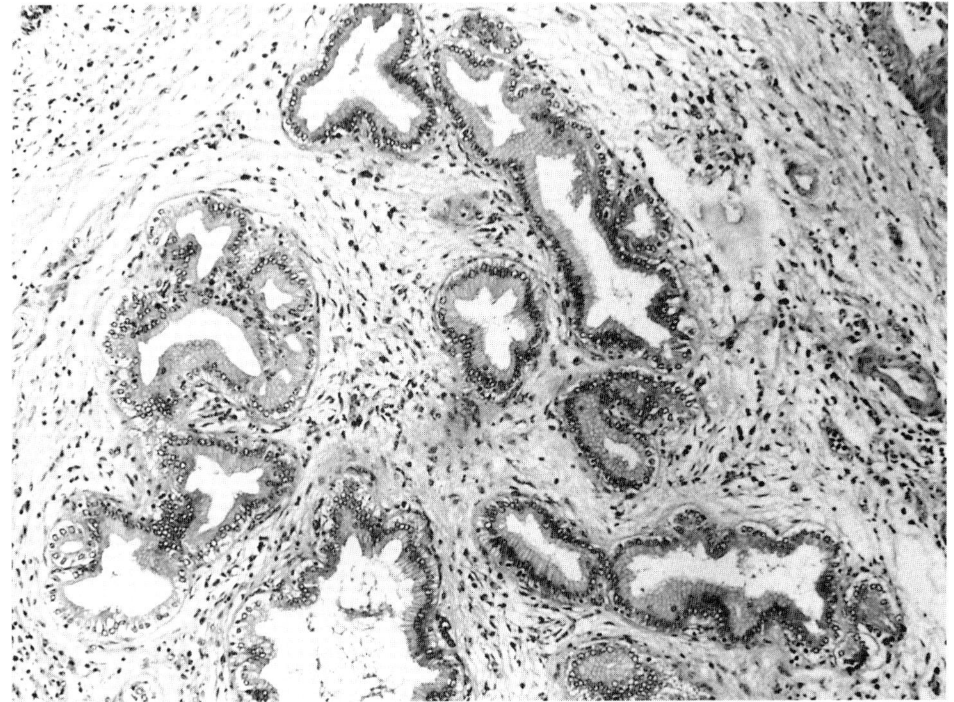

Figure 7-4
CHRONIC PANCREATITIS

This pancreatic tissue shows advanced chronic pancreatitis with replacement of large areas of the acinar parenchyma by sclerotic tissue and lobular aggregation of the irregularly sized remaining ducts.

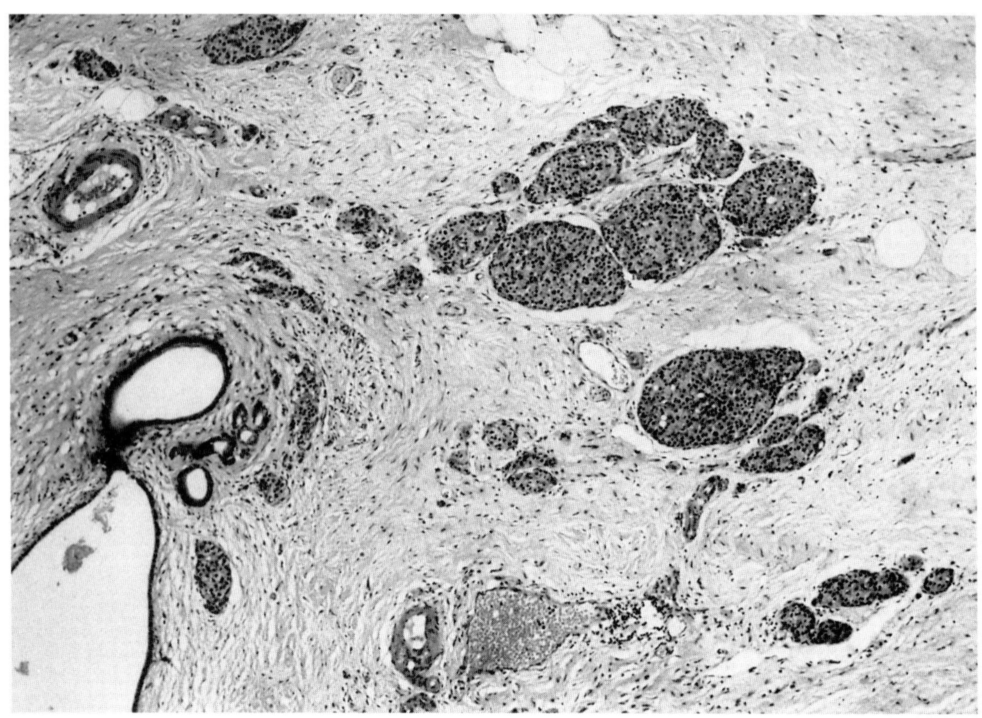

Figure 7-5
CHRONIC PANCREATITIS
Sclerotic area of the pancreas with dilated duct (left) and clusters of remaining islets (right).

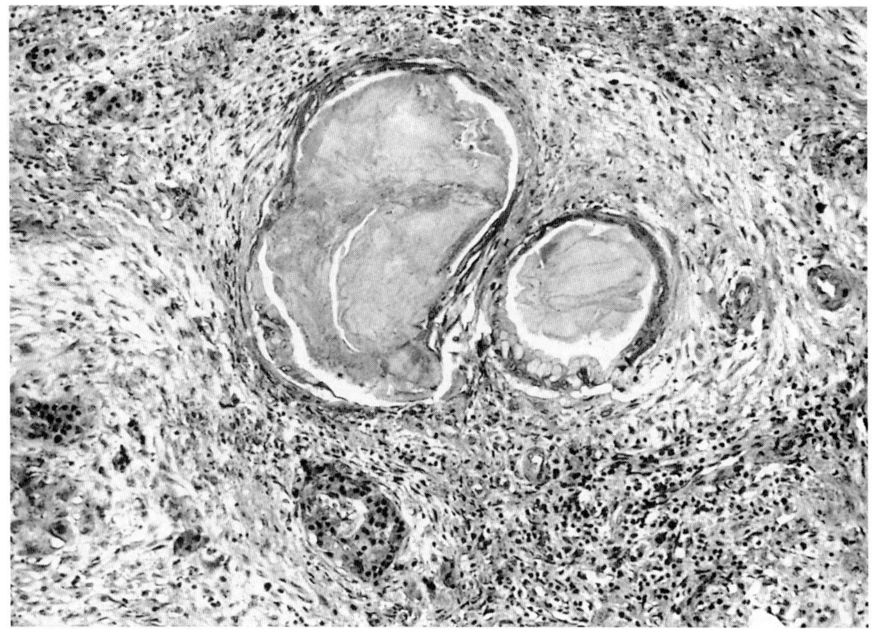

Figure 7-6
CHRONIC PANCREATITIS
Dilated interlobular ducts containing protein plugs. The surrounding tissue shows sclerosis and an inflammatory reaction. Note the small islet at the bottom.

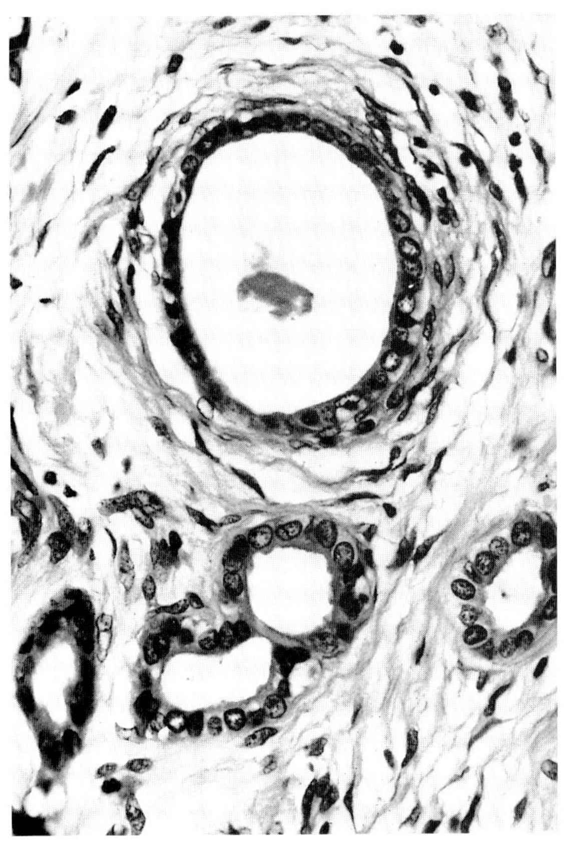
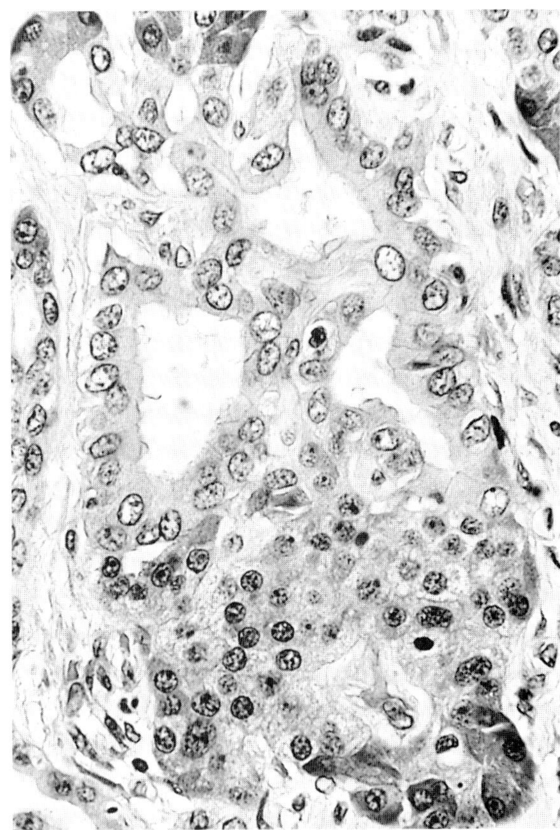

Figure 7-7
DUCTS IN CHRONIC PANCREATITIS
Left: The lining epithelium of these irregularly sized ducts lacks cellular atypia.
Right: Ducts (top) in association with an islet (bottom). Note the benign appearance of the duct cell nuclei.

biopsy specimen it may be difficult to differentiate from ductal adenocarcinoma. In all forms of chronic pancreatitis, even in cases with severe fibrosis, the distorted ductular elements, which may be mistakenly diagnosed as infiltrating ductal adenocarcinoma, are arranged in a lobular pattern and lack clearly atypical nuclei with conspicuous nucleoli (fig. 7-7). Islets, which may become very large and mistaken as small solid tumor nodules, are also arranged in clusters and never show a diffuse and irregular infiltration of the fibrotic tissue. Perineural invasion by ductal elements, a criterion of invasive carcinoma, is not found in chronic pancreatitis, while the presence of calculi usually exclude a carcinoma (see Ductal Adenocarcinoma, Differential Diagnosis). Those rare patients who develop a ductal adenocarcinoma concurrent with chronic calcifying pancreatitis often suffer from a hereditary form of pancreatitis or a sporadic form of the disease which started very early in life (see Ductal Adenocarcinoma, General Features).

## MISCELLANEOUS INFLAMMATORY CHANGES

Sarcoidosis occasionally involves the pancreas and leads to nodular changes due to the development of noncaseating granulomas (38,69). Involvement of the pancreas, with obstruction of the common bile duct and pancreatic duct, was described in a case of idiopathic fibrosis (57). Malakoplakia was found to be the cause of a large lesion in the tail of the pancreas of a 76-year-old man (28). In a 45-year-old woman, malakoplakia of the pancreas was associated with a ductal adenocarcinoma of the head of the pancreas (73). Xanthomatous neuropathy may also involve the pancreas.

## CYSTS

The most common cystic lesions of the pancreas are pseudocysts: they account for approximately 75 percent of pancreatic cystic lesions. Other common pancreatic cystic lesions include neoplastic, retention, and congenital cysts (15).

### Pseudocyst

**Definition.** Pseudocyst is a cystic lesion lined by inflammatory and fibrotic tissue. It occurs within (intrapancreatic) or, more frequently, attached to (extrapancreatic) the pancreas and is due to autodigestive tissue necrosis from acute alcoholic, biliary, or traumatic pancreatitis (25).

**Morphology.** Pseudocysts present as cystic cavities, usually located outside the pancreas, but bound to it by inflammatory tissue. They vary in size (3 to 10 cm) and are filled with necrotic-hemorrhagic material, turbid fluid rich in pancreatic enzymes, or both. The inner surface of the wall has no epithelium and consists of fibrin, granulation tissue (with hemosiderin-filled macrophages), and loose collagen (fig. 7-8). In older cysts, the wall is thicker and has dense collagen. Pseudocysts may communicate with the duct system and may erode into major portal vessels causing thrombosis, bleeding, and, occasionally, disseminated fat necrosis. The pancreatic tissue adjacent to a pseudocyst shows either signs of resolving severe acute pancreatitis or fibrotic changes indicating chronic pancreatitis.

**Differential Diagnosis.** The most common differential diagnosis is with mucinous cystic tumor and solid-pseudopapillary tumor, because the gross appearance of the latter neoplasms may be very similar to that of pseudocysts (see also Differential Diagnosis of these neoplasms). However, the absence of any epithelial lining or epithelial tissue in pseudocysts excludes the diagnosis of a cystic neoplasm. Moreover, mucinous cystic tumor and solid-pseudopapillary tumor predominantly occur in women, whereas pseudocysts are associated with a history of pancreatitis and usually chronic alcoholism and occur more often in men.

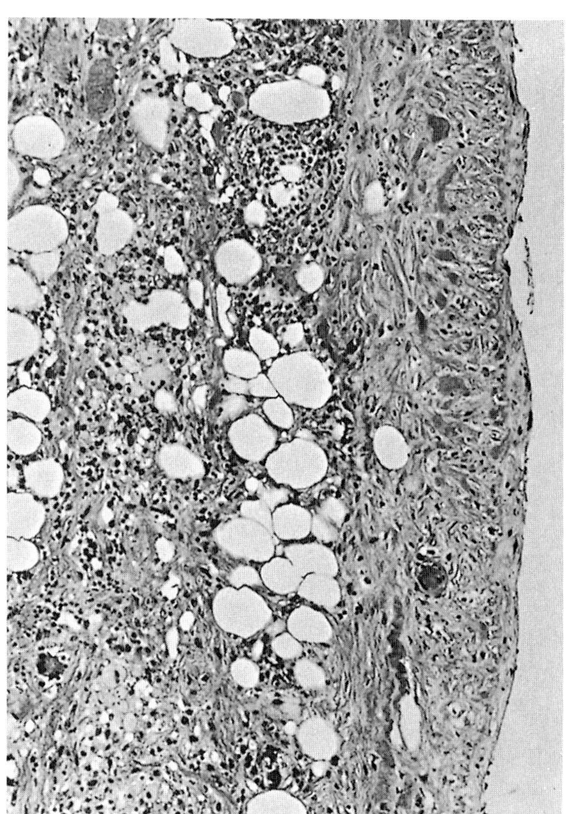

Figure 7-8
PSEUDOCYST: CHRONIC PANCREATITIS
Area of cyst where part of the wall is dense collagen. There is no epithelium lining the inner surface of the cyst wall (right). Deeper in the wall are chronic inflammatory cells and fat (left). (Fig. 45 from Fascicle 19, Second Series.)

### Retention Cyst

**Definition.** Retention cyst is a small cystic structure within the pancreas lined by duct epithelium. It is due to focal ductal obstruction.

**Morphology.** Retention cysts occur in the pancreas upstream of a duct obstruction, either due to tumor, a mucin plug, or a fibrous stricture. Accordingly, the most frequently associated pathologic conditions are carcinoma, cystic fibrosis, or chronic pancreatitis. A retention cyst is a cystically dilated pancreatic duct. Occasionally, part of the epithelium may be replaced by inflammation and necrosis, which is particularly seen in chronic pancreatitis. Because of the small size of this lesion it poses no problem in the differential diagnosis of cystic lesions.

### Parasitic Cyst

This cystic lesion is extremely uncommon and is usually identified as an echinococcal (hydatid) cyst (21).

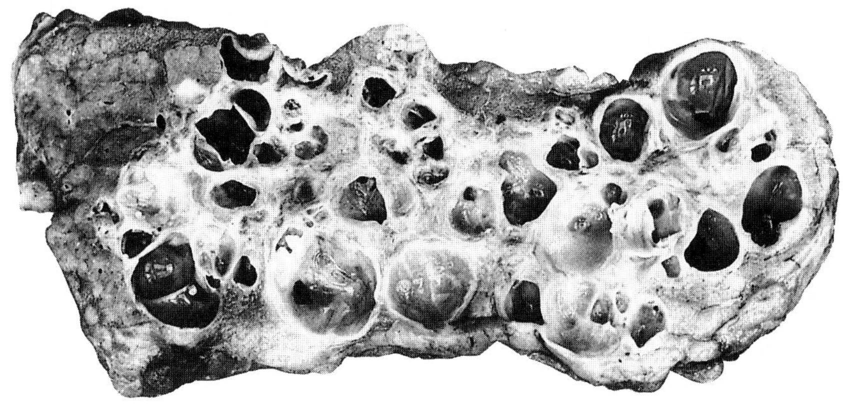

Figure 7-9
CONGENITAL CYST
Multiple congenital cysts transform this pancreas from a patient with von Hippel-Lindau disease into a cystic mass. The cysts are filled with serous fluid. (Fig. 6.1 from Seifert G. Cystic, traumatic and vascular lesions. In: Pancreatic pathology. Klöppel G, Heitz PU, eds. Edinburgh: Churchill Livingstone, 1984:73–8.)

### Congenital Cyst

**Definition.** Congenital (dysgenetic) cyst is an intrapancreatic cystic lesion, noncommunicating with the duct system, and lined by a single layer of flat epithelium. Most of these cysts are multiple and associated with von Hippel-Lindau disease (50) or, rarely, with inherited polycystic kidney disease (53). Large single cysts, unassociated with cystic lesions in other organs, have been reported in children (20,41, 44). Small congenital cysts are incidental findings. Cystic dysplasia of the pancreas is found in a number of malformation syndromes such as the Meckel-Gruber syndrome (20).

**Morphology.** Single congenital cysts are usually small (up to 1 to 2 cm) (65) and only occasionally form a large, unilocular, thin-walled cavity. Multiple congenital cysts may transform the pancreas into a cystic mass studded with numerous small cysts of up to 2 to 3 cm in diameter which are filled with serous fluid (fig. 7-9). The cysts are lined by small nonmucin-producing cuboidal cells and have a fibrous wall (fig. 7-10). Atypical cells are lacking.

**Differential Diagnosis.** The cystic lesions observed in von Hippel-Lindau disease may be difficult to distinguish from serous cystic adenoma (50). Therefore, some authors make no distinction and consider the Hippel-Lindau lesions of the pancreas as manifestations of serous cystic adenoma (see Serous Cystic Adenoma).

### Para-ampullary Duodenal Wall Cyst

**Definition.** Para-ampullary duodenal wall cysts are epithelial-lined cystic lesions occurring in the duodenal submucosa and muscular layer in the vicinity of the ampulla of Vater. They often give rise to secondary inflammation.

It is uncertain whether these cystic lesions are gut duplications in the duodenal wall, or retention cysts resulting from myoadenomatosis in heterotopic pancreas (18,42,66). Clinically, the patients present with symptoms suggestive of pancreatic cancer: pain, vomiting, weight loss, and eventually jaundice.

**Morphology.** The cystic lesions occur either singly or in multiples in the submucosal or intramucosal layers of the duodenum, often in close proximity to the ampulla of Vater and the intrapancreatic portion of the common bile duct (fig. 7-11). Histologically, they are lined by columnar mucin-producing epithelium and may be surrounded by small ductular structures. Some or all of the cystic structures contain eosinophilic hyaline material which is surrounded by leukocytes, macrophages, some foreign body cells, and lymphocytes. The epithelium in contact with the hyaline material is often necrotic. This appears

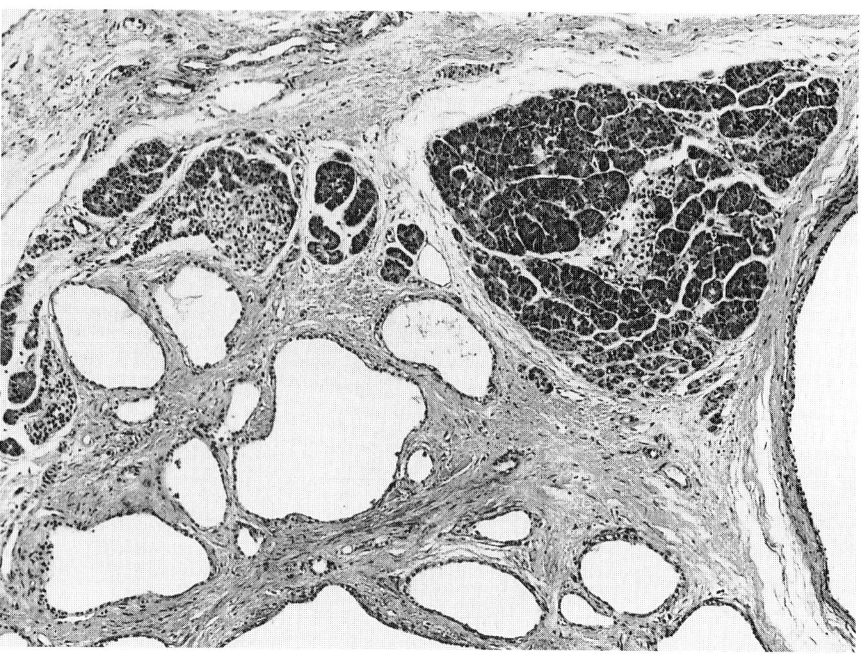

Figure 7-10
CONGENITAL CYST

The cysts are lined by small nonmucin-producing cuboidal cells and are embedded in fibrous tissue.

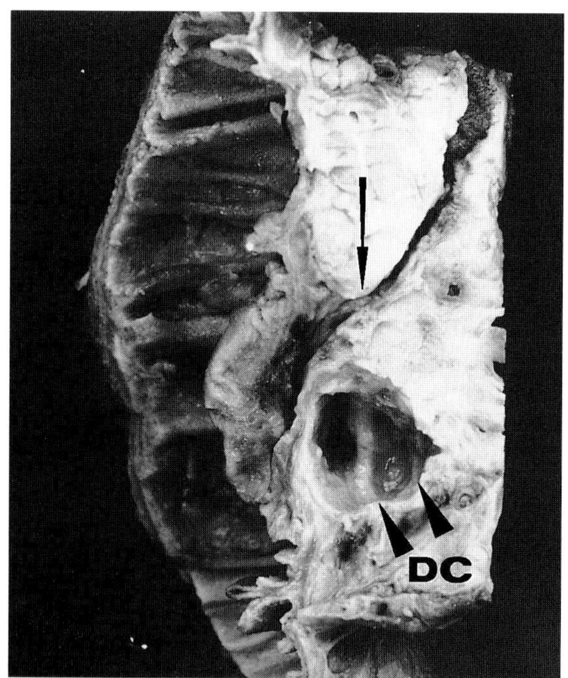


Figure 7-11
DUODENAL WALL CYST

Whipple resection specimen showing a cystic lesion in the wall of the duodenum (DC), in close proximity to the ampulla of Vater and the intrapancreatic portion of the common bile duct (arrow). (Fig. 6.2 from Seifert G. Cystic, traumatic and vascular lesions. In: Pancreatic pathology. Klöppel G, Heitz PU, eds. Edinburgh: Churchill Livingstone, 1984:73–8.)

to induce further inflammation with an intense and sometimes extremely cellular fibrotic reaction, particularly in the area between the duodenum and the pancreas. The fibrotic process then results in compression and tubular stenosis of the common bile duct.

**Differential Diagnosis.** Clinically, the most important differential diagnosis is ductal adenocarcinoma of the pancreas, because most patients present at the same age and with similar symptoms as pancreatic cancer patients. At the morphologic level there is, however, no difficulty in separating the two. The features of cystic structures in the duodenal wall (cystic changes of the duodenum, an intense fibrotic reaction in the area between duodenum and pancreas, and an acute and chronic inflammation) contradict a pancreatic carcinoma.

## Enterogenous Cyst

**Definition.** Enterogenous cyst is a gastrointestinal duplication in the gut wall. If it occurs in a juxtapancreatic position in the duodenal wall, it often communicates with the pancreatic duct system. The lesion is a congenital malformation. It may cause pancreatitis in children (20,30,39).

**Morphology.** The cystic lesions are usually 2 to 4 cm in diameter. Most of them are found in the duodenal wall and only exceptionally occur in the body and tail of the pancreas (54). Some duodenal enterogenous cysts communicate through an ectopic duct with the pancreas. Histologic examination reveals duplicated duodenal or other intestinal mucosa.

**Differential Diagnosis.** Enterogenous cysts have to be distinguished from cystic neoplasms of the pancreas. This is usually easy because of the location of the cystic lesion in the duodenal wall and the intestinal-type lining of mucosa.

### Lymphoepithelial Cyst

**Definition.** Lymphoepithelial cyst is a cystic lesion lined by mature keratinizing squamous epithelium supported by distinct lymphoid tissue. Its histologic features resemble those of the branchial cyst, usually seen in the oral and cervical region. Recently, it has been suggested that it arises from a benign epithelial inclusion in a parapancreatic lymph node (17), but in another report lymphoepithelial cyst is considered to be a dermoid cyst of the pancreas (70). All lesions so far reported occurred in men (age range, 36 to 73 years).

**Morphology.** Grossly, the spherically shaped lesion protrudes from the pancreatic tissue from which it is well demarcated (17,36,56). The cut surface reveals a thin-walled unilocular cyst which is filled with gray-whitish pasty material. Histologically, the cyst is filled with keratin and lined by mature keratinizing squamous epithelium. The epithelium is supported by a small layer of lymphoid tissue containing occasional follicles with germinal centers. Teratoid elements such as skin appendages or mesenchymal tissue are lacking. The surrounding uninvolved pancreatic tissue appears normal.

**Differential Diagnosis.** The differential diagnosis includes all cystic lesions of the pancreas, particularly however, cystic teratoma (dermoid cyst). Absence of skin appendages or mature mesenchymal elements in the cyst wall exclude the latter tumor; presence of a pasty whitish content excludes all other cystic lesions.

### Endometrial Cyst

**Definition.** Endometrial cyst is a manifestation of endometriosis, which is characterized by the presence of endometrial glands and stroma in ectopic sites.

**Morphology.** Endometrial cyst of the pancreas is exceptionally rare. In the single case reported by Marchevsky et al. (40) it presented as a 4-cm, well-circumscribed cyst in the tail of the pancreas of a 36-year-old woman. The cyst wall was smooth and grey-brown, with focal areas of hemorrhage. Histologically, the cyst wall contained endometrial glands admixed with cellular, well-vascularized, spindle cell stroma with foci of hemorrhage, and hemosiderin deposits in macrophages.

**Differential Diagnosis.** Distinguishing this type of cyst from pseudocyst relies on the demonstration of endometrial glands and stroma in the cyst wall. The absence of a continuous epithelial lining separates it from the cystic neoplasms.

## DUCT CHANGES

Duct changes may occur in the normal pancreas or in association with non-neoplastic (pancreatitis) or neoplastic diseases. Five major types of non-neoplastic pancreatic duct changes can be distinguished: squamous metaplasia, mucinous cell hypertrophy (including pyloric gland and goblet cell metaplasia), ductal papillary hyperplasia, and adenomatoid duct hyperplasia. These lesions have to be distinguished from the neoplastic intraductal lesion called severe ductal dysplasia or carcinoma in situ, which is, although without any doubt neoplastic, discussed in this chapter because of its apparently close relationship with mucinous hypertrophy and ductal papillary hyperplasia.

### Squamous Metaplasia

**Definition.** Squamous metaplasia is a replacement of the columnar duct cells by squamous epithelium. Squamous metaplasia is found in 12 to 47 percent of the nontumorous pancreata of middle-aged and elderly patients and in chronically inflamed pancreata (8,23,51,55). No association with pancreatic cancer has been noted.

**Microscopic Findings.** The stratified squamous epithelium that occurs in the duct system is usually patchy (fig. 7-12) and involves mainly the small ducts or ductules. Sometimes the epithelium at the surface of the squamous metaplasia is still mucinous, and occasionally there is a multilayered increase of cuboidal epithelial cells, a few of which have slight squamous differentiation. This change can be regarded as the immature variant of squamous metaplasia; it has also been described

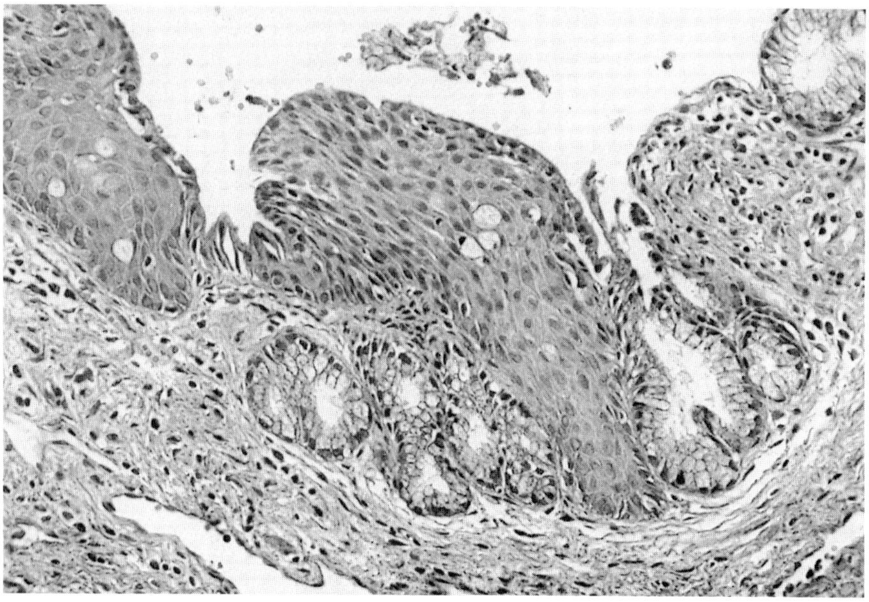

Figure 7-12
SQUAMOUS METAPLASIA
Squamous metaplasia in a patient with chronic pancreatitis. The mucinous epithelial duct cells are partly replaced by squamous epithelium.

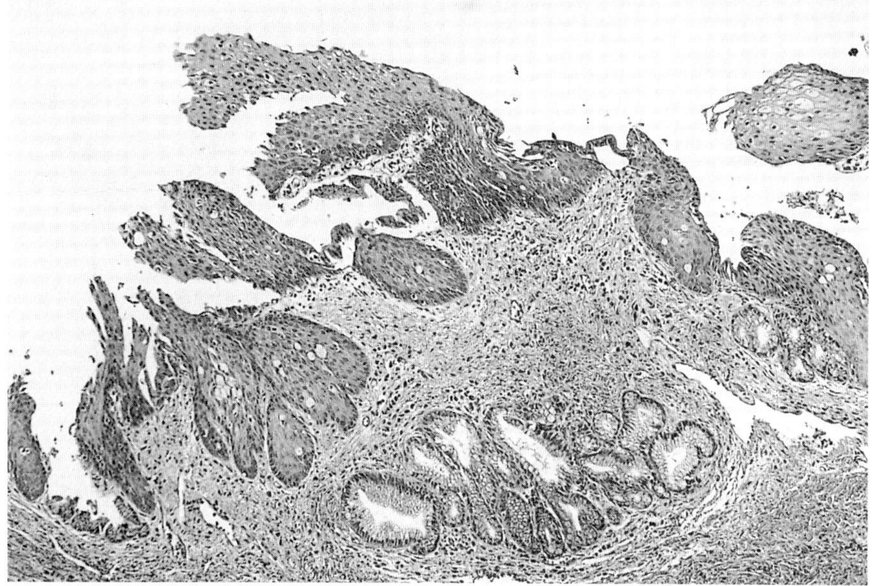

Figure 7-13
SQUAMOUS METAPLASIA
This patient had chronic pancreatitis with calculi and was treated by placing a stent in the main pancreatic duct. The mucinous duct epithelium is almost replaced by squamous epithelium.

under the term *focal atypical epithelial hyperplasia* (9). A marked degree of squamous metaplasia may occur in the main pancreatic duct after prolonged stenting (personal observation) (fig. 7-13) or in association with the presence of *Clonorchis sinensis* worms (6).

### Mucinous Cell Hypertrophy

**Definition.** Mucinous cell hypertrophy is characterized by the replacement of the normal epithelium of the large and medium-sized ducts by tall columnar cells with basal nuclei and considerable supranuclear mucin. These lesions have also been referred to as *mucoid transformation, goblet cell metaplasia, simple hyperplasia,* or *ductal mucinous hyperplasia*. This is the most frequent epithelial change of the pancreatic ducts, and is found in 59 to 90 percent of nontumorous pancreata (7,9,23,27,51,65). It is often seen in association with moderate obstruction and chronic pancreatitis, and occurs in about the same percentage of patients with pancreatic cancer as in

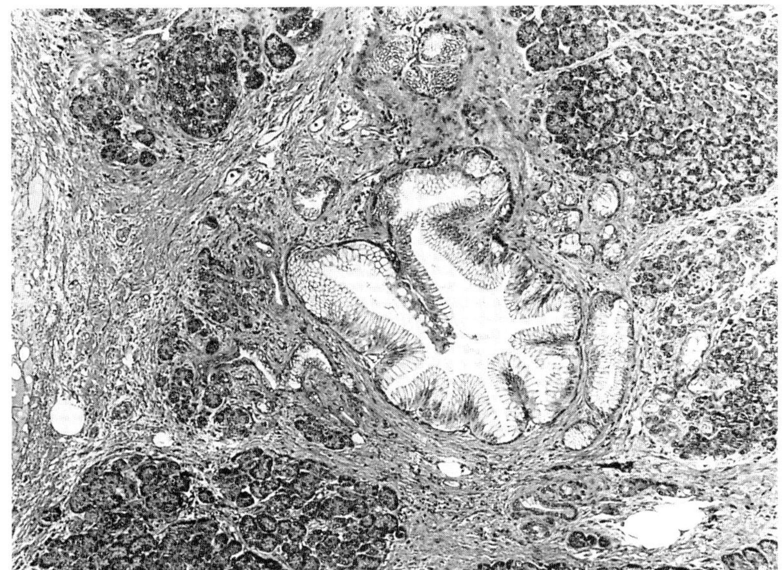

Figure 7-14
MUCINOUS CELL HYPERTROPHY
Nonpapillary epithelial hypertrophy is characterized by the replacement of the normal epithelium of the large and medium-sized ducts by tall mucin-producing columnar cells.

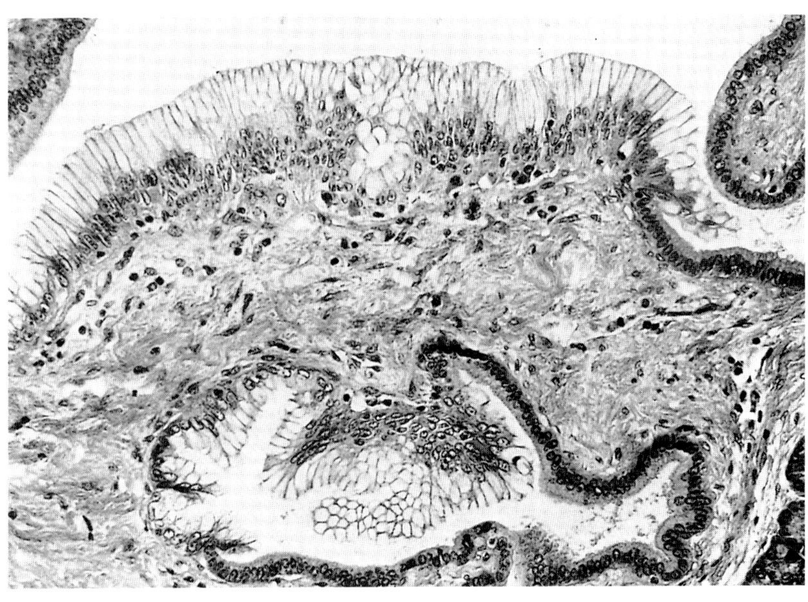

Figure 7-15
MUCINOUS CELL HYPERTROPHY
The lining columnar epithelium shows mild cellular atypia characterized by some crowding of slightly enlarged nuclei. Most nuclei are polarized. The apical portion of the cytoplasm is filled with mucin.

a matched control group of patients with other types of nonpancreatic cancer. In the normal pancreas, mucinous cell hypertrophy occurs more often in the head than the tail, and is more frequent in older patients (27).

**Microscopic Findings.** Mucinous cell hypertrophy is typically focal. The columnar epithelium lining a duct becomes taller because of the increased mucin content of the cells (fig. 7-14). The mucin occupies most of the cytoplasm and pushes the nucleus to the basal pole of the cell (fig. 7-15). Since this change gives the cell a goblet-like appearance, it has also been named goblet cell metaplasia (72). Histochemically, cells with mucinous hypertrophy produce mainly neutral mucin (which stains with combined Alcian blue pH 2.5 and periodic acid–Schiff [PAS]) and sialomucin (which stains with Alcian blue pH 2.5), while sulphated mucin (which stains with combined aldehyde-fuchsin and Alcian blue pH 2.5), normally elaborated in the duct cells, is markedly reduced. Immunohistochemically, the mucin stains for M1 antigen, which is present in gastric superficial epithelium but not in normal

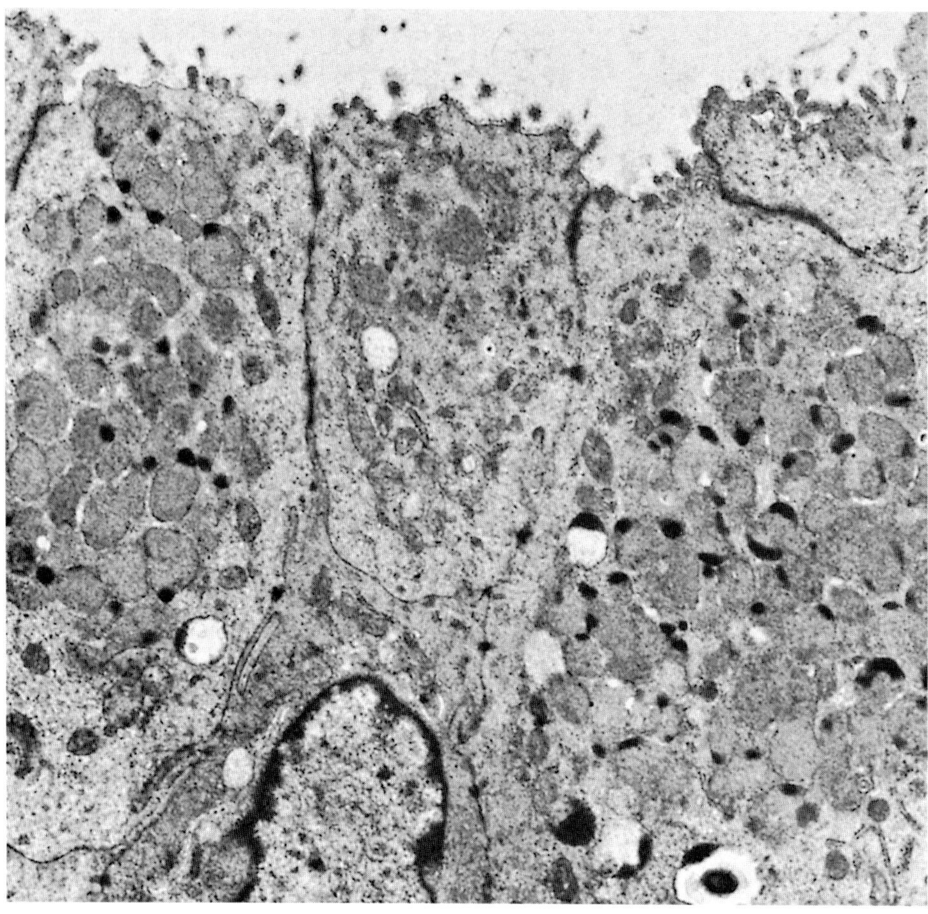

Figure 7-16
MUCINOUS CELL HYPERTROPHY
Electron micrograph of papillary hyperplasia in a patient with cancer of head of pancreas. Mucin granules have an electron-opaque matrix and a darker eccentric core (X12,400). (Fig. 113 from Fascicle 19, Second Series.)

pancreatic duct cells (63). Ultrastructurally, the duct cells with mucinous hypertrophy show punctate cerebroid mucin granules instead of the dense-core granules with a homogeneous inner structure that characterize the mucin granules of the normal large ducts (fig. 7-16) (63). Mucinous cell hypertrophy may be associated with pyloric gland metaplasia (fig. 7-17) (58). In the latter change, which is only revealed by histochemical or immunohistochemical means, the secretion product of the duct cell is similar to the secretion produced by normal juxtapyloric gland cells. It differs from that of normal duct cells by its intense reactivity with PAS and negativity for Alcian blue pH 2.5 (58). These cells are positive for pepsinogen II and cathepsin E (63). Pure metaplastic pyloric-type cell changes are found primarily in small ducts surrounding main or interlobular ducts with mucinous cell hypertrophy or ductal papillary hyperplasia (fig. 7-17).

Mucinous cell hypertrophy is usually associated with a mild epithelial dysplasia characterized by mild cellular atypia with somewhat enlarged and elongated nuclei (fig. 7-15). Focally there may also be slight nuclear stratification. Rarely, there is a moderate degree of dysplasia with more pronounced nuclear crowding and cellular atypia; this change is usually associated with papillary hyperplasia (fig. 7-18).

### Ductal Papillary Hyperplasia

**Definition.** This focal intraductal papillary proliferation of duct cells shows mucinous cell hypertrophy and occasionally pyloric-type metaplasia.

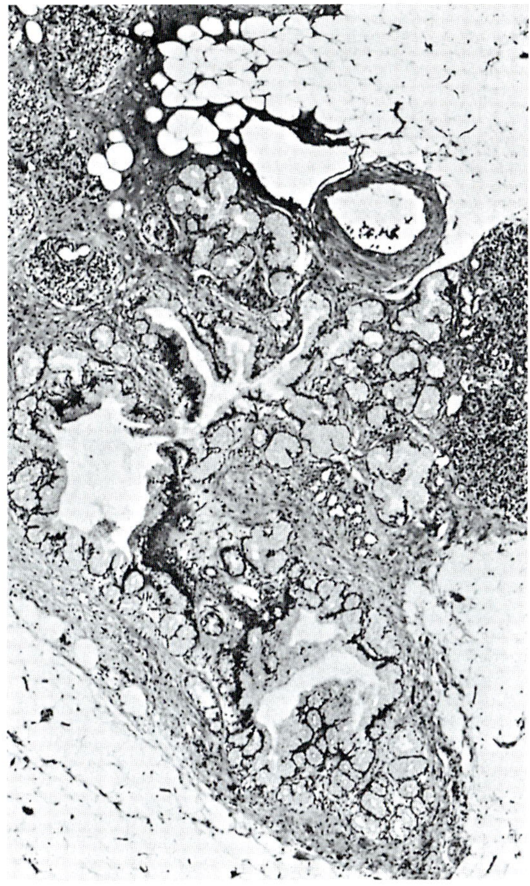

Figure 7-17
MUCINOUS CELL HYPERTROPHY WITH PYLORIC GLAND METAPLASIA

An area of parenchymal atrophy, chronic pancreatitis, and fatty replacement of parenchyma in a patient with carcinoma of the pancreas. There is marked hypertrophy and hyperplasia of mucous glands of the duct epithelium. A diagnosis of pyloric gland metaplasia has to be made histochemically and is suggested when PAS stain is positive and the Alcian blue at pH 2.8 is negative. (Fig. 64 from Fascicle 19, Second Series.)

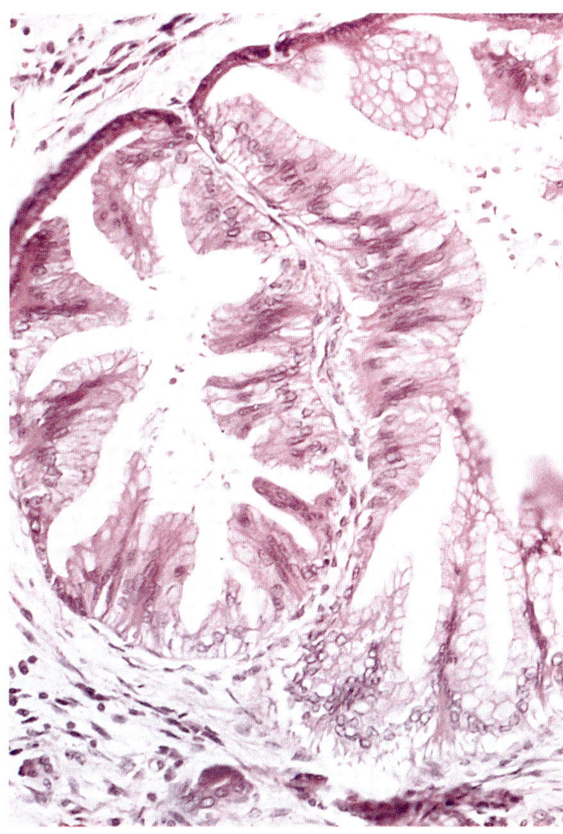

Figure 7-18
TUMOR-LIKE LESIONS: DUCTAL CHANGES

This pancreatic duct shows ductal hyperplasia with mucinous cell hypertrophy and mild to moderate dysplasia. Note the focal nuclear crowding within small papillae.

In the normal pancreas, the incidence of ductal papillary hyperplasia increases with patient age and is greater in the head of the pancreas than in the body and tail (27). It is also more frequent in patients with pancreatic cancer than in those with nonpancreatic cancers (50 versus 12 percent) (7,9,23,27).

**Microscopic Findings.** Ductal papillary hyperplasia is a focal change which occurs in large and medium-sized ducts. The duct epithelium forms papillary folds which protrude into the duct lumen (fig. 7-19). Characteristically, these papillary folds contain a vascular tissue stalk. The papillary duct epithelium shows mucinous cell hypertrophy (with or without pyloric gland metaplasia) (fig. 7-19) and a mild and occasionally moderate cellular atypia, particularly in patients with chronic pancreatitis (fig. 7-20) (71). This implies that the cells contain slightly enlarged and hyperchromatic nuclei which show focal stratification. Mitoses are rare.

Ductal papillary hyperplasia may be combined with focal adenomatoid duct hyperplasia. In elderly patients ductal papillary hyperplasia of secondary ducts may cause duct obstruction. This in turn leads to saccular ductal ectasia upstream to the occlusion, resulting in acinar atrophy and fibrosis of the drained lobule (37,60).

**Differential Diagnosis.** The differential diagnosis of ductal papillary hyperplasia includes severe ductal dysplasia (i.e., carcinoma in situ) and intraductal papillary-mucinous tumor. Severe

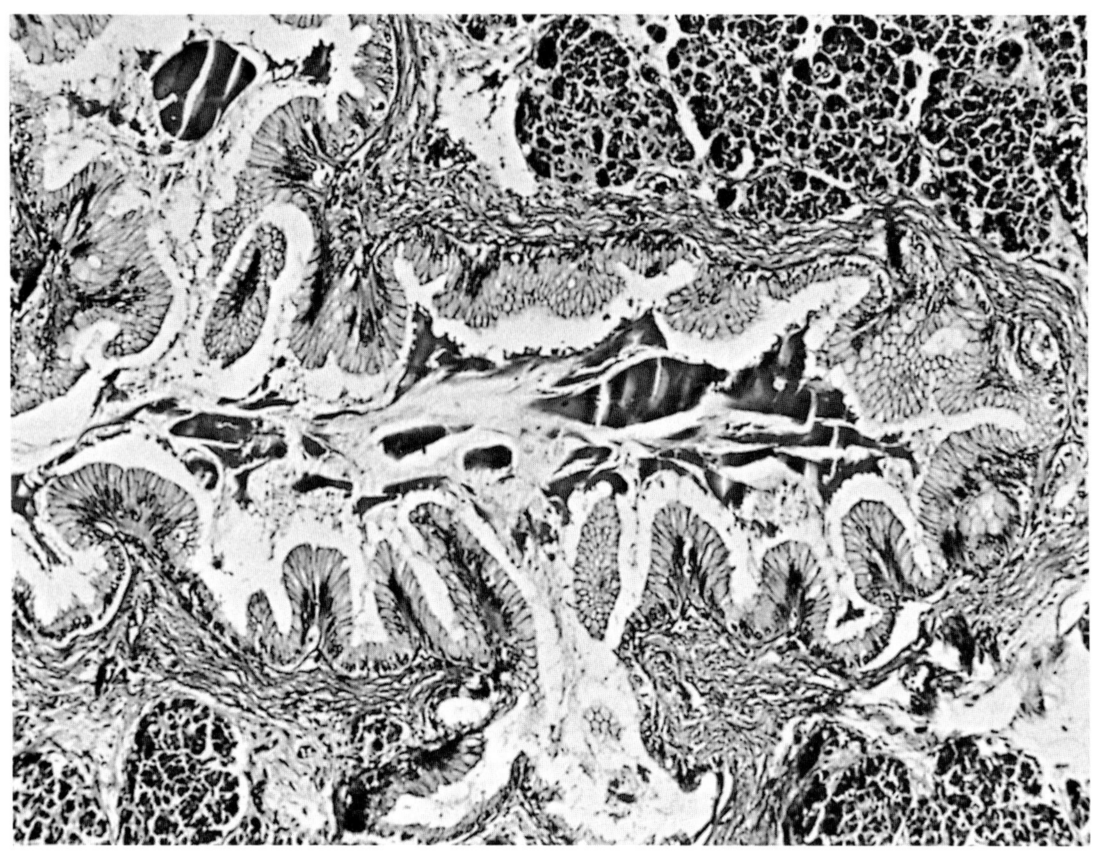

Figure 7-19
DUCTAL PAPILLARY HYPERPLASIA
This patient had marked papillary hyperplasia associated with obstruction to the duct system by pancreatic cancer. Papillae of various sizes, lined with columnar mucinous cells, project into the lumen of main duct, which contains inspissated heavily stained material. A few areas of flat epithelium are present between papillae. (Fig. 60 from Fascicle 19, Second Series.)

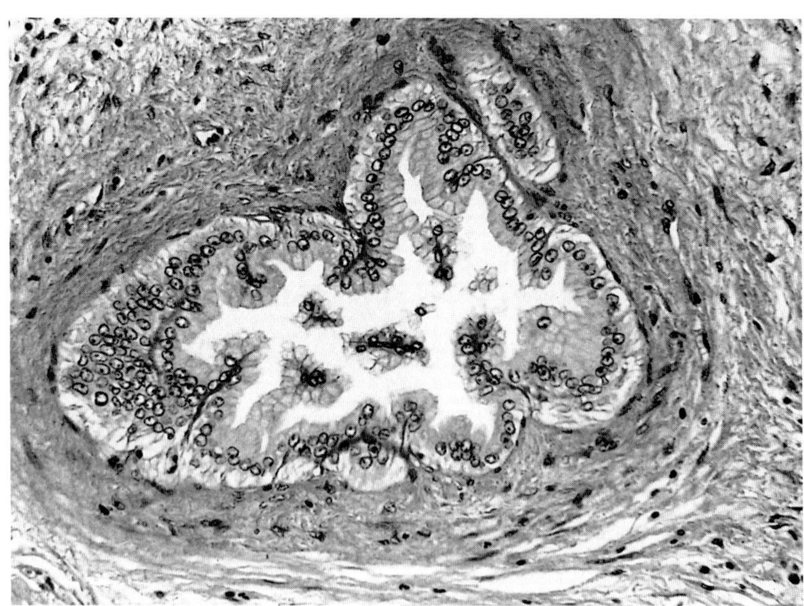

Figure 7-20
DUCTAL
PAPILLARY HYPERPLASIA
This interlobular duct from a pancreas with chronic pancreatitis shows mucous cell hypertrophy and ductular hyperplasia. The epithelium exhibits a slight cellular atypia.

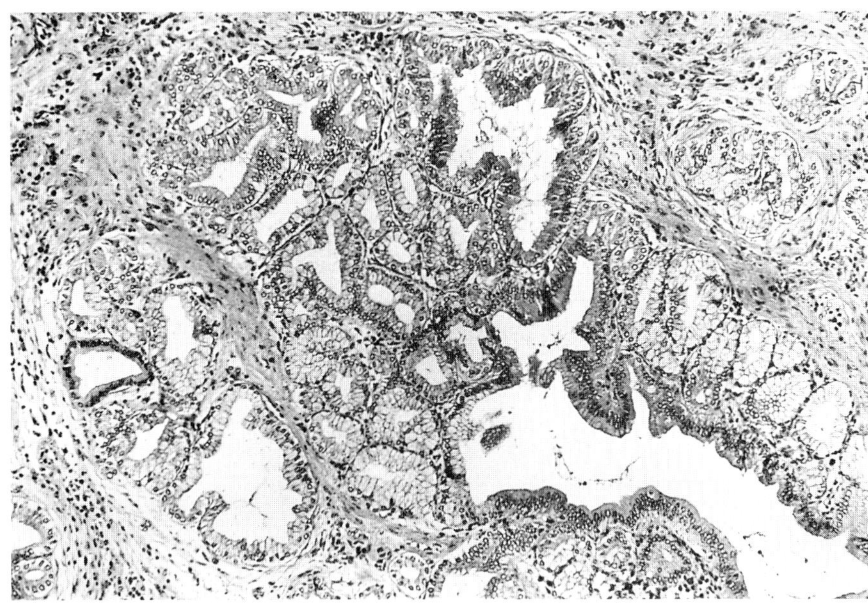

Figure 7-21
ADENOMATOID DUCTAL HYPERPLASIA

The adenomatoid ductal hyperplasia consists of an accumulation of medium-sized pancreatic ducts, ductules, or both embedded in moderately cellular fibrous tissue.

ductal dysplasia is characterized by severe cellular atypia of duct cells: conspicuous pleomorphism and loss of polarity of the nuclei, and high mitotic activity. These cells may form irregularly sized papillae without fibrovascular cores. This change is frequently associated with ductal adenocarcinoma of the pancreas where it occurs in close vicinity to the definitive carcinoma. The involvement of the duct system by intraductal papillary-mucinous tumor is grossly conspicuous because of extreme duct dilatation, either by an intraductal tumor mass or viscous mucin plugs. Ductal papillary hyperplasia, in contrast, is always a microscopic lesion. Histologically, the neoplastic papillary proliferations are much taller and more prominent than the papillae seen in ductal papillary hyperplasia. Moreover, the neoplastic lesion often exhibits severe dysplasia-carcinoma in situ changes not seen in ductal papillary hyperplasia.

### Adenomatoid Ductal Hyperplasia

**Definition.** Adenomatoid (adenomatous) ductal hyperplasia is a focal aggregation of ducts or ductules, usually lined by epithelium, showing mucinous cell hypertrophy and often pyloric gland metaplasia. This lesion is rare in the normal pancreas and shows no preferential localization (23,64). Although its ductal adenoma-like appearance may give the impression of a neoplastic growth, it most likely represents a nonneoplastic proliferation of ducts.

**Microscopic Findings.** The lesions consist of an accumulation of medium-sized pancreatic ducts or ductules embedded in moderately cellular fibrous tissue (fig. 7-21). The lesions are small and rarely exceed 1 mm in diameter. Usually there are single islets and acini between the aggregated ducts. Occasionally, however, the lesions consist of ducts only and are so well demarcated that they resemble adenomas. The cells of the aggregated ducts are well differentiated and often show mucinous hypertrophy and pyloric gland metaplasia. The lining epithelium occasionally consists of eosinophilic epithelial cells (oxyphilic cell metaplasia).

**Differential Diagnosis.** The lesions, particularly if multiple, have to be distinguished from microscopic foci of a well-differentiated ductal adenocarcinoma. This distinction, however, is easy, because adenomatoid ductal hyperplasia lacks any severe cellular atypia and the ducts are of regular size and structure and do not invade the surrounding tissue. Adenomatoid ductal hyperplasia should also be differentiated from lesions called ductular (cystic) hyperplasia (9) or tubular hyperplasia (65), changes seen in chronic pancreatitis. They occur in areas of fibrosis, where the disappearance of the acini has led to a concentration and crowding of small ducts and ductules. The ductular structures in these areas

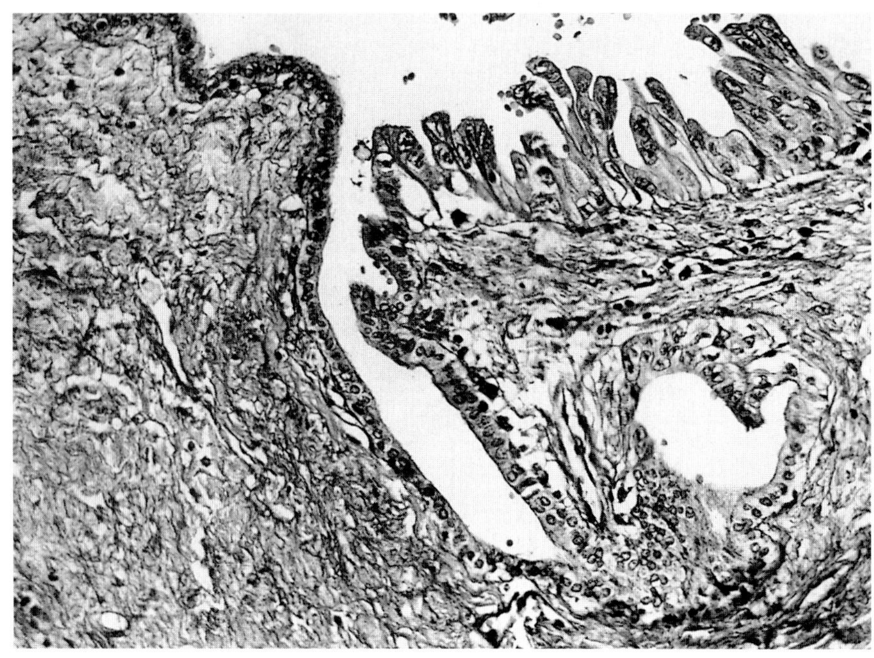

Figure 7-22
SEVERE DUCTAL DYSPLASIA
Note the severe atypia of the duct epithelium (right) which abruptly replaces benign-appearing duct cells.

may be tubular or ectatic, and are lined by cuboidal epithelium resembling ductular epithelium.

## Severe Ductal Dysplasia (Atypical Hyperplasia)

**Definition.** Severe ductal dysplasia defines a severe cellular atypia of the duct epithelium, with or without papillary proliferation. This is a neoplastic lesion and is equivalent to intraductal carcinoma or carcinoma in situ.

The dysplasia is usually found in close proximity to a well-differentiated ductal adenocarcinoma. It may therefore represent intraductal extension from an established invasive carcinoma (see also Ductal Adenocarcinoma) rather than a multicentric tumor focus. Lesions of atypical ductal epithelium that are severe enough to merit the designation carcinoma in situ have been reported in the absence of invasive pancreatic carcinoma (27,55), but are extremely rare.

**Microscopic Findings.** Severe ductal dysplasia is characterized by severe cellular atypia of the duct epithelium. The criteria for severe cellular atypia include irregular cell size, loss of nuclear polarity, marked nuclear pleomorphism, presence of distinct nucleoli, and frequent mitotic figures (fig. 7-22). Usually the atypical cells form small and irregularly sized papillary projections lacking a fibrovascular core but occasionally exhibiting a cribriform pattern (fig. 7-23). The stroma surrounding the involved ducts shows a concentric and cellular desmoplastic reaction.

**Differential Diagnosis.** The differential diagnosis includes intraductal papillary-mucinous tumor and intraductal extension of established invasive carcinoma. In the latter condition, the severe ductal dysplasia can be identified as an intraductal tumor component by tracing the lesion back through serial or step-wise sectioning to the established invasive carcinoma. As for papillary-mucinous tumor, the same diagnostic considerations are applied as discussed above for ductal papillary hyperplasia. The few reports that described severe ductal dysplasia and carcinoma in situ in pancreata without frank carcinoma (11,32, 45,47) have to be interpreted with caution, because the lesions that were illustrated appear to be intraductal papillary-mucinous tumors.

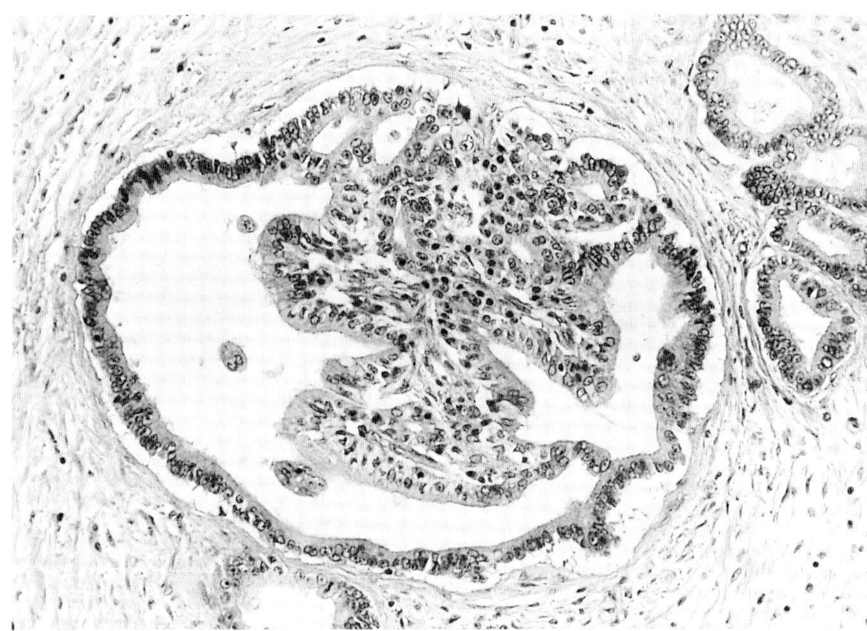

Figure 7-23
SEVERE
DUCTAL DYSPLASIA
This duct is lined by a severely atypical epithelium which forms an irregular papillary projection showing a cribriform pattern and lacking a fibrovascular core. This lesion was found in the vicinity of an invasive ductal adenocarcinoma.

## ACINAR CHANGES

Acinar changes include acinar dilatation (acinar ectasia) and focal transformation of acinar cells (51,65). Within the scope of tumor-like lesions only nodular acinar changes will be considered.

### Focal Acinar Transformation

**Definition.** Focal acinar transformation defines a group of acinar cells with cytoplasmic alterations but almost no nuclear changes. These alterations are of unknown significance and have no clear relationship with any pancreatic diseases. Focal acinar transformation of the pancreas has been described as *eosinophilic degeneration of acinar cells* (65), *acinar adenomatous hyperplasia* (13), *acinar cell dysplasia* (22,33,34), and *hyperplastic acinar cell nodule* (55). Its incidence in the nontumorous pancreas ranges from 1.3 to 43.5 percent (22,33,55,65). So far most studies have failed to identify any clear association between focal acinar cell transformation (which is most likely a degenerative lesion) and acinar cell carcinoma.

**Microscopic Findings.** Focal acinar transformation is only recognized in the well-preserved pancreas. It is characterized by the occurrence of irregularly sized but sharply outlined groups of acinar cells, measuring from 300 to 3000 µm in their greatest dimension. The cytoplasm of the cells often shows a homogeneous eosinophilia or a loss of basophilia (fig. 7-24), but may also be vacuolated, probably due to a marked dilatation of the rough endoplasmic reticulum (26). The cells and their nuclei are similar in size to the surrounding acinar cells, but the nuclei may have denser chromatin. Mitoses are infrequent and inflammatory infiltrates are absent.

## HETEROTOPIC PANCREAS

**Definition.** Heterotopic pancreas (ectopic pancreas, accessory pancreas, and aberrant pancreas) is a developmental anomaly that results in the occurrence of pancreatic tissue at ectopic sites. Pancreatic heterotopia is found in 2 to 15 percent of all autopsies (20). It is usually an incidental finding, but may present as peptic ulceration or intestinal obstruction (3,43). Rarely, it gives rise to malignant transformation (14,68).

**Morphology.** The most frequent sites of heterotopic pancreas are gastric antrum (30 percent), duodenum (30 percent), jejunum (20 percent), and Meckel's diverticulum (5 percent) (10, 20,61). Unusual locations are the colon, spleen, liver, biliary tract, mesentery, and lymph nodes (48). In the gastrointestinal tract, the heterotopic pancreas forms a rounded or lobulated,

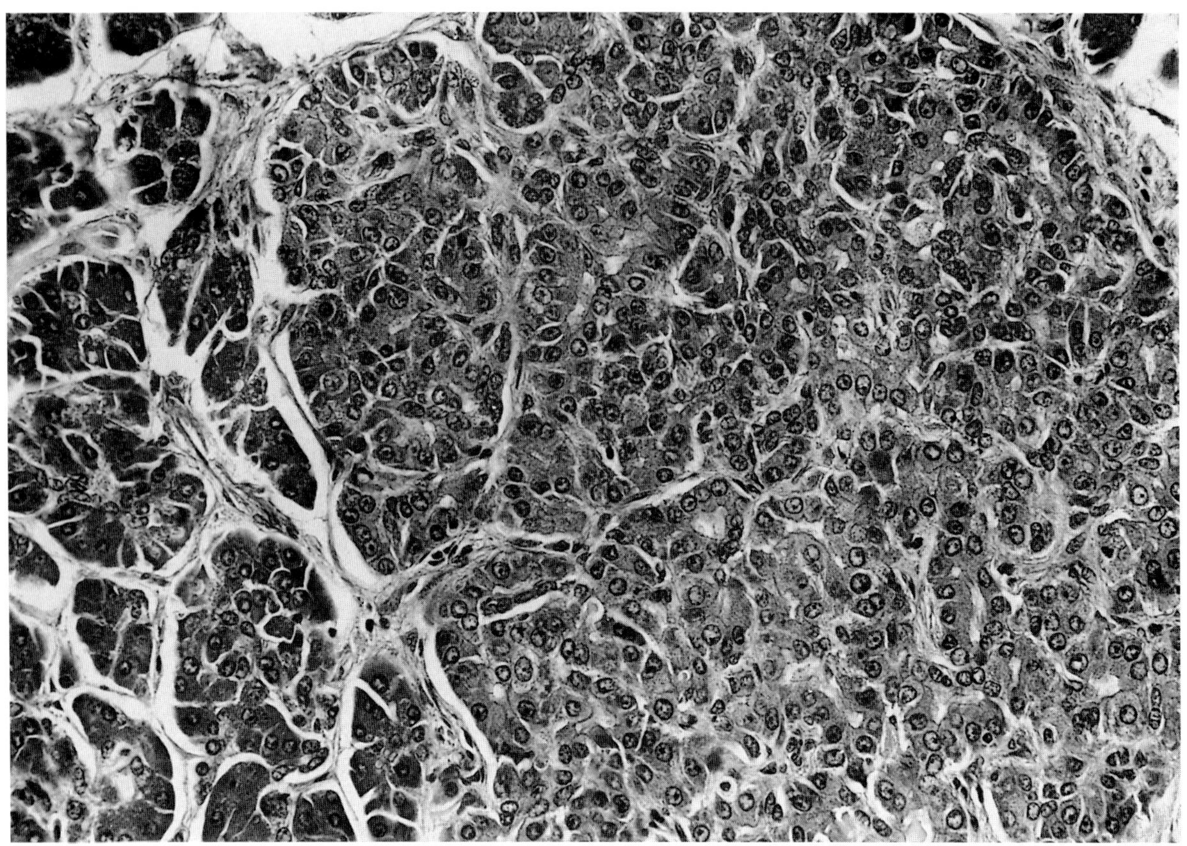

Figure 7-24
FOCAL ACINAR TRANSFORMATION
Well-demarcated focus of acinar cells with eosinophilic-staining cytoplasm. Acini are not as distinct as adjoining normal acini (left), but nuclei and nucleoli are about the same size as those of adjacent normal acinar cells. Ductules and islets are not present. (Fig. 4 from Longnecker DS, Pour P, Klöppel G. Preneoplastic lesions of the exocrine pancreas. In: Atlas of exocrine pancreatic tumors. Pour P, Konishi Y, Klöppel G, Longnecker DS, eds. Tokyo, Springer Verlag, 1994:211–9.)

white or yellowish lump that is usually between 1 to 4 cm in diameter. The mass lies most commonly in the submucosa and often has a centrally ulcerated pit. Sometimes it presents as a subserosal nodule. Histologically, the heterotopic tissue consists of normal-appearing exocrine and endocrine parenchyma or, in about one third of the cases, of a lobular arrangement of ducts with few or even no acinar and endocrine elements (fig. 7-25, top). Occasionally, only ducts or islets are present (fig. 7-25, bottom).

Well-organized pancreatic tissue may be found in mature teratomas, particularly of mediastinal origin (20). Immunohistochemically, all islet cell types are found in regular distribution (67). In two cases, the mediastinal teratoma secreted insulin (19,59).

## HETEROTOPIC (ECTOPIC) SPLEEN

Accessory splenic tissue may be found in the pancreas. It forms a small (range, 0.5 to 4 cm) well-demarcated, red mass that is usually found in the tail of the gland, but has also been observed in the head (29). Recently, an epidermoid cyst of the pancreas thought to be derived from an ectopic spleen was described (46).

## HAMARTOMA AND PSEUDOTUMOR

Pancreatic nodular lesions that have been called hamartomas or pseudotumors have been reported only in a few cases. Burt et al. (5) described a premature infant with refractory hypoglycemia and hypocalcemia whose entire pancreas consisted of noncystic ductal elements

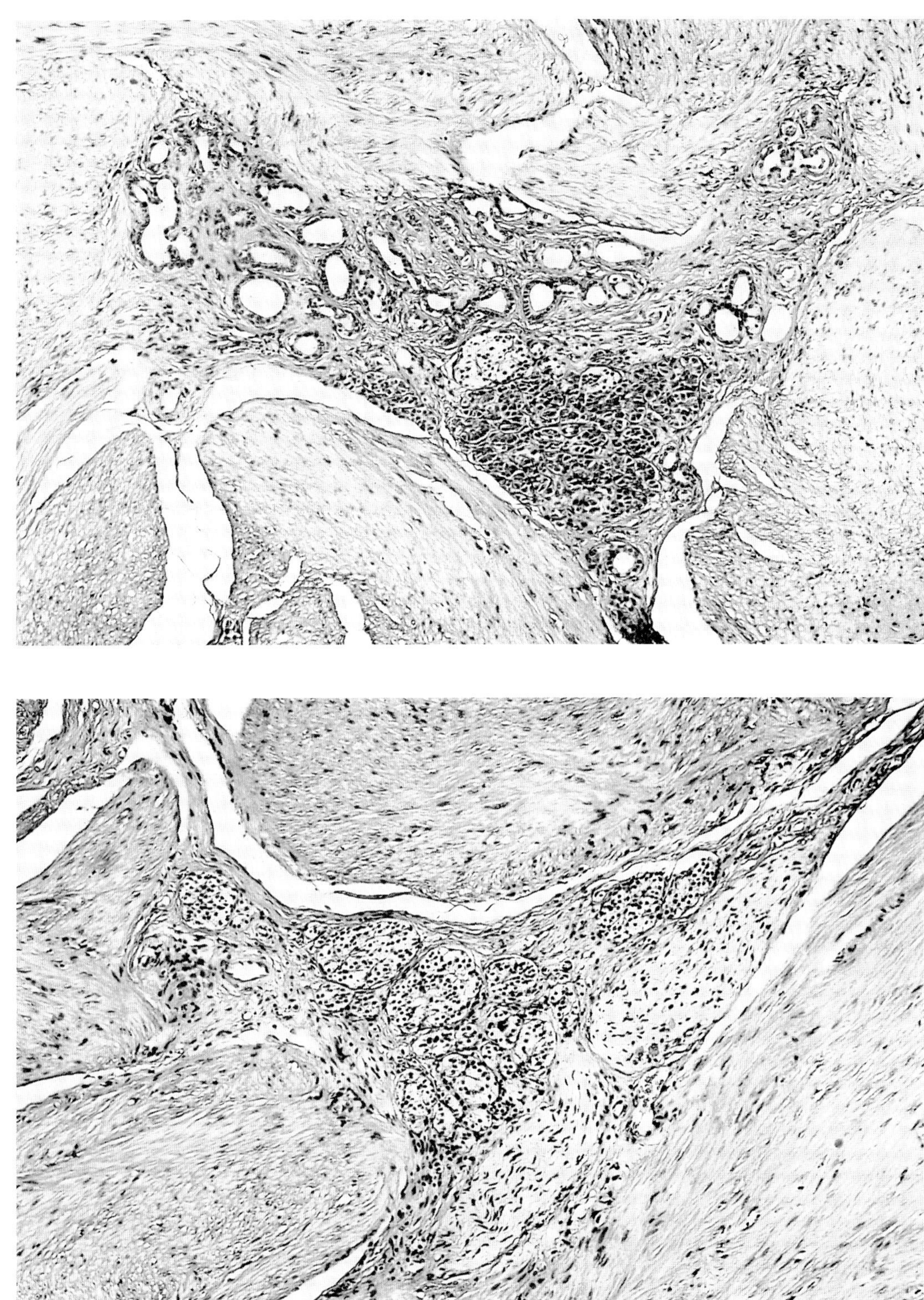

Figure 7-25
HETEROTOPIC PANCREAS

Top: Heterotopic pancreatic tissue in the muscular layer of the stomach composed of ducts, a few islets, and a group of acinar cells.
Bottom: Another nodule of heterotopic pancreatic tissue in the stomach wall consisting exclusively of islets. (Courtesy of Dr. Sören Schröder, Hamburg, Germany.)

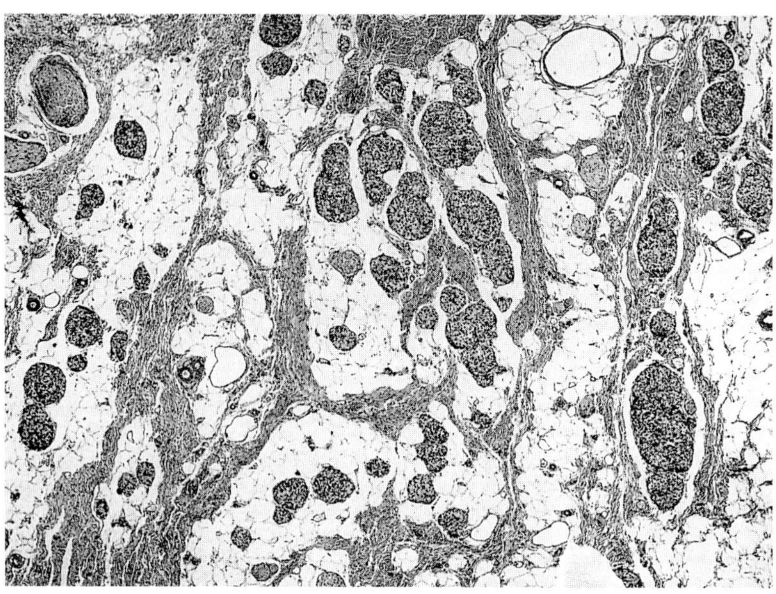

Figure 7-26
PSEUDOLIPOMATOUS HYPERTROPHY
The pancreatic parenchyma consists of mature fatty tissue separated by thin fibrous septa containing isolated clusters of normal islets.

with a minority of well-organized islets and acinar tissue. More recently, Flaherty and Benjamin (12) described a 20-month-old female infant who presented with abdominal distention due to a mass in the head of the pancreas. The resected specimen contained a 9-cm multicystic mass. The mass was composed of cyst-like spaces admixed with acinar tissue but without endocrine elements. Anthony et al. (1) described three patients with focal areas in the pancreas composed of lobulated connective tissue enclosing acinar cells, endocrine cells, and dilated pancreatic ducts in complete disarray. An inflammatory pseudotumor was recently reported by Pallazo and Chang (52).

## PSEUDOLIPOMATOUS HYPERTROPHY

Marked pancreatic lipomatosis may be seen in patients with obstruction of the pancreatic duct due to impacted calculi, carcinoma, or cysts (4). Massive pancreatic lipomatosis may also occur in patients with advanced cystic fibrosis or Shwachman's syndrome (62). Pancreatic lipomatosis as an isolated abnormality is rare. It may be associated with pancreatic exocrine insufficiency (35). Grossly, the pancreas is moderately or markedly enlarged, but maintains its usual shape. Histologically, the parenchyma consists of mature fatty tissue separated by thin fibrous septa containing isolated clusters of normal islets (fig. 7-26).

## PSEUDOLYMPHOMA

Pseudolymphoma is an isolated, localized, non-neoplastic proliferation of lymphoid tissue. The alimentary tract is one of the most common locations, but only three cases have been reported in the pancreas (2,16,49). In two patients the pancreatic tissue contained a soft, yellowish white nodule, 2 to 3 cm in diameter. In one case there was a diffuse thickening of the pancreas. Histologically, the lesions consist of lymphoid follicles with germinal centers, embedded in a dense fibrous stroma containing large ducts.

## REFERENCES


1. Anthony PP, Faber RG, Russell RC. Pseudotumours of the pancreas. Br Med J 1977;1:814–14.
2. Barbaryka I, Thomas E. Pankreatitis lymphomatosa. Zentralbl Allg Pathol 1981;125:315–8.
3. Barbosa JJ, Dockerty MB, Waugh JM. Pancreatic heterotopia: a review of the literature and report of 41 authenticated cases, of which 25 were clinically significant. Surg Gynecol Obstet 1946;82:527–42.
4. Bartholomew LG, Baggenstoss AH, Morlock CG, Comfort MW. Primary atrophy and lipomatosis of the pancreas. Gastroenterology 1959;36:563–72.
5. Burt TB, Condon VR, Matlak ME. Fetal pancreatic hamartoma. Pediatr Radiol 1983;13:287–9.
6. Chan PH, Teoh TB. The pathology of Clonorchis sinensis infestation of the pancreas. J Pathol Bacterial 1967;93:185–9.

7. Chen J, Baithun SI, Ramsay MA. Histogenesis of pancreatic carcinoma: a study based on 248 cases. J Pathol 1985;146:65–76.
8. Cubilla AL, Fitzgerald PJ. Morphological lesions associated with human primary invasive nonendocrine pancreas cancer. Cancer Res 1976;36:2690–8.
9. Cubilla AL, Fitzgerald PJ. Tumors of the exocrine pancreas. Atlas of Tumor Pathology, 2nd Series, Fascicle 19. Washington, D.C.: Armed Forces Institute of Pathology, 1984;71–89.
10. Dolan RV, ReMine WH, Dockerty MB. The fate of heterotopic pancreatic tissue. A study of 212 cases. Arch Surg 1974;109:762–5.
11. Ferrari BT, O'Halloran RL, Longmire WP Jr, Lewin KJ. Atypical papillary hyperplasia of the pancreatic duct mimicking obstructing pancreatic carcinoma. N Engl J Med 1979;301:531–2.
12. Flaherty MJ, Benjamin DR. Multicystic pancreatic hamartoma: a distinctive lesion with immunohistochemical and ultrastructural study. Hum Pathol 1992;23:1309–12.
13. Glenner GG, Mallory GK. The cystadenoma and related nonfunctional tumors of the pancreas. Pathogenesis, classification, and significance. Cancer 1956;9:980–96.
14. Goldfarb WB, Bennett D, Monafo W. Carcinoma in heterotopic gastric pancreas. Ann Surg 1963;158:56–9.
15. Hastings PR, Nance FC, Becker WF. Changing patterns in the management of pancreatic pseudocysts. Ann Surg 1975;181:546–51.
16. Hatzitheoklitos E, Büchler MW, Friess H, et al. Pseudolymphoma of the pancreas mimicking cancer. Pancreas 1994;9:668–70.
17. Hisaoka M, Haratake J, Horie A, Yasunami Y, Kimura T. Lymphoepithelial cyst of the pancreas in a 65-year-old man. Hum Pathol 1991;22:924–6.
18. Holstege, A, Barner S, Brambs HJ, Wenz W, Gerok W, Farthmann EH. Relapsing pancreatitis associated with duodenal wall cysts. Diagnostic approach and treatment. Gastroenterology 1985;88:814–9.
19. Honicky RE, dePapp EW. Mediastinal teratoma with endocrine function. Am J Dis Child 1973;126:650–3.
20. Jaffe R. The pancreas. In: Wigglesworth JS, Singer DB, eds. Textbook of fetal and perinatal pathology, Vol. 2. Boston: Blackwell Scientific, 1991:1021–55.
21. Kattan YB. Hydatid cysts in the pancreas. Br Med J 1975;4:729–30.
22. Kishi K, Nakamura K, Yoshimori M, et al. Morphology and pathological significance of focal acinar cell dysplasia of the human pancreas. Pancreas 1992;7:177–82.
23. Klöppel G, Bommer G, Rückert K, Seifert G. Intraductal proliferation in the pancreas and its relationship to human and experimental carcinogenesis. Virchows Arch [A] 1980;387:221–33.
25. Klöppel G, Maillet B. Pathology of acute and chronic pancreatitis. Pancreas 1993;8:659–70.
24. Klöppel G, Maillet B. The morphological basis for the evolution of acute pancreatitis into chronic pancreatitis. Virchows Arch [A] 1992;420:1–4.
26. Kodama T, Mori W. Atypical acinar cell nodules of the human pancreas. Acta Pathol Jpn 1983;33:701–14.
27. Kozuka S, Sassa R, Taki T, et al. Relation of pancreatic duct hyperplasia to carcinoma. Cancer 1979;43:1418–28.
28. Kulatunga A, Kyllönen AP, Dammert K. Malakoplakia of the pancreas. A case report. Acta Path Microbiol Immunol Scand [Sect A] 1987;95:127–9.
29. Landry ML, Sarma DP. Accessory spleen in the head of the pancreas [Letter]. Hum Pathol 1989;20:497.
30. Lavine JE, Harrison M, Heyman MB. Gastrointestinal duplications causing relapsing pancreatitis in children. Gastroenterology 1989;97:1556–8.
31. Lilja P, Evander A, Ihse I. Hereditary pancreatitis—a report on two kindreds. Acta Chir Scand 1978;144:35–7.
32. Liou TC, Lin XZ, Cahng T, et al. Pancreas division with early pancreatic cancer—presenting as chronic obstructive pancreatitis. Pancreas 1992;2:251–6.
33. Longnecker DS, Hashida Y, Shinozuka H. Relationship of age to prevalence of focal acinar cell dysplasia in the human pancreas. JNCI 1980;65:63–6.
34. Longnecker DS, Shinozuka H, Dekker A. Focal acinar cell dysplasia in human pancreas. Cancer 1980;45:534–40.
35. Lozano M, Navarro S, Pérez-Ayuso R, et al. Lipomatosis of the pancreas: an unusual cause of massive steatorrhea. Pancreas 1988;3:580–2.
36. Lüchtrath H, Schriefers KH. Pankreaszyste unter dem Bild einer sogenannten branchiogenen Zyste. Pathologe 1985;6:217–9.
37. MacCarty RL, Stephens DH, Brown AL, Carlson HC. Retrograde pancreatography in autopsy specimens. Am J Roentgenol Radium Ther Nucl Med 1975;123:359–66.
38. Maher L, Choi H, Dodds WJ. Noncaseating granulomas of the pancreas. Probable sarcoidosis. Am J Gastroenterol 1981;75:222–5.
39. Mahmood K, Butt MM, Haleem A. Duplication of the duodenum exhibiting heterotopia in the pancreas: report of a case. Ann Saudi Med 1989;9:602–4.
40. Marchevsky AM, Zimmerman MJ, Aufses AH, Weiss H. Endometrial cyst of the pancreas. Gastroenterology 1984;86:1589–91.
41. Mares AJ, Hirsch M. Congenital cysts of the head of the pancreas. J Pediatr Surg 1977;12:547.
42. Martin ED. A new aetiology in chronic pancreatitis? The para-ampullary duodenal cysts. Review of 26 cases. Biol Gastroenterol 1976;9:53–4.
43. Matsumoto Y, Kawai Y, Kimura K. Aberrant pancreas causing pyloric obstruction. Surgery 1974;76:827–9.
44. Miles RM. Pancreatic cyst in the newborn: a case report. Ann Surg 1959;149:576–81.
45. Mizumoto K, Inagaki T, Koizumi M, et al. Early pancreatic duct adenocarcinoma. Hum Pathol 1988;19:242–4.
46. Morohoshi T, Hamamoto T, Kunimura T, et al. Epidermoid cyst derived from an accessory spleen in the pancreas. A case report with literature survey. Acta Pathologica Jpn 1991;41:916–21.
47. Mukada T, Yamada S. Dysplasia and carcinoma in situ of the exocrine pancreas. Tohoku J Exp Med 1982;137:115–24.
48. Murayama H, Kikuchi M, Imai T. A case of heterotopic pancreas in lymph node. Virchows Arch [A] 1978;377:175–9.
49. Nakashiro H, Tokunaga O, Watanabe T, Ishibashi K, Kuwaki T. Localized lymphoid hyperplasia (pseudolymphoma) of the pancreas presenting with obstructive jaundice. Hum Pathol 1991;22:724–6.

50. Neumann HP, Dinkel E, Brambs HJ, et al. Pancreatic lesions in the Hippel-Lindau syndrome. Gastroenterology 1991;101:465–71.
51. Oertel JE. The pancreas. Non-neoplastic alterations. Am J Surg Pathol 1989;13:50–65.
52. Palazzo JP, Chang CD. Inflammatory pseudotumor of the pancreas. Histopathology 1993;23:475–7.
53. Pasternack A, Hjelt L. Cystic disease of the kidneys, liver, and pancreas. Annales Paediatrici Finnlandiae 1961;7:138–45.
54. Pilcher CS, Bradley EL III, Majmudar B. Enterogenous cyst of the pancreas. Am J Gastroenterol 1982;77:576–7.
55. Pour PM, Sayed S, Sayed G. Hyperplastic, preneoplastic and neoplastic lesions found in 83 human pancreases. Am J Clin Path 1982;77:137–52.
56. Ramsden KL, Newman J. Lymphoepithelial cyst of the pancreas. Histopathology 1991;18:267–8.
57. Renner IG, Ponto GC, Savage WT III, Boswell WD. Idiopathic retroperitoneal fibrosis producing common bile duct and pancreatic duct obstruction. Gastroenterology 1980;79:348–51.
58. Roberts PF. Pyloric gland metaplasia of the human pancreas. A comparative histochemical study. Arch Pathol 1974;97:92–5.
59. Schlumberger HG. Teratoma of anterior mediastinum in the group of military age: a study of 16 cases, and a review of theories of genesis. Arch Pathol 1946;41:398–444.
60. Schmitz-Moormann P, Hein J. Altersveränderungen des pankreasgangsystems und ihre rückwirkungen auf das parenchym. Virchows Arch [A] 1976;371:145–52.
61. Seifert G. Congenital anomalies. In: Klöppel G, Heitz PH, eds. Pancreatic pathology. Edinburgh: Churchill Livingstone, 1984:22–6.
62. Seifert G. Lipomatous atrophy and other forms. In: Klöppel G, Heitz PH, eds. Pancreatic pathology. Edinburgh: Churchill Livingstone, 1984:27–31.
63. Sessa F, Bonato M, Frigerio B, et al. Ductal cancers of the pancreas frequently express markers of gastrointestinal epithelial cells. Gastroenterology 1990;98:1655–65.
64. Sommers SC, Murphy SA, Warren S. Pancreatic duct hyperplasia and cancer. Gastroenterology 1954; 27:629–40.
65. Stamm BH. Incidence and diagnostic significance of minor pathologic changes in the adult pancreas at autopsy: a systematic study of 112 autopsies in patients without known pancreatic disease. Hum Pathol 1984;15:677–83.
66. Stolte M, Weiss W, Volkholz H, Rösch W. A special form of segmental pancreatitis: groove pancreatitis. Hepatogastroenterology 1982;29:198–208.
67. Suda K, Mizuguchi K, Hebisawa A, Wakabayashi T, Saito S. Pancreatic tissue in teratoma. Arch Pathol Lab Med 1984;108:835–7.
68. Tanimura A, Yamamoto H, Shibata H, Sano E. Carcinoma in heterotopic gastric pancreas. Acta Path Jap 1979;29:251–7.
69. Tsou E, Romano MC, Kerwin DM, Soteropoulos C, Katz S. Sarcoidosis of anterior mediastinal nodes, pancreas, and uterine cervix: three unusual sites in the same patient. Am Rev Resp Dis 1980;122:333–8.
70. Vermeulen BJ, Widgren S, Gur V, Meyer P, Iselin C, Rohner A. Dermoid cyst of the pancreas. Case report and review of the literature. Gastroenterol Clin Biol 1990;14:1023–5.
71. Volkholz H, Stolte M, Becker V. Epithelial dysplasias in chronic pancreatitis. Virchows Arch [A] 1982;396:331–49.
72. Walters MN. Goblet-cell metaplasia in ductules and acini of the exocrine pancreas. J Pathol Bacteriol 1965;89:569–72.
73. Zuk RJ, Neal JW, Baithun SI. Malakoplakia of the pancreas. Virchows Arch [A] 1990;417:181–4.

✧✧✧

# 8

# TUMOR-LIKE LESIONS OF THE ENDOCRINE PANCREAS

Tumor-like lesions of the endocrine pancreas include islet hyperplasia, nesidioblastosis, and islet dysplasia. Islet hyperplasia and nesidioblastosis may coexist in the same pancreas, especially of newborns and infants, where patterns of endocrine tissue structure and distribution resembling those of nesidioblastosis are found normally; the two lesions are also observed independently of each other.

## ISLET HYPERPLASIA

**Definition.** This is an increase in pancreatic islet mass resulting from an absolute increase in islet size or number. The volume density of the endocrine component is clearly in excess of corresponding values for age-matched controls: 1 to 2 percent of total pancreatic volume in adults and 10 percent in newborns (6). In hyperplasia, islets are over 250 μm in diameter (normal is up to 225 μm) and in children more than 15 percent of the islets measure more than 200 μm (5). Islet hyperplasia should not be mistaken for the islet crowding resulting from exocrine tissue atrophy, a frequent finding in chronic pancreatitis (see preceding chapter).

**Incidence.** Islet hyperplasia has been sporadically reported as an unexpected finding in asymptomatic subjects, in patients with alpha-1-antitrypsin deficiency (7), or as a cause of hyperfunctional syndromes such as hyperinsulinism (13), Zollinger-Ellison syndrome (2), and Verner-Morrison syndrome (12). However, the occurrence of islet hyperplasia in Zollinger-Ellison and Verner-Morrison syndromes has been questioned, due to lack of confirmation by other studies and lack of morphometric data. In addition, there has been no direct evidence of gastrin or vasoactive intestinal polypeptide (VIP) production by these "hyperplastic" islets (9,10). Hyperinsulinemic hypoglycemia not due to tumor may be caused by islet changes and are described as "nesidioblastosis" or islet hyperplasia due to an increased number of B cells (3). Islet hyperplasia due to an increased number of B cells has been documented in newborns and infants as a result of (or in association with) maternal diabetes, erythroblastosis fetalis, hereditary tyrosinemia of hepatorenal type (4), Zellweger's cerebro-hepato-renal syndrome (14), and leprechaunism (8); features of the latter are characteristic facies, hirsutism, prominent external genitalia, and reduced muscle mass (3). Islet hyperplasia associated with malformative changes is found in the Beckwith-Wiedemann syndrome (11), which is characterized by macroglossia, omphalocele, visceromegaly, gigantism, kidney dysplasia, and increased tumor incidence. All these conditions may be associated with hypoglycemia and hyperinsulinism.

**Microscopic Findings.** Histologically, islet hyperplasia is especially prominent in patients with Beckwith-Wiedemann syndrome (11). Abnormally large and apparently confluent islets accumulate in the center of the lobules leaving only narrow rims of acinar tissue at some sites (fig. 8-1). The normal distribution of the four main cell types inside the islets is retained. However, in Beckwith syndrome pancreatic polypeptide (PP)-rich (irregular) islets and PP-poor (regular) islets are not segregated into two embryologically distinct portions (of ventral and dorsal pouch origin, respectively), in keeping with the multiple malformative components of the syndrome. Some fetal-type bipolar islets in which B and non-B cells are separated are found throughout the gland. The absolute volume, in decreasing order of magnitude, of the insulin, PP, glucagon, and somatostatin cells, is increased several times, with an obvious relative increase in number of B cells and decrease in D cells. In addition to increased size and number of islets, hypertrophy of B cells may be present in all the hypoglycemic conditions. However, this is never as prominent as in the majority of neonatal nesidioblastosis cases.

Coexisting signs of chronic pancreatitis and, especially, close topographic association with atrophy of acinar tissue, allow in most cases separation of passive islet crowding secondary to parenchymal collapse from true, active hyperplasia. However, in some cases the morphologic features, including patterns of nesidioblastosis and increase in endocrine tissue, suggest the

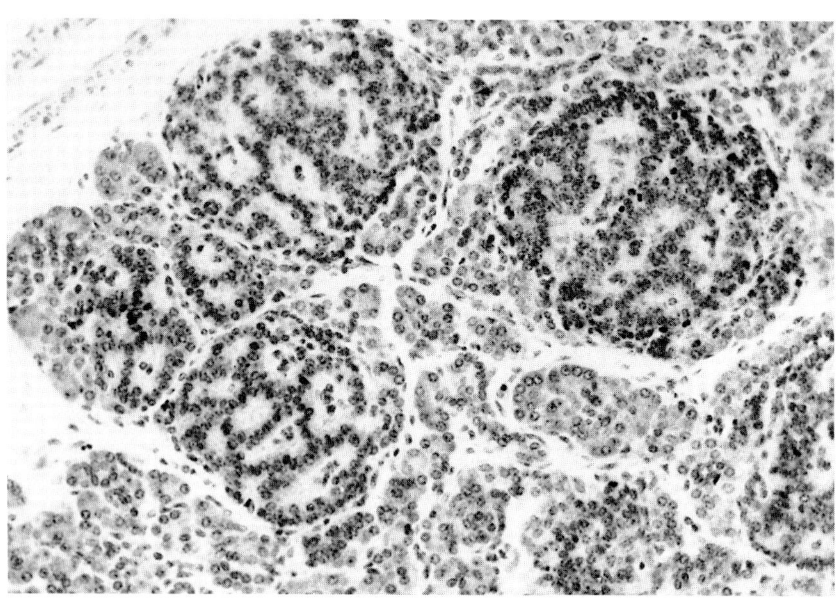

Figure 8-1
ISLET HYPERPLASIA OF BECKWITH-WIEDEMANN SYNDROME

Note crowding without fusion of islets inside pancreatic lobules. (Courtesy of Dr. Cesare Bordi, Parma, Italy.)

concurrence of an active process of endocrine neogenesis (3); this interpretation is also supported by occasional signs of endocrine hyperfunction. When prominent endocrine neogenesis occurs in areas of sclerosis, small endocrine nests and cords dispersed in the desmoplastic tissue may give an appearance suggestive of stromal invasion and, occasionally, perineural space invasion (1). In such cases only unequivocal findings, such as a morphologically distinct proliferation of cells especially from a single population (monotypic), a significant extension into regional tissues, or metastatic disease, should be taken as evidence of neoplasia (1).

## NESIDIOBLASTOSIS

This is a hyperfunctional disorder of pancreatic insulin-producing cells characterized by hypertrophic B cells within enlarged or normal-appearing islets, small scattered endocrine cell clusters, and ductuloinsular complexes. These changes cause persistent hyperinsulinemic hypoglycemia in neonates; in adults, hyperinsulinemic hypoglycemia is only exceptionally caused by nesidioblastosis and is usually due to an insulinoma. Nesidioblastosis is also called *diffuse hyperplasia, nesidiodysplasia, endocrine cell dysplasia, microadenomatosis, focal islet cell adenomatosis, neonatal islet cell tumor,* and *congenital insulinoma.*

### Persistent Neonatal Hyperinsulinemic Hypoglycemia

Persistent neonatal hyperinsulinemic hypoglycemia (PNHH) is a rare clinical syndrome characterized by hypoglycemia-related symptoms including pallor, sweating, hypotonia, somnolence, ataxia, seizures, and obesity. The syndrome starts within the first days after birth in more than 70 percent of patients and is rarely seen in patients older than 1 year. Although rare, PNHH is the most frequent cause of neonatal and infantile hyperinsulinism, insulinoma being exceptional at this age: PNHH accounts for almost 50 percent of all cases of persistent neonatal hypoglycemia. Other causes are panhypopituitarism, growth hormone deficiency, Addison's disease, hypothyroidism, glycogen storage disease, and ketotic hypoglycemia (29).

The most important laboratory finding for establishing the diagnosis of PNHH is an elevated serum insulin level (more than 10 μU/ml) despite the presence of hypoglycemia, which requires an intravenous glucose infusion rate above 15 mg/kg/min to prevent symptoms of hypoglycemia. Although most PNHH cases occur sporadically, familial cases have been recorded, with a hereditary pattern suggestive of an autosomal recessive disorder (28), which has been recently mapped to chromosome 11p14-15.1 (19a). All familial cases are of the diffuse type of pancreatic nesidioblastosis; in the remaining

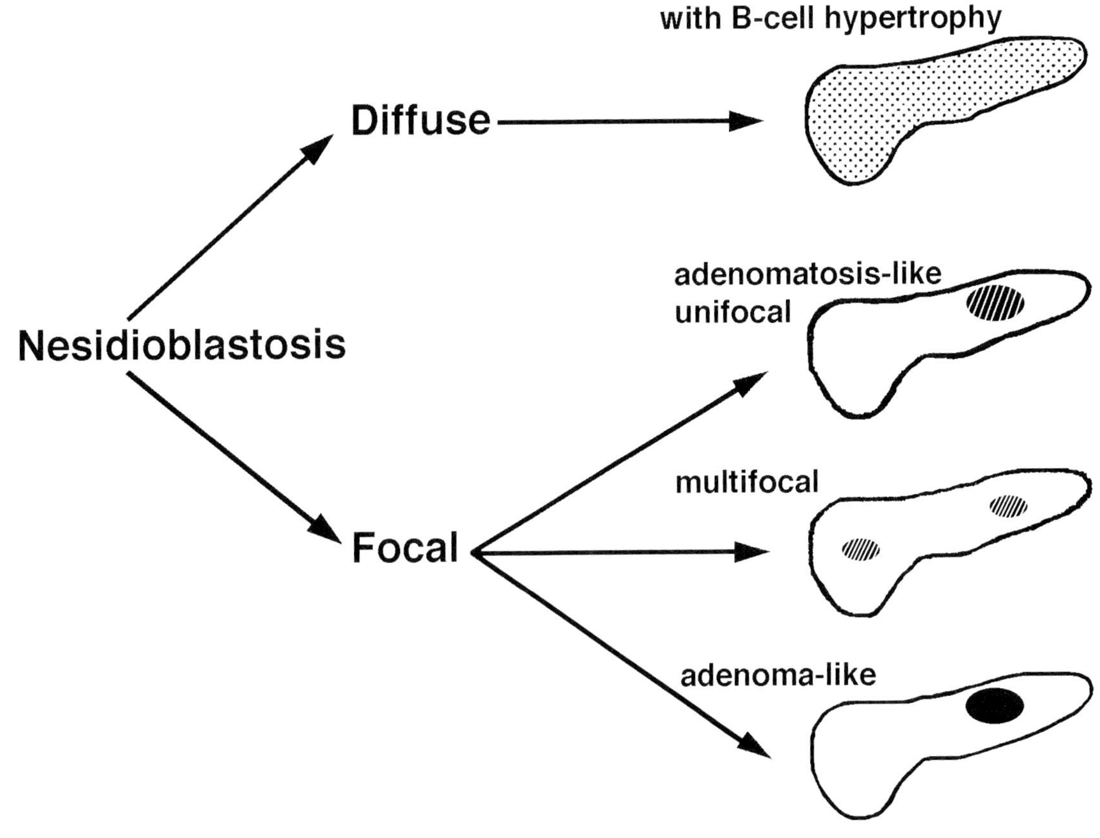


Figure 8-2
TYPES OF NESIDIOBLASTOSIS IN INFANTS
(Adapted and revised from Fig. 6 in Goossens A, Gepts W, Saudubray JM, et al. Diffuse and focal nesidioblastosis. A clinicopathological study of 24 patients with persistent neonatal hyperinsulinemic hypoglycemia. Am J Surg Pathol 1989;13:766–75.)

cases the etiology and pathogenesis of the disease are obscure.

**Pathology.** The morphologic changes of PNHH affect the pancreas either focally or diffusely (fig. 8-2) (20). *Focal nesidioblastosis* accounts for one fourth to half of the PNHH cases; only one lesion is found in three quarters of these cases (unifocal nesidioblastosis), preferentially located in the tail or body. In the multifocal form two or more sites are involved in any part of the gland. The size of the lesion in focal nesidioblastosis ranges from 2 to 10 mm. With smaller lesions the pancreas appears grossly normal; larger lesions may present as an ill-defined area of increased consistency, which occasionally protrudes from the surface as a tumor-like nodule (fig. 8-3).

Histologically, focal nesidioblastosis is characterized by an ill-defined accumulation of partly confluent, islet-like cell clusters separated from each other by rims of acinar cells or thin strands of connective tissue (fig. 8-4). Ductuloinsular complexes and polyploid nuclei twice as large as normal are regularly found inside the lesion (fig. 8-5). Hormone immunohistochemistry shows the presence of insulin, glucagon, somatostatin, and PP cells that retain their normal spatial arrangement inside the islet-like clusters (21). However, the proportion of insulin-immunoreactive B cells is higher than normal, corresponding to 70 to 90 percent of the whole endocrine cell population (versus about 50 percent in normal newborns), and includes most of the hypertrophic cells with enlarged nuclei.

In focal nesidioblastosis the endocrine pancreas outside the focal lesions is morphologically normal. Because of their small size (2 to 4 mm),

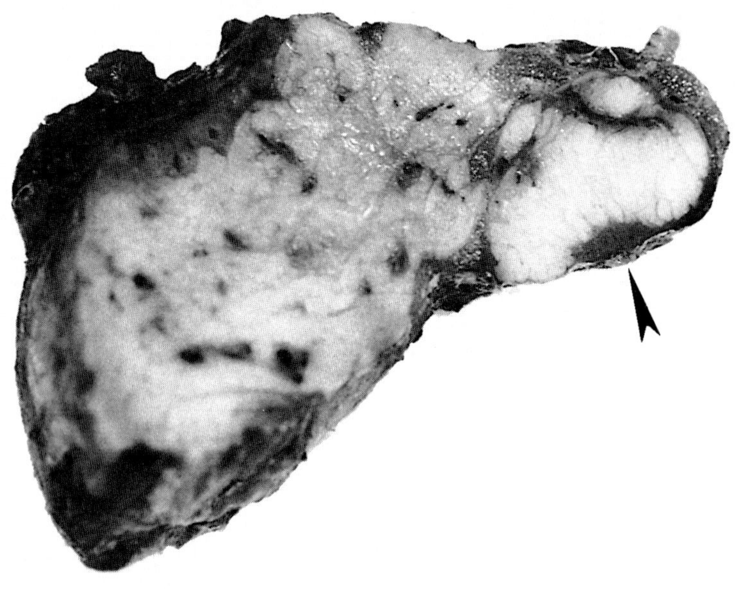

Figure 8-3
FOCAL NESIDIOBLASTOSIS

Cut surface of a protruding focal lesion (arrowhead) in a 9-month-old girl with persistent neonatal hyperinsulinemic hypoglycemia (PNHH). (Fig. 5 from Goossens A, Heitz PU, Klöppel G. Pancreatic endocrine cells and their non-neoplastic proliferations. In: Dayal Y, ed. Endocrine pathology of the gut and pancreas. Boca Raton: CRC Press, 1991:69–104.)

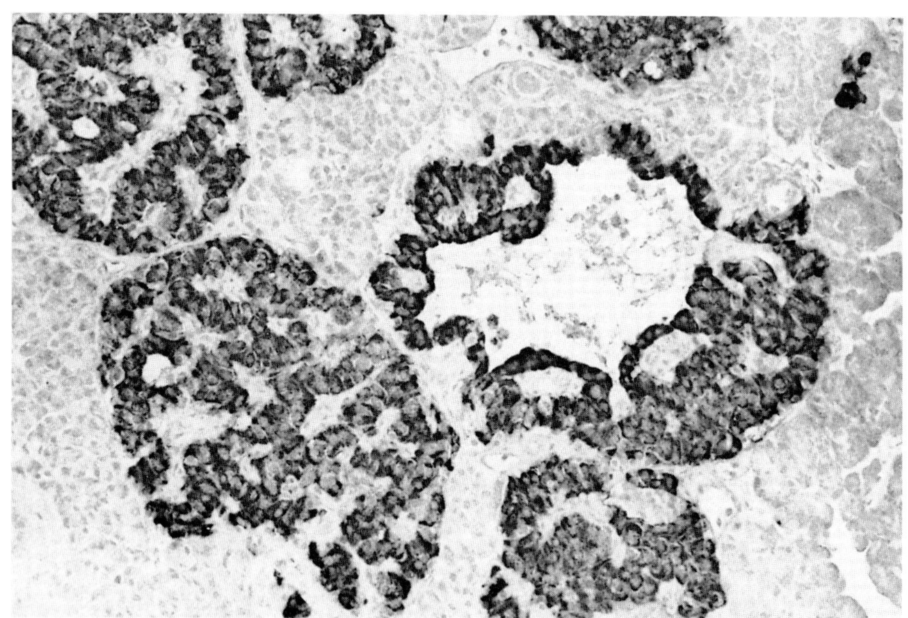

Figure 8-4
FOCAL NESIDIOBLASTOSIS IN PNHH

Focal accumulation of islet-like cell clusters separated by thin rims of acinar cells and thin strands of connective tissue. (Insulin immunostaining) (Figures 8-4 and 8-5 are from the same patient.)

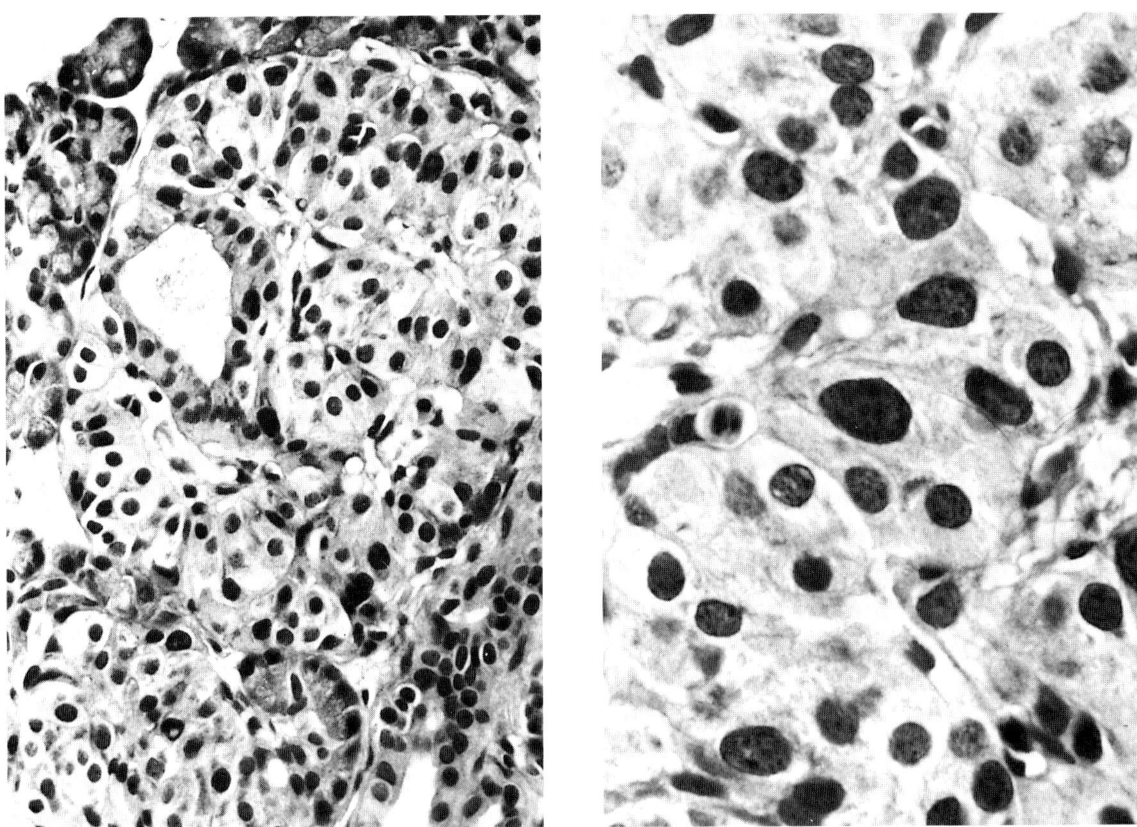

Figure 8-5
FOCAL NESIDIOBLASTOSIS IN PNHH
Ductuloinsular complex (left) and polyploid nuclei (right).

many focal lesions may easily escape macroscopic detection and systematic investigation of serial sections of all available pancreatic tissue is mandatory in PNHH cases in which the histology is nondiagnostic.

At the ultrastructural level signs of functional hyperactivity, with increased, well-organized endoplasmic reticulum and prominent Golgi complex, are regularly found in the B cells of focal nesidioblastosis. A, D, and PP cells usually have a normal structure (25).

A rarely occurring histologic variant of focal nesidioblastosis is a well-circumscribed adenoma-like lesion composed of endocrine clusters separated by thin fibrovascular septa without acinar tissue (fig. 8-6) (16,18). The normal spatial arrangement of the four endocrine cell types inside the islet-like clusters suggests a hyperplastic, rather than neoplastic, nature of this adenomatoid variant of focal nesidioblastosis.

*Diffuse nesidioblastosis* is found in about three quarters of infants with PNHH. Grossly, the pancreas shows no abnormality. Microscopically, the morphologic features of nesidioblastosis are present throughout the entire pancreas. Increased variability of islet size (often larger than normal so as to suggest islet hyperplasia/hypertrophy) and shape; presence of abundant, scattered endocrine cell clusters or individual cells; prominent ductuloinsular complexes; and B-cell hypertrophy are the hallmarks of the lesion (fig. 8-7) (17,20,22,24). However, some of these changes may be also found in the pancreas of normoglycemic newborns and infants. B cells with enlarged nuclei and prominent ductuloinsular complexes are the most useful diagnostic findings for PNHH (fig. 8-8). A 40 percent increase in nuclear volume compared to age-matched controls has been recorded by morphometric studies. No other consistent differences

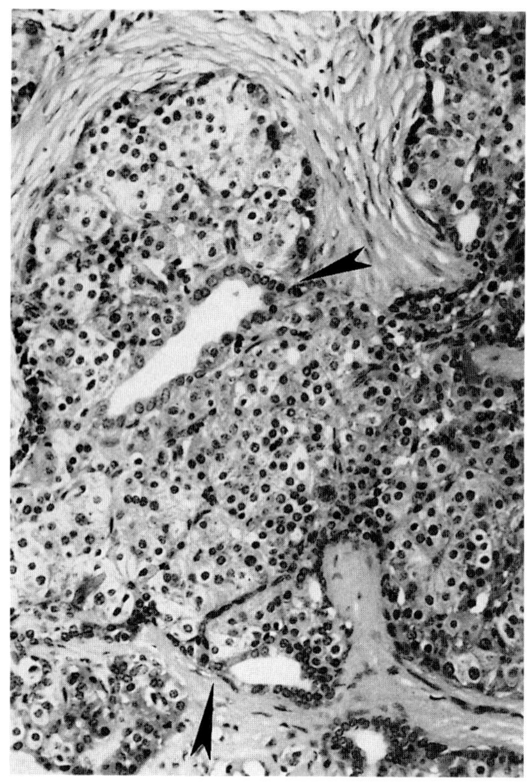

Figure 8-6
ADENOMA-LIKE FOCAL NESIDIOBLASTOSIS IN PNHH

Interconnecting clusters of endocrine cells separated by strands of fibrous tissue without interposition of acinar parenchyma. Note the ductuloinsular complexes (arrows). (Fig. 13 from Goossens A, Heitz PU, Klöppel G. Pancreatic endocrine cells and their non-neoplastic proliferations. In: Dayal Y, ed. Endocrine pathology of the gut and pancreas. Boca Raton: CRC Press, 1991:69–104.)

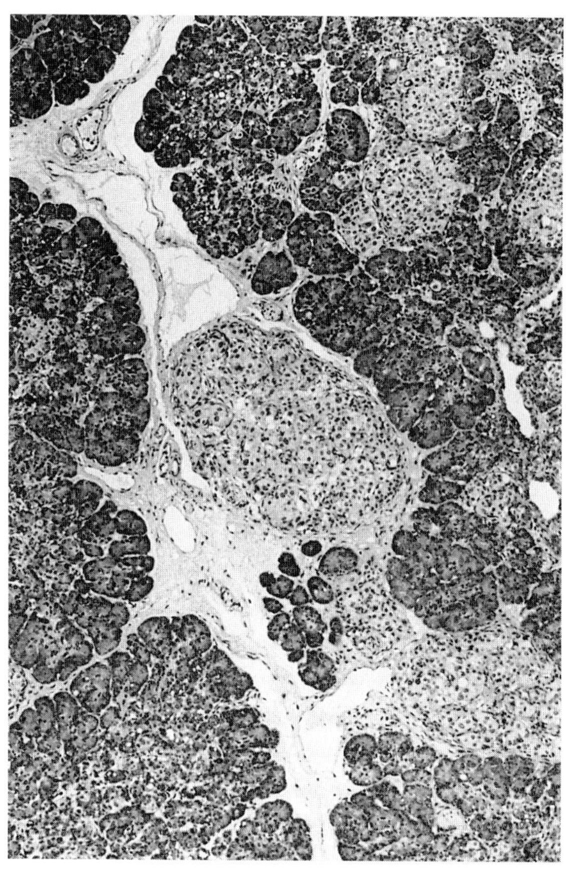

Figure 8-7
DIFFUSE NESIDIOBLASTOSIS IN PNHH

Variably sized islets irregularly distributed in the acinar tissue and interlobular stroma. (Fig. 15 A from Goossens A, Heitz PU, Klöppel G. Pancreatic endocrine cells and their non-neoplastic proliferations. In: Dayal Y, ed. Endocrine pathology of the gut and pancreas. Boca Raton: CRC Press, 1991:69–104.)

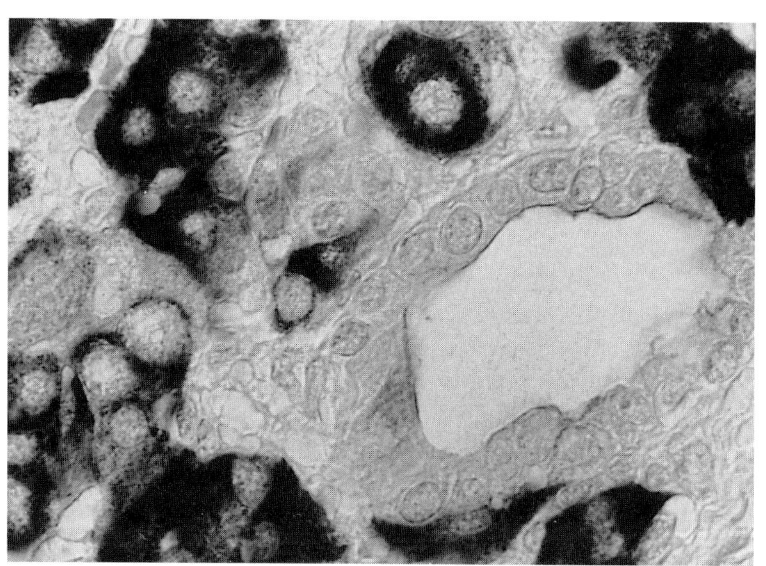

Figure 8-8
INSULIN CELL HYPERTROPHY IN PNHH

Diffuse nesidioblastosis with hypertrophy of insulin-storing cytoplasm and giant unstained nuclei. Note the intrainsular ductule. (Insulin immunostaining in Nomarski optics) (Fig. 18 from Goossens A, Heitz PU, Klöppel G. Pancreatic endocrine cells and their non-neoplastic proliferations. In: Dayal Y, ed. Endocrine pathology of the gut and pancreas. Boca Raton: CRC Press, 1991:69–104.)

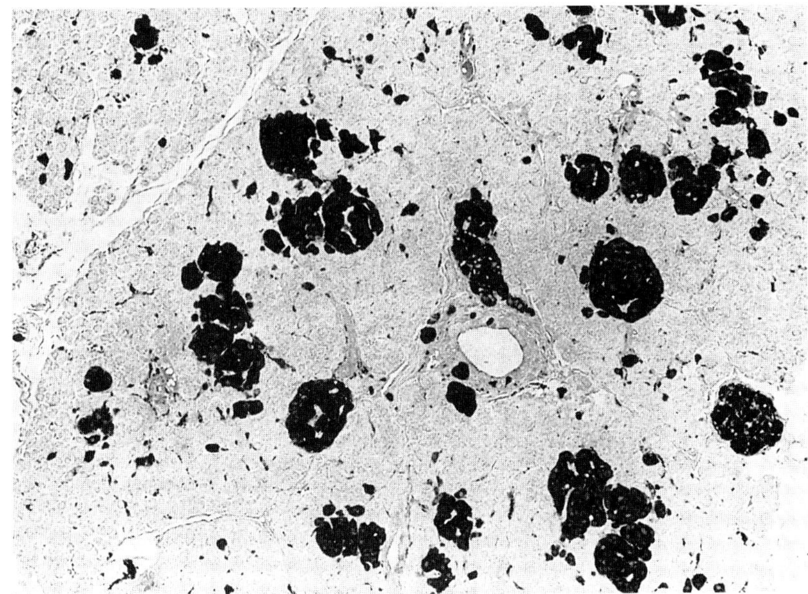

Figure 8-9
HAPHAZARD DISTRIBUTION OF ISLETS IN PNHH

Irregular dissemination of islets, small endocrine cell clusters, and individual endocrine cells in a 1-month-old infant with PNHH in the absence of insulin cell hypertrophy. (Immunostaining for synaptophysin) (Fig. 19 from Goossens A, Heitz PU, Klöppel G. Pancreatic endocrine cells and their non-neoplastic proliferations. In: Dayal Y, ed. Endocrine pathology of the gut and pancreas. Boca Raton: CRC Press, 1991:69–104.)

have been observed, although in some studies there is a tendency for increased B cells and decreased D cells, with an increased B to D cell ratio (30,32). A tetraploid pattern of DNA content has been found in enlarged B-cell nuclei (19).

For some PNHH patients who lack signs of islet hyperplasia, routine histology fails to reveal abnormalities despite systematic investigation of serial sections. Only immunohistochemistry reveals the subtle differences in the endocrine pancreas. Dissemination of individual and clustered endocrine cells throughout the exocrine tissue in excess of those found in age-matched controls is the most frequent, though not universally accepted, finding (fig. 8-9) (20,32). Ductuloinsular complexes are present but are not prominent, while large islets and hypertrophied B cells with giant nuclei are lacking. The proportion of endocrine tissue, or its B-cell fraction, to the remaining gland tissue is not increased (24). Fewer glucagon (26) and somatostatin cells (30) have been reported in some cases but this finding has not been confirmed in larger series investigated (20,22,24,32).

Signs of active protein synthesis, such as a well-developed endoplasmic reticulum and prominent Golgi complex, are found in many B cells. Mixed acinar-endocrine (composite or amphicrine) cells have been also reported, with coexistent zymogen and endocrine granules, mostly of beta (insulin) and alpha (glucagon) type. Such cells with hybrid differentiation may be the site of inappropriate insulin secretion (22,24,32).

**Prognosis and Treatment.** The severe, prolonged hypoglycemia caused by PNHH is resistant to medical therapy and may lead to permanent neurologic and cardiac damage. For patients with unifocal nesidioblastosis, whose lesions are usually located in the tail or body of the pancreas, the prognosis is favorable after partial (distal, 75 to 80 percent) pancreatectomy. However, after the same surgical treatment recurrence of hypoglycemia is the rule for patients with diffuse and multifocal nesidioblastosis. Postoperative treatment with diazoxide may prevent severe hypoglycemia in some of the patients. Repeat surgery, with extension of the pancreatectomy to 95 percent of the gland (near-total pancreatectomy), is required for most patients. This is often followed by an insulin-dependent diabetes which occasionally subsides in a few months. It has been reported that when near-total pancreatectomy is performed as the primary procedure, it is more effective and results in postoperative normoglycemia (31). In most cases it is impossible to distinguish preoperatively between focal and diffuse nesidioblastosis. When a nodule is visualized or a focal increase in consistency is palpated by the surgeon intraoperatively, a partial pancreatectomy is indicated. If the pancreas appears grossly normal at inspection and palpation, a near-total pancreatectomy is the treatment of choice (27,31).

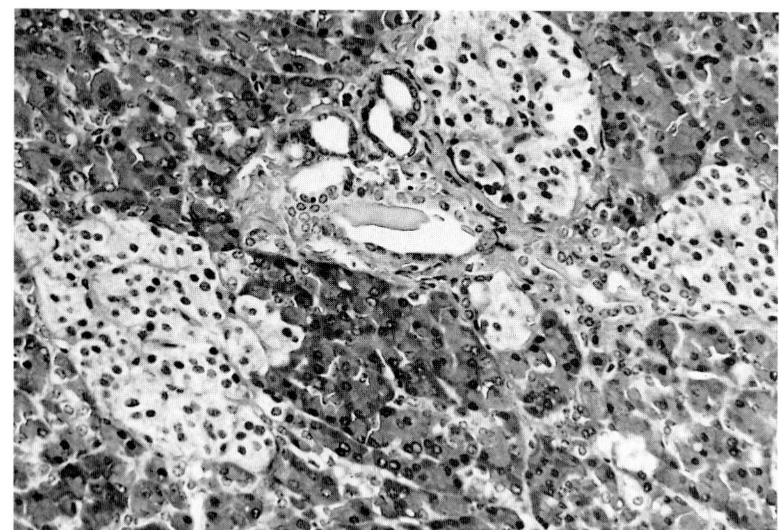

Figure 8-10
NESIDIOBLASTOSIS IN AN ADULT WITH PAHH

Clustering of irregular islets in the vicinity of small ductules. Patient had persistent adult hyperinsulinemic hypoglycemia (PAHH).

### Persistent Hyperinsulinemic Hypoglycemia in Adults

Nesidioblastosis in adults rarely causes persistent hyperinsulinemia and hypoglycemia (PAHH), in the absence of an insulinoma. There have been 22 cases in world literature (21). Clinically, there are hypoglycemia-related neuropsychiatric symptoms (fainting, confusion, dizziness, visual disturbances) which are precipitated by fasting, exercise, or stress. The symptoms usually begin in adulthood and only rarely in adolescence. Inappropriately elevated blood insulin levels during fasting hypoglycemia, in the absence of an insulin-secreting tumor, is suggestive of PAHH. Step sectioning of the pancreas, with systematic histologic investigation, is necessary to exclude a minute insulinoma.

The most relevant histologic finding is the presence of endocrine cells, especially insulin and glucagon cells, scattered as single elements or small clusters in the exocrine tissue, in direct connection with (or in close apposition to) ductules (fig. 8-10). The nuclei of B cells may be slightly enlarged, but they are less prominent than in newborns. The islets show increased variability in shape, size, and distribution. Some are localized in the connective tissue surrounding the interlobular ducts, a pattern absent in the normal adult pancreas and only seen in fetuses. There is no increase in volume density of the total endocrine tissue or in B cells compared to age-matched controls (15).

The treatment of choice for PAHH associated with nesidioblastosis is subtotal (75 to 90 percent) pancreatectomy, although recurrent hypoglycemia or diabetes mellitus are frequent complications (23).

## DYSPLASIA

Nontumor dysplasia of the endocrine pancreas is defined by a lesion which resembles normal or hyperplastic islets in size and shape, but 1) deviates structurally (often in a trabecular manner) from the microlobular architecture of normal islets; 2) loses the normal topographic and quantitative relationships between the four main islet cell types, with sharp prevalence of one type; and 3) has some (generally mild) cellular atypia (fig. 8-11). This definition covers microscopic lesions of questionable neoplastic potential; growths of at least 0.5 mm are considered microadenomas. Both minute microadenomas and dysplasias (i.e., moderately atypical lesions less than 0.5 mm in size) are frequently detected in the pancreas of patients with type 1 multiple endocrine neoplasia (MEN 1), and are rare in non-MEN pancreata (33–35). The term dysplasia should not be used to label some histologic, possibly malformative, aspects of PNHH unless proof of some kind of neoplastic potential is obtained.

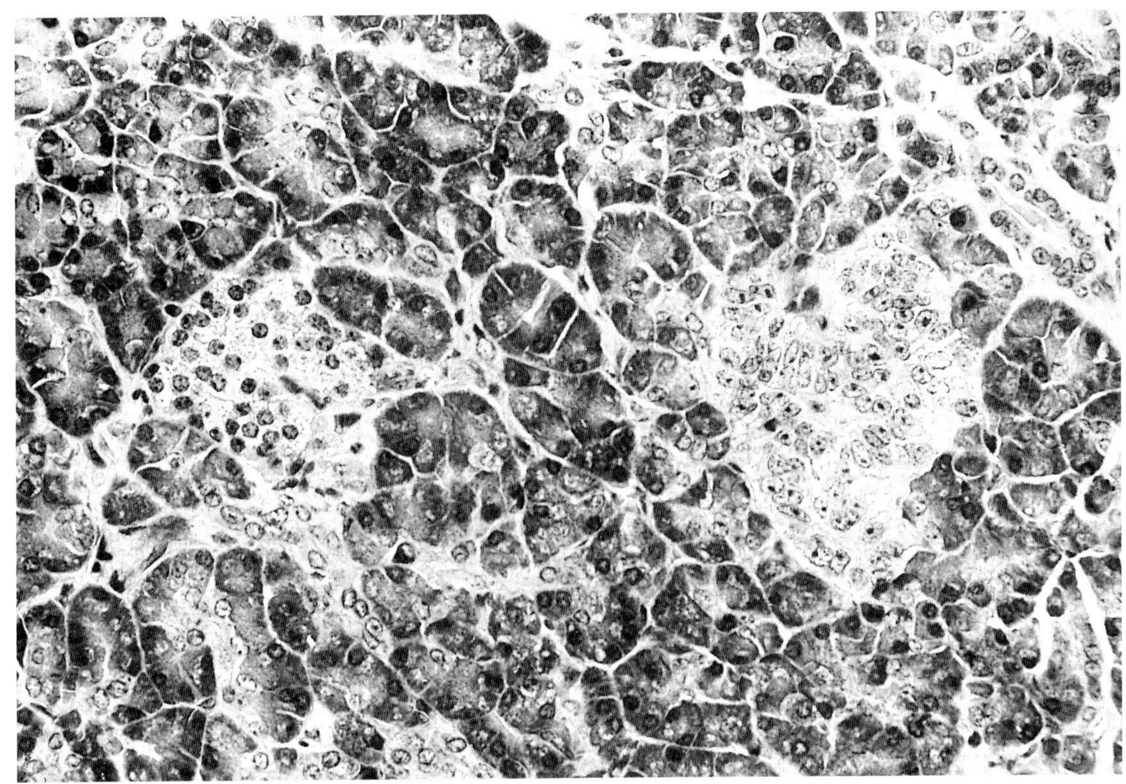

Figure 8-11
PANCREATIC ENDOCRINE DYSPLASIA

Pancreatic tissue from a patient with combined ZES-MEN 1 showing pancreatic adenomatosis, duodenal gastrinoma, and hyperparathyroidism. Cells with enlarged nucleus and prominent nucleolus are seen in the small dysplastic growth on the right, to be compared with cells of a normal islet on the left. Note associated hyperplasia of centroacinar and ductular cells, a frequent finding in patients with ZES, likely due to their enhanced secretin release. (Fig. 5 from Solcia E, Sessa F, Rindi G, Bonato M, Capella C. Pancreatic endocrine tumors: general concepts; nonfunctioning tumors and tumors with uncommon function. In: Dayal Y, ed. Endocrine pathology of the gut and pancreas. Boca Raton: CRC Press, 1991:105–31.)

## REFERENCES

### Islet Hyperplasia


1. Bartow SA, Mukai K, Rosai J. Pseudoneoplastic proliferation of endocrine cells in pancreatic fibrosis. Cancer 1981;47:2627–33.
2. Ellison EH, Wilson SD. The Zollinger-Ellison syndrome updated. Surg Clin North Am 1967;47:1115–24.
3. Goossens A, Heitz PU, Klöppel G. Pancreatic endocrine cells and their non-neoplastic proliferations. In: Dayal Y, ed. Endocrine pathology of the gut and pancreas. Boca Raton: CRC Press, 1991:69–104.
4. Hardwick DF, Dimmick JE. Metabolic cirrhosis of infancy and early childhood. In: Rosenberg HS, Bolande RP, eds. Perspectives in Pediatric Pathology, Vol. 3 Chicago: Year Book Med Publ, 1976;103.
5. Jaffe R, Hashida Y, Yunis EJ. Pancreatic pathology in hyperinsulinemic hypoglycemia of infancy. Lab Invest 1980;42:356–65.
6. Rahier J, Goebbels RM, Henquin JC. Cellular composition of the human diabetic pancreas. Diabetologia 1983;24:366–71.
7. Ray MB, Zumwalt R. Islet-cell hyperplasia in genetic deficiency of alpha-1-proteinase inhibitor. Am J Clin Pathol 1986;85:681–7.
8. Rosenberg AM, Haworth JC, Degroot W, Trevenen L, Rechler M. A case of leprechaunism with severe hyperinsulinemia. Am J Dis Child 1980;134:170–5.
9. Solcia E, Capella C, Buffa R, Tenti P, Rindi G, Cornaggia M. Antigenic markers of neuroendocrine tumors: their diagnostic and prognostic value. In: Fenoglio CM, Weinstein RS, Kaufman N, eds. New concepts in neoplasia as applied to diagnostic pathology. Baltimore: Williams & Wilkins, 1986:242–61.

10. Solcia E, Capella C, Riva C, Rindi G, Polak JM. The morphology and neuroendocrine profile of pancreatic epithelial VIPomas and extrapancreatic, VIP-producing, neurogenic tumors. Ann NY Acad Sci 1988;527:508–17.
11. Stefan Y, Bordi C, Grasso S, Orci L. Beckwith-Wiedemann syndrome: a quantitative, immunohistochemical study of pancreatic islet cell populations. Diabetologia 1985;28:914–9.
12. Verner JV, Morrison AB. Endocrine pancreatic islet disease with diarrhea. Report of a case due to diffuse hyperplasia of nonbeta islet tissue with a review of 54 additional cases. Arch Intern Med 1974;133:492–9.
13. Weidenheim KM, Hinchey WW, Campbell WG Jr. Hyperinsulinemic hypoglycemia in adults with islet-cell hyperplasia and degranulation of exocrine cells of the pancreas. Am J Clin Pathol 1983;79:14–24.
14. Zellweger H. Cerebro-hepato-renal syndrome. In: Bergsma D, ed. Birth defects compendium, 2nd ed.New York: Alan R Liss, 1979:178–96.

**Nesidioblastosis**

15. Albers N, Löhr M, Bogner U, Loy V, Klöppel G. Nesidioblastosis of the pancreas in an adult with persistent hyperinsulinemic hypoglycemia. Am J Clin Pathol 1989;91:336–40.
16. Bordi C, Ravazzola M, Pollak A, Lubec G, Orci L. Neonatal islet cell adenoma: a distinct type of islet cell tumor? Diabetes Care 1982;5:122–5.
17. Dahms BB, Landing BH, Blaskovics M, Roe TF. Nesidioblastosis and other islet cell abnormalities in hyperinsulinemic hypoglycemia of childhood. Human Pathol 1980;11:641–9.
18. Dahms BB, Lippe BM, Dakake CH, Fonkalsrud EW, Mirra JM. The occurrence in a neonate of a pancreatic adenoma with nesidioblastosis in the tumor. Am J Clin Pathol 1976;65:462–6.
19. Falkmer S, Askensten U. Disturbed growth of the endocrine pancreas. In: Lefebvre PJ, Pipeleers DG, eds. The pathology of the endocrine pancreas in diabetes. Berlin: Springer-Verlag, 1988;125–40.
19a. Glaser B, Chiu KC, Anker R, et al. Familial hyperinsulinism maps to chromosome 11p14-15.1, 30cM centromeric to the insulin gene. Nat Genet 1994;7:185–8.
20. Goossens A, Gepts W, Saudubray JM, et al. Diffuse and focal nesidioblastosis. A clinicopathological study of 24 patients with persistent neonatal hyperinsulinemic hypoglycemia. Am J Surg Pathol 1989;13:766–75.
21. Goossens A, Heitz PU, Klöppel G. Pancreatic endocrine cells and their non-neoplastic proliferations. In: Dayal Y, ed. Endocrine pathology of the gut and pancreas. Boca Raton: CRC Press, 1991:69–104.
22. Gould VE, Memoli VA, Dardi LE, Gould NS. Nesidiodysplasia and nesidioblastosis of infancy: structural and functional correlations with the syndrome of hyperinsulinemic hypoglycemia. Pediatr Pathol 1983;1:7–31.
23. Harness JK, Geelhoed GW, Thompson NW, et al. Nesidioblastosis in adults. A surgical dilemma. Arch Surg 1981;116:575–80.
24. Jaffe R, Hashida Y, Yunis EJ. Pancreatic pathology in hyperinsulinemic hypoglycemia of infancy. Lab Invest 1980;42:356–65.
25. Klöppel G, Altenähr E, Menke B. The ultrastructure of focal islet cell adenomatosis in the newborn with hypoglycemia and hyperinsulinism. Virchows Arch [A] 1975;366:223–36.
26. Kollee LA, Monnens LA, Cecjka V, Wilms RM. Persistent neonatal hypoglycemia due to glucagon deficiency. Arch Dis Child 1978;53:422–4.
27. Kramer JL, Bell MJ, De Schrijver K, Bower RJ, Ternberg JL, White NH. Clinical and histologic indications for extensive pancreatic resection in nesidioblastosis. Am J Surg 1982;43:116–9.
28. Mathew PM, Young JM, Abu-Osba YK, et al. Persistent neonatal hyperinsulinism. Clin Pediatr 1988;27:148–51.
29. Pagliara AS, Karl IE, Haymond M, Kipnis DM. Hypoglycemia in infancy (parts 1 and 2). J Pediatr 1973;82:365–79 and 558–77.
30. Rahier J, Falt K, Müntefering H, Becker K, Gepts W, Falkmer S. The basic structural lesion of persistent neonatal hypoglycemia with hyperinsulinism: deficiency of pancreatic D cells or hyperactivity of the B cells? Diabetologia 1984;26:282–9.
31. Spitz L, Buick RG, Grant DB, Leonard JV, Pincott JR. Surgical treatment of nesidioblastosis. Pediatr Surg Int 1986;1:26–9.
32. Witte DP, Greider MH, Deschrijver-Kecskemeti K, Kissane JM, White MH. The juvenile human endocrine pancreas: normal versus idiopathic hyperinsulinemic hypoglycemia. Sem Diagn Pathol 1984;1:30–42.

**Dysplasia**

33. Klöppel G, Willemer S, Stamm B, Häcki WH, Heitz PU. Pancreatic lesions and hormonal profile of pancreatic tumors in multiple endocrine neoplasia type I. An immunocytochemical study of nine patients. Cancer 1986;57:1824–32.
34. Pilato FP, D'Adda T, Banchini E, Bordi C. Nonrandom expression of polypeptide hormones in pancreatic tumors. An immunohistochemical study in a case of multiple islet cell neoplasia. Cancer 1988;61:1815–20.
35. Solcia E, Sessa F, Rindi G, Bonato M, Capella C. Pancreatic endocrine tumors: general concepts; nonfunctioning tumors and tumors with uncommon function. In: Dayal I, ed. Endocrine pathology of the gut and pancreas. Boca Raton: CRC Press, 1991:105–31.

# 9
# DIAGNOSIS OF PANCREATIC TUMORS

## CLINICAL, LABORATORY, AND RADIOLOGIC EVALUATION

It is difficult to diagnose a pancreatic mass because the pancreas is hidden in the retroperitoneum and is closely associated with adjacent organs. The recently available diagnostic techniques of ultrasonography, endoscopic retrograde cholangiopancreatography (ERCP), computed tomography (CT) (1,3), and serum tumor markers (6) are superior to other nonsurgical screening tests in detecting pancreatic lesions. In a recent analysis of the diagnostic accuracy of various techniques, ERCP provided a sensitivity of 92 percent; CT, 83 percent; and ultrasound, 74 percent. The specificity of all three imaging techniques exceeded 90 percent. However, ERCP is of value only for ductal adenocarcinomas and intraductal papillary mucinous tumors, and may fail to detect other tumor types. Selective angiography and scintigraphy with octeotride (a long-acting somatostatin analogue which binds somatostatin receptors present on endocrine tumor cells) are particularly useful in detecting primary endocrine tumors of the pancreas as well as their liver metastases (2,4). Serum determination of CA19-9, a gastrointestinal cancer antigen (initially abbreviated as GICA) specifically recognized by monoclonal antibodies and developed by Koprowski et al. (5), is 83 percent sensitive. This is higher than for carcinoembryonic antigen (CEA) and various other tumor markers. The combination of CA19-9 and ultrasound improves the sensitivity of each test performed alone by 10 to 15 percent (7). Pathologic verification of tumor diagnosis obtained by imaging and tumor markers is required to avoid unnecessary diagnostic laparotomy and to classify the type of tumor precisely before major surgical pancreatic resection, notorious for its morbidity and mortality. Pathologic evaluation is based on tissue biopsies, fine-needle cytologic aspirates, and endoscopic cytologic aspirates.

## TISSUE BIOPSIES AND FROZEN SECTIONS

All biopsy methods described allow a histodiagnosis. A core needle biopsy can be obtained preoperatively with an 18-gauge needle guided by ultrasonography, CT, or angiography, or perioperatively with a Silverman or similar "thick" needle under the visual control of the surgeon. A possible complication of this biopsy technique is the seeding of malignant cells through the needle tract. Wedge biopsy can be obtained only perioperatively and is suitable for frozen section diagnosis. Visually directed biopsies can be obtained preoperatively under laparoscopy (9), a technique also used to define the extent of the disease and monitor results of treatment (10).

The major criteria of malignancy in ductal adenocarcinomas, regardless of the type of biopsy, are: increase in the number of glandular structures with irregular distribution in both intralobular and interlobular areas, ductal structures larger than benign ducts, more irregularly branched ducts exhibiting partial or incomplete lumens or cribriform patterns, perineural invasion, necrotic material (amorphous debris and degenerating cells) within glandular lumens, invasion of duodenal muscle fascicles by single glands unaccompanied by connective tissue, variation in nuclear size of 4 to 1 or greater between ductal epithelial cells, huge irregular epithelial nucleoli, and glandular mitoses. The haphazard appearance of multiple glands with irregular shape and distribution, and nuclear changes are the two criteria needed to make a diagnosis of ductal adenocarcinoma. These criteria are also relevant for the frozen section diagnosis of a pancreatic duct cell adenocarcinoma (8). Chronic pancreatitis, especially when associated with ductal epithelial hyperplasia, is the nonmalignant disease most frequently mistaken for duct cell adenocarcinoma in biopsy material. In chronic pancreatitis, however, duct distribution is fairly regular and necrotic glandular debris is not seen, despite fibrosis.

According to the literature, the rate of correct diagnoses (number with positive histology/number with proven malignancy) is 67 percent (range, 50 to 78 percent) for Vim-Silverman biopsies (129 cases), and 76 percent (range, 43 to 89 percent) for wedge biopsies (253 cases) (11). For laparoscopy, positive biopsy rates approximate

75 percent for lesions of the head and 85 percent for those in the tail (9). False negative results are either due to sampling errors or to underevaluation of morphologic patterns. An important pitfall is a sample of sclerotic and inflammatory tissue which macroscopically mimics pancreatic cancer in coexistent carcinoma and pancreatitis. Errors in the diagnosis of pancreatic carcinoma usually arise when well-differentiated duct carcinomas are embedded in sclerotic tissue.

The safety of intraoperative core needle biopsy and wedge resection has been matter of controversy for many years because they may cause fistulae, hemorrhage, pancreatitis, and peritonitis. Fine-needle biopsy, which is especially used for deeply located lesions, has a higher incidence of complications (16 of 220 cases) than wedge biopsy (15 of 470 cases) which is used for more superficial lesions (12).

## FINE-NEEDLE ASPIRATION CYTOLOGY OF THE PANCREAS: PREOPERATIVE OR PERCUTANEOUS

Aspiration cytology is performed with a nontraumatic 20- to 23-gauge needle (fine needle). There are two main approaches to the diagnostic aspiration of the pancreas: 1) intraoperative aspiration under direct visualization of the pancreas or, when necessary, guided by intraoperative ultrasound (17); 2) percutaneous transabdominal aspiration under the guidance of ultrasound, CT, ERCP, and selective angiography. ERCP permits visualization of pancreatic ducts; small carcinomas of the pancreas can be detected by the localized stricture or obstruction of the pancreatic ducts. Selective angiography of the celiac artery may visualize an encasement of blood vessels by a tumor growth. Improved ultrasonography with a special biopsy transducer has become the routine method of imaging of the pancreas for localization and aspiration biopsy because of its simplicity and accuracy in obtaining representative samples. CT is also often used, especially if the first attempt under the guidance of ultrasound is unsuccessful.

Normal pancreatic tissue obtained by fine-needle aspiration usually contains numerous acinar cells, a few fragments of ductal epithelium, and sheets of mesothelial and endothelial cells. Hepatocytes appear in the smear when the lesion is located in the head and the needle passes through the liver. Islet cells are an infrequent finding and difficult to identify in aspirate smears; special stains such as Grimelius silver or chromogranin may help in their identification. Acinar cells occur singly or in small clusters, and are often arranged as spherical, tridimensional structures (fig. 9-1). They have round nuclei with uniformly distributed, finely granular chromatin in an abundant granular or vacuolated cytoplasm. Ductal epithelium is seen as cohesive sheets of uniform columnar or cuboidal cells (fig. 9-2). The cytoplasm is relatively scanty, faintly vacuolated, and poorly defined, and the nuclei are spherical and of even size with a fine chromatin pattern and inconspicuous nucleoli.

The aspirate from well-differentiated ductal adenocarcinoma is usually cellular. Tumor cells tend to form large, tightly packed cell clusters and flat sheets, resembling, at first glance, those of normal duct epithelium. Within the clusters the cells are generally significantly larger than normal duct cells and have large nuclei of variable size and irregular contour, dark chromatin, and distinct single or multiple nucleoli. The cytoplasm is relatively scanty in most cuboidal or columnar tumor cells but may be abundant and vacuolated in some, indicating mucin secretion. Cells displaying some irregularity and variation in size are difficult to distinguish from cells of well-differentiated ductal adenocarcinoma, and are often seen in cases of chronic pancreatitis (24). Criteria that differentiate epithelial reactive cells of a chronic inflammatory condition from truly malignant cells are a lack of three-dimensional, tightly packed cell clusters; a preserved nuclear/cytoplasmic ratio; and the frequent presence of many inflammatory cells (Table 9-1) (24). In a recent study based on stepwise logistic regression analysis, anisonucleosis, large nuclei, and nuclear molding were identified as significant cytologic features of pancreatic carcinoma (15). In combination, these three criteria have a sensitivity of 98 percent and a specificity of 100 percent.

In aspirate smears, tumor cells from moderately differentiated ductal adenocarcinoma form cohesive clusters, noncohesive groups of various size, or occur singly. The cells in groups show nuclear crowding and overlapping (fig. 9-3). Cancer cells are markedly pleomorphic, with irregular nuclei and prominent nucleoli. The cytoplasm

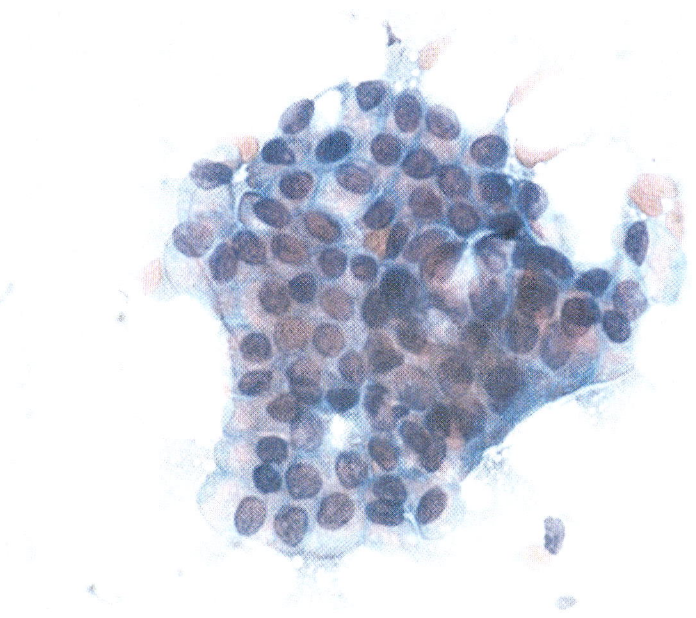

Figure 9-1
FINE-NEEDLE
ASPIRATION CYTOLOGY
OF THE PANCREAS
Normal pancreatic acinar cells with eccentrically located round nuclei and abundant cytoplasm.

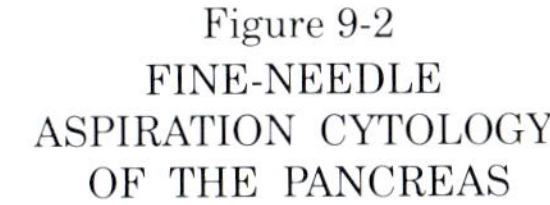

Figure 9-2
FINE-NEEDLE
ASPIRATION CYTOLOGY
OF THE PANCREAS
Normal ductal cells, in a sheet arrangement, showing round nuclei and relatively scarce cytoplasm.

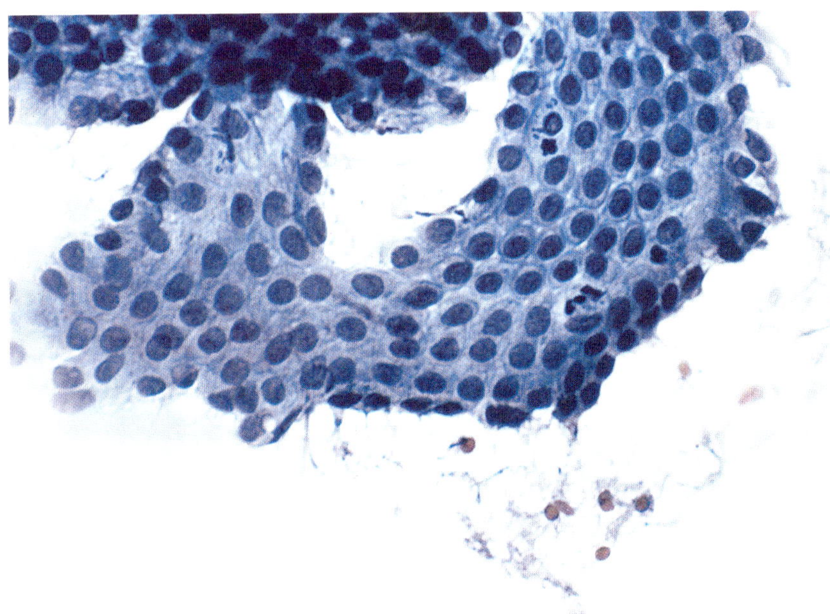

varies from scant to abundant. Mucin-secreting cells are rare, and mitotic figures are common.

Cytologic preparations of poorly differentiated ductal adenocarcinoma show cancer cells forming noncohesive groups or lying singly. The cytoplasm is scant and poorly defined. The nuclei are round and have coarsely granular chromatin and prominent nucleoli. Positive immunostaining for cytokeratin or carcinoembryonic antigen, which are epithelial markers, is helpful in differentiating these tumors from malignant lymphomas of the immunoblastic type (24).

Aspirated tumor cells from small cell carcinomas are seen singly or in small loose clusters (16). They have ill-defined, very scanty cytoplasm and round, heavily stained nuclei with inconspicuous nucleoli. Nuclear stripping and molding may be seen. Undifferentiated (anaplastic) carcinoma

Table 9-1

**DIFFERENT CYTOLOGIC PATTERNS IN CHRONIC PANCREATITIS AND WELL- DIFFERENTIATED DUCTAL ADENOCARCINOMA**

| | Chronic Pancreatitis | Well-Differentiated Ductal Adenocarcinoma |
|---|---|---|
| Number of groups | Few | Often numerous |
| Outline of groups | Regular, loose, monolayer | Irregular, tight, three-dimensional |
| Irregular nuclear contours | Absent | Present |
| Size of nuclei | Normal | Enlarged |
| Anisonucleosis | Absent or slight | Apparent in most groups |
| Nucleoli | Tiny | Small, readily visible |
| Single, large atypical cells | Absent | Present |

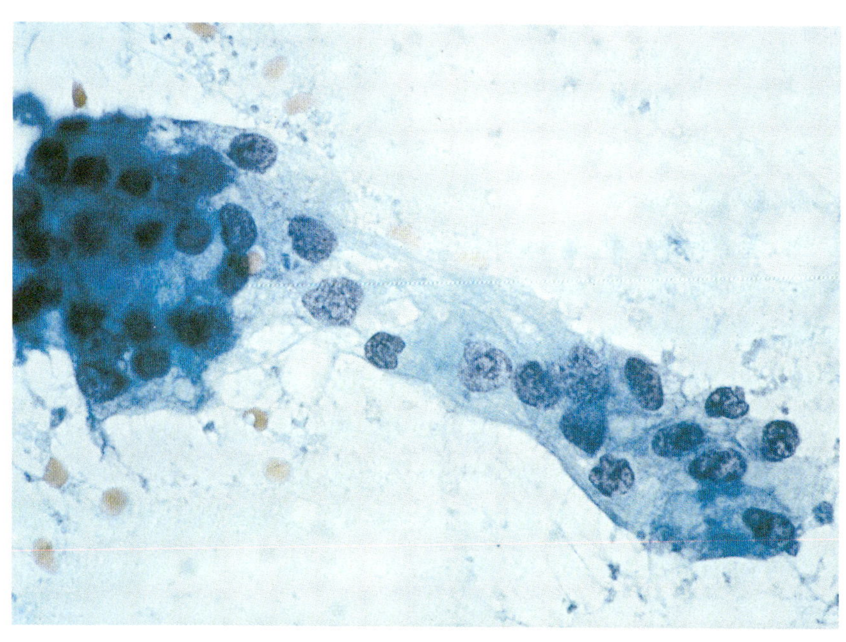

Figure 9-3
FINE-NEEDLE ASPIRATION CYTOLOGY OF THE PANCREAS
Moderately differentiated duct cell adenocarcinoma of the pancreas. The cells are in cohesive groups and have large, pleomorphic nuclei and a moderate amount of cytoplasm.

aspirates contain epithelial tumor cells that vary greatly in size and shape: cells with squamoid features and large multinucleated and spindle-shaped cells may be seen. Giant cell carcinomas with osteoclast-like cells contain malignant epithelial cells singly or in clusters and benign-looking, osteoclast-type, multinucleated giant cells with fairly regular nuclei (19,26). Aspiration cytology of adenosquamous carcinoma is characterized by a dual population: adenocarcinoma cells showing secretory activity and squamous carcinoma cells with evidence of keratinization (28). The aspirate material of mucinous cystadenocarcinoma and borderline or benign cystadenoma is mucoid and cells are scanty. There may be a few large groups of columnar epithelium cells with regular, round to ovoid nuclei in a palisading arrangement and abundant vacuolated cytoplasm. In some tumors, in addition to these benign-looking duct epithelial cells, there are tridimensional fragments containing crowded, irregular nuclei with clumps of chromatin, indicative of malignant transformation from a benign precursor (25). Aspirates of serous cystadenoma consist of watery fluid. In most cases smears made from the sediment of the cyst content show numerous duct

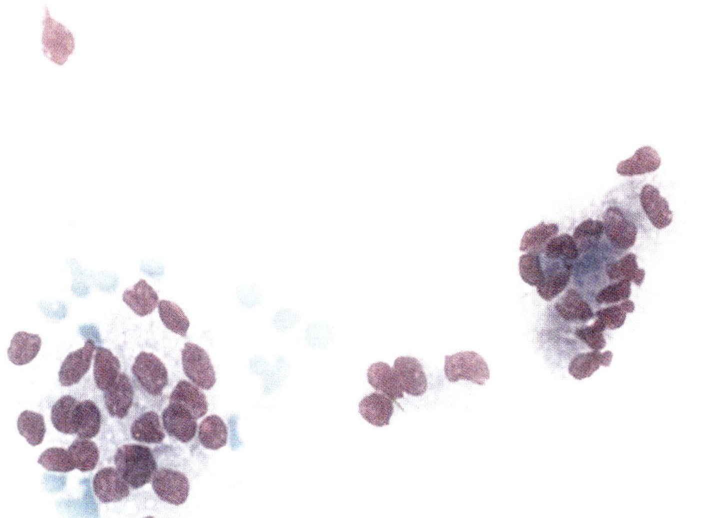

Figure 9-4
FINE-NEEDLE ASPIRATION CYTOLOGY OF THE PANCREAS
Endocrine tumor of the pancreas. Tumor cells have round nuclei and scanty, poorly defined cytoplasm.

epithelial cells, occurring either singly or in cohesive sheets. The cells are columnar or cuboidal, have scanty cytoplasm, and have regular nuclei with indistinct nucleoli (24). Diagnostic cytologic features of solid-pseudopapillary tumor include: large tight cell clumps with a perivascular, branching, papillary appearance; cells with scanty nonsecretory cytoplasm; uniform and regular nuclei of round or ovoid shape showing occasional grooves; inconspicuous nucleoli; and absence of necrotic debris, mitotic figures, or significant pleomorphism (14,29). Aspirated material from a pure acinar cell carcinoma shows irregular clusters of large monomorphic polygonal cells, with pale and abundant granular and occasionally foamy cytoplasm, and vesicular nuclei with prominent nucleoli, singly or in small groups (18,21).

The cytopathologic features of well-differentiated endocrine tumors (fig. 9-4) include: highly cellular smears; single cells in noncohesive clusters; a fairly uniform population of small cells; round, uniform, eccentric nuclei with a characteristic granular chromatin pattern; inconspicuous, small nucleoli; and scanty granular cytoplasm clustering around segments of capillaries. The main differential diagnostic consideration is well-differentiated adenocarcinoma (Table 9-2) and acinar cell carcinoma. The distinction between these tumors is important, since the biologic behavior, management, and prognosis of these lesions are extremely different (see pertinent chapters). Endocrine tumors can be distinguished from well-differentiated duct cell carcinomas by purely cytomorphologic criteria: a three-dimensional, irregular, cohesive grouping; ovoid nuclei with prominent nucleoli; and well-defined, vacuolated cytoplasm favor the diagnosis of adenocarcinoma and exclude endocrine tumors. The cells of acinar cell carcinoma differ from those of endocrine tumors since they are larger and have vesicular nuclei with prominent nucleoli. Confirmation is provided by immunohistochemistry and special stains. Chromogranin, PGP9.5, and neuron-specific enolase are positive in the cytoplasm of at least some cells from pancreatic endocrine tumors (13,23). Endocrine tumor cells may also display Grimelius silver–positive granules. However, the argyrophil reaction is negative or relatively weak in comparison with corresponding histologic sections; the most positive reaction is seen in formalin-fixed cellular samples (27).

In aspirate preparations, it is not always possible to differentiate islet cell "hyperplasia" resulting from islet crowding due to acinar atrophy from a well-differentiated endocrine tumor. The main cytologic features of islet cell hyperplasia are scant cellularity, small clusters of cells, absence of isolated cells, and the associated presence of a large number of benign exocrine pancreatic cells (21). These findings differ from those

Table 9-2

**DIFFERENT CYTOLOGIC FEATURES IN WELL-DIFFERENTIATED DUCT CELL ADENOCARCINOMA AND ENDOCRINE TUMORS OF THE PANCREAS**

| | Well-Differentiated Adenocarcinoma | Well-Differentiated Endocrine Tumors |
|---|---|---|
| Configuration of clusters | Three-dimensional cohesive groups with irregular contours | Noncohesive groups |
| Nuclei | Ovoid, irregular, prominent nucleoli in some cells | Round, uniform, regular, inconspicuous nucleoli |
| Cytoplasm | Well-defined, variable amount of mucin vacuoles in some cells | Scanty, poorly defined, nonvacuolated |

of well-differentiated endocrine tumors, which, as reported above, are characterized by highly cellular aspirates with large numbers of isolated cells. Identification of non-neoplastic endocrine cells in a pancreatic fine-needle biopsy is important for differentiating chronic pancreatitis and pancreatic ductal adenocarcinoma: the presence of endocrine cells in needle aspirates from different parts of the pancreas, in the absence of malignant epithelial cells, favors the diagnosis of chronic pancreatitis (20).

Due to the similarity between cells of malignant and apparently benign well-differentiated endocrine tumors, the prediction of tumor behavior is impossible on a cytologic basis alone. However, in frankly malignant endocrine tumors (small cell or intermediate endocrine carcinomas) the overall cytologic findings are highly suggestive of malignancy and include: variation in nuclear size, significant increase in average nuclear size, large cells with moderate to scarce well-defined cytoplasm, mitotic figures, multinucleated tumor cells, and necrotic tumor debris. According to Tao (24), any endocrine tumor with four of these five cytologic features should be considered malignant.

Preoperative fine-needle aspiration biopsy provides a positive cytologic diagnosis of malignant cells in 83 percent of patients with pancreatic carcinoma (data from 614 cases reported in the literature [22]). The specificity is 99 percent, with only rare mention of false positive results. This implies that this method has an advantage over all other biopsy methods. However, the disadvantage is that percutaneous aspiration, especially under the guidance of ultrasound, can only be applied to advanced pancreatic carcinomas, since the size of the tumor usually has to exceed 2 cm to be detectable. CT is more useful as a guide to aspiration of small pancreatic lesions and with this guidance procedure for needle biopsy the accuracy rate can increase to 94 percent (24). In about 10 percent of patients, fine-needle biopsy is inadequate and a cytologic diagnosis is not possible. However, fine-needle biopsies can be repeated until sufficient cytologic material is obtained. In most cases, the aspirated material not only permits recognition of malignant cells, but also allows distinction of adenocarcinomas from endocrine tumors, and with the help of immunohistochemistry, identification of different types of exocrine and endocrine tumors. Due to its high specificity, especially in distinguishing between chronic pancreatitis and cancer, this technique is of great help in avoiding most diagnostic laparotomies, especially in patients with nonresectable tumors.

Nontraumatic fine needles for intraoperative aspiration biopsy, guided by intraoperative ultrasound, are safer and diagnostically more accurate than intraoperative biopsies, either wedge or large needle. With fine-needle aspiration the direct biopsy risks of hemorrhage, fistulae, abscess formation, pancreatitis, and subphrenic abscess can be avoided and multiple aspirations from different areas can be safely done. This reduces the sampling error inherent to blind biopsy, in which no intraoperative ultrasound guidance is available. Intraoperative fine-needle aspiration provides precise differentiation between chronic pancreatitis and pancreatic carcinoma in 95 to 100 percent of cases (22). As a consequence, fine-needle aspiration is considered the safer and more accurate diagnostic technique for intraoperative evaluation of a pancreatic mass, especially when it is deeply situated in the gland.

## PANCREATIC JUICE CYTOLOGY

ERCP is the most sensitive imaging technique for diagnosing pancreatic duct cell adenocarcinoma and intraductal papillary mucinous tumors. Because of the increasing number of physicians experienced in this technique, ERCP-guided aspiration cytology is now easily available. Pancreatic fluid can be collected in ice-cooled tubes by continuous aspiration with a syringe. With this method well-preserved cells are obtained by cytocentrifugation of large quantities of pancreatic fluid (1 to 4 ml). An additional cytologic sampling technique during ERCP uses a special device for direct brush cytology (32).

The cells most frequently observed in the smears are benign duct cells with round to oval, often polarized, regular nuclei and absent or inconspicuous nucleoli. The cytoplasm is well defined and sometimes displays mucus-containing vacuoles. Normal duct cells frequently form groups or sheets with regular contours. Other duct cells may show larger, more central nuclei and more eosinophilic cytoplasm indicating a squamous metaplasia, or pyknotic nuclei suggestive of regressive changes. The main cytologic criteria for the diagnosis of duct cell adenocarcinoma are disoriented or crowded cells in three-dimensional groups, nuclear enlargement with an irregular nuclear contour, anisonucleosis, unevenly distributed chromatin, and prominent nucleoli.

A major limitation of ERCP-guided aspiration is that cannulation of the ampulla of Vater requires a great deal of time and experience. The overall sensitivity of cytologic analysis is limited (average accuracy, 60 to 70 percent) because false negative results may be obtained when the tumors are peripherally located, or when only a small volume of pancreatic fluid can be aspirated due to complete obstruction of the pancreatic duct (31). In fact, the sensitivity of cytology is higher for lesions in the head in comparison to lesions in the body and tail by a ratio of about 2 to 1. The yield of positive cytology can be improved by aspirating more than 3 ml of fluid, which can be obtained by inserting the cannula 2 to 3 cm within the pancreatic duct (30). No serious complications have been observed with this cytologic sampling method.

## DIAGNOSTIC GUIDELINES

In summary, for a rational approach to the diagnosis of pancreatic tumors ultrasound should be the first imaging method used. Radioimmunoassay of CA19-9, which is the most suitable serum marker, is useful for determining whether a negative ultrasound should be followed by CT or other investigations. A circumscribed mass identified by ultrasound or CT should be biopsied by percutaneous fine-needle aspiration to identify tumor type. Positive ultrasound or CT followed by a positive fine-needle biopsy eliminates additional diagnostic procedures, including ERCP. ERCP is reserved for cases in which ultrasound and CT coupled with fine-needle aspiration fail to clarify the diagnosis. Laparoscopy may be useful in detecting abdominal metastases not shown by CT and ultrasound. Diagnostic laparotomy with intraoperative fine-needle aspiration should be reserved for the few patients in whom imaging techniques have failed to localize a cancer despite clinical signs suspicious for pancreatic carcinoma and an elevated CA19-9 in serum. In such cases, resection of the pancreas is not justified unless a cytologic or histologic diagnosis of cancer is made.

## PROCEDURES FOR PATHOLOGIC EXAMINATION

### Macroscopic

Proper handling of pancreatectomy specimens is important in order to assure precise location, size, and stage as well as correct diagnosis and adequate treatment of pancreatic tumors. This is especially true for the localization of ductal adenocarcinoma. Examination of the pancreas requires knowledge of the anatomic relationship between the common bile duct, pancreatic duct, and ampulla of Vater, and of the major types of operative procedures for resection. The following are the types of pancreatectomies that have to be considered.

The *Whipple procedure* is a partial pancreatectomy with resection of the head of the pancreas, the duodenum, and the distal stomach.

A *distal pancreatectomy* is a partial ("left-sided") pancreatectomy with resection of the body and/or tail of the pancreas and splenectomy. A *near total pancreatectomy* is an extended left-sided partial pancreatectomy with removal of 80 to 90 percent of the pancreas (tail, body, and part of the head) up to the common bile duct in the head of the gland. A *total pancreatectomy* is a total resection of the gland with distal gastrectomy, duodenectomy, and splenectomy.

For adequate examination of a tumor in the head of the pancreas removed either by a Whipple procedure or a total pancreatectomy the following guidelines are helpful:

1. Describe the surface appearance of the specimen and particularly of the tumor; measure the external size of the specimen; and determine possible invasion into the surrounding tissue.

2. Identify lymph nodes that are attached to the specimen according the anatomic-topographic classification shown in figure 1-9. If lymph nodes are not definitely identifiable, submit the nodule, fat, or other tissue suspected of containing tumor tissue for microscopic examination.

3. Take cut sections from the resection margin of the common bile duct and (in the case of a Whipple specimen) the pancreas for microscopic examination.

4. Open the stomach through the greater curvature; then open the duodenum at the opposite side of the ampulla of Vater. Identify the ampulla and describe changes in the duodenum (ulcer, polyp, tumor, diverticula, heterotopic pancreas).

5. Approach the common bile duct by opening the duct proximal to the tumor and probe it from its proximal margin through the ampulla of Vater. Probe the main pancreatic duct from the body through the ampulla. Once both ducts are probed and shown to be patent, or obstructed, cut the whole pancreatic specimen horizontally (pancreas lying flat, anterior surface uppermost), exposing the duct systems by opening the common bile duct and, if possible, also the pancreatic duct along the probes. State whether there is obstruction to either or both ducts. Look for calculi in the main pancreatic duct and the ampulla. Try to determine if there is a separate opening for the Santorini duct in the duodenum and note whether there is a minor ampulla. Describe the relation of the tumor to the bile duct, the pancreatic duct, and the ampulla. Describe color, consistency, and other features of the tumor and measure its diameter in two or three axes. Describe whether there is only one nodule or multiple nodules, cyst formation, necrosis, hemorrhage, mucoid appearance, calcification, and other changes.

6. Take cross sections from the ampulla of Vater to the end of the specimen at right angle to the longitudinal axes of the common bile duct and the pancreatic duct to determine extent of tumor invasion. The cross sections should include the parapancreatic fatty tissue and the vessels attached to the pancreas. The sections should be numbered. In the case of small tumors (1 to 2 cm), all sections containing tumor tissue should be processed for microscopic examination. In larger tumors, a minimum of six blocks of tumor should be obtained. Also obtain at least two blocks of nontumor-involved pancreatic tissue from a Whipple resection and four blocks from a total pancreatectomy.

For examination of a tumor in the body or tail of the pancreas removed by a left-sided distal pancreatectomy, the specimen should be serially (0.5-cm intervals) sectioned at right angle to the main pancreatic duct. Sections from the resection margin, the tumor, and the uninvolved pancreatic tissue should be taken for microscopic examination.

For special studies concerning localization, size, and spread of the tumor or tumor-associated lesions the whole specimen may be fixed for 24 hours in formalin prior to dissection. To improve tissue preservation and visibility of the duct systems formalin should be injected into the unopened common bile duct, pancreatic duct, and duodenum. The fixed pancreas is then dissected horizontally at the level of the common bile duct and the pancreatic duct. Instead of a horizontal cutting the fixed pancreatic specimen may also be sliced perpendicular to the axis of the duct systems (cephalo-caudal axis).

### Microscopic

**Tissue Processing.** Histologic specimens from pancreatic tumor as well as surrounding nontumor tissue should be fixed in formalin (4 percent formaldehyde), neutral or weakly acidic. In the case of suspected endocrine tumor, small tumor pieces may be fixed in Bouin's fluid fixation. Ideally, a tumor sample should be frozen for extraction and analysis of DNA, RNA, proteins, or hormones. Small fresh samples should also be fixed in a glutaraldehyde or formaldehyde-glutaraldehyde mixture for electron microscopy. However, in most cases. formalin fixation is perfectly adequate for diagnostic as well as research purposes. Indeed, a variety of "unmasking" treatments, especially with the help of a microwave oven, may restore a number of immunoreactivities in formalin-fixed paraffin-embedded tissues, while most DNA technology can be easily applied to such tissues. This reduces the need for frozen material and opens the way to reinvestigation of archival material. Use of relatively short fixation times (6 to 24 hours, depending on specimen size) and lower (52 to 54 CÉ) melting point paraffins may prevent or reduce protein and nucleic acid denaturation as well as the need for unmasking treatments.

**Choice of Stains and Histochemical Tests.** In the majority of cases, hematoxylin-eosin and Alcian blue–periodic acid-Schiff based stains (AB-PAS) are sufficient to reveal an appropriate diagnosis, including separation of ordinary ductal cancer from uncommon types of exocrine tumors and from endocrine tumors. Immunohistochemical tests for pancreatic enzymes (lipase, amylase, and trypsin) are needed to conclusively prove a diagnosis of acinar cell carcinoma, to separate it unquestionably from endocrine tumors with a solid-trabecular and microacinar structure, and to help diagnose pancreatoblastoma (see Table 3-1). On the other hand, chromogranin A or synaptophysin immunohistochemistry, or at least Grimelius silver, confirm the endocrine nature of tumors showing endocrine-like histology. In addition, at least insulin, gastrin, glucagon, pancreatic polypeptide, and somatostatin antibodies should be tested to adequately type the tumor cells. When dealing with tumors showing histologic patterns of poorly differentiated endocrine neoplasia and no or poor reactivity for all general endocrine markers and hormones, neuron-specific enolase (NSE) and protein gene product (PGP) 9.5 may also be tested. However, both of these may be positive in some nonendocrine tumors, notably solid-pseudopapillary tumors, from which small cell endocrine carcinoma must be separated on histologic and, especially, cytologic grounds. Alpha-1-antitrypsin immunostaining in the absence of endocrine (except NSE), acinar cell, and ductal carcinoma markers (mucin staining, carcinoembryonic antigen [CEA], DuPan 2, and M1) supports the histologic diagnosis of solid-pseudopapillary and serous cystic tumors (see Table 3-1).

**Electron Microscopy.** Present availability of reliable, selective histochemical markers for the different types of pancreatic cells and their tumor equivalents has greatly reduced the need of more costly and time-consuming ultrastructural investigation. However, in the absence of conclusive histologic or histochemical evidence, electron microscopy may still be contributive to tumor cell typing and precise assessment of phenotype. The goals of electron microscopy are recognition of the endocrine nature of small cell carcinoma and appropriate identification of acinar cell carcinoma, solid-pseudopapillary tumors, and nonfunctioning endocrine tumors. Functional typing of endocrine tumors can only be done in well-differentiated cases, with special reference to insulin, glucagon, and a few gastrin cell tumors.

## STAGING AND GRADING OF CARCINOMAS

Systems for staging and grading pancreatic tumors have only been developed and, to some extent, validated for ductal adenocarcinoma (see pertinent chapter). Criteria for grading other tumors (e.g., endocrine tumors) have been discussed in relevant sections. However, organization of a workable and useful grading system remains to be done. In principle, the staging system for ductal adenocarcinoma could be applied to other pancreatic tumors as far as identification of progression steps, organic barriers, and ways of diffusion of the tumor growth are concerned. In practice, the manyfold qualitative and quantitative differences between various tumors with respect to local growth (infiltrative or expansive), invasion pattern (capsular, angio-lympho-perineural, parapancreatic), and spread (lymphatic, hematogenous) require adaptation of the system to each tumor type, and tumor assessment in terms of clinical parameters such as patient survival or indication for surgery.

## REFERENCES

### Clinical, Laboratory, and Radiologic Evaluation


1. Campbell JP, Wilson SR. Pancreatic neoplasms: how useful is evaluation with US? Radiology 1988;167:341–4.
2. Doppman JL, Shawker TH, Miller DL. Localization of islet cell tumors. Gastroenterol Clin North Am 1989;18:793–804.
3. Freeny PC, Marks WM, Ryan JA, Traverso WL. Pancreatic ductal adenocarcinoma: diagnosis and staging with dynamic CT. Radiology 1988;166:125–33.
4. Krenning EP, Bakker WH, Breeman WA, et al. Localization of endocrine related tumors with radioiodinated analogue of somatostatin. Lancet 1989;1:242–4.
5. Magnani JL, Steplewsksi Z, Koprowski H, Ginsburg V. Identification of the gastrointestinal and pancreatic cancer-associated antigen detected by monoclonal antibody CA 19-9 in the sera of patients as a mucin. Cancer Res 1983;43:5489–92.
6. Malesci A, Tommasini MA, Bonato C, et al. Determination of CA 19-9 antigen in serum and pancreatic juice for differential diagnosis of pancreatic adenocarcinoma from chronic pancreatitis. Gastroenterology 1987;92:60–7.
7. Niederau C, Grendell JH. Diagnosis of pancreatic carcinoma. Imaging techniques and tumor markers. Pancreas 1992;7:66–86.


### Tissue Biopsies and Frozen Sections


8. Hyland C, Kheir SM, Kashlan MB. Frozen section diagnosis of pancreatic carcinoma: a prospective study of 64 biopsies. Am J Surg Pathol 1981;5:179–91.
9. Ishida H. Peritoneoscopy and pancreas biopsy in the diagnosis of pancreatic diseases. Gastrointest Endosc 1983;29:211–8.
10. Ishida H, Dohzono T, Furukawa Y, Kobayashi M, Tsuneoka K. Laparoscopy and biopsy in the diagnosis of malignant intra-abdominal tumors. Endoscopy 1984;16:140–2.
11. Klöppel G. Pancreatic biopsy. In: Klöppel G, Heitz PU, eds. Pancreatic pathology. Edinburgh: Churchill Livingstone, 1984:114–22.
12. Reuben A, Cotton PB. Operative pancreatic biopsy: a survey of current practice. Ann Royal Coll Surg Engl 1978;60:53–7.


### Fine-Needle Aspiration Cytology of the Pancreas: Preoperative or Percutaneous


13. Al-Kaisi N, Weaver MG, Abdul-Karim FW, Siegler E. Fine needle aspiration cytology of neuroendocrine tumors of the pancreas. A cytologic, immunocytochemical and electron microscopic study. Acta Cytol 1992;36:655–60.
14. Chen KT, Workman RD, Efird TA, Cheng AC. Fine-needle aspiration cytology diagnosis of papillary tumor of the pancreas. Acta Cytol 1986;30:523–7.
15. Cohen MB, Egerter DP, Holly EA, Ahn DK, Miller TR. Pancreatic adenocarcinoma: regression analysis to identify improved cytologic criteria. Diagn Cytopathol 1991;7:341–5.
16. Frable WJ. Thin needle aspiration biopsy. Philadelphia: WB Saunders, 1983:222–51.
17. Hastrup J, Thommesen P, Frederiksen P. Pancreatitis and pancreatic carcinoma, diagnosed by preoperative fine needle aspiration biopsy. Acta Cytol 1977;21:731–3.
18. Ishiara A, Sanda T, Takanari H, Yatani R, Lin PI. Elastase-1-secreting acinar cell carcinoma of the pancreas. A cytologic, electron microscopic and histochemical study. Acta Cytol 1989;33:157–63.
19. Manci EA, Gardner LL, Pollack WJ, Dowling EA. Osteoclastic giant cell tumor of the pancreas: aspiration cytology, light microscopy, and ultrastructure with review of the literature. Diagn Cytopathol 1985;1:105–10.
20. Nguyen GK. Cytology of hyperplastic endocrine cells of the pancreas in fine needle aspiration biopsy. Acta Cytol 1984;28:499–502.
21. Nguyen GK. Percutaneous fine-needle aspiration cytology of the pancreas. Pathol Ann 1985;20:221–38.
22. Niederau C, Grendell JH. Diagnosis of pancreatic carcinoma. Imaging techniques and tumor markers. Pancreas 1992;7:66–86.
23. Shaw JA, Vance RP, Geisinger KR, Marshall RB. Islet cell neoplasms. A fine-needle aspiration cytology study with immunocytochemical correlations. Am J Clin Pathol 1990;94:142–9.
24. Tao LC. Transabdominal fine-needle aspiration biopsy. New York: Igaku-Shoin, 1990:133–78.
25. Vellet D, Leiman G, Mair S, Bilchik A. Fine needle aspiration cytology of mucinous cystadenocarcinoma of the pancreas. Further observations. Acta Cytol 1988;32:43–8.
26. Walts AE. Osteoclast-type giant cell tumor of the pancreas. Acta Cytol 1983;27:500–4.
27. Wilander E, Norheim I, Oberg K. Application of silver stains to cytologic specimens of neuroendocrine tumors metastatic to the liver. Acta Cytol 1985;29:1053–7.
28. Wilcyznski SP, Valente BF, Atkinson BF. Cytodiagnosis of adenosquamous carcinoma of the pancreas. Use of intraoperative fine needle aspiration. Acta Cytol 1984;84:733–6.
29. Wilson MB, Adams DB, Garen PD, Gansler TS. Aspiration cytologic, ultrastructural, and DNA cytometric findings of solid and papillary tumor of the pancreas. Cancer 1992;69:2235–43.

**Pancreatic Juice Cytology**

30. Goodale RL, Gail-Peczalska K, Dressel T, Samuelson J. Cytologic studies for the diagnosis of pancreatic cancer. Cancer 1981;47:1652–5.
31. Klöppel G. Pancreatic biopsy. In: Klöppel G, Heitz PU, eds. Pancreatic pathology. Edinburgh: Churchill Livingstone, 1984:114–22.
32. Osnes M, Serck-Hanssen A, Kristensen O, Swensen T, Aune S, Myren J. Endoscopic retrograde brush cytology in patients with primary and secondary malignancies of the pancreas. Gut 1979;20:279–84.

# INDEX*



*Numbers in boldface indicate table and figure pages.

✧✧✧